D1223386

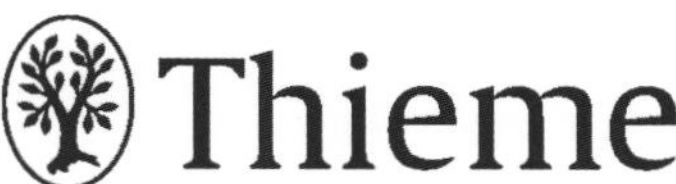
Thieme

Facial Nerve Disorders and Diseases: Diagnosis and Management

Orlando Guntinas-Lichius, MD
Professor and Chairman
Department of Otorhinolaryngology and Facial Nerve Center
Jena University Hospital
Jena, Germany

Barry M. Schaitkin, MD
Professor
Facial Nerve Center
Department of Otolaryngology
University of Pittsburgh Medical Center
Pittsburgh, Pennsylvania, USA

264 illustrations

Thieme
Stuttgart • New York • Delhi • Rio de Janeiro

Library of Congress Cataloging-in-Publication Data
is available from the publisher.

Thieme Publishers Stuttgart
Rüdigerstrasse 14, 70469 Stuttgart, Germany
+49 [0]711 8931 421, customerservice@thieme.de

Thieme Publishers New York
333 Seventh Avenue, New York, NY 10001 USA
+1 800 782 3488, customerservice@thieme.com

Thieme Publishers Delhi
A-12, Second Floor, Sector-2, Noida-201301
Uttar Pradesh, India
+91 120 45 566 00, customerservice@thieme.in

Thieme Publishers Rio, Thieme Publicações Ltda.
Edifício Rodolpho de Paoli, 25º andar
Av. Nilo Peçanha, 50 – Sala 2508
Rio de Janeiro 20020-906 Brasil
Tel: +55 21 3172-2297 / +55 21 3172-1896

Cover design: Thieme Publishing Group
Typesetting by Ditech Process Solutions

Printed in Germany by Aprinta GmbH, Wemding 5 4 3 2 1

ISBN 978-3-13-175181-2

Also available as an e-book:
eISBN 978-3-13-175191-1

Important note: Medicine is an ever-changing science undergoing continual development. Research and clinical experience are continually expanding our knowledge, in particular our knowledge of proper treatment and drug therapy. Insofar as this book mentions any dosage or application, readers may rest assured that the authors, editors, and publishers have made every effort to ensure that such references are in accordance with **the state of knowledge at the time of production of the book.**

Nevertheless, this does not involve, imply, or express any guarantee or responsibility on the part of the publishers in respect to any dosage instructions and forms of applications stated in the book. **Every user is requested to examine carefully** the manufacturers' leaflets accompanying each drug and to check, if necessary in consultation with a physician or specialist, whether the dosage schedules mentioned therein or the contraindications stated by the manufacturers differ from the statements made in the present book. Such examination is particularly important with drugs that are either rarely used or have been newly released on the market. Every dosage schedule or every form of application used is entirely at the user's own risk and responsibility. The authors and publishers request every user to report to the publishers any discrepancies or inaccuracies noticed. If errors in this work are found after publication, errata will be posted at www.thieme.com on the product description page.

Some of the product names, patents, and registered designs referred to in this book are in fact registered trademarks or proprietary names even though specific reference to this fact is not always made in the text. Therefore, the appearance of a name without designation as proprietary is not to be construed as a representation by the publisher that it is in the public domain.

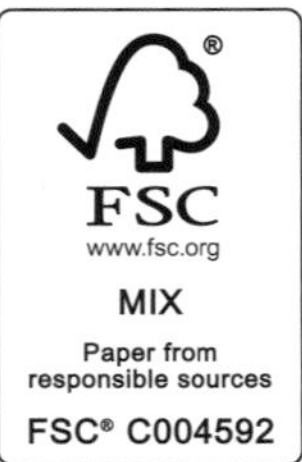

Contents

Part VII: Diseases Other Than Peripheral Facial Palsy

Part VIII: Miscellaneous

Videos

Video 3.1: Slow-motion video of a rat with facial–facial nerve suture on the right side showing poor recovery of the whisking on the right side compared to normal whisking on the left side.

Video 15.1: Placement of blue "eye" recording electrodes just above the brow.

Video 15.2: Placement of red "mouth" recording electrodes along the nasolabial groove.

Video 15.3: Placement of green ground and white anode electrode. The anode represents the return of the stimulus current.

Video 15.4: Final electrode positions secured with clear adhesive tape. These electrical wires will be led off the table to be connected into the headbox. Electrode wires should be kept distant from electrocautery cables in order to reduce artifact as well as the risk of burn injuries.

Video 15.5: Proper color-coded connection of recording electrodes into the headbox. A black-colored sterile cable is used to routinely attach the stimulator on the field to the headbox. The stimulus can be delivered using dedicated monopolar or bipolar probes, or Kartush Stimulating Instruments that allow simultaneous surgical dissection with monopolar stimulation.

Video 15.6: Placement of all electrodes is demonstrated using standardized color-coding to minimize errors.

Video 15.7: Prior to sterile draping of the patient, a "tap test" is performed to confirm that there are auditory and visual responses elicited by tapping adjacent to the electrodes. Note that this is an artifact, not a true EMG response which can be elicited even when muscle relaxants are present. Therefore, while this test provides critical information, it is not by itself sufficient to demonstrate a fully functioning monitoring set-up.

Video 15.8: An NIM monitor is used to demonstrate proper pre-check assessments of output volume and electrode impedance.

Video 15.9: A novel method to confirm both stimulus and recording functionality is demonstrated by stimulating the facial nerve transcutaneously prior to sterile draping.

Video 15.10: A variety of NIM response tones are demonstrated including responses to electric stimulation and trauma: electrically triggered responses, bursts, and trains.

Video 15.11: Obtaining an early baseline EMG response to electrical stimulation is critical to exclude neuromuscular blockade or temporary paralysis of the facial nerve by local anesthetics.

Video 15.12: The response to stimulus-evoked facial nerve responses are demonstrated during acoustic tumor resection.

Video 15.13: An increased EMG baseline is demonstrated when the depth of anesthesia becomes too light.

Video 15.14: EMG train of responses is demonstrated following stretching of the facial nerve. Note that interpretation of EMG trains can only be properly performed when the interpreting professional is aware of the ongoing real-time surgical events.

Video 15.15: Proper electrode removal is critical to minimize post-monitoring ecchymoses and trauma to the eye. The eyelids must remain taped shut until the electrodes are off the field.

Foreword

The first parotidectomy I ever saw was during my fellowship with Dr. John Conley in 1968. He felt that "parotidectomy is surgery of the facial nerve." Watching him expose the facial nerve and dissecting it made me think of Michelangelo painting the Sistine Chapel. When I was appointed Chairman of the Department of Otolaryngology at the University of Pittsburgh in 1972 I quickly became the "go-to guy" for patients who required parotid surgery. Why? Because other surgeons in our region were not interested in being involved with the facial nerve in the litigious society that we live in. In those days parotid surgery was not well taught, and attempts by those who were inadequately trained often eventuated in disastrous results, in particular facial nerve paralysis. I estimate that I have performed more than 1,500 parotidectomies in my career. The majority of these were for tumor resections.

In 1991, Dr. Barry M. Schaitkin had just completed his residency, and he came to Pittsburgh and applied for a position on our faculty. Unfortunately for us, but fortunately for him, there was no position available. He went into practice with Dr. Mark May who had moved to Pittsburgh in the 1970s and later established a facial nerve center in a nearby community hospital. Dr. Schaitkin acquired substantial experience in facial nerve surgery, and when Dr. May retired in 1996, Dr. Schaitkin became a member of our full-time faculty where he is Professor of Otolaryngology and Director of our Residency Program. He has contributed to the literature on facial nerve and coedited the 2000 edition of Dr. May's book *The Facial Nerve*. Dr. Schaitkin was recently approached by Dr. Orlando Guntinas-Lichius from Germany, who had just published a prize-winning book on salivary gland disorders with Dr. Patrick Bradley, and realized that there was no current textbook devoted entirely to disorders of the facial nerve. This transatlantic connection combines both American and European thinking on this topic. For example, this book includes the extracapsular approach to tumors of the parotid gland; this has not been well accepted in the United States but is popular in the United Kingdom and Germany.

There is much to like about this book. It is a scholarly work, as comprehensive in scope as a book can be but not intimidating to the reader. While diagnostic and surgical procedures are appropriately described in detail, the authors have used contemporary devices such as checklists, algorithms, and "pop-up" boxes to highlight the main take-home message of a section or paragraph, and these make the important points very accessible to the reader. There are multiple authors from several countries, experts in their respective fields, including basic science and modern diagnostic surgical and reconstructive methods. Topics not usually included in surgical texts, yet invaluable to the patient, include the very humanistic topics of the diagnostic and therapeutic approaches to the emotional and social impairment in patients with facial nerve paralysis. The last section of the book brings us back to the stark reality of surgery on the facial nerve with a section on medicolegal aspects of iatrogenic facial nerve paralysis.

The text is beautifully illustrated with color photos and drawings done with great precision also in color, which provides great clarity on the concepts discussed in the book. The book is adequately but not overly referenced and is up to date. The book is all encompassing in the field with topics that will be helpful in everyday surgical practice, such as the checklist for measures that help avoid facial paralysis during and after surgery, to a chapter on the very contemporary and somewhat controversial topic of facial transplantation.

Many advances have been made since I first learned surgery of the facial nerve. Residents now in training are regularly exposed to the diagnosis and management of patients with facial nerve problems. Technical improvements have been made, including diagnostics, facial nerve monitoring, free flaps, free nerve grafts, and Botox. The readers will benefit from using this book to supplement their clinical experience, and this will be to the benefit of the patient.

Eugene N. Myers, MD, FACS, FRCS Hon (Edin)

Foreword

The language of facial expression is of highest importance for every human being (Prof. Dr. A. Miehlke, 1973). Facial expression, which may reflect our deepest emotions, is only possible through the integrity of the central and peripheral portions of the facial nerve and mimic musculature. Although in many cases it is not a life-threatening disease, facial palsy is a psychologically devastating event and certainly life altering. Therefore, when spontaneous resolution of facial palsy is not expected, the patient is very motivated to undergo many investigations and various medical treatments or surgical procedures with the aim of restoring facial function and quality of life. The medical specialist should be well aware of state-of-the-art diagnostic and prognostic investigations, medical and surgical treatments available, and the contribution of rehabilitation procedures and psychological support. This book, *Facial Nerve Disorders and Diseases: Diagnosis and Management*, will support the specialist in making decisions as it provides a systematic and comprehensive up-to-date review, covering all aspects of both conventional and contemporary topics of the facial nerve (and its disorders) in 8 sections, comprising 29 chapters. The key information is tabulated in a logical fashion at the end of each chapter for quick reference. When relevant, algorithms or flowcharts are added to enable the specialist to choose the best pathway for optimal management. Each chapter is well referenced, providing the most recent information. The traditional chapters dealing with embryology, anatomy, physiology, and nerve regeneration contain a wealth of scientific information. For the first time in a textbook, the significance of ultrasound as a diagnostic tool for facial nerve disorders is systematically elucidated in the chapter on imaging. The review of facial nerve function following face transplantation, for 30 cases operated worldwide, is impressive, giving insight into this challenging surgery. The chapters entitled Pediatric Facial Nerve Palsies, Intraoperative Facial Nerve Monitoring, and Grading deserve particular attention. Developments in the treatment of facial palsy have taken place in the field of surgery and in the use of Botox for the contractures and synkinesis. These topics are extensively reviewed and well illustrated.

This book provides a greater understanding of the scientific and clinical issues of the facial nerve and its disorders. This will aid skillful management of the patient to obtain the best results and the highest quality of life.

The editors are to be congratulated as they have been successful in bringing together the most recent scientific and clinical data from experts in this field.

Johannes J. Manni, MD, PhD

Preface

This book is the outcome of our inspiration to create a modern, complete facial nerve textbook comprising a mixed European and American authorship. We were fortunate enough to attract current experts from both continents. They have provided us with a state-of-the-art, in-depth perspective on current approaches to facial nerve problems.

The book allows one to consult it à la carte on topics of basic science, diagnosis, testing, and treatment. However, the chapters build on each other and are cross-referenced so that reading the book in order will give the reader a much better insight into our current successes and limitations.

In addition to covering the required information for a facial nerve textbook, we have brought in entirely new topics that we hope you will find interesting and useful. For example, we include chapters on face transplant and medicolegal aspects of facial nerve care.

We hope that you will not only learn from the information provided by the authors and editors, but that you will appreciate our limitations, and through your own exploration and documentation help us move the treatment of these patients further toward their goal of cosmesis and function.

Orlando Guntinas-Lichius, MD
Barry M. Schaitkin, MD

Dedication and Acknowledgments

This book is dedicated to two of my teachers and mentors. I thank Prof. Wolfram F. Neiss (Cologne) for teaching me how to work scientifically, soundly, and validly, and for encouraging me to pursue a clinical career in otolaryngology, head and neck surgery. I thank Prof. Eberhard Stennert (Cologne) for teaching me everything about the facial nerve and for his iron will to constantly evolve surgical procedures.

I would like to dedicate this book to all my patients, whom it has been a privilege to treat, and their parents; to my medical colleagues and the multidisciplinary team, without whom nothing would have been achieved; to my scientific colleagues; and the endless possibilities I have had to explore the world.

My thanks also go to my parents, Ursula and Jaime Guntinas, for giving me the basis of freedom of thought and action. Special thanks are due to my wife, Julia Warnking, for keeping me constantly in intellectual and spiritual dynamics; and to my children Josephine, Mathilda, and Felicia for keeping me grounded.

Orlando Guntinas-Lichius

This book is dedicated to the key individuals who started me on the right path and most significantly impacted my growth as a human being and physician. I would like to thank my mother and father, Madeline and Edward Schaitkin, for teaching me kindness and respect. To Dr. George Conner, I greatly appreciate you sharing your incredible insights into the qualities of patience and teaching techniques, and for being the first one to introduce me to the facial nerve.

To Dr. Eugene Myers and Dr. Jonas Johnson, thank you for expanding my professional life immensely by bringing me into the nurturing and academically rich environment of the University of Pittsburgh's Department of Otolaryngology. I most especially recognize and thank Dr. Mark May for selflessly sharing with me his vast knowledge of the facial nerve and for being my eternal sounding board, confidante, and friend. I am also very grateful to Ms. Susan Klein, MA, CCC-A. She has invested considerable time and expertise in evaluating, testing, and counseling facial nerve patients and makes the facial nerve database possible. Each of my patients has taught me something about the facial nerve, and I am so grateful that they trusted me to do my very best for them.

Tremendous thanks are also due to my wife and partner, Dr. Sally E. Carty, for her wisdom and encouragement towards my work and life; to my children Hope, Simon, and Iris for all the joy they bring me and all they have taught me; and to Thea for being nice.

Barry M. Schaitkin

Contributors

Doychin N. Angelov, MD, PhD
Professor
Institute of Anatomy
The University Hospital of Cologne
Cologne, Germany

Farhad Ardeshirpour, MD
Fellow
Division of Facial Plastic and Reconstructive Surgery
Department of Otolaryngology
University of Washington School of Medicine
Seattle, Washington, USA

Caroline A. Banks, MD
Facial Plastic and Reconstructive Surgery Fellow
Department of Otolaryngology—Head and Neck Surgery
Massachusetts Eye and Ear Infirmary/Harvard Medical School
Boston, Massachusetts, USA

Brent J. Benscoter, MD
Michigan Ear Institute
Farmington Hills, Michigan, USA

Gregory H. Borschel, MD
Assistant Professor
Division of Plastic and Reconstructive Surgery
Hospital for Sick Children
University of Toronto
Toronto, Canada

Derald E. Brackmann, MD
Associate
House Clinic
Los Angeles, California, USA

Hartmut Peter Burmeister, MD
Assistant Medical Director
Institute of Radiology, Neuroradiology and Nuclear Medicine
Bremerhaven Reinkenheide Hospital
Bremerhaven, Germany

Kristen M. Davidge, MD, MSc
Staff Surgeon
Division of Plastic and Reconstructive Surgery
Hospital for Sick Children
University of Toronto
Toronto, Canada

Christian Dobel, PhD
Professor
Department of Otorhinolaryngology and Facial Nerve Center
Jena University Hospital
Jena, Germany

Mira Finkensieper, MD
Clinical Fellow
Department of Otorhinolaryngology
St. Anna Hospital
Wuppertal, Germany

Bahar Bassiri Gharb, MD
Clinical Fellow
Cleveland Clinic Foundation
Dermatology and Plastic Surgery Institute
Cleveland, Ohio, USA

John C. Goddard, MD
Associate
House Clinic
Los Angeles, California, USA

Orlando Guntinas-Lichius, MD
Professor and Chairman
Department of Otorhinolaryngology and Facial Nerve Center
Jena University Hospital
Jena, Germany

Tessa A. Hadlock, MD
Director
Division of Facial Plastic and Reconstructive Surgery and Facial Nerve Center
Department of Otolaryngology—Head and Neck Surgery
Massachusetts Eye and Ear Infirmary/Harvard Medical School
Boston, Massachusetts, USA

J. Michael Hendry, MD, MSc
Resident
Division of Plastic and Reconstructive Surgery
Hospital for Sick Children
University of Toronto
Toronto, Canada

Barry E. Hirsch, MD
Professor
Department of Otolaryngology
University of Pittsburgh Medical Center
Pittsburgh, Pennsylvania, USA

Andrey Irintchev, MD, PhD
Associate Professor
Department of Otorhinolaryngology
Jena University Hospital
Jena, Germany

Robert K. Jackler, MD
Sewall Professor and Chair
Department of Otolaryngology—Head and Neck Surgery
Stanford University
Stanford, California, USA

Markus Jungehülsing, MD
Professor
Department of Otorhinolaryngology
Ernst von Bergmann Hospital
Berlin, Germany

Jack M. Kartush, MD
Professor Emeritus
Michigan Ear Institute
Farmington Hills, Michigan, USA

Matthew L. Kircher, MD
Assistant Professor
Department of Otolaryngology—Head and Neck Surgery
Loyola University Medical Center
Chicago, Illinois, USA

Carsten M. Klingner, MD
Clinical Fellow
Hans Berger Clinic for Neurology
University Hospital Jena
Jena, Germany

John P. Leonetti, MD
Professor and Vice Chairman
Department of Otolaryngology—Head and Neck Surgery
Loyola University Medical Center
Chicago, Illinois, USA

Sam J. Marzo, MD
Professor
Department of Otolaryngology—Head and Neck Surgery
Loyola University Medical Center
Chicago, Illinois, USA

Jacob Seth McAfee, MD
Neurotology Fellow
University of Pittsburgh Medical Center
Pittsburgh, Pennsylvania, USA

Eva Maria Miltner
Certified Physical Therapist
Department of Otolaryngology
Jena University Hospital
Jena, Germany

Wolfgang H. R. Miltner, PhD
Professor
Department of Biological and Clinical Psychology
Friedrich Schiller University
Jena, Germany

Kris S. Moe, MD, FACS
Professor and Chief
Division of Facial Plastic and Reconstructive Surgery
Departments of Otolaryngology—Head and Neck Surgery and Neurological Surgery
University of Washington School of Medicine
Seattle, Washington, USA

Howard S. Moskowitz, MD, PhD
Assistant Professor
Department of Otorhinolaryngology—Head and Neck Surgery
Montefiore Medical Center
New York, New York, USA

Peter L. Santa Maria, MBBS, PhD
Instructor
Department of Otolaryngology—Head and Neck Surgery
Stanford University
Stanford, California, USA

Barry M. Schaitkin, MD
Professor
Facial Nerve Center
Department of Otolaryngology
University of Pittsburgh Medical Center
Pittsburgh, Pennsylvania, USA

Hans-Christoph Scholle, PhD
Professor
Department of Trauma, Hand and Reconstructive Surgery
Jena University Hospital
Jena, Germany

Nikolaus-Peter Schumann, PhD, MD
Department of Trauma, Hand and Reconstructive Surgery
Jena University Hospital
Jena, Germany

Maria Z. Siemionow, MD, PhD, DSc
Professor
Department of Orthopedics
University of Illinois at Chicago
Chicago, Illinois, USA

Eric L. Slattery, MD
Fellow
Michigan Ear Institute
Farmington Hills, Michigan, USA

Eric Smouha, MD
Associate Professor
Department of Otolaryngology—Head and Neck Surgery
Icahn School of Medicine at Mount Sinai
New York, New York, USA

Elizabeth Toh, MD
Director, Balance and Hearing Implant Center
Co-Director, Center for Cranial Base Surgery
Department of Otolaryngology—Head and Neck Surgery
Lahey Hospital and Medical Center
Burlington, Massachusetts, USA

Courtney C. J. Voelker, MD, PhD
Clinical Fellow
House Clinic
Los Angeles, California, USA

Gerd Fabian Volk, MD
Clinical Fellow
Department of Otorhinolaryngology and Facial Nerve Center
Jena University Hospital
Jena, Germany

Thomas Weiss, MD, PhD
Professor
Department of Biological and Clinical Psychology
Friedrich Schiller University
Jena, Germany

Otto W. Witte, MD
Professor and Chairman
Hans Berger Clinic for Neurology
Jena University Hospital
Jena, Germany

Claus Wittekindt, MD
Associate Professor
Department of Otorhinolaryngology—Head and Neck Surgery
Justus Liebig University School of Medicine
Giessen, Germany

Ronald Zuker, MD, FRCS(C), FACS, FAAP
Professor
Division of Plastic and Reconstructive Surgery
Hospital for Sick Children
University of Toronto
Toronto, Canada

Part I

Embryology, Anatomy, Physiology, and Applied Basic Sciences

1 Embryology and Anatomy of the Facial Nerve: Correlates of Misdirected Reinnervation and Poor Recovery of Function after Lesions

Doychin N. Angelov

1.1 Introduction

The facial nerve is the most frequently damaged nerve in head and neck trauma. Apart from traffic-accident injuries (temporal bone fractures, or lacerations of the face), most facial nerve lesions are postoperative (removal of cerebellopontine angle tumors, parotid resections). Despite the use of fine microsurgical techniques for repair of interrupted nerves, recovery of voluntary movements of all 42 facial muscles and emotional expression of the face remain poor; the occurrence of "postparalytic syndrome," including paresis, abnormally associated movements, and altered reflexes, is inevitable.

This insufficient recovery has been attributed to many factors; more details are given in Chapters 2 and Chapter 3. However, three of these factors (misdirected regrowth of axons towards "inappropriate" muscle targets, extensive collateral branching of axons at the lesion site, and vigorous intramuscular sprouting of axons in the facial muscles) are of crucial importance for recovery of facial motor function.

Due to a common neural and muscular nature of these factors, the reasons for their occurrence should be sought in the intimately associated and synchronous embryonic development of the facial nerve and muscles. In this very short synopsis, the author tries to convey several key moments in their ontogenesis. In this way the author hopes to improve the general understanding of pathogenesis, mechanisms of functional recovery, and reasonable therapeutic approaches.

1.2 Neural Plate, Neural Crest, Ectodermal Placodes

The entire nervous system originates from three sources, each derived from specific regions of the *neural ectoderm*. The first source is the *neural plate* that forms the central nervous system, the somatic motor nerves, and the preganglionic autonomic nerves. The second source is cells located at the periphery of the neural plate (*neural crest*) that migrate away from the plate just before its fusion into a neural tube. The third source is the *ectodermal placodes*: groups of cells at the edge of the neural plate that remain there after neural tube formation and after the neural crest cells have started their migration.[1] The ectodermal placodes contribute to the somatic sensory ganglia of the cranial nerves, to the hypophysis cerebri, and to the inner ear (otic placode).[1]

1.3 Neural Folds, Neural Tube, Rhombomeres, Roof and Floor Plates

The neural plate consists of thickened epithelium whose lateral edges elevate as *neural folds*, approach one another, and fuse in the dorsal midline as the *neural tube* (neurulation). Just prior to closure of the neural tube, the neural folds expand in the head region as the first indication of a brain. Subsequent to the closure of the tube, these regional expansions (primary cerebral vesicles) give rise to the *prosencephalon* or forebrain, the *mesencephalon* or midbrain, and the *rhombencephalon* or hindbrain.[1]

In addition to these gross divisions, the neural tube manifests a number of ridges and depressions that subdivide it further. Prominent among these are serial bulges that appear very early especially in the rhombencephalon —the so-called rhombomeres—that apparently constitute the primary units of the later regional patterning. Recent studies have shown that the rhombomeres represent rostrocaudal domains of different gene expression that have characteristic fates. Each rhombomere is characterized by a unique combination of *Hox* genes.[1–3] The nucleus of origin of the facial nerve develops from the fourth and fifth rhombomeres.[4,5]

During neurulation the neural tube becomes subdivided in the dorsoventral axis into a *floor plate* (a ventral midline region with non-neuronal cells that are able to induce motor neurons). As the neural tube closes, cells from the edges of the neural folds form a distinct transitory population—the *neural crest*—in the dorsal midline. The derivatives of the neural crest include the sensory ganglia of the cranial and spinal nerves, the autonomic ganglia and nerves, the Schwann cells, and ectomesenchyme cells of the pharyngeal arches, as described in The Second Pharyngeal Arch. The "departure" of the neural crest is followed by the formation of another specialized non-neuronal region, the *roof plate*.[1]

1.4 First Differentiation into Motor and Sensory Cells

As the lateral walls of the neural tube gradually thicken, the central canal widens and a longitudinal *sulcus limitans* develops on each side. This sulcus divides the lateral wall into a ventrolateral lamina and a dorsolateral lamina, a division that indicates a fundamental functional difference: the ventral lamina is concerned with motor function as it contains the cell bodies of motor neurons, while the dorsal lamina receives inflow from the sensory ganglia (▶ Fig. 1.1a).[6] In the head, the cranial nerves form a continuation to the series of spinal nerves.[1]

1.5 Primordial Tissues of the Facial Nerve Occur at the End of the 3rd Week

The future facial and acoustic nerves occur together as a group of cells dorsolateral to the rhombencephalon and just rostral to the otic placode as early as the end of the 3rd week (embryo is 3 mm long). These cells build the so-called facioacoustic primordium (▶ Fig. 1.1b). Very soon (4th week) the facial portion extends ventrally and reaches a placode located on the upper portion of the second pharyngeal arch, which is described in The Second Pharyngeal Arch. Later, during the 5th week, a group of cells appears in the facial portion of the common primordium; these cells are derived from the placode and will develop into the geniculate ganglion. The distal segment of this primordium divides into two equally thick branches: the first courses caudally to the mesenchyma of the second pharyngeal arch, and represents the *main trunk of the facial nerve*; the second curves rostrally towards the first arch and develops into the *chorda tympani*.[5]

!

The embryological development of the facial nerve starts during the 3rd to 5th week of gestation.

1.6 The Second Pharyngeal Arch

In all vertebrate embryos, after the head fold formation, the mandibular region and the whole neck are still absent. They will be formed soon by the appearance and modification of six paired pharyngeal arches, which develop in the lateral aspects of the head adjacent to the hindbrain.[7,8]

The second pharyngeal arch is especially important for the purpose of this monograph. This arch (called also postmandibular or hyoid) is seen at first on days 23 to 25 after fertilization (▶ Fig. 1.2a).[8] Like most pharyngeal arches, it is composed of: (1) ectoderm (external epithelial covering originating from a strip lateral to the rhombencephalic neural fold); (2) pharyngeal endoderm (internal covering); and (3) mesenchyme (derived from the neural crest, angiogenic and paraxial mesodermal cell populations).[3] From these disparate cell populations develop:

- Specific motor and sensory nerves (e.g., the facial nerve for the second arch).
- An arch artery from the angiogenic mesenchyme (mesoderm derived).
- Associated striated muscles from the paraxial mesenchyme (mesoderm derived).[7]

!

The proximity in the development of the facial nerve and adjacent arteries—basilar, posterior inferior cerebellar, anterior inferior cerebellar, labyrinthine—may cause later nerve compression during its course between the brain stem and the porus acusticus internus, and this is one of the possible mechanisms of *hemifacial spasm*.

The muscles of the second arch derive from the fourth and fifth somitomeres (portions of the paraxial mesenchyme beneath the neural plate). Most of them migrate widely (▶ Fig. 1.2b), but retain their innervation by the facial nerve. The facial nerve enters the primordial muscle mass before it begins to differentiate, and it then migrates with the developing muscles, and divides when they divide (▶ Fig. 1.3). In this way the facial nerve “follows” the muscles and achieves its typical fan-shaped appearance (▶ Fig. 1.1c).[4,7,8]

This migration of muscles is facilitated by the early obliteration of the first branchial groove and its internal counterpart the first pharyngeal sac or pouch (grooves and pouches lie between the pharyngeal arches and demarcate zones where the ectoderm and endoderm are in virtual contact).[4,7,8]

!

The facial nerve and the facial muscles arise synchronously and influence the growth and development of each other. This could at least partially explain the poor navigation of injured and regrowing “adult” facial axons toward a target muscle that has already accomplished its development.

1.7 Development of the Intraparenchymal Portion of the Facial Nerve

At the end of the 5th gestational week, the facial motor nucleus can be recognized. It arises from neuroblasts

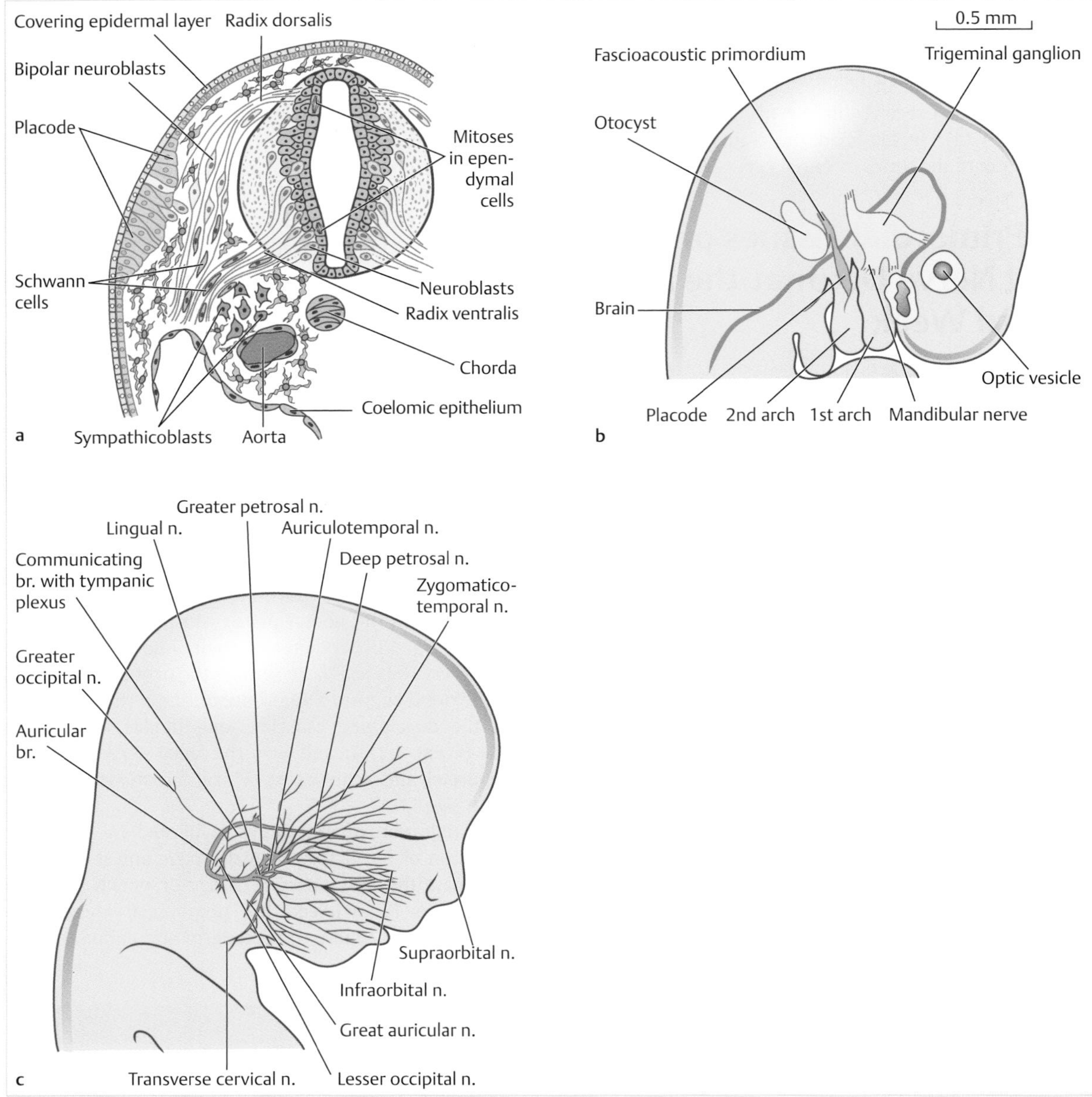

Fig. 1.1 Parallel development of the facial nerve branches (this figure) and the muscles of facial expression (▶ Fig. 1.2). Development of the facial nerve branches. **(a)** Schematic drawing of the early histogenesis in the spinal cord indicating the site of origin of motoneurons and their axons in the ventral radix (from the neural tube), the bipolar neuroblasts of the dorsal ganglia, and the Schwann cells (from the neural crest and the placode). (Adapted with permission from Starck D, ed. Embryologie. Ein Lehrbuch auf allgemein biologischer Grundlage. Stuttgart: Georg Thieme Verlag; 1965.) **(b)** Configuration of the facioacoustic primordium and the second branchial arch at the end of the 4th week of gestation (28 days). (Adapted with permission from May M, Schaitkin BM, eds. The Facial Nerve. New York, NY: Thieme Medical Publishers; 2000.) **(c)** Configuration of the facial nerve at 12 weeks of gestation. All peripheral branches are present and most of their connections to the trigeminal, glossopharyngeal, vagal, and cervical cutaneous nerves are established. (Adapted with permission from May M, Schaitkin BM, eds. The Facial Nerve. New York, NY: Thieme; 2000.)

located in the third metencephalic (the metencephalon is a part of the rhombencephalon that includes the cerebellum and pons) rhombomere. The facial nucleus lies initially in close proximity to the abducens nucleus. As the metencephalon (i.e., pons) elongates and expands, the abducens nucleus ascends and displaces the facial axons. In this way the internal genu of the facial nerve as well as the colliculus facialis in the fossa rhomboidea are formed.[5]

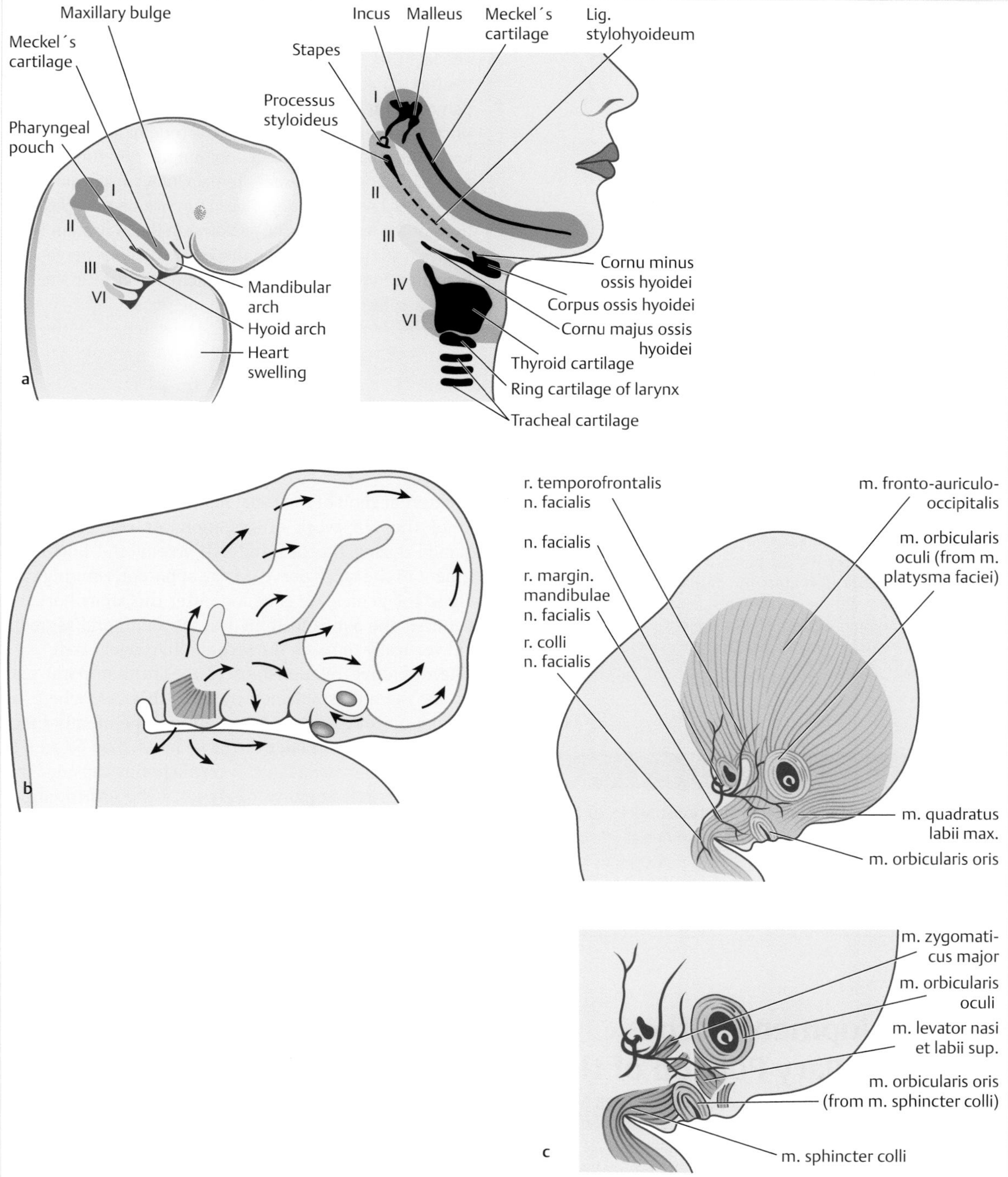

Fig. 1.2 Parallel development of the facial nerve branches (▶ Fig. 1.1) and the muscles of facial expression (this figure). Development of the muscles of facial expression.**(a)** Schematic drawing of the position of the second (hyoid) branchial arch (blue) in the whole embryo (left panel) and the close relation of its derivatives to those stemming from the adjacent arches. (Adapted with permission from Sadler TW. Medizinische Embryologie. Die normale menschliche Entwicklung und ihre Fehlbildungen. 11 Auflage. Stuttgart, New York: Georg Thieme Verlag; 2008.) **(b)** Schematic drawing of the spreading of the facial muscles from the second branchial arch. (Adapted with permission from Clara M, ed. Entwicklungsgeschichte des Menschen. Leipzig: Georg Thieme Verlag; 1966.) **(c)** Differentiation of the superficial (top panel) and deep (bottom panel) facial muscles. (Adapted with permission from Clara M, ed. Entwicklungsgeschichte des Menschen. Leipzig: Georg Thieme Verlag; 1966.)

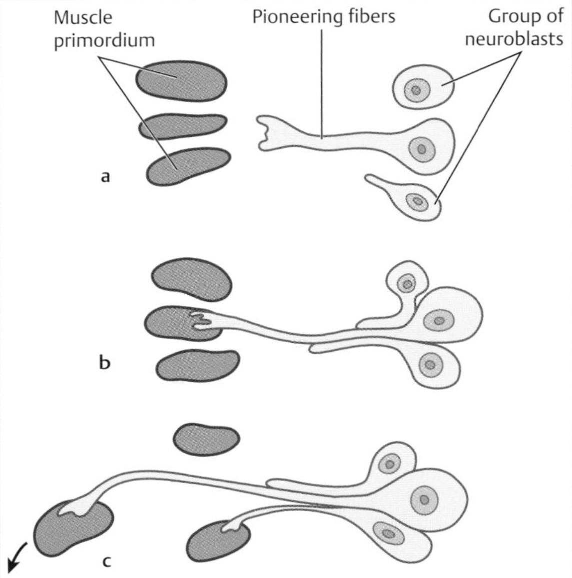

Fig. 1.3 Illustration of the very close relations between developing muscles and growing nerve fibers. **(a)** Neuroblasts grow initially separately from muscle primordia. **(b)** Axons of motoneurons reach and contact the muscles. **(c)** Muscles migrate together with the nerve fibers. (Adapted with permission from Starck D, ed. Embryologie. Ein Lehrbuch auf allgemein biologischer Grundlage. Stuttgart: Georg Thieme Verlag; 1965.)

!

The close relationship between the motor nuclei of the sixth and seventh cranial nerves determines at least in part the pathology of congenital disorders such as Möbius syndrome, as well as that of acquired inflammatory, vascular, and neoplastic disorders.

1.8 Development of the Extramedullary Portion of the Facial Nerve

The facial nerve roots (sensory and motor) become distinguishable near the end of the 7th gestational week synchronously with the ganglion geniculi. The nervus intermedius (sensory root) arises from the ganglion and passes between the motor facial root and the vestibulocochlear nerve. The motor root fibers pass mainly caudal to the geniculate ganglion.[5]

!

The fact that sensitivity develops independently from the motor pathway allows patients with congenital facial palsy to have intact tearing and taste. Furthermore, since most sensory branches of the trigeminal nerve follow routes that are different and remote from those of the facial nerve, they usually remain intact after traumatic facial nerve injuries. This in turn allows manipulations of the lesioned facial perikarya in the brainstem by applying stimulations along the axis: trigeminal nerve branches, trigeminal ganglion, trigeminal nuclei in the pons, and facial motor nucleus in the pons.

1.9 Development of the Pars Intratemporalis

The external genu of the facial nerve begins to form at the end of the 5th week of gestation. As the ear region expands during the 6th and 7th weeks, the horizontal segment of the facial nerve is very apparent, running caudally to the geniculate ganglion. After this short horizontal course, the axons forming the intratemporal segment bend vertically to reach the second pharyngeal arch.[5]

The definitive relationships of the intratemporal portion are mainly established by the 8th week when the cartilaginous otic capsule forms around the membranous labyrinth. Two weeks later the facial nerve may be seen to course in a deep sulcus in the cartilaginous capsule. This capsule does not begin to ossify until the 4th month of gestation and bone does not begin to enclose the nerve until the end of the 5th month.[5]

!

It is important to note that even at birth the canal is not yet completely enclosed by bone. The ossification proceeds in an anterior-to-posterior direction as two periosteal shelves of bone gradually surround the facial nerve. Thus, fallopian canal dehiscences are not congenital anomalies, but variations of normal development.

1.10 Development of Facial Nerve Branches

Facial nerve intratemporal branches form and course into regions that appear to be expanding peripheral to the nerve. The first branch of the intratemporal portion that develops is the *chorda tympani*, followed closely by the *n. petrosus major*. The chorda tympani courses rostrally from the facial nerve trunk as the first and second arches expand in the rostrocaudal plane. Likewise, the greater petrosal nerve (n. petrosus major) forms as the region rostral to the geniculate ganglion expands.[9] The *n. stapedius* can be detected as a discrete nerve only after the target muscle has increased in size sufficiently (8th week of gestation).[5]

The extratemporal branches initially "disappear" into the surrounding mesenchymal cells of the second pharyngeal arch. The proximal branches form before the distal ones: for example, the *ramus auricularis posterior* is the first that can be recognized, followed by the *branch to m. digastricus*. Both branches can be identified by the 6th week of embryonic life. The most peripheral small fascicles of the nerve become evident near the end of the 7th week and the temporofacial and cervicofacial subdivisions become evident in the beginning of the 8th week. Finally, all five major peripheral branches are present as tiny fascicles at the end of the 8th week.[5]

1.11 Development of Intratemporal Communications

The facial nerve *communication to the tympanic plexus* (built by the glossopharyngeal nerve) begins with a tiny branch arising from the geniculate ganglion that joins the upper ganglion of the glossopharyngeal nerve. Another small nerve, the auricular branch of the vagus nerve, which innervates the skin over the external auditory canal (Arnold's nerve), also communicates with the facial nerve. Numerous aberrant sensory fibers from the tympanic plexus have been reported to enter the facial nerve near the stapedial branch.[5]

!

The communications to sensory fibers of, for example, the tympanic plexus may play an important role in the development of viral facial nerve palsy because most viruses have an affinity for afferent fibers.

1.12 Development of Extratemporal Communications

The cutaneous branches of the second and third cervical spinal nerves establish communication with the facial nerve in the 7th week of embryonic life as connections between the *great auricular nerve* and the *transversus colli* nerve, and also between the *posterior auricular branch* and the *cervical branch* of the facial nerve. During the following 8th week, communications are established with the *auriculotemporal*, *infraorbital*, *buccal*, and *mental* branches of the trigeminal nerve.[5]

!

The facial nerve has the largest number of communications with other nerves. This fact may account for the wide variety of neurological signs associated with the viral inflammatory types of nerve palsy, e.g., herpes zoster cephalicus and Bell's palsy.

1.13 Relationships to Developing Facial Muscles

The facial muscles start to develop between the 3rd and 8th weeks of gestation when the mesoderm of the second branchial arch starts to thicken just caudal to the first branchial groove. There is a close relationship between the muscles and the nerve during their formation. The facial muscles develop synchronously with the extratemporal facial nerve branches, i.e., the facial nerve branches form at the same time as the muscles form (▶ Fig. 1.2c). In most areas of the face, the branches are located deep to the facial muscles.[10,11]

!

The muscles of the face are part of the superficial musculoaponeurotic system (SMAS). The terminal branches of the facial nerve are located deep to the SMAS and turn superficially to innervate the facial muscles entering their deep surface. However, the nerve branches for the m. buccinator, m. mentalis, and m. levator anguli oris enter these muscles from their superficial surface and can thus be damaged.[12,13]

During the 7th and 8th gestational weeks, sheet-like collections of premyoblasts and early myoblasts extend from this attenuated mesenchyme of the second pharyngeal arch to form five laminae on each side of the face that extend into the superficial portions of the future temporal, occipital, cervical, and mandibular regions. On each side of the face, the infraorbital lamina and the occipital platysma are the first laminae to appear.[1,14]

In the later part of the 8th week, an infraorbital lamina of myoblasts appears, and by the 12th gestational week all facial muscles can be identified in their definitive positions. Some of these muscles (the orbicularis oculi and the corrugator supercilii) are functional between the 8th and 9th weeks, and others (the orbicularis oris) between the 10th and 11th weeks. The angle of the mouth and the wings of the nose can be elevated at the 12th week.[1,14]

The infraorbital lamina forms the zygomaticus major, the zygomaticus minor, the levator labii superioris, the levator labii superioris alaeque nasi, the superior part of orbicularis oris, the compressor naris, the dilator naris, the depressor septi, the orbicularis oculi, the frontal belly of the occipitofrontalis, the corrugator supercilii, and the procerus muscles.[1,14]

!

The zygomaticus major muscle is a very important surgical landmark. With the exception of lower orbicular branch (which crosses the zygomaticus major at its superficial surface) all facial nerve branches in this region pass deep to it. Therefore skin incisions over the zygomaticus major muscle should be performed superficially to protect the lower orbicular branch.[13]

The occipital lamina forms the occipital belly of the occipitofrontalis muscle. Each temporal lamina gives rise to the superior auricular muscles. Each mandibular lamina forms the mandibular part of the platysma, the depressor labii inferioris, the mentalis, the risorius, the depressor anguli oris, the buccinator, and the levator anguli oris muscles. Mesenchymal cells adjacent to the first branchial cleft form the anterior auricular muscle on each side of the face.

The deep muscles form separately from the mesoderm, and these muscles comprise the posterior belly of the digastric muscle, the digastric tendon, the stapedius muscle, and the stylohyoid muscle on each side of the face.

1.14 Axonal Growth and Guidance

According to the classic view of neural tube histogenesis, neuroblasts are the progenitors of neurons, and spongioblasts of glial cells (astrocytes and oligodendrocytes). Facial motor neurons originate from the neuroepithelium (neural plate); its Schwann cells develop from the neural crest and the placodes.[14]

Initially neuroblasts are round or fusiform (▸ Fig. 1.1a). As maturation proceeds they send out fine cytoplasmic processes (axons) containing neurofilaments and microtubules, whose expanded end—the growth cone—is the principle sensory organ of the neuron. The growth cone is constantly active, changing shape, and extending and withdrawing small filopodia and lamellipodia that apparently “explore” the local environment for a suitable surface along which axonal extension may occur. The molecular basis of this behavior is the scaffolding of microtubules and neurofilaments within the axon. Growing neuroblasts have a cortex rich in actin, associated with the plasma membrane, and a core of centrally located microtubules and neurofilaments.[6]

During development, the growing axons of neuroblasts navigate with precision over considerable distances, often pursuing complex courses to reach their targets (▸ Fig. 1.3). The mechanism of axonal guidance has been demonstrated by two principal theories: (1) neurotropism (chemotropism); and (2) the contact guidance theories. The former proposes that growing fibers are guided by some form of attraction, presumably chemical, which emanated from the target area to be innervated. The second view holds that pioneer axons are guided to their destination by preferential growth along pathways dictated exclusively by the structures with which the growth cone is in direct contact.[6]

Once growth cones arrive in their target area, there occurs the additional problem of forming synapses. If an axon fails to make the correct contacts, its parent soma atrophies and dies, probably due to the failure of neurons to acquire sufficient amounts of varying trophic factors (e.g., nerve growth factor, brain-derived neurotrophic factor, ciliary ganglion trophic factor, fibroblast-like growth factor, glial cell line trophic factor, neurotrophin 3, neurotrophin 4, etc).[3]

In addition to receiving trophic support, the nervous tissue also influences the metabolism of its targets. The most obvious example is the mutual dependence of motor neurons and muscles. If, during development, a nerve fails to connect its muscle, both degenerate. Initially the nerve appears to have no influence on the early stages of development of the end organ (i.e., the facial muscles). However, histological differentiation of the muscles may occur only after innervation (i.e., the trophic influence by nerves is essential for the persistence of muscle tissue).[6]

1.15 Postnatal Development

At birth and until 4 years of age the facial nerve is extremely vulnerable to injury: its trunk lies just under the skin (the mastoid process is absent) and the marginal mandibular branch lies over the mandible.

!

These factors account for the high incidence of facial nerve injury during surgery in the parotid region of infants and young children. The motor fibers of the facial nerve get myelinated between birth and the 4th year. After 40 years of age, the number of myelinated axons decreases. Probably this is why clinical observations indicate that nerve regeneration occurs more readily in young children following nerve injury.

1.16 Intracranial Portion of the Facial Nerve

The facial motor nucleus contains about 7,000 to 10,000 motoneuronal perikarya seated in the lower third of the pons beneath the fourth ventricle. These neuronal cell somata are mytopically organized into four major subnuclei. Motoneurons of the medial and ventral subnuclei innervate the muscles of the auricle and the platysma, respectively. The lateral facial subnucleus innervates the perioral muscles. The dorsal subnucleus innervates the frontalis and orbicularis oculi muscles. The orbicularis oculi motor pool is sometimes called the intermediate nucleus.[15]

The motoneurons of the facial nucleus receive a strong bilateral projection from the motor cortex. The face area of the primary motor cortex, the dorsal and ventral premotor cortex, and the caudate cingulate motor area project to the contralateral lateral subnucleus, which innervates the perioral muscles. The projection of the supplementary motor area is bilateral and targets motoneurons of the medial subnucleus innervating the muscles of the ear. The rostral cingulate motor area provides the motoneurons of the orbicularis oculi with a bilateral innervation.[15]

Impulses from the contralateral cortical motor facial area (middle portion of the gyrus precentralis in the frontal lobe) are carried through the tractus corticobulbaris (corticonuclearis) via the knee of the capsula interna and crus cerebri to the lower brainstem where they synapse on motoneurons of the facial nucleus. Whereas corticobulbar axons arising from the cortical representation of the upper face area project bilaterally (crossed and uncrossed), those to the lower face motoneurons are crossed only.

Two classical clinical observations on (1) sparing of the upper facial muscles in a supranuclear palsy and on (2) preservation of emotional facial expression (smiling and laughing) in certain cases of facial paralysis have been reevaluated recently. Sparing of the upper facial muscles may not be due to a bilateral primary motor cortex projection to the motoneurons supplying these muscles, as previously assumed, but rather it may be the consequence of a bilateral projection of the rostral cingulate motor area. Preserved cingulate motor areas, with projections to upper facial and perioral muscles, in patients who have had a stroke, represent a possible substrate for the presence of emotional facial expression, as discussed in Chapter 27.

The axons of the facial motoneurons do not leave the brain parenchyma along the shortest possible ventrolateral way, but project initially in the dorsomedial direction, pass around the nucleus of n. abducens building the internal facial knee (which causes a "swelling" on the floor of the fourth ventricle called the facial colliculus), and leave the ventrolateral surface of the brainstem at the cerebellopontine angle.[12]

In its intra-arachnoidal segment, the facial nerve is void of epineurium, covered by pia mater, and bathed in cerebrospinal fluid.[12,16] The average distance between the point where the facial nerve exits the brainstem and enters the porus acusticus internus is 15.8 mm. Large pathologies at the cerebellopontine angle (temporal bone fractures, acoustic schwannomas, meningiomas, primary cholesteatomas) can compress the facial nerve.[12]

!

As an acoustic neuroma (also known as vestibular schwannoma, which constitutes about 6–10% of all primary intracranial tumors) grows, the facial nerve is at first merely displaced from its anatomical position. Subsequently, it becomes progressively compressed, ribboned, and splayed on the tumor surface. The compression may cause acute inflammation and herniation of the nerve fibers from the bony canal. This condition places the nerve in great jeopardy, since the protuberant portion can easily be shaved off inadvertently when the surgeon removes the tumor.[13] Nevertheless, despite careful surgical technique that preserves the facial nerve 98% of the time, postoperative peripheral facial nerve palsy (immediate or delayed) may occur in 20–40% of patients with cerebellopontine angle (CPA) tumors.[17] During CPA tumor surgery, exerting a medial pull on the tumor and the attached facial nerve (toward the brainstem) is a common mistake that causes paralysis. Therefore facial nerve injury is usually avoided by using the translabyrinthine approach: after the facial nerve has been identified near the brainstem, dissection should be continued from medial to lateral direction (i.e., toward the point of adherence of the facial nerve at the porus acusticus internus). Dissecting in this direction avoids pulling on the facial nerve as it exits the internal auditory canal. In its labyrinthine segment, the facial nerve occupies the rostrodorsal portion of the meatus and practically lies in a groove over the cochlear and vestibular nerves. It leaves the fundus through a singular foramen. Thus it has little direct stabilizing contact with the dura mater and can be easily displaced and damaged.[2,18]

1.17 Surgical Anatomy of the Facial Nerve Trunk and its Branches

The *facial nerve trunk* emerges from the base of the skull through the stylomastoid foramen. At this point it lies about 9 mm away from the posterior belly of the digastric muscle and 11 mm below the bony external acoustic meatus.[14]

> !
>
> Since these points are difficult to determine, three surgical maneuvers are used to identify the facial nerve trunk as it exits the stylomastoid foramen[14]
>
> - First, the blood-free plane immediately in front of the cartilaginous external acoustic meatus can be opened up by blunt dissection. This leads the surgeon to the skull base just superficial to the styloid process and the stylomastoid foramen. This plane in turn can be gently opened up in an inferior direction by further blunt dissection until the trunk of the facial nerve is encountered
> - Second, the trunk of the facial nerve can be identified by exposing the anterior border of the sternocleidomastoid muscle just below its insertion into the mastoid process. Retracting the muscle posteriorly, the surgeon reaches the posterior belly of m. digastricus, which is then traced upwards and backward to the mastoid process. This point lies immediately below the stylomastoid foramen and the facial nerve trunk
> - A third option is to find a terminal branch of the facial nerve peripherally—commonly the marginal mandibular branch—and to trace it back centripetally until the facial nerve trunk is identified.

Thereafter the facial nerve runs in an arciform course that is concave upward and medianward. It passes in front of the posterior belly of m. digastricus, and lateral to the styloid process, the external carotid artery, and the posterior facial vein. When the nerve reaches the posterior border of the mandible ramus it turns forward at almost a right angle, splitting into its terminal branches, which then course to the muscles of facial expression.[14]

Although most of the following branches contain only motor axons, the facial nerve has been shown to contain some sensory cutaneous fibers. They accompany the auricular branch of the vagus nerve and innervate the skin on both lateral and cranial auricular surfaces including the conchal depression of the auricle and its eminence on the cranial aspect.

Close to the stylomastoid foramen the facial nerve gives off the *posterior auricular branch*, which supplies the occipital belly of the occipitofrontalis, some of the auricular muscles, and the posterior belly of the digastricus and stylohyoideus muscles.

The facial nerve then enters the parotid gland high up on its posteromedial surface and passes forward and downward behind the mandible ramus. Within the substance of the gland the facial nerve branches into a larger temporofacial trunk and a smaller cervicofacial trunk. This division, located just behind (about 5 mm) the retromandibular vein, occurred in every one of 350 cervicofacial dissections done by Davies et al[19] as well as in all 130 dissections performed by D. N. Angelov and B. Spacca (unpublished data). In about 90% of patients both trunks lie superficial to the vein, in intimate contact with it. Occasionally the trunks pass beneath the retromandibular vein (temporofacial trunk in about 9% of patients, cervicofacial trunk in about 2%).[14]

The *temporofacial* and *cervicofacial trunks* branch further to form a parotid plexus, which exhibits variations in branching pattern. Five main terminal branches arise from the plexus and diverge within the gland. They leave the parotid gland by its anteromedial surface, medial to its anterior margin, and supply the muscles of facial expression. Whereas the temporofacial trunk has a plexiform arrangement formed by dichotic and anastomotic divisions, the cervicofacial trunk resembles merely a simple large loop.[14]

The *temporal branches* (*rr. temporales*) are generally multiple and pass across the zygomatic arch towards the temple to supply the anterior and superior auricular muscles. More exactly described, they course along a line from a point 0.5 cm below the inferior edge of the tragus to a point about 2.0 cm above the lateral portion of the eyebrow. The temporal branches join with the zygomaticotemporal branch of the maxillary nerve and the auriculotemporal nerve of the mandibular nerve. The more anterior branches supply m. occipitofrontalis (frontal belly), m orbicularis oculi, and m. corrugator supercilii. Finally, the temporal branches join r. supraorbitalis and r. lacrimalis of the ophthalmic nerve.[14]

> !
>
> Injury to the temporal branches will result in paralysis of the forehead with secondary ptosis of the brow and loss of mimetic function ipsilaterally.

The *zygomatic branches* (*rr. zygomatici*) are also generally multiple and cross the zygomatic bone to the lateral canthus of the eye. They supply m. orbicularis oculi and join the lacrimal nerve as well as the zygomaticofacial branch of the maxillary nerve. These branches may also partially supply muscles associated with the buccal branch of the facial nerve.[14]

The *buccal branch* (*r. buccalis*) has a variable origin and passes horizontally to a distribution below the orbit and around the mouth. It is usually single, but two branches occur in 15% of patients. The buccal branch has a close relationship to the parotid duct and usually lies below it. Its superficial branches run deep to subcutaneous fat, the superficial musculoaponeurotic system, and m. procerus. They join the infratrochlear and external nasal nerves. The upper deep branches pass under m. zygomaticus major and m. levator labii superioris, and supply them and form an infraorbital plexus with the superior labial branches of the infraorbital nerve. Some of these branches also supply m. levator anguli oris, m. zygomaticus minor, m. levator anguli oris alaeque nasi, and the small nasal muscles, and are also frequently referred to as lower zygomatic branches. The lower deep branches supply the buccinator and the orbicularis oris and join the buccal branch of the mandibular nerve.[14]

!

The buccal branch of the facial nerve is deep to the superficial musculoaponeurotic system, but 20 mm lateral to the angle of the mouth it becomes superficial and travels subcutaneously.

The *marginal mandibular branches* (usually two) run forward toward the angulus mandibulae under the platysma, at first superficially in the trigonum submandibulare (trigonum digastricum), then turning upward and forward across the corpus mandibulae to pass under the depressor anguli oris. The branches supply m. risorius and the muscles of the lower lip and chin, and join the mental nerve.

The *cervical branch* issues from the lower part of the parotid gland and runs anteroinferiorly under m. platysma to the front of the neck. It supplies the platysma and communicates with the transverse cutaneous cervical nerve. In 20% of the cases there are two branches.

!

The marginal mandibular branch has an important surgical relationship with the lower border of the mandible (basis mandibulae) and may pass below it with a reported incidence varying between 20 and 50%, the furthest distance being 12 mm.

The peripheral branches of the facial nerve are joined by numerous anastomotic arcades between adjacent branches to form the parotid nerve plexus, which shows considerable variations. Six distinctive anastomotic patterns were described originally by Davis et al[19] in 350 cervicofacial halves. These observations were generally confirmed in 130 cranial halves by ongoing work at the Department of Anatomy, University of Cologne, Germany. The six patterns are as follows:

- Type I. There are no anastomoses between the facial nerve branches. The primary division takes place in a dichotic fashion, the branches thereof spread outward like the "spokes of a wheel" (▶ Fig. 1.4). The incidence rate described by Davis et al[19] is 13%, while Angelov and Spacca report 14.61%.
- Type II. The distinguishing feature of this type is the presence of an anastomotic connection between the

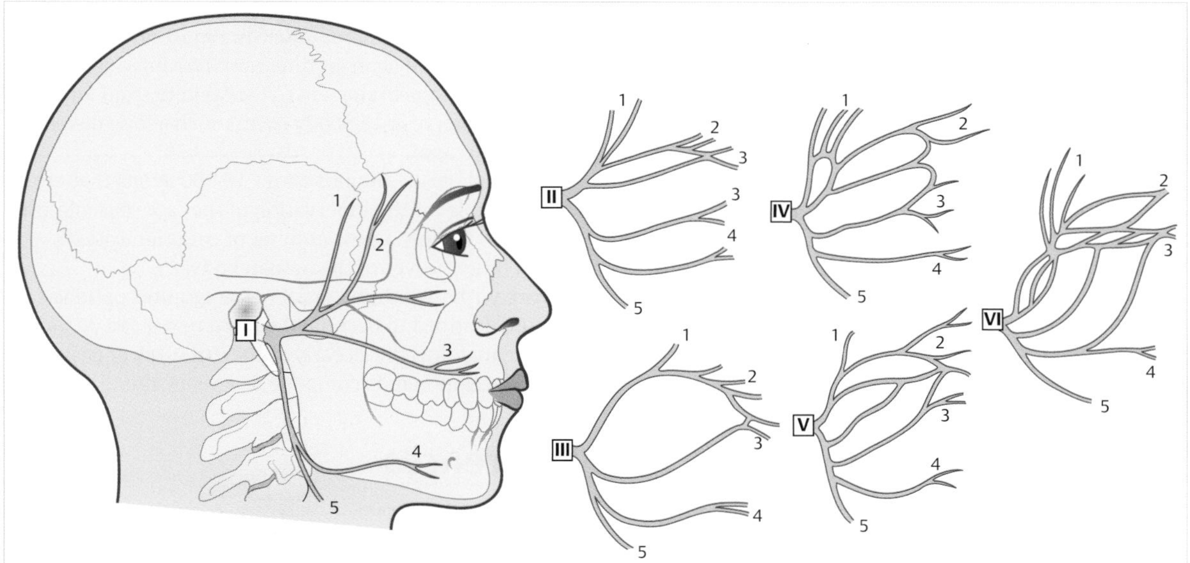

Fig. 1.4 Types of facial nerve branching described in 350 cervicofacial halves by Davis et al[19] and in 130 halves by Angelov and Spacca:
• Type I is characterized by the absence of anastomoses between the two main divisions: temporofacial and cervicofacial divisions of the facial nerve. Incidence 13 to 14.61%.
• Type II is characterized by anastomoses within the temporofacial division of the facial nerve. Incidence 17.69 to 20%.
• Type III displays anastomoses between the main divisions. Incidence 26.15 to 28%.
• Type IV is characte.rized by two anastomotic loops in the temporofacial division. Incidence 18.46 to 24%.
• Type V displays two loops in the cervicofacial division intervened with branches of the temporofacial main branch. Incidence 9 to 14.61%.
• Type VI displays a very extensive intermixture of facial nerve branches. Incidence 8 to 8.46%. (Reproduced from Bradley PJ, Gutinas-Lichius O. Salivary Gland Disorders and Diseases: Diagnosis and Management. Stuttgart, New York: Thieme; 2011.)

various components within the temporofacial division (▶ Fig. 1.4). The temporofacial division splits into two large portions: one directed transversely, the other anterosuperiorly. The latter ramus then splits into branches, some of which are directed to the muscles about the eye, while the more inferior branches run directly across the face. These inferior branches then anastomose with the main transverse ramus, generally beyond the anterior border of the gland; they give off branches to the buccal and zygomatic regions. The incidence rate of this type described by Davis et al[19] is 20%, while Angelov and Spacca report 17.69%.

- Type III. This type is characterized by a single anastomosis between the two main cervicofacial and temporofacial divisions (▶ Fig. 1.4). Usually one branch arises from the cervical division immediately distal to the point of bifurcation of the main trunk; this offshoot then follows an oblique course upward to join the zygomatic branch. The anastomosis occurs beyond the anterior border of the gland and generally over the parotid duct. In all instances, the upward-arching contribution of the cervicofacial division follows one of two schemes: one in which a large-caliber cervicofacial portion supplies the buccal region, and then sends a relatively small anastomotic branch to the zygomatic ramus; the other scheme is an arrangement whereby a small-size cervicofacial contribution forms a rather large loop and then joins the zygomatic ramus; multiple smaller branches emerge from this anastomosis and get distributed to zygomatic and buccal regions. The incidence rate of this type described by Davis et al[19] is 28%, while Angelov and Spacca report 26.15%.
- Type IV. This pattern is a summation of types II and III, with anastomoses between the temporal and zygomatic branches, as well as connections between the cervicofacial division and the zygomatic or buccal rami (▶ Fig. 1.4). The incidence rate of this type described by Davis et al[19] is 24%, while Angelov and Spacca report 18.46%.
- Type V. In this type there are two anastomotic rami that pass from the cervicofacial division to intervene with the branches of the temporofacial division (▶ Fig. 1.4). The contribution from the cervicofacial division may be buccal in origin or it may arise from the point at which the main facial trunk divides, and then follow a transverse course on the way to a junction with the buccal and zygomatic branches at the periphery of the gland. The incidence rate of this type described by Davis et al[19] is 9%, while Angelov and Spacca report 14.61%.
- Type VI. This type is characterized by a richly plexiform arrangement and is encountered less frequently. Separate large branches are missing, and small branches dominate. The transverse branch (which is zygomatic and buccal in distribution) consists actually of series of smaller rami and filaments (▶ Fig. 1.4). This type represents the most complex pattern of anastomosis; only in specimens of this type does the mandibular branch join any member of the temporofacial division. The incidence rate of this type described by Davis et al[19] is 8%, while Angelov and Spacca report 8.46%.

!

These anastomoses are important because they explain why accidental or essential division of a small branch often fails to result in the expected facial muscle weakness. Alternatively, although all branches of the facial nerve are preserved during surgery, there is often postoperative facial weakness caused by bruising and ischemia of the nerve. This may often result in a temporary and reversible demyelination of the nerve fibers (axons). Although this can affect all branches of the facial nerve, the weakness is often confined to the territory innervated by the marginal mandibular branch and is manifested by a weakness of the lower lip on the affected side. This is because anastomotic arcades between the marginal mandibular branch and other branches of the facial nerve are relatively rare.[14]

1.18 Key Points

- Work on the injured facial nerve demands extreme caution because proper reinnervation of original muscle targets after any kind of injury is almost impossible.
- The facial nerve changes direction five times during its course from the brainstem to the stylomastoid foramen.
- No other nerve in the body covers such a long distance in a bony canal.
- The facial nerve contains about 10,000 axons that are responsible for the innervation of the face musculature, and also for the largest number of communications with other nerves of the human body.
- Work with the injured facial nerve requires patience: tissue destined to become the facial nerve can be identified anatomically as early as the 3rd week of gestation and development is complete at 4 years after birth.

References

[1] Collins P. Development of the nervous system and special sense organs. In: Williams PL, ed. Gray's Anatomy. 38th ed. New York: Churchill Livingstone; 1995:217–298

[2] Nieuwenhuys R, Voogd J, van Huijzen C. Development. In: Nieuwenhuys R, Voogd J, van Huijzen C, eds. The Human Central Nervous System. Berlin: Springer; 2008:7–66

[3] Som PM, Streit A, Naidich TP. Illustrated review of the embryology and development of the facial region, part 3: an overview of the molecular interactions responsible for facial development. AJNR Am J Neuroradiol 2014; 35: 223–229

[4] Clara M. Die Entwicklung der Organsysteme. In: Clara M, ed. Entwicklungsgeschichte des Menschen. Leipzig: Georg Thieme Verlag; 1966:200–433

[5] Gasser FR, May M. Embryonic development. In: May M, Schaitkin BM, eds. The Facial Nerve. New York, NY: Thieme Medical Publishers; 2000:1–17

[6] Starck D. Die Entwicklung des Nervensystems und Sinnesorgane. In: Starck D, ed. Embryologie. Ein Lehrbuch auf allgemein biologischer Grundlage. Stuttgart: Georg Thieme Verlag; 1965:350–356

[7] Moore KL. The branchial apparatus and the head and neck. In: KL Moore, ed. The Developing Human. Philadelphia: WB Saunders Co; 1982

[8] Sadler TW. Medizinische Embryologie. Die normale menschliche Entwicklung und ihre Fehlbildungen. 11th ed. Stuttgart, New York: Georg Thieme Verlag; 2008:354–355

[9] Gasser RF, Hendrickx AG. The development of the facial nerve in baboon embryos (Papio sp.). J Comp Neurol 1969; 129: 203–218

[10] Gasser RF. The development of the facial muscles in man. Am J Anat 1967; 120: 357–375

[11] Hinrichsen K. The Early Development of Morphology and Patterns of the Face in the Human Embryo. Berlin, Heidelberg, New York, Tokyo: Springer Verlag; 1985

[12] May M. Anatomy for the clinician. In: May M, Schaitkin BM, eds. The Facial Nerve. New York, NY: Thieme Medical Publishers; 2000:19–56

[13] Vuyk HD, D'Souza AR, Vermeersch HFE. Forehead, temple and scalp reconstruction. In: Vuy HD, Lohuis PJFM, eds. Facial Plastic and Reconstructive Surgery. New York: Hodder Arnold Publishers; 2006:423–435

[14] Berkovitz BKB. Face and scalp. In: Standring S, ed. Gray's Anatomy. 39thed. Edinburgh: Elsevier Churchill Livingstone; 2005:513–515

[15] Nieuwenhuys R, Voogd J, van Huijzen C. Motor systems. In: Nieuwenhuys R, Voogd J, van Huijzen C, eds. The Human Central Nervous System. Berlin: Springer; 2008:865–867

[16] Klein CM. Diseases of the seventh cranial nerve. In: Dyck PJ, Thomas PK, eds. Peripheral Neuropathy. 4th ed. Elsevier; 2005:1219–1252

[17] Glockner FX, Hopf HCh. N. facialis: (VII) Fazialisparesen. In: Hopf HCh, Kömpf D, eds. Erkrankungen der Hirnnerven. Stuttgart: Thieme; 2006:133–148

[18] Brackmann DE. Otoneurosurgical procedures. In: May M, Schaitkin BM, eds. The Facial Nerve. New York: Thieme; 2000:515–533

[19] Davis RA, Anson BJ, Budinger JM, Kurth LR. Surgical anatomy of the facial nerve and parotid gland based upon a study of 350 cervicofacial halves. Surg Gynecol Obstet 1956; 102: 385–412

2 Physiology of the Facial Motor System

Andrey Irintchev

2.1 Introduction

The facial muscular system is one of the most complex motor systems in mammals. It controls muscles surrounding the mouth, nostrils, eyes, and ears, and is involved in numerous behaviors including simple protective responses (e.g., blink reflex), more complex functions performed in cooperation with other motor and sensory systems (respiration, ingestion, tactile perception, and sound localization), and social communication (vocalization, facial expression).

2.2 Muscles

Most muscles in the human body span joints and control movement and position in space of body segments. In contrast, facial muscles move soft tissues in relation to the skull and, thus, do not contribute to posture and movements of the body (▶ Table 2.1). The functional demands on the facial musculature as a whole, and on individual muscle groups and even single muscles, for example the orbicularis oculi, vary considerably—from a fast defense response such as rapid eyelid closure, through a rhythmic motor behavior such as spontaneous blinking, to a coordinated motor activity pattern generating a smile. All these functions require a precisely controlled rather than a powerful motor output. Fine grading of force in the thin facial muscles is enabled by a high, relative to muscle mass, number of small motor units (a motoneuron and the muscle fibers it innervates). For example, the estimated average motor unit size in the human platysma is 25 muscle fibers as opposed to almost 2,000 fibers in the powerful medial gastrocnemius muscle, while the motor unit numbers per muscle are 1,100 and 580 respectively.[1] In addition, human facial muscle fibers have average diameters that are about twice as small as fibers in limb muscles and can, therefore, develop less maximum tension.[2–4] Accordingly, the motor unit action potentials are of short duration and small amplitude.[5] While the functional (e.g., speed of contraction) and biochemical properties (e.g., myosin heavy chain [MHC], expression profile) of muscle fibers in one motor unit are similar, different motor units differ in these characteristics and each facial muscle is composed of a mixture of different motor unit types. Analysis of MHC expression in humans has revealed that most facial muscles are composed predominantly (72–86%) of fast-twitch muscle fibers, suggesting fast contractile properties (▶ Fig. 2.1).[6] Indeed, fast contractile properties have been confirmed in vitro and fast contraction times have been recorded in such muscles in vivo, e.g., 43 milliseconds in the orbicularis oculi muscle (85% fast-twitch, type II fibers), which is almost three times faster than in the slow human soleus (120 millisecond contraction time, 0% type II fibers).[4,7,8] Such fast contractions are mandatory for efficient defense responses such as eyelid closure. Higher proportions of slow-twitch (type I) muscle fibers

Table 2.1 Characteristic features of facial muscles as opposed to limb musculature

Feature	Differences of facial muscles when compared with limb muscles
Anatomy	Mostly poorly defined flat muscles embedded in connective tissue, no bone origin and insertion (superficial musculoaponeurotic system)
Actions	Soft tissue movements versus joint movements
Muscle fiber diameters	Smaller
Muscle fiber composition	Mostly fast-twitch muscle fibers Presence of tonic fibers
Contraction time	Faster
Motor unit size	Smaller
Muscle spindles	Absent
γ-Motoneuron innervation	Absent

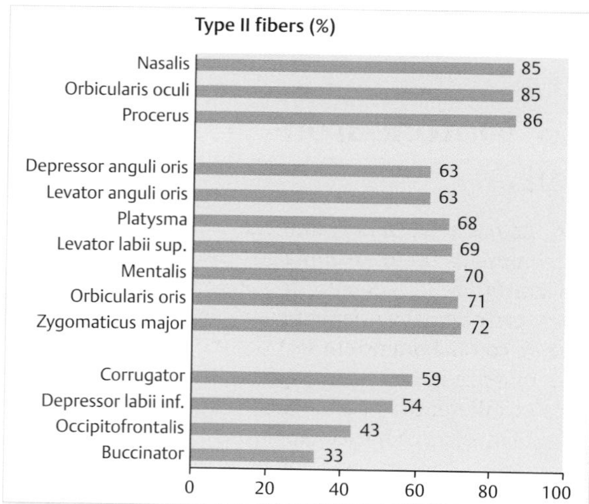

Fig. 2.1 Percentage of fast-twitch (type II) muscle fibers in different facial muscles of humans. (Data from Freilinger et al.[6])

in other muscles (41–67% of the corrugator supercilii, depressor labii inferioris, occipitofrontalis, and buccinators; ► Fig. 2.1) indicate that the phenotype of these muscles is adapted to perform more sustained or frequent contractions also. In general, faster muscles such as the orbicularis oculi are composed of thinner muscle fibers and have a lower capillary density than muscles with a predominance of slow fibers such as the corrugator supercilii.[6,9] As estimated by electromyography (EMG), muscles with moderate and high proportions of type I fibers, such as orbicularis oris (29%), zygomaticus (28%), and frontalis (57%) (► Fig. 2.1), fatigue considerably less during repeated brief contractions (25 × 3 seconds, 4–12% decline in EMG activity) than after sustained contractions (1 × 10 seconds, 23–35%).[10]

In addition to slow-twitch and fast-twitch muscle fibers, each of which is innervated by a single end plate and contracts in response to action potentials propagated along the muscle fiber length, a significant proportion (26%) of muscle fibers sampled from 11 different human facial muscles are innervated by two to five end plates separated by distances of 10 to 500 µm.[11] In such multiply innervated mammalian muscle fibers, observed also in laryngeal and extraocular muscles, contractions may be entirely or in part coupled to focal depolarizations in the muscle fiber rather than to propagated action potentials that would enable slow tonic contractions resembling these in tonic amphibian fibers.[12,13]

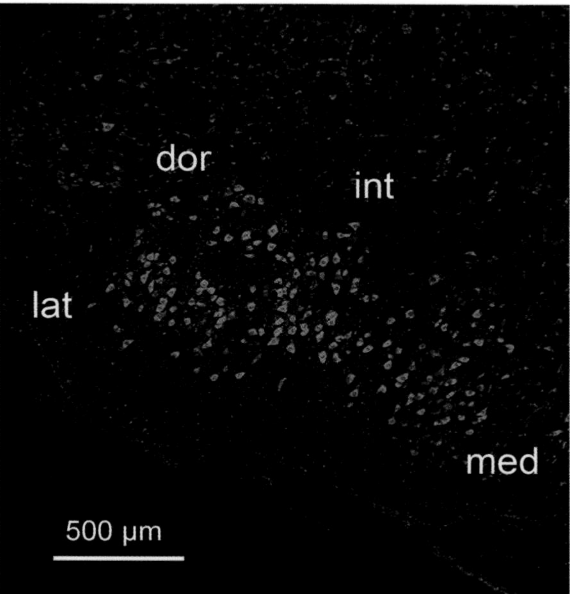

Fig. 2.2 The facial nucleus is a conspicuous group of large-diameter cells that may be subdivided in medial (med), lateral (lat), dorsal (dor), and intermediate (int) subnuclei. Note that the boundaries between subnuclei are not well defined. Coronal section through the rat brainstem stained with a Nissl-like fluorescence dye.

> **!**
>
> Small motor unit size in facial muscles enables precisely graded control of motor output. A mixture of fast-twitch and slow-twitch motor unit phenotypes and presence of slow toniclike fibers enables fast phasic contractions as well as slower rhythmic or sustained muscle responses.

2.3 Motoneurons and Glial Cells

The motoneurons innervating the superficial (mimetic) facial musculature of mammals are localized in the facial nucleus (► Fig. 2.2). Similar to spinal motoneurons, they form rostrocaudally oriented motor columns ("subnuclei" seen in coronal brainstem sections, ► Fig. 2.2) that innervate muscles in a musculotopic fashion. Although interspecies differences and variability in nomenclature are present, a general musculotopic pattern across different mammalian species including humans is apparent: the rostrocaudal axis of the facial musculature is represented in the mediolateral axis of the facial nucleus.[14] For example, muscles surrounding ear, eye, and mouth are innervated by motoneurons in the medial, intermediate/dorsal, and lateral subdivisions of the nucleus, respectively. The number of facial motoneurons in humans is about 10,000 per nucleus.[14]

Facial motoneurons are large cholinergic neurons (► Fig. 2.3) with fusiform or multipolar cell bodies (diameters of 15–60 µm, average 30 µm, cat),[15] which are smaller than those of spinal α-motoneurons (40–80 µm, average 50 µm, cat ankle extensors).[16] Soma surface area of facial motoneurons is positively correlated with mean diameter of dendrites, axon conduction velocity, and rheobase, and negatively correlated with motoneuron input resistance.[15] It is tempting to speculate that the size of a motoneuron, in conjunction with other characteristics like afterhyperpolarization duration, is correlated with motoneuron excitability, discharge frequencies, and metabolic profile, and, thus, with a specific activity pattern that in turn governs the functional properties (type) of the muscle fibers in its motor unit; however, evidence for such relationships in the facial system have not been presented. It can be currently assumed that the facial motor system controls muscle contraction force by the two mechanisms known for spinal systems: increase in motoneuron firing rate (rate modulation)[17] and orderly motor unit recruitment (size principle).[18]

The dendritic trees of the facial motoneurons are inconspicuous and possess several (4–10) primary dendrites and a few orders of dendritic branching.[15,19,20]

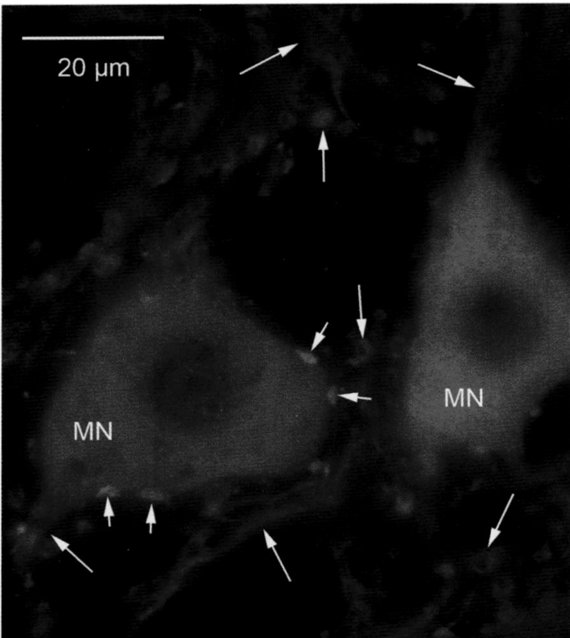

Fig. 2.3 Choline acetyltransferase (ChAT) staining of rat facial motoneurons. The cholinergic marker enzyme is detectable in the cytoplasm of motoneuronal cell bodies (MN), motoneuronal dendrites (*long arrows*), and large perisomatic synaptic terminals (*short arrows*). Pale areas in the centers of the cell bodies (MN) are occupied by nuclei. In addition to the structures indicated in this figure, MN axons and their terminal arborizations at end plates are ChAT positive (see ▶ Fig. 2.5).

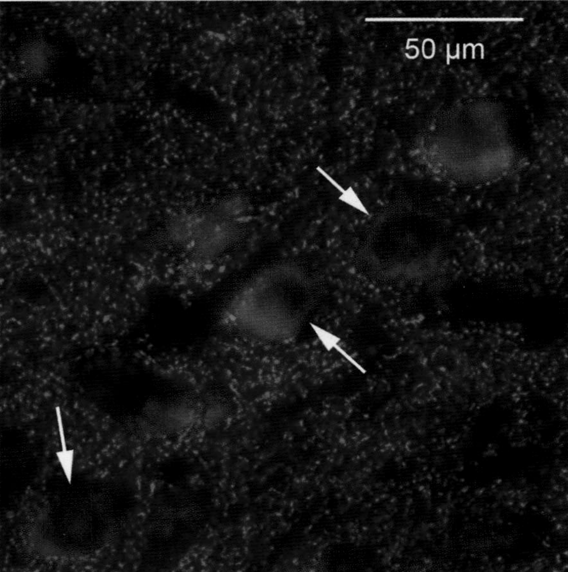

Fig. 2.4 Distribution of excitatory presynaptic terminals in the facial nucleus of rat. Immunofluorescence staining with an antibody against VGLUT2 (red), which is a vesicular glutamate transporter expressed in excitatory facial afferents. Motoneuron cell bodies (*arrows*) are visualized by a fluorescence Nissl stain. Note that the vast majority of the VGLUT-positive terminals is localized in the neuropil where the dendrites of the motoneurons (unstained by the Nissl dye) reside.

Similar to other α-motoneurons, these dendrites are spineless and harbor the vast majority of the excitatory and inhibitory terminals targeting the cell (▶ Fig. 2.4).[15,19] The axons of the facial motoneurons are myelinated and of moderate caliber (mostly 3–6 µm, cat) and moderate conduction velocities (25–75 m/s, cat).[21,22] Normally, α-motor axons branch only intramuscularly and each of them innervates a group of muscle fibers (motor unit) by forming only one synapse (end plate) per fiber (▶ Fig. 2.5). This monosynaptic pattern of innervation is predominant in facial muscles but, as mentioned previously, a significant proportion of muscle fibers are innervated by multiple end plates suggesting that their contractions are controlled by the nervous system in a different, as of yet nonclarified, way compared with mono-innervated twitch fibers.[11]

The facial nucleus is composed exclusively of α-motoneurons and morphological evidence for existence of associated γ-motoneurons or Renshaw cells has not been found.[14] γ-Motoneurons control the sensitivity of muscle spindles and, thus, contribute to stretch reflexes, muscle tone, and voluntary movement. The notion that the facial nucleus is devoid of γ-motoneurons is in line with the finding that facial muscles essentially lack spindles[9,23–25] and monosynaptic reflexes cannot be elicited by muscle stretch or electrical nerve stimulation.[26] These observations indicate that proprioceptive control in the facial system is enabled by extramuscular receptors, as described in Proprioception).

Renshaw interneurons, located in lamina VII of the spinal cord close to motoneurons (lamina IX), regulate the firing rate of spinal α-motoneurons by recurrent inhibition, which is manifested by a long-lasting (60–80 ms) silent period after antidromic nerve stimulation. Such inhibition is not observed after facial nerve stimulation indicating, along with lack of morphological evidence for Renshaw interneurons in or close to the facial nucleus, that recurrent inhibition is absent.[27] Considering the lack of muscle proprioceptors in the system, absence of the feedback inhibitory (Renshaw) loop is not very surprising as it seems to be, in the spinal cord, functionally coupled to the proprioceptive feedback system.[28]

!

In contrast to spinal motoneurons, the facial motoneurons are not functionally coupled to γ-motoneurons and feedback inhibitory (Renshaw) interneurons.

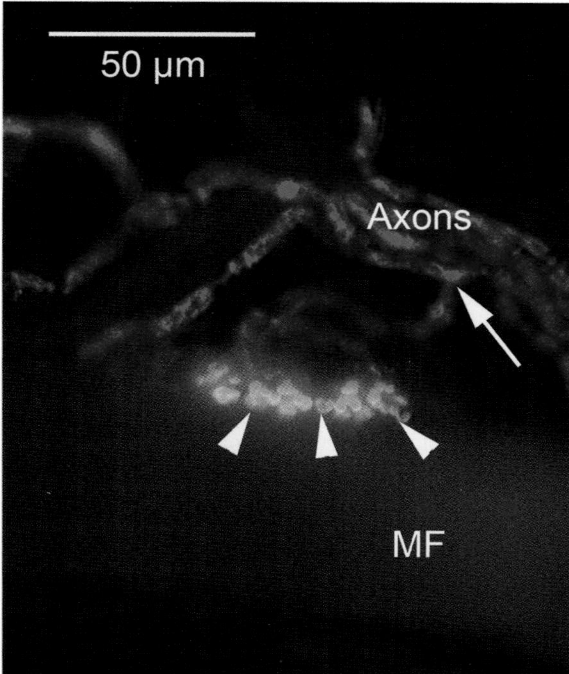

Fig. 2.5 A neuromuscular synapse (end plate) in the levator labii superioris of rat. A bundle of axons (red, choline acetyltransferase staining) is seen on the right. One of the axons branches (*arrow*) and one of its branches innervates, by several collaterals, an end plate (*arrowheads*, green staining of postsynaptic acetylcholine receptors using fluorescein-conjugated α-bungarotoxin) on a muscle fiber (MF, light green background staining).

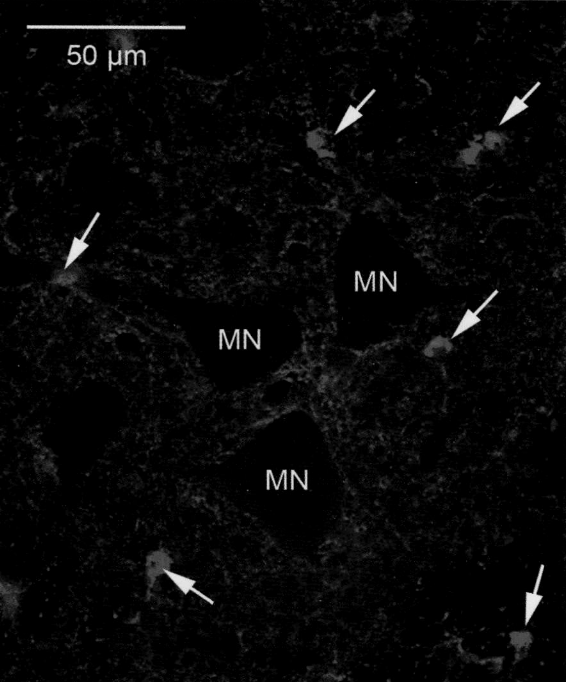

Fig. 2.6 Astrocytes in the facial nucleus of rat visualized using immunofluorescence staining with an antibody against S-100 protein. The cell bodies (*arrows*) are inconspicuous and randomly distributed within the nucleus. A dense network of astrocytic processes fills the neuropil among motoneuronal cell bodies (MN).

Of the four types of glia present in the facial nucleus—astrocytes (▶ Fig. 2.6), microglia (▶ Fig. 2.7), oligodendrocytes, and NG2 glia—the former two types have received most attention because of their involvement in synaptic remodeling after axotomy.[29,30] Also, under physiological conditions, astrocytes and microglia are involved, among other functions, in the maintenance, surveillance, and/or functional regulation of synapses including synaptic plasticity. In rats, the facial nucleus comprises 4,800 motoneurons and contains approximately 12,000 astrocytes and 11,000 microglial cells, i.e., an "average" motoneuron is supported by more than two astrocytes and two microglial cells.[19]

2.4 Proprioception

Information about movements or posture, required for efficient and accurate motor performance, is provided to the central nervous system by proprioceptors: mechanoreceptors in muscles, tendons, joints, and skin. Facial muscles lack tendons and muscle proprioceptors (muscle spindles and Golgi tendon organs) and do not perform movements on joints. Therefore, sensory feedback can be supplied by only trigeminal mechanoreceptors densely innervating the human facial skin and oral cavity.[31,32] In line with this notion are observations that: (1) trigeminal mechanoreceptors respond to deformations (strain) of the facial skin and mucosa during natural behaviors like chewing, swallowing, or licking, to contacts between lips, and to air pressure generated to produce sounds[33,34]; and (2) abrupt changes in the perioral skin strain leads to compensatory muscle contractions.[35–37] Facial mechanoreceptors activated upon skin deformations and facial muscle contractions are highly sensitive to dynamic changes in stimulus intensity but respond, even the slowly adapting receptors, little or not at all to sustained stimuli.[32,38] All these findings indicate that the sensory feedback regulating the facial motor output is limited to information on dynamic changes in muscle length, in contrast to limb muscles where muscle proprioceptors constantly monitor muscle length and tension. Lack of muscle proprioception could explain why it is difficult for healthy individuals to precisely reproduce a voluntary facial expression in the absence of visual control, and why patients with hyperkinesis after degeneration and regeneration of the facial nerve see their eye as narrow or their cheek as swollen but don't really sense the increased resting tone of the face as tight.

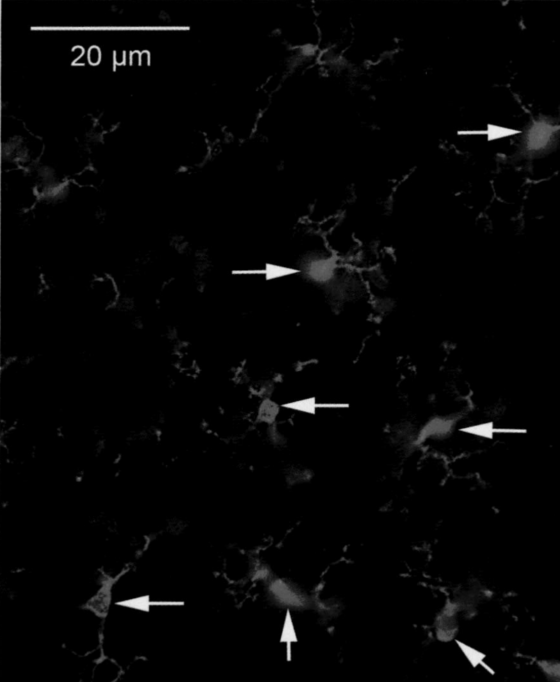

Fig. 2.7 Microglial cells in the facial nucleus of rat visualized using immunofluorescence staining with an antibody against the microglial marker Iba1. Similar to astrocytes, the cell bodies (*arrows*) are randomly distributed within the nucleus. The cell processes emerging from the cell bodies are slender and ramified.

!

The proprioceptive control of facial muscle contractions depends primarily on information from trigeminal skin mechanoreceptors. Lack of muscle proprioceptors results in a relatively imprecise control of prolonged voluntary contractions.

2.5 Reflex Responses and Automatic Motor Behaviors

While monosynaptic stretch reflexes cannot be elicited in facial muscles, they respond to a variety of stimuli in stereotypic fashions. Among these responses, of clinical value are two trigeminofacial defense reactions: the blink and the corneal reflex.[26,39,40] The clinical application of the blink reflex is presented in Chapter 6. Electrical current applied to the supraorbital nerve or a tap on the skin around the eye leads to activation of the ipsilateral orbicularis oculi muscle. The eyelid closure is evoked by two waves of facial motoneuron discharges registered in EMG recordings as a short-latency (8–12 ms) R1 and a long-latency (25–35 ms) R2 response. The reflex pathway underlying the R1 response is most likely composed of (1) an A-β trigeminal (cutaneous) afferent, (2) an interneuron in the principal trigeminal nucleus or its vicinity, and (3) a facial motoneuron. While the R1 response is present ipsilaterally to the stimulation site, the R2 wave is bilateral and is conducted through the ipsilateral caudal spinal trigeminal nucleus, the ipsilateral lateral tegmental field in the medulla, and a bilaterally projecting trigeminofacial connection ascending from the medulla to the facial nucleus in the pons. The blink reflex shows habituation, particularly the polysynaptic R2 response, upon repetitive stimulation and is a part of a more complex motor behavior including, apart from the orbicularis oculi muscle activation contralaterally, contraction of the lip, relaxation of the perioral muscle musculature, and inhibition of the orbicularis oculi antagonist, the levator palpebrae muscle, innervated by the oculomotor nerve. The corneal reflex differs from the blink reflex in that (1) it is evoked by stimulation of A-δ afferents in the ophthalmic division of the trigeminal nerve, (2) it does not have an R1 component, and (3) it is less prone to suprabulbar influences, e.g., from the motor cortex and basal ganglia.[39] Similar to the blink reflex is a protective cutaneous trigeminofacial reflex known as the perioral reflex: a tap on the lips evokes contraction of the orbicularis oris muscle associated with an early (R1) and a late (R2) response.[35]

Blink reflex responses are not strictly linked to "local" stimuli such as tap of the periocular skin and stimulation of the trigeminal afferents in the supraorbital nerve. Electrical stimulation of the infraorbital nerve and low-intensity stimuli (tap or electrical shock) applied over a wide area of the facial skin effectively evoke blink responses.[40] A blink response is also produced upon electrical stimulation of spinal nerves, e.g., the median nerve (somatosensory blink reflex), and by acoustic stimuli (acoustic blink reflex), both considered to be parts of generalized startle responses.[39] Another blink reflex is the bilateral eyelid closure following retinal light stimulation.[41] These examples indicate that facial defense responses are of low threshold and can be evoked by stimulation of different modalities.

In addition to "simple" reflexes, facial muscles are involved in a variety of more complex "automatic" motor behaviors. For example, children and adult humans respond to gustatory and olfactory stimuli with stereotyped responses like brow lowering, raising of the upper lip, and depression of the lip corner (negative facial displays) upon presentation of unpleasant tastes and odors.[42] Breathing and feeding behaviors are further examples of facial muscle involvement requiring rhythmic temporally coordinated activity in different motor and sensory systems.[43] Interestingly, the rhythmical activity pattern imposed onto one and the same muscles may differ considerably in different motor behaviors, as observed for perioral muscles of macaques during lip smacks versus ingestion.[44] It is apparent that facial reflex responses are parts of diverse stereotyped motor behaviors, diversity requiring multiple subcortical centers of motor control.

> **!**
>
> Facial reflexes are of complex nature. Even "simple" responses like eyelid closure are typically integrated in more sophisticated coordinated motor patterns involving different facial muscles and often different motor and sensory systems.

2.6 Central Pattern Generators

Autonomous motor behaviors such as locomotion, defense reactions, swallowing, and breathing are generated by central pattern generators (CPGs), which are interneuron networks that produce fundamental rhythms driving motoneurons even in the absence of sensory and cortical input.[45] These rhythms are modulated by feedback systems to adapt them to different functional demands. Several CPGs underlying rhythmic and coordinated activities of facial muscles have been identified. Spontaneous *blinking* in rats appears to arise from a "blink generator" in the spinal trigeminal complex that is modulated by corneal afferents and indirect basal ganglia inputs.[46] The minimal network sufficient to generate *whisking*, rhythmic movements of the tactile (vibrissal) hairs in the rat, consists of vibrissal motoneurons of the facial nucleus and serotonergic premotoneurons that are likely to be localized in the lateral paragigantocellularis nucleus.[47] In addition, neurons in the intermediate band of the reticular formation provide rhythmic input to the facial motoneurons that drive the vibrissal protractions (forward movement).[48] The CPG for *mastication*, i.e., rhythmic opening and closing of the jaws accompanied by coordinated movements of the tongue, cheeks, and lips, is localized, in rabbits and rodents, in a segment of the brainstem between the facial and trigeminal motor nuclei.[49,50] It comprises neurons with intrinsic burst properties in the principal trigeminal nucleus and several nuclei at the medullary—pontine border that project to the trigeminal motor nucleus and the facial and hypoglossal nuclei. The CPG of *respiration* is localized in the brainstem and is driven by neurons in the pre-Bötzinger complex in the ventral medulla.[48,51]

Mastication, swallowing, and respiration all use jaw, facial, and tongue muscles, and the CPGs underlying these behaviors must, therefore, interact. Interactions between mastication and swallowing and between swallowing and respiration, but not between mastication and respiration, have been identified.[49] Coordinated activity of left and right CPGs is enabled by reciprocal and bilateral connections of the interneuron pools. Recent findings suggest that the pre-Bötzinger respiratory complex plays a central role in coordinating orofacial behaviors in the rat.[48] A respiratory master clock in this complex ensures that different behaviors like whisking and sniffing, which coordinate with breathing and share muscle groups, do not impede each other.

> **!**
>
> Rhythmic coordinated motor behaviors such as respiration, swallowing, and mastication that involve facial muscles are produced by central pattern generators, which are interneuron circuitries in the hindbrain modulated by feedback systems.

2.7 Voluntary Motor Control

The powerful influence of the cerebral cortex on facial voluntary movements is well recognized. Anatomical and functional analyses have shown that in higher mammals, humans, and nonhuman primates, multiple cortical areas send direct projections to facial motoneurons (▶ Fig. 2.8).[52,53] These areas include the facial representation in the primary motor cortex (M1—areas F1 and F4), the ventral lateral premotor cortex (VLPCv—area 6V), the supplementary motor cortex (M2—area 6m), the rostral cingulate motor cortex (M3—area 24c), and the caudal cingulate motor cortex (M4—area 23c). All these five areas are interconnected through topographically organized corticocortical projections and most areas possess incomplete "maps" of the face,

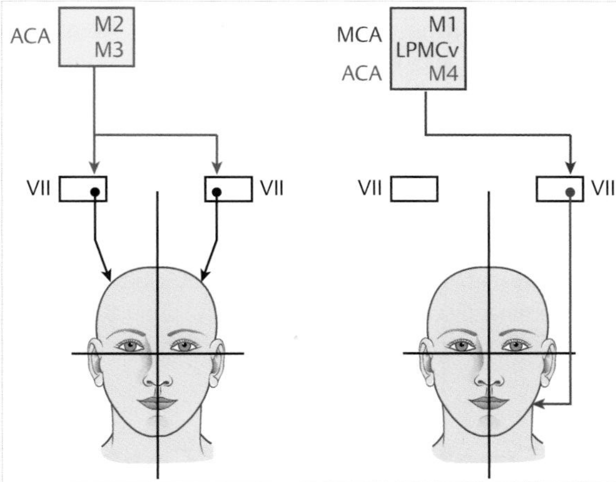

Fig. 2.8 Cortical projections to the upper and lower facial musculature. The motoneurons innervating upper face muscles receive bilateral projections from the supplementary motor area (M2) and the rostral cingulate motor area (M3). The cortical projections to motoneurons of lower face muscles are contralateral and arise from the primary motor cortex (M1), the ventral lateral premotor cortex (LPMCv), and the caudal cingulate motor cortex (M4). M2, M3, and M4 receive a vascular supply from the anterior cerebral artery (ACA), while M1 and LPMCv are in the territory of the middle cerebral artery (MCA). (Adapted from Morecraft et al.[52])

i.e., not all facial motoneuron groups receive innervation from each cortical representation. The facial representations in M1, LPMCv, and M4 are bilateral but asymmetric, with predominance for the contralateral lateral facial subnucleus, i.e., for motoneurons innervating the contralateral lower face.[53,54] M2 and M3 give bilateral symmetric projections to motoneurons of the upper face musculature.[53] These results indicate that a highly interconnected, multifocal network underlies the wide spectrum of facial expressions. Each of the facial motor representations is likely to have specific duties in relation to facial functions.[53,55] M1 is involved in sensorimotor integration, modulation of automatic movements (e.g., mastication), and voluntary face movements. M2 may play a role in movement planning and control of eye movements, speech, and laughter. And M3 and M4 possibly function as mediators between association cortical areas related to emotion, attention, and decision making, on the one hand, and facial motoneurons on the other hand, i.e., they could be involved in higher-order facial responses.

The existence of several cortical motor representations with different projection patterns to motoneurons and localized in cortical areas supplied by different blood vessels has led to a novel interpretation of the differential impairment of upper and lower face musculature after medial cerebral artery infarction in humans.[53] Such infarction leads to destruction of the M1 and VLPCv representations that are in the vascular supply territory of the medial cerebral artery, but leaves M2, M3, and M4, supplied by the anterior cerebral artery, intact. The consequence is paralysis of the contralateral lower face muscles, receiving input predominantly from (the destroyed) M1 and VLPCv, but sparing of the upper face muscles that are bilaterally innervated by M2 and M3.

!

Voluntary control of facial movements is enabled by a complex neuronal network localized in five cortical motor representations giving rise to symmetric bilateral or predominantly contralateral corticofacial projections.

2.8 Emotional Motor Control

Facial movements associated with emotions such as fear, sadness, or surprise are generated to a large extent by the limbic system and appear to use different pathways down to the facial motoneurons compared with those used for voluntary motor control.[56] As indicated by results of animal experiments, the limbic structures involved in emotional facial expressions include the central nucleus of the amygdala, the lateral hypothalamus, the bed nucleus of the stria terminalis, and the periaqueductal grey. These structures innervate facial motoneurons indirectly, via premotoneurons in the brainstem. The best proof of separate voluntary and emotional systems controlling facial motor behavior in humans are isolated voluntary and emotional facial palsies after localized central nervous system lesions; for example, loss of voluntary control over the lower face musculature but preserved emotional responses (e.g., smiling to a funny story) in the same muscles after destruction of the corticofacial projections.[56] However, involvement of cortical control in emotional expression in healthy individuals and in neurological disorders cannot be ruled out and the roles of subcortical structures such as basal ganglia, hypothalamus, and trigeminal complex in voluntary and emotional facial expression remain to be elucidated.[53]

!

Emotional face expressions are generated by limbic structures.

2.9 Key Points

- The facial motor system differs in its anatomy and function from other motor systems, in particular spinal nerves.
- The facial muscles are composed of different types of muscle fibers and their motor units are small allowing fine grading and varying duration and speed of muscle contractions.
- Muscle proprioceptors and reciprocal inhibition are missing in the system and the proprioceptive information supplied by cutaneous trigeminal afferents is insufficient for precise voluntary control of prolonged muscle contractions.
- Motor patterns underlying automatic coordinated rhythmic behaviors are generated in multiple interacting brainstem pattern generators.
- The voluntary control of facial expression is under a powerful control of multiple interconnected brain representations.
- Control of emotional face expressions is largely independent from that of voluntary movements and exerted mainly by subcortical limbic areas.

References

[1] Feinstein B, Lindegard B, Nyman E, Wohlfart G. Morphologic studies of motor units in normal human muscles. Acta Anat (Basel) 1955; 23: 127–142

[2] Happak W, Burggasser G, Gruber H. Histochemical characteristics of human mimic muscles. J Neurol Sci 1988; 83: 25–35

[3] Schwarting S, Schröder M, Stennert E, Goebel HH. Enzyme histochemical and histographic data on normal human facial muscles. ORL J Otorhinolaryngol Relat Spec 1982; 44: 51–59

[4] Campbell SP, Williams DA, Frueh BR, Lynch GS. Contractile activation characteristics of single permeabilized fibres from levator palpebrae superioris, orbicularis oculi and vastus lateralis muscles from humans. J Physiol 1999; 519: 615–622

[5] Papagianni AE, Kokotis P, Zambelis T, Karandreas N. MUAP values of two facial muscles in normal subjects and comparison of two methods for data analysis. Muscle Nerve 2012; 46: 346–350

[6] Freilinger G, Happak W, Burggasser G, Gruber H. Histochemical mapping and fiber size analysis of mimic muscles. Plast Reconstr Surg 1990; 86: 422–428

[7] Buller AJ, Dornhorst AC, Edwards R, Kerr D, Whelan RF. Fast and slow muscles in mammals. Nature 1959; 183: 1516–1517

[8] McComas AJ, Thomas HC. Fast and slow twitch muscles in man. J Neurol Sci 1968; 7: 301–307

[9] Goodmurphy CW, Ovalle WK. Morphological study of two human facial muscles: orbicularis oculi and corrugator supercilii. Clin Anat 1999; 12: 1–11

[10] Brach JS, VanSwearingen J. Measuring fatigue related to facial muscle function. Arch Phys Med Rehabil 1995; 76: 905–908

[11] Happak W, Liu J, Burggasser G, Flowers A, Gruber H, Freilinger G. Human facial muscles: dimensions, motor endplate distribution, and presence of muscle fibers with multiple motor endplates. Anat Rec 1997; 249: 276–284

[12] Jacoby J, Chiarandini DJ, Stefani E. Electrical properties and innervation of fibers in the orbital layer of rat extraocular muscles. J Neurophysiol 1989; 61: 116–125

[13] Hess A, Pilar G. Slow fibres in the extraocular muscles of the cat. J Physiol 1963; 169: 780–798

[14] Sherwood CC. Comparative anatomy of the facial motor nucleus in mammals, with an analysis of neuron numbers in primates. Anat Rec A Discov Mol Cell Evol Biol 2005; 287: 1067–1079

[15] Nishimura Y, Asahara T, Yamamoto T, Tanaka T. Observations on morphology and electrophysiological properties of the normal and axotomized facial motoneurons in the cat. Brain Res 1992; 596: 305–310

[16] Burke RE, Dum RP, Fleshman JW et al. A HRP study of the relation between cell size and motor unit type in cat ankle extensor motoneurons. J Comp Neurol 1982; 209: 17–28

[17] Monster AW, Chan H. Isometric force production by motor units of extensor digitorum communis muscle in man. J Neurophysiol 1977; 40: 1432–1443

[18] Henneman E, Somjen G, Carpenter DO. Functional significance of cell size in spinal motoneurons. J Neurophysiol 1965; 28: 560–580

[19] Raslan A, Ernst P, Werle M et al. Reduced cholinergic and glutamatergic synaptic input to regenerated motoneurons after facial nerve repair in rats: potential implications for recovery of motor function. Brain Struct Funct 2014; 219: 891

[20] Perez-Torrero E, Torrero C, Salas M. Effects of perinatal undernourishment on neuronal development of the facial motor nucleus in the rat. Brain Res 2001; 905: 54–62

[21] Kitai ST, Tanaka T, Tsukahara N, Yu H. The facial nucleus of cat: antidromic and synaptic activation and peripheral nerve representation. Exp Brain Res 1972; 16: 161–183

[22] Van Buskirk C. The seventh nerve complex. J Comp Neurol 1945; 82: 303–333

[23] Lovell M, Sutton D, Lindeman RC. Muscle spindles in nonhuman primate extrinsic auricular muscles. Anat Rec 1977; 189: 519–523

[24] Stål P, Eriksson PO, Eriksson A, Thornell LE. Enzyme-histochemical and morphological characteristics of muscle fibre types in the human buccinator and orbicularis oris. Arch Oral Biol 1990; 35: 449–458

[25] Kadanoff D. Sensitive nerve endings in human mimic muscles [in German]. Z Mikrosk Anat Forsch 1956; 62: 1–15

[26] Kugelberg E. [Facial reflexes] Brain 1952; 75: 385–396

[27] Fanardjian VV, Manvelyan LR, Kasabyan SA. Mechanisms regulating the activity of facial nucleus motoneurones—1. Antidromic activation. Neuroscience 1983; 9: 815–822

[28] Windhorst U. Muscle proprioceptive feedback and spinal networks. Brain Res Bull 2007; 73: 155–202

[29] Moran LB, Graeber MB. The facial nerve axotomy model. Brain Res Brain Res Rev 2004; 44: 154–178

[30] Blinzinger K, Kreutzberg G. Displacement of synaptic terminals from regenerating motoneurons by microglial cells. Z Zellforsch Mikrosk Anat 1968; 85: 145–157

[31] Siemionow M, Gharb BB, Rampazzo A. The face as a sensory organ. Plast Reconstr Surg 2011; 127: 652–662

[32] Nordin M, Thomander L. Intrafascicular multi-unit recordings from the human infra-orbital nerve. Acta Physiol Scand 1989; 135: 139–148

[33] Trulsson M, Johansson RS. Orofacial mechanoreceptors in humans: encoding characteristics and responses during natural orofacial behaviors. Behav Brain Res 2002; 135: 27–33

[34] Johansson RS, Trulsson M, Olsson KA, Abbs JH. Mechanoreceptive afferent activity in the infraorbital nerve in man during speech and chewing movements. Exp Brain Res 1988; 72: 209–214

[35] Abbs JH, Gracco VL. Control of complex motor gestures: orofacial muscle responses to load perturbations of lip during speech. J Neurophysiol 1984; 51: 705–723

[36] Andreatta RD, Barlow SM, Biswas A, Finan DS. Mechanosensory modulation of perioral neuronal groups during active force dynamics. J Speech Hear Res 1996; 39: 1006–1017

[37] Ito T, Ostry DJ. Somatosensory contribution to motor learning due to facial skin deformation. J Neurophysiol 2010; 104: 1230–1238

[38] Nordin M, Hagbarth KE. Mechanoreceptive units in the human infraorbital nerve. Acta Physiol Scand 1989; 135: 149–161

[39] Aramideh M, Ongerboer de Visser BW. Brainstem reflexes: electrodiagnostic techniques, physiology, normative data, and clinical applications. Muscle Nerve 2002; 26: 14–30

[40] Shahani B. The human blink reflex. J Neurol Neurosurg Psychiatry 1970; 33: 792–800

[41] Yates SK, Brown WF. Light-stimulus-evoked blink reflex: methods, normal values, relation to other blink reflexes, and observations in multiple sclerosis. Neurology 1981; 31: 272–281

[42] Weiland R, Ellgring H, Macht M. Gustofacial and olfactofacial responses in human adults. Chem Senses 2010; 35: 841–853

[43] Miller AJ. Oral and pharyngeal reflexes in the mammalian nervous system: their diverse range in complexity and the pivotal role of the tongue. Crit Rev Oral Biol Med 2002; 13: 409–425

[44] Shepherd SV, Lanzilotto M, Ghazanfar AA. Facial muscle coordination in monkeys during rhythmic facial expressions and ingestive movements. J Neurosci 2012; 32: 6105–6116

[45] Arshavsky YI, Deliagina TG, Orlovsky GN. Pattern generation. Curr Opin Neurobiol 1997; 7: 781–789

[46] Kaminer J, Powers AS, Horn KG, Hui C, Evinger C. Characterizing the spontaneous blink generator: an animal model. J Neurosci 2011; 31: 11256–11267

[47] Cramer NP, Li Y, Keller A. The whisking rhythm generator: a novel mammalian network for the generation of movement. J Neurophysiol 2007; 97: 2148–2158

[48] Moore JD, Deschênes M, Furuta T et al. Hierarchy of orofacial rhythms revealed through whisking and breathing. Nature 2013; 497: 205–210

[49] Lund JP, Kolta A. Brainstem circuits that control mastication: do they have anything to say during speech? J Commun Disord 2006; 39: 381–390

[50] Barlow SM, Estep M. Central pattern generation and the motor infrastructure for suck, respiration, and speech. J Commun Disord 2006; 39: 366–380

[51] Tan W, Janczewski WA, Yang P, Shao XM, Callaway EM, Feldman JL. Silencing preBötzinger complex somatostatin-expressing neurons induces persistent apnea in awake rat. Nat Neurosci 2008; 11: 538–540

[52] Morecraft RJ, Louie JL, Herrick JL, Stilwell-Morecraft KS. Cortical innervation of the facial nucleus in the non-human primate: a new interpretation of the effects of stroke and related subtotal brain trauma on the muscles of facial expression. Brain 2001; 124: 176–208

[53] Morecraft RJ, Stilwell-Morecraft KS, Rossing WR. The motor cortex and facial expression: new insights from neuroscience. Neurologist 2004; 10: 235–249

[54] Pilurzi G, Hasan A, Saifee TA, Tolu E, Rothwell JC, Deriu F. Intracortical circuits, sensorimotor integration and plasticity in human motor cortical projections to muscles of the lower face. J Physiol 2013; 591: 1889–1906

[55] Avivi-Arber L, Martin R, Lee JC, Sessle BJ. Face sensorimotor cortex and its neuroplasticity related to orofacial sensorimotor functions. Arch Oral Biol 2011; 56: 1440–1465

[56] Holstege G. Emotional innervation of facial musculature. Mov Disord 2002; 17 Suppl 2: S12–S16

3 Applied Basic Science: Improvement of Nerve Regeneration

Andrey Irintchev and Doychin N. Angelov

3.1 Introduction

In humans, peripheral nerve injuries leading to disruption of axons, myelin, and connective tissue sheaths (neurotmesis) are typically associated with incomplete functional recovery even in cases of optimal surgical repair and subsequent abundant muscle reinnervation.[1,2] Characteristic for facial nerve neurotmesis is the appearance, after target reinnervation, and persistence thereafter of a postparalytic syndrome characterized by synkinesis, myokymia, and hemifacial mass contractions.[3] Effective treatments for these symptoms are still not available and it remains a major challenge for experimental researchers to further clarify the reasons for functional deficits and test novel therapeutic approaches with translational potential.

Many molecular and cellular aspects of peripheral nerve regeneration have been clarified by experimental research. In this chapter the authors address the questions of whether and how this knowledge could contribute to progress in the clinical management of peripheral nerve injuries.

3.2 Clinical Relevance of Animal Models

The most widely used model to study facial nerve regeneration is the laboratory rat, although genetically manipulated mice attract increasing attention.[4] After surgical reconstruction of the rat facial nerve, complete muscle reinnervation is accomplished within 2 months.[5] Despite rapid reinnervation, persistent face asymmetry is apparent for months after injury (▶ Fig. 3.1) indicating "faulty regeneration" also seen, for example, in humans with facial nerve repair. In contrast to humans, motor deficits in the animal model can be estimated numerically in a precise way. The most widely used approach is kinematics of exploratory whisking, the rhythmic movement of the vibrissae to acquire tactile information, allowing assessment of amplitude, velocity, acceleration, and frequency of movement during spontaneous[6,7] or forced whisking behavior.[8] Kinematics shows that the functional outcome after facial nerve repair in rodents is poor (▶ **Video 3.1**), reaching, for example, about 30% of the control values for whisking amplitude at ≥ 2 months.[9] Quantitative analyses also reveal considerable residual deficits in eyelid closure[10] and high frequencies of synkinesis.[8]

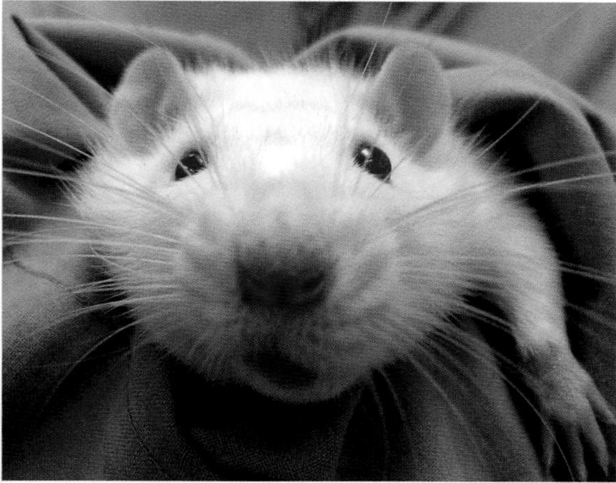

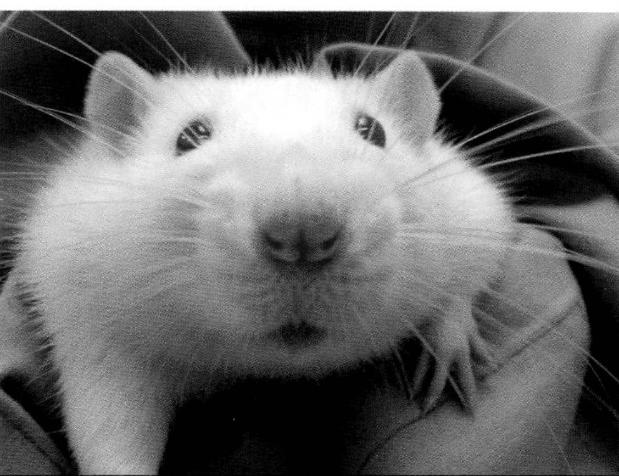

Fig. 3.1 Facial asymmetry 4 months after right facial nerve transection and suture in an adult rat (top panel). Note narrowing of the right eye. A noninjured littermate is shown in the bottom panel.

> **!**
>
> Despite species differences, rodent models of facial nerve injuries resemble the pathology and residual deficits seen in human patients.

3.3 Factors Limiting Recovery

Experimental studies have identified several potential causes of incomplete functional restoration in cases of good reinnervation of peripheral targets. These factors (▶ Table 3.1) are:

- Misdirected regrowth of axons into inappropriate targets[11] including branching of single axons to more than one muscle (▶ Fig. 3.2).[12]
- Diminished trophic support by Schwann cells in the distal stump.[13]
- Poor myelination and aberrant functional properties of regenerated axons.[14,15]
- Polyneuronal innervation of muscle fibers (▶ Fig. 3.3).[5]
- Reduced synaptic input to motoneurons after muscle reinnervation.[16,17]

Table 3.1 Factors limiting motor recovery after nerve repair and abundant muscle reinnervation

Factors	Origins and functional consequences
Misdirected regrowth and branching of axons (see also ▶ Fig. 3.2)	Nerve transection leads to disruption of endoneural tubes[a], the pathways guiding regenerating axons to peripheral targets. Since pathway choice is nonspecific, some axons emerging from the proximal nerve stump choose wrong pathways in the distal nerve stump and reach false muscles while others find the correct pathway and reach their "own" muscle. Severed axons produce multiple permanent branches (sprouts) at the site of injury and, therefore, one axon may reinnervate more than one muscle. Thus individual muscles receive innervation by own and foreign MNs and functionally different muscles share MN pools. The functional consequences of such faulty rewiring would be, in the absence of compensatory CNS responses, undesired involuntary muscle contractions accompanying voluntary movements (synkinesis) that impair precision of motor control, for example, during face expression and skilled hand movements
Diminished support by Schwann cells	Schwann cells in the denervated (distal) nerve stump guide regrowing axons and vigorously support axonal elongation by growth-promoting trophic factors, cytokines, and extracellular matrix molecules. This support becomes increasingly limited after several months of denervation (absence of axons in the distal nerve segment) in experimental animals. Since the axonal regrowth along the distal nerve segment in human patients often requires 6 to 12 months or even longer, the progressive loss of trophic support by Schwann cells may become significant and additionally delay and worsen muscle fiber reinnervation, i.e., significantly contribute to unfavorable functional outcomes in humans
Aberrant properties of regenerated axons	Regenerated axons in peripheral nerves have smaller diameters than normal axons and thinner, relative to axon thickness, myelin sheaths. Reduction in axonal diameters leads to slower propagation of action potentials (reduced conduction velocity) and, possibly, to propagation failures at some branching points. Abnormal myelination (e.g., short distorted intermodal sheaths) may result in abnormal current flows in the extracellular space and "cross-talk" between axons, i.e., ectopic generation of nerve impulses in neighboring axons (ephaptic excitation). Such abnormal coactivation of motor units may underlie or contribute to synkinesis
Polyinnervation of muscle fibers (see also ▶ Fig. 3.3)	Adult mammalian muscle fibers are normally "mono-innervated", i.e., their bear one end plate innervated by an axon collateral of an MN. Polyneuronally innervated muscle fibers, receiving input from ≥ 2 MNs, are observed only transiently during normal development but they persist, often in high numbers, for long time periods after muscle reinnervation in adults. Since simultaneous control of muscle fiber force output by more than one MN is functionally unfavorable, persistent polyinnervation may significantly contribute to motor dysfunctions after muscle reinnervation
Deafferentation of MNs	Deafferentation of MNs (synaptic stripping), in particular loss of inhibitory synapses on their cell bodies, has been proposed to underlie facial MN hyperexcitability in the early phases of regeneration. Chronic deficits in cholinergic and glutamatergic inputs to facial MNs may reduce the motor drive and, thus, contribute to residual deficits after nerve repair

Abbreviations: CNS, central nervous system; MN, motoneuron.
[a]Basal laminae of individual axons with surrounding connective tissue containing chains of proliferated Schwann cells, the bands of Büngner.

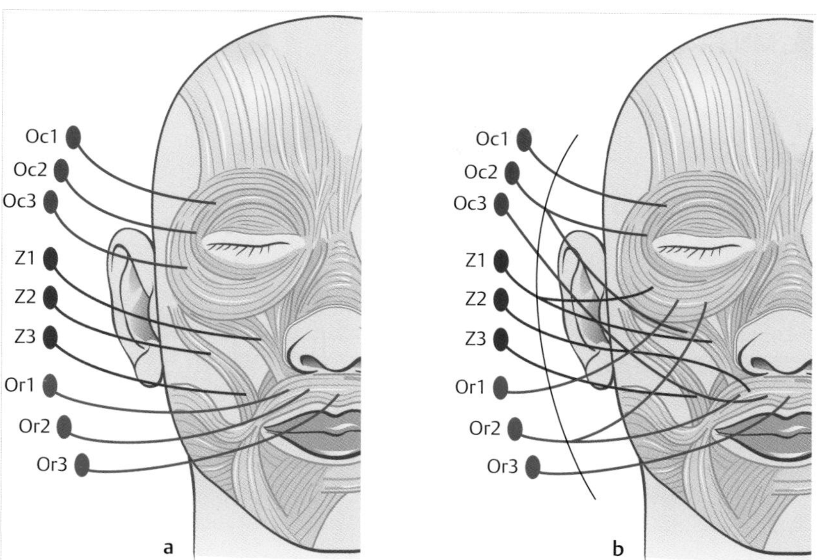

Fig. 3.2 False targeting of regenerated motor axons after facial nerve regeneration. **(a)** Normally, distinct motoneuron (MN) pools innervate individual facial muscles in adults. The illustration shows three MNs in the orbicularis oculi (Oc), zygomatic (Z), and orbicularis oris (Or) pool that extend unbranched axons along the facial nerve to their target muscles. Recruitment of MNs in one pool, for example Oc, leads to contraction in the target muscle (orbicularis oculi) only. **(b)** After neurotmesis, intraneural axonal branching (sprouting) occurs at the site of injury (*vertical gray line*) and many sprouts reach the distal stump guided by Schwann cells but show no selectivity for the growth pathway. Sprouting and initial axonal regrowth are followed by pruning of axon collaterals, and the three variables, sprouting, pruning, and random regrowth, produce variable reinnervation patterns: some MN axons (Oc1, Z3, Or3) find the correct pathways and reinnervate the originally innervated muscles. Other MNs are guided along false pathways and reinnervate inappropriate targets (Oc3, Z2, Or1). And yet other MNs produce and permanently maintain collaterals each of which innervates: (1) an appropriate and an inappropriate target (Oc2, Z1, Or2), (2) the appropriate muscle (not shown), or (3) inappropriate muscles (not shown). The apparent functional consequence of such abnormal rewiring is that recruitment of one MN pool, for example Oc, would lead to synkinesis, which is desired contraction of orbicularis oculi accompanied by undesired contractions of the zygomaticus and orbicularis oris. This simplified presentation does not, however, take into account that the MN pool recruitment is under powerful and versatile suprabulbar control. For example, even if the final motor pathways are separated, different MN pools and muscles are, as a rule, simultaneously activated during normal facial reflex responses or facial expressions, i.e., synkinesis is frequent in the healthy facial motor system; see Chapter 2.5. This illustration also does not consider the possibility that, after regeneration, central nervous system plasticity could compensate for aberrant peripheral rewiring.

The most widely accepted and easily comprehensive cause of functional deficits is axonal misdirection (▶ Fig. 3.2). Experimental evidence for the exceptional role of axonal misdirection is, however, not convincing and normal muscle function has been observed in rats with high degrees of axonal misdirection after facial nerve repair.[5,7] Similar to misdirection, the contributions of the other potential factors in the periphery to failures of functional restoration remain uncertain. The matter becomes even more complicated when considering the immense complexity of central nervous system (CNS) reorganizations after peripheral nerve injury[18] including alterations in cortical motor representations[19] and loss of connectivity.[16,17,20] Promoting CNS plasticity by removal of growth-inhibitory molecules leads to better functional outcome after nerve injuries, which indicates that CNS mechanisms significantly contribute to failure of functional restitution.[21,22]

!

Multiple mechanisms, central and peripheral, contribute to the success or failure of motor recovery after nerve injury.

3.4 Therapeutic Approaches

Extensive experimental work has been devoted to "improvement of nerve regeneration" including that of the facial nerve. However, many studies have used inadequate outcome measures, for example number of axons as a functional index. Here, the authors consider experimental work providing evidence in favor or against the efficacy of therapeutic interventions in animal models based mostly on functional analyses.

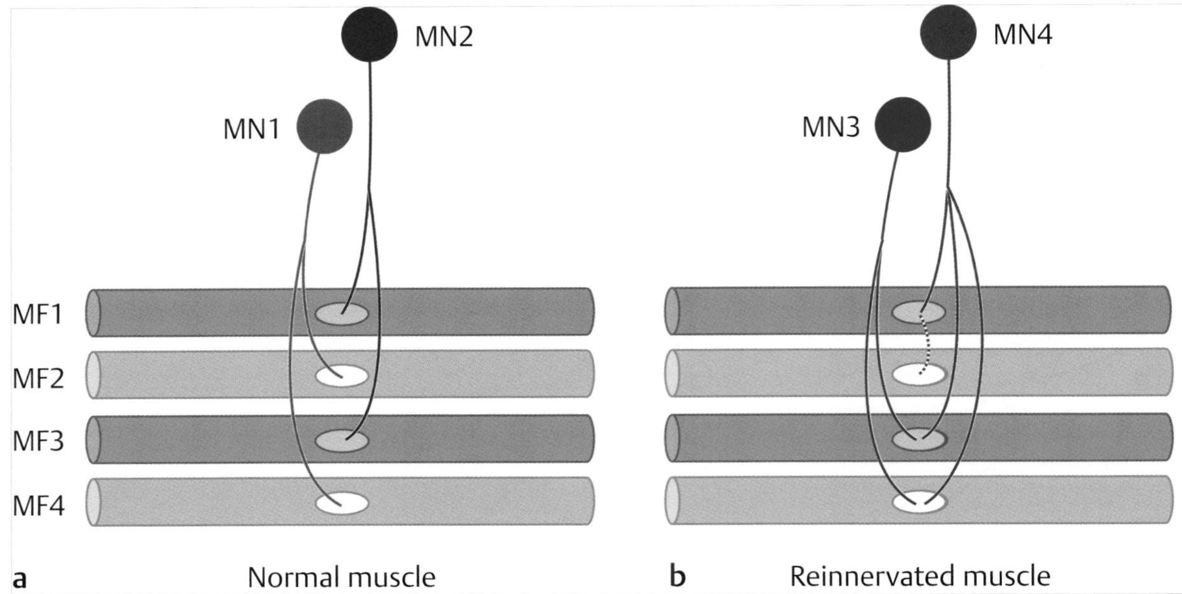

Fig. 3.3 Aberrant reinnervation of muscle fibers. **(a)** In normal muscles, individual motoneurons (e.g., MN1) innervate groups of muscle fibers (MF2 and MF4) by intramuscular branches terminating at end plates (ellipses in the middle of the fibers). Each muscle fiber has only one end plate innervated by one axon terminal. **(b)** After transection and surgical repair of the nerve, motor axons that find their way back to the muscle produce intramuscular axonal branches (sprouts) and reinnervate denervated end plates. Most MNs build contacts on "foreign" muscle fibers, i.e., fibers previously innervated by other MNs (e.g., MF3 and MF4 initially innervated by MN1 and MN2 become reinnervated by MN3 and MN4). Some end plates may remain denervated (not shown), others receive mononeuronal innervation (MF1), and yet other end plates are polyneuronally reinnervated (MF3 and MF4). The presence of denervated end plates may induce a third form of sprouting: terminal sprouting. In this case, axon collaterals arise from the terminal arborization of the end plate and, guided by terminal Schwann cells, reach neighboring denervated end plates (*dotted line* from end plate MF1 to MF2). Functional consequences: presence of moderate amounts of denervated fibers in one muscle can be well compensated by hypertrophy of the innervated fibers. Persistence of polyneuronal innervation is, however, functionally unfavorable since the motor output of the muscle fiber is inefficient when controlled by asynchronous input by two or more MNs. Muscle fibers in a normal motor unit (MN1 and MN2 in **(a)**) are innervated in a parallel circuitry mode that ensures simultaneous depolarization of the end plates and simultaneous muscle fiber contractions in the motor unit. Terminal sprouts form an additional circuitry in series leading to asynchronous contractions in the motor unit. In the case of MN4 in **(b)**, an action potential in the MN will lead to simultaneous contractions of MF1, MF3, and MF4, and a slightly delayed contraction of MF2. Reinnervation by terminal sprouts is detectable in EMG recordings of motor units but does not have any noticeable functional disadvantages. In contrast, terminal sprouting is a major reinnervation mechanism leading to good functional recovery after partial muscle denervation (e.g., in poliomyelitis) and botulinum toxin paralysis.

3.4.1 Targeting Axonal Misdirection

Application of bone-marrow-derived mesenchymal stem cells to the proximal stump of the transected facial nerve in rats failed to reduce collateral axonal branching at the lesion site and did not improve the quality of muscle reinnervation (mono- versus polyinnervated muscle fibers) or recovery of function.[23] Reduction of axonal misdirection and improved functional recovery have been achieved by stimulation of the trigeminal afferents,[24,25] application of olfactory mucosa at the site of nerve injury,[26] and by stabilization of microtubules in the proximal nerve stump with taxol.[27] Axonal branching and false targeting have also been reduced by topical application of growth factor–neutralizing antibodies, but the functional effects in these cases are unsatisfactory.[12]

!

Polyneuronal reinnervation of end plates—rather than collateral axonal branching at the lesion site—may be a critical limiting factor for restoration of facial motor function. Because polyneuronal innervation of muscle fibers is activity dependent and can be manipulated, these findings raised hopes that clinically feasible and effective therapies could be soon designed and tested; see Manual Stimulation Reduces Polyinnervation of Muscle Fibers.

3.4.2 Electrical Stimulation to Counteract Denervation Atrophy and Accelerate Reinnervation

Electrical stimulation of muscles has been widely used as a rehabilitation treatment of human patients with peripheral nerve injuries.[28] A major assumption behind the use of electrical stimulation (ES) is that it could counteract disuse-related alterations such as loss of muscle fiber excitability and muscle atrophy in the denervation period, and thus promote functional recovery.[29,30]

While some experimental studies have shown small-to-moderate beneficial effects of chronic ES such as increased muscle weight, decreased fatigue, and increased muscle strength,[31] and improved functional recovery,[32] reduced muscle atrophy, and increased oxidative capacity,[33] many other investigations report no effects.[34–36] Multiple, in part counteracting, effects of ES may underlie its low efficacy. For example, ES of denervated muscle inhibits intramuscular sprouting of ingrowing axons and could thus delay reinnervation but promote recovery by diminishing subsequent polyinnervation of muscle fibers.[37,38] ES can have adverse effects in partially denervated muscles by stimulating overuse of innervated muscle fibers and suppressing the production of chemical mediators required for reinnervation of denervated muscle fibers.[39] Based on animal experiments, chronic ES cannot be recommended. Similar to chronic ES, a recently introduced form of ES, brief intraoperative ES of the proximal nerve stump (1 × 1 hour, 20 Hz),[40] accelerates recovery but does not improve the final outcome of facial and femoral nerve injury in rodents.[41,42]

> !
>
> Electrical muscle stimulation is widely used in clinical rehabilitation, but there is no convincing experimental evidence for its efficacy in treatment of nerve injuries.

3.4.3 Manual Stimulation Reduces Polyinnervation of Muscle Fibers

Before reinnervation, the denervated muscle undergoes progressive changes including muscle fiber atrophy, reduced blood supply, and fibrosis.[43,44] Based on clinically established benefits of soft tissue massage, supposed to promote muscle blood flow and possibly counteract atrophy and fibrosis,[45] several groups have tested the effects of manual mechanical stimulation of denervated vibrissal muscles after facial nerve repair in the rat.[7,10,46–49] By stroking the whisker pad, the fine vibrissal muscle slings are stimulated leading to enhanced recovery of vibrissal motor performance and reduction of polyinnervated end plates. The effects of manual stimulation could be explained by reduction of intramuscular sprouting by the artificially imposed muscle activity during the phase of synaptic formation and consolidation.[39]

> !
>
> Soft tissue massage (manual muscle stimulation) may be a simple and effective way to improve the functional outcome after facial nerve injury.

3.4.4 Growth Factors to Promote Axonal Growth

Many neurotrophic factors produced at the lesion site and distal nerve stump of the injured nerve are potent stimulators of axon growth, and modulation of their levels has been considered a promising way to improve nerve regeneration and recovery of function.[50] However, these factors also promote axonal branching, a phenomenon that might attenuate or even overrule positive functional effects.[50] Studying the time course of the expression of several neurotrophic factors (nerve growth factor, brain-derived neurotrophic factor, basic fibroblast growth factor, glial cell derived neurotrophic factor, ciliary neurotrophic factor, and insulin-like growth factor 1) in a semiquantitative approach, Streppel et al[12] found a very rapid, many-fold increase in their expression at the lesion site.

The Basic Fibroblast Growth Factor

Jungnickel et al[51] performed sciatic nerve lesions and functional tests in transgenic mice overexpressing basic fibroblast growth factor (FGF-2). They proposed that endogenously synthesized FGF-2 influenced early peripheral nerve regeneration by regulating Schwann cell proliferation, axonal regrowth, and remyelination.

The Insulin-Like Growth Factors

Lewis et al[52] found that subcutaneous injections of insulin-like growth factor 1 (IGF-1) accelerate functional recovery following sciatic nerve crush in mice and attenuate the peripheral motor neuropathy induced by chronic administration of the cancer chemotherapeutic agent vincristine. In contrast, Lutz et al[53] report that systemically applied IGF-1 fails to improve motor recovery and accuracy of reinnervation following transection and epineural repair of rat median nerve.

Ciliary Neurotrophic Factor

Ciliary neurotrophic factor has been observed in vivo to increase the rate of axonal elongation, axonal sprouting, and end-plate reinnervation, and it improved functional recovery.[54]

Manipulation of neurotrophic factor levels in the injured nerve has not yet become a promising treatment approach perhaps because of the multifunctional properties of the neurotrophic factors.

3.4.5 Mimetic Peptides Improve Diameters and Myelination of Regenerated Axons

A novel approach for treatment of nerve injuries uses peptide mimetics of glycans, which are carbohydrate moieties on protein or lipid molecules. Glycans are essential for the functional properties of the carrier proteins and increasing evidence indicates that these carbohydrates are beneficial for neural repair.[55] The human natural killer (HNK) cell glycan known as HNK-1 epitope has been associated with proper targeting of regenerating motor axons.[56] Application of peptides that mimic the functional properties of the HNK-1 epitope to the injured femoral nerve of adult mice and nonhuman primates improves diameters and myelination of regenerating axons and functional (gait) recovery.[57,58] Application of a mimetic of another glycan involved in nerve regeneration, α2,8 polysialic acid, leads to improved gait and better axonal myelination after femoral nerve injury in mice.[59]

Use of mimetic peptides appears to be an attractive perspective for treatment of nerve injuries, but additional knowledge of the mechanisms of action is required.

3.4.6 Cell-Based Approaches for Axonal Growth Enhancement across a Nerve Prosthesis

In cases requiring bridging by nerve conduits, nerve regeneration is particularly poor primarily due to poor regrowth of axons across the gap. For this reason, tissue engineering approaches using cells capable of promoting axonal growth is attracting increased attention. Schwann cell–filled conduits can promote regeneration and functional recovery but the clinical feasibility of this approach is limited by cell availability.[60] Embryonic and mesenchymal stem cells of different origins, capable of differentiating into Schwann-like cells, also have positive functional effects but the efficacy of such approaches is still low and issues such as cell availability, post-transplantation survival, homing, proliferation, and differentiation have to be optimized with regard to clinical feasibility.[61]

Cell-replacement therapies for long-gap nerve injuries are of promise but currently these approaches cannot compete with standard autologous grafting.

3.5 Key Points

- None of the potential therapies for nerve repair suggested by basic research has been translated into clinical practice. This shortage cannot be attributed to use of inadequate models and methods in basic research.
- Translation is hampered in part by some unresolved issues such as clinical feasibility, mechanisms of action, and potential side effects. Beyond these limitations, however, failure of translation can be primarily related, similar to central nervous system lesions, to the complex pathophysiology of peripheral nerve injuries.
- Potential therapeutic targets, among others, appear to be aberrant polyinnervation of muscle fibers, insufficient axonal myelination, and reduced axonal diameters of regenerated axons.
- The improvement of any single structural aberration after nerve regeneration could be expected to produce moderate functional benefits and the search for efficient combinatorial treatments in experimental studies could provide the key to successful cure of regeneration-related movement disorders.

References

[1] Lundborg G, Rosén B. Hand function after nerve repair. Acta Physiol (Oxf) 2007; 189: 207–217

[2] Guntinas-Lichius O, Straesser A, Streppel M. Quality of life after facial nerve repair. Laryngoscope 2007; 117: 421–426

[3] Valls-Solé J, Montero J. Movement disorders in patients with peripheral facial palsy. Mov Disord 2003; 18: 1424–1435

[4] Moran LB, Graeber MB. The facial nerve axotomy model. Brain Res Brain Res Rev 2004; 44: 154–178

[5] Guntinas-Lichius O, Irintchev A, Streppel M et al. Factors limiting motor recovery after facial nerve transection in the rat: combined structural and functional analyses. Eur J Neurosci 2005; 21: 391–402

[6] Tomov TL, Guntinas-Lichius O, Grosheva M et al. An example of neural plasticity evoked by putative behavioral demand and early use of vibrissal hairs after facial nerve transection. Exp Neurol 2002; 178: 207–218

[7] Angelov DN, Ceynowa M, Guntinas-Lichius O et al. Mechanical stimulation of paralyzed vibrissal muscles following facial nerve injury in adult rat promotes full recovery of whisking. Neurobiol Dis 2007; 26: 229–242

[8] Hadlock TA, Kowaleski J, Lo D, Mackinnon SE, Heaton JT. Rodent facial nerve recovery after selected lesions and repair techniques. Plast Reconstr Surg 2010; 125: 99–109

[9] Angelov DN, Guntinas-Lichius O, Wewetzer K, Neiss WF, Streppel M. Axonal branching and recovery of coordinated muscle activity after transection of the facial nerve in adult rats. Adv Anat Embryol Cell Biol 2005; 180: 1–130

[10] Bischoff A, Grosheva M, Irintchev A et al. Manual stimulation of the orbicularis oculi muscle improves eyelid closure after facial nerve injury in adult rats. Muscle Nerve 2009; 39: 197–205

[11] Sumner AJ. Aberrant reinnervation. Muscle Nerve 1990; 13: 801–803

[12] Streppel M, Azzolin N, Dohm S et al. Focal application of neutralizing antibodies to soluble neurotrophic factors reduces collateral axonal branching after peripheral nerve lesion. Eur J Neurosci 2002; 15: 1327–1342

[13] Fu SY, Gordon T. The cellular and molecular basis of peripheral nerve regeneration. Mol Neurobiol 1997; 14: 67–116

[14] Mert T, Gunay I, Daglioglu YK. Role of potassium channels in the frequency-dependent activity of regenerating nerves. Pharmacology 2004; 72: 157–166

[15] Hildebrand C, Kocsis JD, Berglund S, Waxman SG. Myelin sheath remodelling in regenerated rat sciatic nerve. Brain Res 1985; 358: 163–170

[16] Raslan A, Ernst P, Werle M et al. Reduced cholinergic and glutamatergic synaptic input to regenerated motoneurons after facial nerve repair in rats: Potential implications for recovery of motor function. Brain Struct Funct 2014; 219: 891–909

[17] Hundeshagen G, Szameit K, Thieme H et al. Deficient functional recovery after facial nerve crush in rats is associated with restricted rearrangements of synaptic terminals in the facial nucleus. Neuroscience 2013; 248: 307–318

[18] Navarro X, Vivó M, Valero-Cabré A. Neural plasticity after peripheral nerve injury and regeneration. Prog Neurobiol 2007; 82: 163–201

[19] Franchi G. Changes in motor representation related to facial nerve damage and regeneration in adult rats. Exp Brain Res 2000; 135: 53–65

[20] Blinzinger K, Kreutzberg G. Displacement of synaptic terminals from regenerating motoneurons by microglial cells. Z Zellforsch Mikrosk Anat 1968; 85: 145–157

[21] Galtrey CM, Asher RA, Nothias F, Fawcett JW. Promoting plasticity in the spinal cord with chondroitinase improves functional recovery after peripheral nerve repair. Brain 2007; 130: 926–939

[22] Guntinas-Lichius O, Angelov DN, Morellini F et al. Opposite impacts of tenascin-C and tenascin-R deficiency in mice on the functional outcome of facial nerve repair. Eur J Neurosci 2005; 22: 2171–2179

[23] Grosheva M, Guntinas-Lichius O, Arnhold S et al. Bone marrow-derived mesenchymal stem cell transplantation does not improve quality of muscle reinnervation or recovery of motor function after facial nerve transection in rats. Biol Chem 2008; 389: 873–888

[24] Angelov DN, Skouras E, Guntinas-Lichius O et al. Contralateral trigeminal nerve lesion reduces polyneuronal muscle innervation after facial nerve repair in rats. Eur J Neurosci 1999; 11: 1369–1378

[25] Bendella H, Pavlov SP, Grosheva M et al. Non-invasive stimulation of the vibrissal pad improves recovery of whisking function after simultaneous lesion of the facial and infraorbital nerves in rats. Exp Brain Res 2011; 212: 65–79

[26] Guntinas-Lichius O, Wewetzer K, Tomov TL et al. Transplantation of olfactory mucosa minimizes axonal branching and promotes the recovery of vibrissae motor performance after facial nerve repair in rats. J Neurosci 2002; 22: 7121–7131

[27] Grosheva M, Guntinas-Lichius O, Angelova SK et al. Local stabilization of microtubule assembly improves recovery of facial nerve function after repair. Exp Neurol 2008; 209: 131–144

[28] Kern H, Salmons S, Mayr W, Rossini K, Carraro U. Recovery of long-term denervated human muscles induced by electrical stimulation. Muscle Nerve 2005; 31: 98–101

[29] Ashley Z, Sutherland H, Russold MF et al. Therapeutic stimulation of denervated muscles: the influence of pattern. Muscle Nerve 2008; 38: 875–886

[30] Salmons S, Jarvis JC. Functional electrical stimulation of denervated muscles: an experimental evaluation. Artif Organs 2008; 32: 597–603

[31] Cole BG, Gardiner PF. Does electrical stimulation of denervated muscle, continued after reinnervation, influence recovery of contractile function? Exp Neurol 1984; 85: 52–62

[32] Williams HB. A clinical pilot study to assess functional return following continuous muscle stimulation after nerve injury and repair in the upper extremity using a completely implantable electrical system. Microsurgery 1996; 17: 597–605

[33] Marqueste T, Decherchi P, Desplanches D, Favier R, Grelot L, Jammes Y. Chronic electrostimulation after nerve repair by self-anastomosis: effects on the size, the mechanical, histochemical and biochemical muscle properties. Acta Neuropathol 2006; 111: 589–600

[34] Diels HJ. Current concepts in non-surgical facial nerve rehabilitation. In: Beurskens CHG, van Gelder RS, Heymans PG, Manni JJ, Nicolai JPA, eds. The Facial Palsies. Complementary Approaches. Utrecht: Lemma Publishers; 2005:275–283

[35] Dow DE, Carlson BM, Hassett CA, Dennis RG, Faulkner JA. Electrical stimulation of denervated muscles of rats maintains mass and force, but not recovery following grafting. Restor Neurol Neurosci 2006; 24: 41–54

[36] Sinis N, Horn F, Genchev B et al. Electrical stimulation of paralyzed vibrissal muscles reduces endplate reinnervation and does not promote motor recovery after facial nerve repair in rats. Ann Anat 2009; 191: 356–370

[37] Love FM, Son YJ, Thompson WJ. Activity alters muscle reinnervation and terminal sprouting by reducing the number of Schwann cell pathways that grow to link synaptic sites. J Neurobiol 2003; 54: 566–576

[38] Brown MC, Holland RL, Ironton R. Nodal and terminal sprouting from motor nerves in fast and slow muscles of the mouse. J Physiol 1980; 306: 493–510

[39] Tam SL, Archibald V, Jassar B, Tyreman N, Gordon T. Increased neuromuscular activity reduces sprouting in partially denervated muscles. J Neurosci 2001; 21: 654–667

[40] Al-Majed AA, Neumann CM, Brushart TM, Gordon T. Brief electrical stimulation promotes the speed and accuracy of motor axonal regeneration. J Neurosci 2000; 20: 2602–2608

[41] Ahlborn P, Schachner M, Irintchev A. One hour electrical stimulation accelerates functional recovery after femoral nerve repair. Exp Neurol 2007; 208: 137–144

[42] Skouras E, Merkel D, Grosheva M et al. Manual stimulation, but not acute electrical stimulation prior to reconstructive surgery, improves functional recovery after facial nerve injury in rats. Restor Neurol Neurosci 2009; 27: 237–251

[43] Eccles JC. Investigations on muscle atrophies arising from disuse and tenotomy. J Physiol 1944; 103: 253–266

[44] Sunderland S. Capacity of reinnervated muscles to function efficiently after prolonged denervation. AMA Arch Neurol Psychiatry 1950; 64: 755–771

[45] Hovind H, Nielsen SL. Effect of massage on blood flow in skeletal muscle. Scand J Rehabil Med 1974; 6: 74–77

[46] Guntinas-Lichius O, Hundeshagen G, Paling T et al. Manual stimulation of facial muscles improves functional recovery after hypoglossal-facial anastomosis and interpositional nerve grafting of the facial nerve in adult rats. Neurobiol Dis 2007; 28: 101–112

[47] Hadlock T, Lindsay R, Edwards C et al. The effect of electrical and mechanical stimulation on the regenerating rodent facial nerve. Laryngoscope 2010; 120: 1094–1102

[48] Lindsay RW, Heaton JT, Edwards C, Smitson C, Vakharia K, Hadlock TA. Daily facial stimulation to improve recovery after facial nerve repair in rats. Arch Facial Plast Surg 2010; 12: 180–185

[49] Heaton JT, Knox CJ, Malo JS, Kobler JB, Hadlock TA. A system for delivering mechanical stimulation and robot-assisted therapy to the rat whisker pad during facial nerve regeneration. IEEE Trans Neural Syst Rehabil Eng 2013; 21: 928–937

[50] Klimaschewski L, Hausott B, Angelov DN. The pros and cons of growth factors and cytokines in peripheral axon regeneration. Int Rev Neurobiol 2013; 108: 137–171

[51] Jungnickel J, Haase K, Konitzer J, Timmer M, Grothe C. Faster nerve regeneration after sciatic nerve injury in mice over-expressing basic fibroblast growth factor. J Neurobiol 2006; 66: 940–948

[52] Lewis ME, Neff NT, Contreras PC et al. Insulin-like growth factor-I: potential for treatment of motor neuronal disorders. Exp Neurol 1993; 124: 73–88

[53] Lutz BS, Wei FC, Ma SF, Chuang DC. Effects of insulin-like growth factor-1 in motor nerve regeneration after nerve transection and repair vs. nerve crushing injury in the rat. Acta Neurochir (Wien) 1999; 141: 1101–1106

[54] Sendtner M, Dittrich F, Hughes RA, Thoenen H. Actions of CNTF and neurotrophins on degenerating motoneurons: preclinical studies and clinical implications. J Neurol Sci 1994; 124 Suppl: 77–83

[55] Irintchev A, Schachner M. The injured and regenerating nervous system: immunoglobulin superfamily members as key players. Neuroscientist 2012; 18: 452–466

[56] Martini R, Xin Y, Schmitz B, Schachner M. The L2/HNK-1 carbohydrate epitope is involved in the preferential outgrowth of motor neurons on ventral roots and motor nerves. Eur J Neurosci 1992; 4: 628–639

[57] Simova O, Irintchev A, Mehanna A et al. Carbohydrate mimics promote functional recovery after peripheral nerve repair. Ann Neurol 2006; 60: 430–437

[58] Irintchev A, Wu M-M, Lee HJ et al. Glycomimetic improves recovery after femoral injury in a non-human primate. J Neurotrauma 2011; 28: 1295–1306

[59] Mehanna A, Mishra B, Kurschat N et al. Polysialic acid glycomimetics promote myelination and functional recovery after peripheral nerve injury in mice. Brain 2009; 132: 1449–1462

[60] Walsh S, Midha R. Use of stem cells to augment nerve injury repair. Neurosurgery 2009; 65 Suppl: A80–A86

[61] Ren Z, Wang Y, Peng J, Zhao Q, Lu S. Role of stem cells in the regeneration and repair of peripheral nerves. Rev Neurosci 2012; 23: 135–143

Part II

Diagnostics

4 Clinical Examination

Gerd Fabian Volk, Orlando Guntinas-Lichius, and Barry M. Schaitkin

4.1 Introduction

Any diagnosis of diseases related to the facial nerve is a diagnostic challenge. Most patients seek early medical attention when they have a facial palsy. Therefore, this chapter will focus mainly on clinical examination for these patients. Special diagnostic procedures needed to address patients with rarer diseases such as facial dystonia or facial spasms are presented in detail in Chapter 28. The basis on which to elucidate the cause of a facial palsy relies most importantly on a careful history and examination of the patient. It is always important to remember that although idiopathic palsies are a common diagnosis not all acute palsies are idiopathic (Bell's).[1] An idiopathic palsy still is a diagnosis of exclusion; because idiopathic palsy is such an important topic, Chapter 8 will also address in detail when to make such an exclusion. Every effort must be made to determine the etiology of the underlying disease, especially for patients with acute palsy secondary to a treatable cause, to allow for prompt initiation of treatment. The most common causes of a facial palsy are listed in ▶ Table 4.1. The physical examination includes a basic otorhinolaryngologic and a gross

Table 4.1 Causes of facial palsy

	Possible cause of facial palsy
Birth	• Molding • Forceps delivery • Dystrophia myotonica • Möbius syndrome
Trauma	• Basilar skull fractures • Facial injuries • Penetrating injury to middle ear • Slag injury to middle ear • Altitude paralysis (barotrauma) • Scuba diving (barotrauma) • Lightning • Nose-blowing palsy • Reactive neuroma
Neurologic	• Opercular syndrome (cortical lesion in facial motor area) • Millard–Gubler syndrome (abducens palsy with contralateral hemiplegia due to lesion in base of pons) • Cephalic tetanus • Wernicke–Korsakoff syndrome • Pseudotumor cerebri • Lacunar syndrome
Infection	• External otitis • Otitis media • Mastoiditis • Chicken pox • Herpes zoster cephalicus • Encephalitis • Poliomyelitis (type 1 poliovirus) • Mumps • Mononucleosis • Leprosy • Influenza • Coxsackie virus • Malaria • Syphilis • Scleroma • Tuberculosis • Botulism • Acute hemorrhagic conjunctivitis • Gnathostomiasis • Mucormycosis • Lyme disease • Cat scratch disease • AIDS • Sinus thrombosis • Acute suppurative parotitis
Metabolic	• Diabetes mellitus • Hyperthyroidism • Hypothyroidism • Pregnancy • Hypertension • Acute porphyria • Vitamin A deficiency
Neoplastic	• Cholesteatoma • Seventh nerve tumor • Glomus jugulare tumor • Leukemia • Meningioma • Hemangioblastoma • Sarcoma • Carcinoma (invading or metastatic) • Anomalous sigmoid sinus • Carotid artery aneurysm • Hemangioma of tympanum • Hydradenoma • Schwannoma • Teratoma • Histiocytosis • Fibrous dysplasia • von Recklinghausen disease • Benign parotid gland lesions • Temporal bone myeloma • Endolymphatic sac tumors • Malignant parotid lesions • Fibrosarcoma • Ossifying hemangioma • Granular cell myoblastoma

Table 4.1 continued

	Possible cause of facial palsy
Toxic	• Thalidomide • Misoprostol • Tetanus • Diphtheria • Carbon monoxide • Ethylene glycol • Arsenic intoxication • Alcoholism
Iatrogenic	• Mandibular block anesthesia • Antitetanus serum • Vaccine for rabies • Postimmunization • Parotid surgery • Temporal bone surgery • Post-tonsillectomy and adenoidectomy • Iontophoresis • Embolization • Dental • Sagittal split osteotomy
Idiopathic	• Bell's palsy • Melkersson–Rosenthal syndrome • Hereditary hypertrophic neuropathy Charcot–Marie–Tooth disease, Dejerine–Sottas disease • Autoimmune syndrome • Temporal arteritis • Thrombotic thrombocytopenic purpura • Periarteritis nodosa • Landry–Guillain–Barré syndrome • Multiple sclerosis • Myasthenia gravis • Amyloidosis • Sarcoidosis • Osteopetrosis • Osteogenesis imperfecta

Source: Adapted with permission from Schaitkin et al 2000.[37]

neurologic examination. Depending on preliminary diagnosis, the basic clinical examination is completed by further diagnostics such as topodiagnostic tests and ultrasound of the neck. Based on the results of the history and of first examinations, further more elaborate diagnostic investigations are planned if needed (▶ Fig. 4.1). Treatment and follow-up is finally determined.

4.2 Patient History

The patient's history, especially the onset and progression of the facial palsy (See Box 4.1 (p. 33)), and accompanying conditions such as trauma, surgery, pregnancy, systemic illness, or history of malignancy are important hints to determine the proper work-up and possible etiologies. A recurrence of a palsy, an alternating palsy, or a bilateral palsy is a special situation limiting the differential diagnosis.

Box 4.1 Factors of patient's history and diagnostic factors in evaluating facial palsy

- Date of onset
- Progressive versus sudden onset
- Incomplete versus complete palsy
- First bout versus recurrence
- Same side versus alternating
- Facial twitching
- Mass in head or neck
- Recent viral infection or exposure
- Pain or numbness
- Ear infection, drainage, surgery, tinnitus
- Hearing change: decreased or hyperacusis
- Dizziness
- Tearing changes: increased or absent
- Taste: decreased or absent
- Vesicles and location
- Trauma: describe
- Family history of facial paralysis
- Pregnancy
- Systemic illness
- Malignancies (breast, lung, thyroid, genitourinary)
- Medications: isonicotinylhydrazine (isoniazid)
- Signs of immunodeficiency (AIDS)

4.2.1 Time Course

One cannot determine the etiology of facial paralysis merely from its onset. Whether incomplete, complete, sudden, or delayed, each pattern can be seen in a wide variety of pathology including idiopathic Bell's palsy, herpes zoster cephalicus, temporal bone fractures, iatrogenic, infection, and neoplasms. However, while the type of onset is not diagnostic, it is certainly often prognostic. When the cause of incomplete palsy is idiopathic, trauma, or infection, and the patient does *not* go on to a complete facial paralysis, then the likelihood of a satisfactory recovery is extremely high. If the facial nerve remains incompletely involved with Bell's palsy for 14 days or more, there is also a very high satisfactory recovery rate. However, if a patient with incomplete recovery does not begin to recover within 3 to 6 weeks or if the paresis continues to progress for more than 3 weeks, then a tumor must be considered as a possible underlying cause and proper imaging should be obtained. More importantly, the occurrence of a slowly progressive facial paralysis always dictates the need for evaluation for possible neoplasm involving the facial nerve; see Chapter 15.

Although slow progression beyond 3 weeks is diagnostic of a tumor, progression that occurs within the first 10 days of onset has been noted with idiopathic (Bell's) palsy, external blunt trauma, and surgical trauma to the facial nerve within the parotid, temporal bone, or

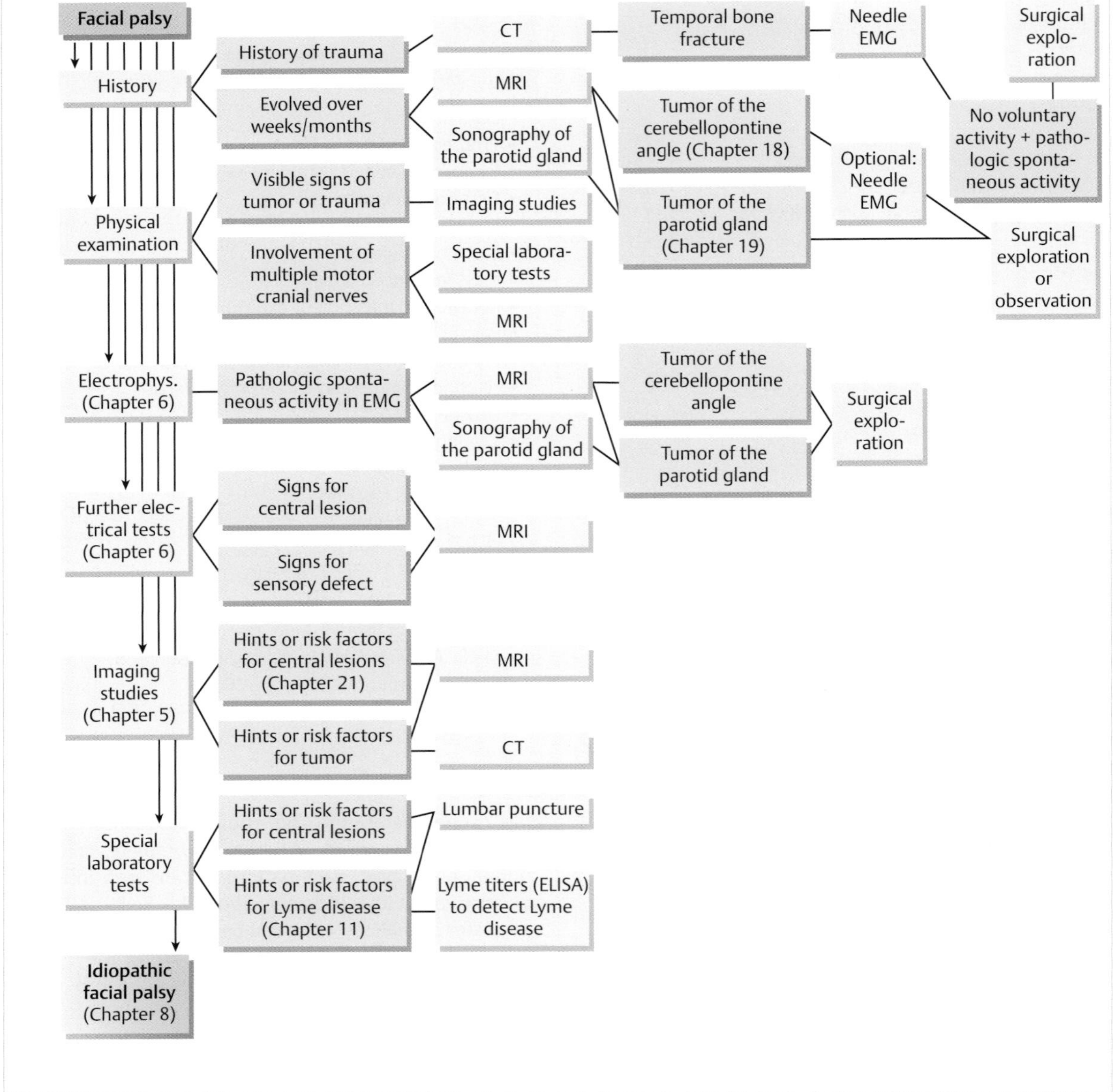

Fig. 4.1 Algorithm showing the diagnostic work-up for a patient presenting with a facial palsy. CT, computed tomography; Electrophys., electrophysiology; ELISA, enzyme-linked immunosorbent assay; EMG, electromyography; MRI, magnetic resonance imaging.

posterior fossa. Slow progression implies that the injury is initially incomplete and additional injury is either secondary to edema or due to compression of the blood supply to the facial nerve. However, slow progressive onset of idiopathic (Bell's) palsy may still have a favorable prognosis for satisfactory recovery providing that involvement of the facial nerve remains incomplete during this 10-day window. Bell's should never progress beyond 10 days and usually is maximum by day 5. However, if the paresis progresses to total paralysis, the likelihood of a satisfactory recovery falls. Herpes zoster cephalicus differs from Bell's in that progression may continue up to 14 to 21 days; see Chapter 10. A slow onset of palsy due to trauma carries a favorable prognosis because 90% of patients with such paresis will have a satisfactory recovery; see Chapter 9.

However, this is not true with tumors. In the case of slow-growing neoplasms, whether benign or malignant, the nerve is slowly replaced and compressed by the enlarging mass. Despite this, the nerve may survive and function until a critical number of axons are destroyed. Although the time factor is variable, as the injury to the nerve progressively worsens, the prospects for complete recovery become more unlikely. Of the patients with Bell's palsy seen by the authors, about 57% present with sudden complete onset of facial paralysis. This type of presentation has a worse prognosis than presentation with incomplete onset of paralysis. Half of the patients with complete onset of palsy will have a less than complete recovery. However, although half of the patients with Bell's palsy present with sudden complete onset of facial paralysis, this is not diagnostic of Bell's palsy because the onset is sudden and complete in about one-quarter of patients with confirmed tumors involving the facial nerve. Important hints to consider a nonidiopathic palsy in a patient with acute facial palsy are listed in Box 4.2 (p. 35). A sudden complete onset associated with trauma may indicate that the facial nerve has been transected, whereas a history of a delayed onset or a slowly progressive onset would rule out nerve transection. Even though sudden complete onset of facial paralysis following trauma determines the time of injury, only by appropriate electrical tests and sometimes imaging studies can the occurrence of an actual transection be established. When dealing with traumatic facial paralysis, the onset is only one of various factors that must be considered. For further discussion on the approach to patients with a facial paralysis after trauma see Chapter 9.

Box 4.2 Idiopathic (Bell's) palsy diagnosis of exclusion: when to suspect non-Bell's diagnosis

- Visible signs of tumor
- Bilateral simultaneous palsy
- Vesicles
- Involvement of multiple motor cranial nerves
- History and findings of trauma
- Ear infection
- Signs of central nervous system lesion
- Facial palsy noted at birth
- Triad of infectious mononucleosis (fever, sore throat, cervical lymphadenopathy)

In patients with a slowly progressive facial paralysis an evaluation for possible neoplasm involving the facial nerve is mandatory.

4.2.2 Recurrence

The patient who shows a recurrence of facial paralysis deserves special attention. A recurrence has been noted with Bell's palsy, Melkersson–Rosenthal syndrome,[2,3] and tumors. The incidence of recurrent facial paralysis is about 10 to 15%, with about one-third of cases on the same side, and two-thirds on the opposite side. A mean interval of about 10 years (range: 1 month to 43 years) between recurrence of Bell's palsy has been reported.[4] A recurrence is about 2.5 times more likely to have a positive family history. It is important to note that although Bell's palsy may be recurrent, herpes zoster cephalicus can also be recurrent. Recurrence is a common finding of herpes simplex type 1 and rare with varicella zoster; suggesting that recurrent Bell's palsy may be due to a herpes simplex infection; see Chapter 8 and Chapter 10. Recurrent herpes zoster cephalicus is so unusual that one must be certain that the cause is not herpes simplex, which at times may be difficult to distinguish clinically from varicella zoster. If it is determined that herpes zoster has recurred, one must be certain to rule out an underlying immunodeficiency or malignancy because it might be associated with recurrent herpes zoster.

Ipsilateral recurrence may be caused by a tumor involving the facial nerve. It has been reported that in case of recurrence on the same side, a tumor involving the facial nerve was ultimately found in about one-third of patients.[5] Therefore, it is recommended that a tumor be suspected of being the cause of all ipsilateral recurrent facial palsies and that a diagnostic tumor work-up be considered in all such cases.

!

The onset of facial palsy is not in itself diagnostic. Tumors can, just as with Bell's palsy, present with incomplete, complete, sudden, delayed, or recurrent ipsilateral peripheral facial paralysis.

4.2.3 Recurrent Alternating Palsy

In contrast to recurrent facial paralysis on the same side, recurrence involving the opposite side is almost always diagnostic of idiopathic (Bell's) palsy because alternating recurrent facial paralysis has been noted only rarely with other disorders. Melkersson–Rosenthal syndrome is the most common example of a rare disorder that is characterized by recurrent alternating facial palsy.[3] This syndrome can be distinguished from idiopathic palsy by its very specific identifying features:

- Recurrent alternating facial palsy.
- Recurrent orofacial edema.
- Cheilitis.
- Fissured tongue.

Most authors agree that the presence of any two of these four manifestations permits the diagnosis, but painless, nonpitting edema of the lips is most common. The edema is short lived, usually less than 48 hours; however, over time, a chronic brawny deformity may ensue. The syndrome may be accompanied by migraine phenomena and have a positive family history. The facial weakness is indistinguishable from idiopathic palsy and may be partial, complete, and occasionally bilateral. Histology is characterized by multinucleated Langerhans' giant cells and noncaseating granulomas. The clinical impression can be confirmed with a lip biopsy.

!

Melkersson–Rosenthal syndrome is the most common example of a rare disorder that is characterized by recurrent alternating facial palsy.

4.2.4 Bilateral Simultaneous Palsy

Bilateral facial nerve paresis may be a medical emergency and presents special diagnostic and therapeutic challenges (▶ Fig. 4.2 and ▶ Fig. 4.3). The differential diagnosis of bilateral facial paralysis is listed in Box 4.3 (p. 36). These patients require an aggressive and appropriate diagnostic work-up to allow for the initiation of appropriate therapy. Less than 2% of all patients presenting with facial palsy have bilateral facial palsy. The patients normally present during the acute onset. Excluding the diagnostically obvious congenital processes and iatrogenic or acquired traumatic insults, there are patients who present with bilateral simultaneous facial palsy who require immediate medical attention. Examples include patients with Guillain–Barré syndrome, Lyme disease, as described in Chapter 11, acute leukemia, and a patient with bulbar palsy caused by to rabies immunization. In some epidemic regions, Lyme disease is the most frequent reason for bilateral palsy.[6] To date, no one has presented with bilateral simultaneous herpes zoster cephalicus. The term bilateral simultaneous facial palsy has been expanded in most series to include patients who develop facial paralysis involving the initially spared side within 4 weeks after onset. Based on these criteria, less than 1% of patients with Bell's palsy have bilateral simultaneous onset of facial palsy. When the paralysis is incomplete but bilateral, it may be difficult to appreciate the less involved side. However the recognition of bilateral involvement is imperative given the diagnostic possibilities just discussed. Although the patients will commonly have a profound involvement of both sides, creating a masklike face, the patients must be scrutinized for bilaterality. Normally a patient should be able to squeeze the eyelids tightly so that wrinkles from and the eyelashes become buried in the folds of the orbicularis oculi muscle. In addition, with a smile, the patient should be able to show the upper and lower teeth on the intact side. Loss of flaring of the nostrils, a blink lag, and inability to close the eyelid against the examiner's finger resistance will detect a paresis on what seems to be the intact side.

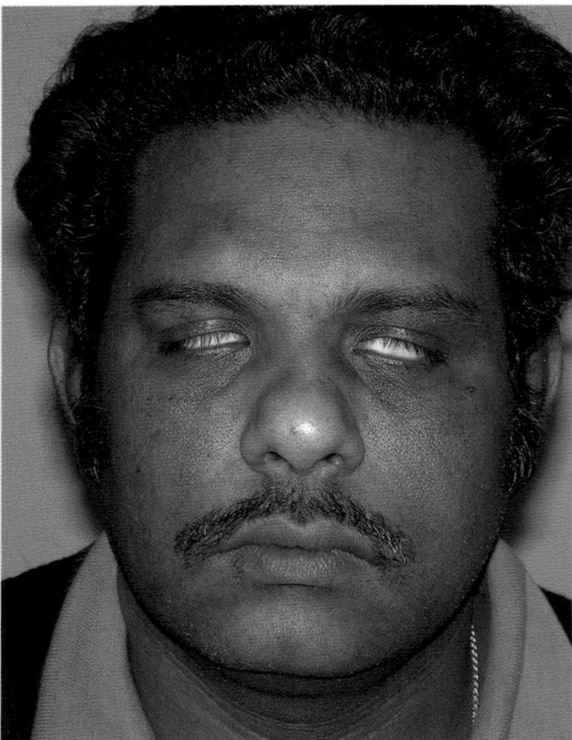

Fig. 4.2 Bilateral facial palsy with bilateral Bell's phenomenon 2 weeks after onset, due to Lyme disease.

Box 4.3 Differential diagnosis of bilateral simultaneous facial palsy

- Guillain–Barré syndrome
- Möbius syndrome
- Sarcoidosis (Heerfordt's syndrome)
- Myotonic dystrophia
- Skull trauma
- Infectious mononucleosis
- Cytomegalovirus
- Acute porphyrias
- Botulism
- Herpex simplex virus infection
- Bone disorder (dysplasia, dysostosis, osteogenesis imperfecta)
- Hypothyroidism
- Charcot–Marie–Tooth syndrome
- Myasthenia gravis
- Bilateral acute or chronic otitis media

To see a bilateral facial palsy can be more difficult than a unilateral palsy, especially in incomplete cases as the asymmetry is missing.

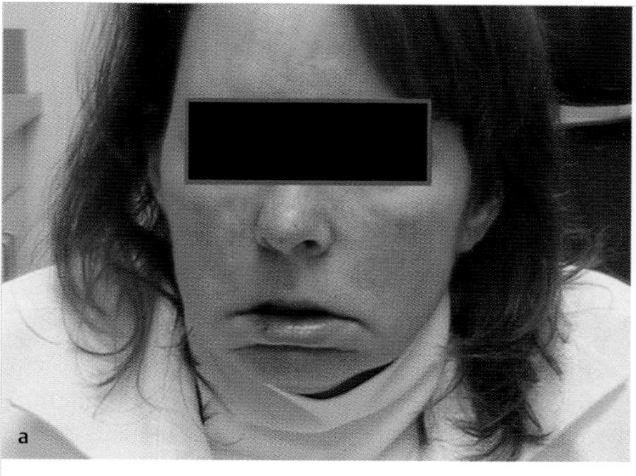

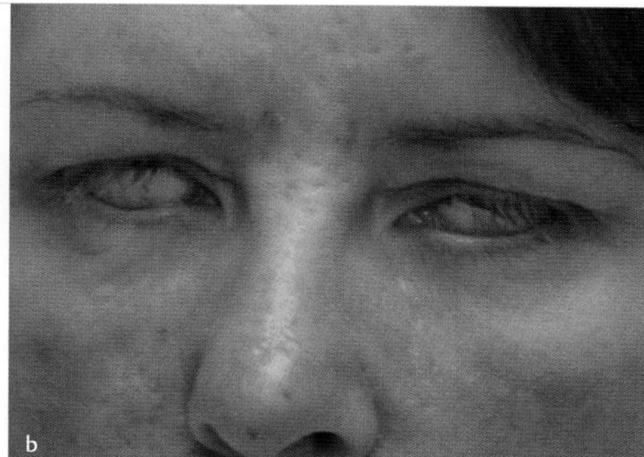

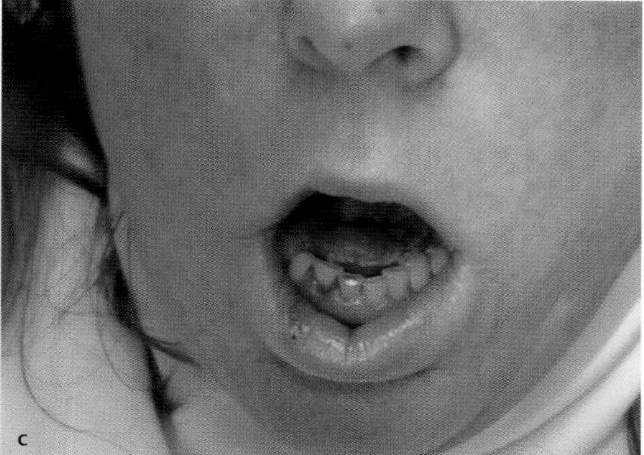

Fig. 4.3 (a–c) Bilateral facial palsy with bilateral Bell's phenomenon, due to postviral encephalitis.

4.2.5 Conditions Associated with Facial Nerve Palsy

Guillain–Barré Syndrome

Guillain–Barré syndrome (GBS) is an acute inflammatory demyelinating polyradiculopathy. It is characterized by an acute progressive ascending paresthesia, weakness, and areflexia. The incidence of GBS is estimated to be 0.5 to 2.0 cases per 100,000.[7] The origin of GBS is thought to be an autoimmune or hypersensitivity reaction involving cell-mediated and humoral mechanisms directed against peripheral myelin. Approximately half of the patients with this disorder give a history of an antecedent acute infectious illness that is usually cleared by the time neuropathic symptoms begin. The onset of symptoms is subacute, and its evolution is complete within 2 weeks in about 80% of cases, after 3 weeks in over 80%, and after 4 weeks in over 90%. A satisfactory recovery occurs in 85% of cases by the end of 4 to 6 months, although the majority of patients show permanent deficits of varying severity. Patients with GBS present with ascending motor paralysis that may progress rapidly to tetraplegia and respiratory failure. The severity of motor weakness covers a wide continuous spectrum from mild to total paralysis of every motor and cranial nerve. In most instances, it is noticed first in the legs, but it can begin in the arms. Facial nerve weakness is the most common cranial neuropathy. It occurs in approximately 50% of cases and is frequently bilateral. The other cranial nerves, seen in order of decreasing frequency, include the extraocular muscles and cranial nerves V, VIII, X, XI, and XII. GBS begins in the cranial nerves in less than 5% of cases. Associated sensory symptoms can also be seen. Abnormal cerebrospinal fluid (CSF) findings are characteristic of this disorder, although in the first few days they may be absent. After several days, the protein value begins to rise and may become very high and peak at approximately 4 to 6 weeks after the onset of clinical symptoms. Cells in the CSF are not prominent. The absence of cells in conjunction with an elevated protein level is the "albuminocytologic dissociation" that at one time was thought to be characteristic of the disease. In a few cases, lymphocytes, up to 20 to 30 cells/μL, may be seen in the CSF specimen. It is imperative that the physician recognizes this disorder in its earliest stages so that patients can be hospitalized and observed for progression of neurologic deficits, in particular for the possible need of respiratory support. GBS presenting as acute bilateral vocal cord paralysis has also been reported. The prognosis for spontaneous recovery in GBS is not dissimilar from Bell's palsy. In addition to EMG, other electrical tests are of limited value because of the bilaterality of disease: that is, the response may be equal on both sides of the face yet be significantly reduced from normal. Despite this, absolute reduction in response to needle EMG is the important prognostic sign; see Chapter 5. Plasma exchange or intravenous immunoglobulins are the treatment of choice for GBS.[8]

!

Facial nerve weakness is the most common cranial neuropathy in patient with Guillain–Barré syndrome.

Infectious Mononucleosis

Mononucleosis is characterized by fluctuating fever, sore throat, and lymphadenopathy. It is uncommon for unilateral, recurrent, or simultaneous bilateral facial paralysis to be caused by this disorder.[9] The syndrome of infectious mononucleosis, caused by the Epstein–Barr virus, has a classical presentation that can often be diagnosed on clinical grounds. The prodrome lasts from 3 to 5 days and consists of headache, malaise, myalgia, and fatigue. Sore throat occurs in the first week and is the most common feature of infectious mononucleosis. A grayish-white exudative tonsillitis is practically pathognomonic. Palatal petechiae located near the border of the hard and soft palate are observed in about one-third of patients. Lymph node enlargement is also characteristic. At times, it may be difficult to distinguish mononucleosis from the early stages of other forms of febrile exudative tonsillitis such as streptococcal infections and exudative tonsillitis of viral etiology. The differentiation depends on the results of throat cultures as well as hematologic and serologic features characteristic of infectious mononucleosis. Increased lymphocytes and the presence of atypical lymphocytes in peripheral blood are suggestive of mononucleosis. Positive results of a monospot serological test document rising titers for the heterophile antibodies.

!

Infectious mononucleosis can rarely present with unilateral, recurrent, or simultaneous bilateral facial paralysis.

Cytomegalovirus

Cytomegalovirus (CMV), a member of the herpes virus group, is capable of involving the facial nerve, producing a picture similar to infectious mononucleosis although sore throat and cervical adenopathy are usually absent.[10] CMV is excreted in the urine, and a rising compliment fixation antibody can usually be demonstrated.

Sarcoidosis

A patient presenting with bilateral facial paralysis and uveitis should be suspected of having sarcoidosis.[11] The diagnosis should certainly be suggested if in addition there is bilateral tender parotid enlargement due to parotitis (Heerfordt's syndrome). Sarcoidosis is a granulomatous disease of undetermined origin that involves multiple systems. Although there is no single laboratory test that is absolutely diagnostic, sarcoidosis is characterized by an elevation in serum and urinary calcium levels, an increase in serum globulin, and an elevated level of serum angiotensin-converting enzyme. Chest radiographs may demonstrate the characteristic hilar adenopathy or diffuse pulmonary infiltrates. An examination of the eye grounds may indicate uveitis, supporting the diagnosis. The diagnosis is made on the basis of clinical findings together with biopsy of tissue involved by sarcoid. Such tissue will contain characteristic noncaseating granulomas with multinucleate giant cells. In the head and neck, the disease may involve cervical lymph nodes as well as salivary tissue. The mucus membranes of the nose, mouth, tonsil, and larynx may be involved less commonly. Facial palsy is the most commonly seen clinical neurologic deficit to accompany sarcoidosis. Uveitis occurs four times more often in patients with neurologic symptoms than in those without symptoms. The peripheral neuropathy associated with sarcoidosis has been shown to be due to perineural inflammatory changes. The nerve fibers themselves are undamaged, which might account for the favorable prognosis in patients with sarcoid when treated with systemic steroids.

!

A patient with facial palsy and bilateral tender parotid enlargement due to parotitis is suspicious for a special form of sarcoidosis, i.e., Heerfordt's syndrome.

Acute Porphyrias

Another disorder that might rarely present as bilateral facial paralysis is acute porphyria.[12] Acute porphyrias are a group of disorders characterized by various abnormalities in the synthesis of heme, each of which results in an accumulation of heme precursors. Clinical manifestations usually include abdominal pain as the initial and most prominent symptom. In addition, photosensitivity and very often acute neurologic crisis may occur and result in serious morbidity and mortality. This crisis may be precipitated by a number of different medications including sulfonamides and barbiturates. The diagnosis is confirmed by noting elevated urinary and stool porphyrins and a markedly increased urinary porphobilinogen level.

Amyloidosis

Amyloid is a proteinaceous substance that is deposited in a variety of tissues. The cause of primary amyloidosis is unknown. Secondary amyloidosis may result from tuberculosis, rheumatoid arthritis, or multiple myeloma. Amyloidosis rarely causes facial palsy.[13] The diagnosis of amyloidosis is normally made by biopsy of the affected area. When the facial nerve is affected there is axonal neuropathy with deposits of amyloid in the perineurium. Histopathology uses polarizing microscopy to demonstrate the classic green birefringence with Congo red stain. Electrophysiologic studies should document the axonal lesion.

Sclerosing Bone Dysplasia

Sclerosing bone dysplasia is a severe, progressive, autosomal-recessive craniotubular hyperostosis. This disorder, which may become apparent at age 10 years or earlier, is frequently associated with bilateral facial weakness, progressive loss of hearing, and progressive loss of facial nerve function.[14] The hyperostosis and sclerosis are most prominent in the skull and tubular bones. Impairment of vision and severe headaches frequently develop in early childhood, and death may result suddenly from the compression of the medulla oblongata.

Botulism

Uncommonly, bilateral facial paralysis may be caused by botulism.[15] This disease may be recognized clinically by a red parched tongue, oropharynx, hypopharynx, and larynx associated with bilateral cranial nerve deficits. Early diagnosis is critical because respiratory collapse may be eminent. The diagnosis is confirmed by isolating botulinum toxin from a stool specimen.

Lyme Disease

Lyme disease is an important cause of facial palsy, especially in epidemic regions and children. The disease is discussed in detail in Chapter 11, and Lyme disease in children is addressed in Chapter 12. Lyme disease has also been reported to cause bilateral facial paralysis.

This spirochete disorder is transmitted by the tick. Successful transmission of the spirochete requires attachment of an infected tick for over 12 hours. The disease is characterized by the erythema chronicum migrans skin lesion that begins as a red macule or papule and expands to form a large bull's eye–shaped rash. This lesion typically lasts about 3 weeks. Associated symptoms include malaise, fatigue, chills and fever, headaches, stiff neck, backache, myalgias, nausea, vomiting, and sore throat. Some patients may develop a spectrum of neurologic symptoms, including meningitis, encephalitis, chorea, cerebellar ataxia, cranial neuritis (including bilateral facial palsy), motor and sensory radiculoneuritis, mononeuritis multiplex, and myelitis.

The clinical course of Lyme disease is broken down into three stages.

- During stage 1, erythema chronica migrans is reported in 60 to 80% of patients. This is the hallmark of stage 1 Lyme disease.
- It is during stage 2 when neurologic symptoms ensue that patients are likely to see an otolaryngologist; 15 to 20% of patients have been reported to develop neurologic complications with facial paralysis being the most common. About 10% of patients with Lyme disease have a facial paralysis, and, of these, up to 25% have bilateral paralysis.[16] Any cranial nerve can be involved as nerve involvement has nothing to do with the site of inoculation. Neuro-otologic symptoms are frequently associated with Lyme disease: about half of the patients have hearing abnormalities and four of five patients show vestibular symptoms. Fifty percent of these patients have also a facial paralysis.[17]
- Stage 3 can occur months to years after infection. The hallmarks of this stage are oligoarthritis, monarthritis, psychiatric changes, profound fatigue, permanent paralysis, and chronic dermatologic syndromes such as acrodermatitis chronicum atrophicans.

The diagnosis of Lyme disease can be quite easy to make if the characteristic skin lesion is present and an otolaryngologist sees the patient early in their disease course. A specific enzyme-linked immunosorbent assay (ELISA) is currently the preferred test to measure exposure to the spirochete. False-negative results are possible in the first few weeks of infection. Also, patients who have been treated in the early courses of the infection may fail to mount an antibody response. The treatment of the infection varies with the stages of the disease; for details see Chapter 11.

> **!**
>
> A patient with acute facial palsy should always, not only in epidemic regions, be asked for recent tick bites and/or occurrence of an erythema migrans.

Minor Trauma

If the patient had a severe trauma, for instance a temporal bone fracture, and develops immediately a facial palsy, the relation is obvious. The treatment of traumatic facial palsies is presented in Chapter 9. However, a patient may have sustained a minor accident and might not associate the incident with the onset of the facial paralysis or even be aware that a recent injury occurred. Such situations emphasize the importance of detecting subtle physical abnormalities and eliciting the pertinent history to avoid making an erroneous diagnosis of idiopathic (Bell's) palsy.

4.2.6 Family History and Congenital Facial Palsy

Apparently there is a genetic predisposition to Bell's palsy.[18] The incidence of a positive family history for Bell's palsy is 5 to 20%. Based on this, a positive family history is strongly suggestive but not diagnostic of Bell's palsy; the reason for this is that patients refer to all causes of facial palsy as Bell's palsy. A patient must be questioned carefully to be certain that the facial paralysis that involved a family member was truly of the idiopathic type. Further, the fact that a family member had Bell's palsy does not eliminate the possibility that the patient's palsy may have a treatable cause.

Hereditary congenital facial palsy (HCFP) is a very rare disease.[19] HCFP belongs to the congenital cranial dysinnervation disorders.[20] Symptoms of HCFP1 are an asymmetric, mostly bilateral, weakness of some or all facial muscles. A unilateral or bilateral facial palsy often combined with hearing loss or congenital deafness is typical for HCFP2. The lifetime prevalence in western Europe and the United States reaches about 0.6%. The incidence has been estimated to be 10 to 50 cases per 100,000 of population. A family history is found in 2 to 28% of all cases.[21] Recurrence in familial facial palsy is frequent, especially if the first episode occurs during childhood. The mode of inheritance in idiopathic familial facial palsy is possibly of autosomal dominance with low penetrance. The genetic factors that can lead to neuropathy of the intratemporal facial nerve or increase the individual's susceptibility to facial palsy are unknown. Inheritance of HCFP is autosomal dominant with a penetrance of 95% in HCFP1 and 60% in HCFP2. Two loci have been identified: one on chromosome 3q21.2-q22.1 (HCFP1) and one on chromosome 10q21.3-q22.1 (HCFP2). Although the cause remains unknown, recent evidence suggests a possible association with a reactivation of an infection by herpes simplex virus in some cases that has been shown to be latent in a high proportion of seventh-nerve ganglia. Probably, the infection leads to a viral inflammation and edema of the nerve. Due to its complicated course through a narrow bone channel within the temporal bone, the edema causes rapid impact on the nerve's vascular supply, particularly in the labyrinthine segment. The prevailing notion is that the inflammation is variably accompanied by autoimmune processes related to herpes simplex virus.[22] The result is nerve damage of various degrees with or without nerve degeneration and regeneration. HCFP is probably caused by maldevelopment of the facial nucleus and/or the facial nerve.

4.2.7 Pregnancy

Whether the incidence of facial paralysis is higher among pregnant women compared with nonpregnant women of the same age is a matter of debate, as study results are controversial.[23] There might be an indirect effect: chronic hypertension and obesity are independent risk factors for Bell's palsy. Bell's palsy during pregnancy is significantly associated with severe pre-eclampsia.[24] In addition, if a facial palsy occurs during pregnancy, this does not automatically mean that the diagnosis is Bell's palsy. These women need a thorough evaluation to rule out other diagnoses, as with any new patient with facial paralysis. It is important to limit any studies involving radiation, even though this can be an important limitation during the diagnostic work-up. Consultation with the obstetrician is recommended regarding invasive diagnostic testing and possible treatment. Outcome for idiopathic palsy may be poorer in pregnant patients, although historically, unnecessarily, conservative treatment with corticosteroids given to other patients is often withheld from these patients.[23]

!

A pregnancy itself may not be a risk factor for facial palsy. After discussion with the responsible obstetrician, Bell's palsy should ideally be treated as in nonpregnant patients.

4.2.8 Systemic Illnesses

Several systemic disorders may present with peripheral neuropathies including, for instance, diabetes, alcoholism, collagen vascular disorders, hypothyroidism, amyloidosis, and hypertension. The mechanism leading to facial palsy with hypertension is presumed to be hemorrhage into the fallopian canal.[25] Although facial paralysis occurs in patients with these disorders, one should not assume, in the presence of one or more of these disorders, that the cause of palsy is known without undertaking a thorough evaluation.

4.2.9 Drugs

There are some case reports describing drugs leading to facial palsy. For instance, isoniazid prescribed as a treatment for tuberculosis can be neurotoxic and involve cranial nerves, particularly the ophthalmic division of the fifth nerve. Isoniazid can also lead to a facial palsy. A unilateral facial paralysis has also been described secondary to arsenic toxicity. Thalidomide is also known to lead to malformation associated with a facial palsy. Misoprostol misused for abortion is related to congenital malformations of the child after abortion failure, and these children in particular have a high risk of being born with Möbius syndrome.[26]

4.2.10 Immunizations

Bell's palsy, bulbar palsy involving multiple cranial nerves, and GBS have been noted following vaccination against tick-borne encephalitis (▶ Fig. 4.4), polio, rabies, and influenza. However, such reports are rare. Therefore, there are doubts whether there is an association between immunization and idiopathic facial palsy.[27]

4.2.11 Malignancies

A history of cancer in general, and particularly involving the skin of the face and scalp, upper aerodigestive tract, parotid, thyroid, breast, lung, kidney, ovary, or prostate, associated with a facial paralysis suggests that a metastatic lesion is causing the palsy. Appropriate radiographic and laboratory studies are indicated to search for the primary site as well as to localize the site of facial nerve involvement.

4.2.12 Idiopathic (Bell's) Palsy

Finally, one must consider a diagnosis of idiopathic (Bell's) palsy for those patients in whom no cause of facial palsy can be found despite the implementation of intensive diagnostic measures suggested in ▶ Table 4.2 and described in detail in Chapter 8.

4.3 Clinical Examination

▶ Table 4.2, ▶ Table 4.3, Box 4.1 (p. 33), Box 4.2 (p. 35) and Box 4.3 (p. 36) list the most important symptoms and related examinations that should be considered in a patient with facial palsy. Regarding the possible topographical lesion sites, ▶ Table 4.3 lists the most important diseases and related symptoms. An optimal examination room is shown in ▶ Fig. 4.5.

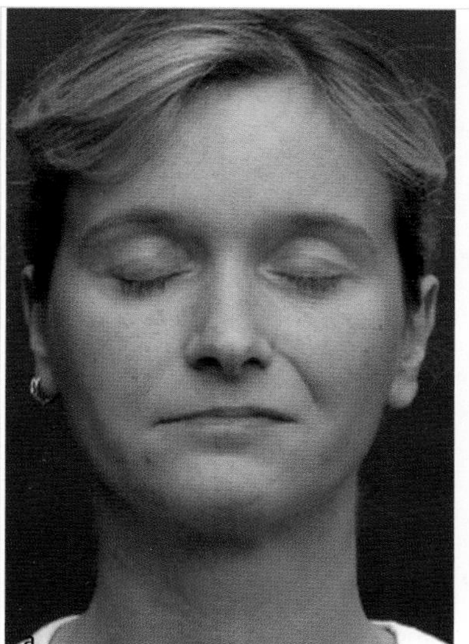

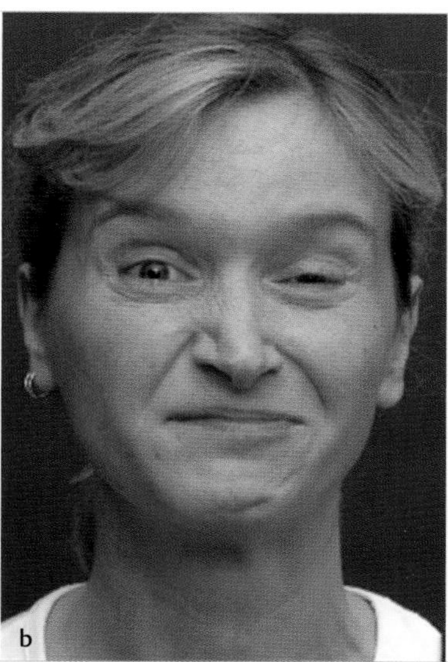

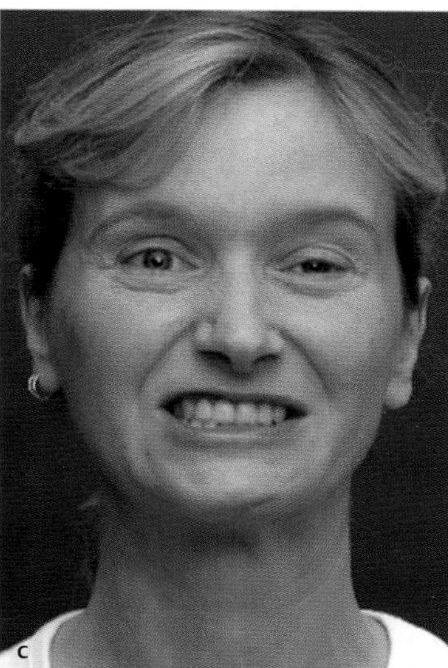

Fig. 4.4 (a–c) Defective healing of the left side 2 years after immunization against tick-borne encephalitis. A complete facial palsy developed 2 weeks after immunization. There has been stable defective healing since 1 year postimmunization. The diagnosis is facial paralysis secondary to vaccination damage.

Table 4.2 Diagnostic evaluation of facial palsy

Diagnostic evaluation	Specific test
History	
Physical examination	
Topognostic tests	• Hearing and balance tests • Schirmer's test • Stapedial reflex • Taste test
Imaging studies; see Chapter 5	• Chest radiographic survey to detect sarcoidosis, lymphoma, carcinoma • CT of brainstem, cerebellopontine angle, temporal bone, skull base; contrast sialography of parotid • MRI of brainstem, brain, cerebellopontine angle, temporal bone, and parotid gland • Sonography of the parotid gland, the face and the facial muscles
Electrical tests; see Chapter 6	• Blink reflex • Electroneurography • Magnetic evoked potentials • Needle electromyography • Surface electromyography
Grading and documentation; Chapter 7	
Surgical exploration	
Special laboratory tests	• Lumbar puncture (cerebrospinal fluid) to detect meningitis, encephalitis, Guillain–Barré syndrome, multiple sclerosis, meningeal carcinomatosis • Complete white blood cell count and differential to detect infectious monucleosis, leukemia • Monospot test to detect infectious mononucleosis • Fluorescent treponemal antibody titer to detect syphilis • Erythrocyte sedimentation rate to detect sarcoidosis, collagen vascular disorders • Urine and fecal examination: • Acute porphyria: elevated porphyrins and urinary porphobilinogen • Botulism: *Clostridium botulinum* toxin in stool specimen • Sarcoidosis: urinary calcium • Cytomegalovirus in urine • Serum cryoglobulins and immune complexes to detect Lyme disease • Serum globulin level to detect sarcoidosis • Serum and urine calcium determinations to detect sarcoidosis • Serum angiotensin-converting enzyme level to detect sarcoidosis • Serum antinuclear antibody test and rheumatoid factor to detect collagen vascular disorders (periarteritis nodosa) • Bone marrow examination to detect leukemia, lymphoma • Glucose tolerance test to detect diabetes mellitus • Lip biopsy to detect Melkersson–Rosenthal syndrome • Surgical biopsy to detect amyloidosis • Lyme titers (ELISA testing) to detect Lyme disease • Drug testing to detect isoniazid toxicity, alcohol, arsenic • Blood test to detect HIV • Psychological exploration; see Chapter 13

Source: Adapted with permission from Schaitkin et al 2000.[37]

4.3.1 Facial Muscle Weakness and Facial Palsy

The motor deficit can be very variable, and depends on whether the patient presents with an acute or chronic facial palsy, be it incomplete or complete palsy (▶ Fig. 4.6, ▶ Fig. 4.7, ▶ Fig. 4.8 and ▶ Fig. 4.9). The presence of facial weakness and numbness may be the first sign of the disease. A physician should be consulted as soon as possible after developing a facial palsy. A facial weakness and numbness can also be a sign of a tumor located in the course of the facial nerve and deserves evaluation and periodic reassessment. Facial weakness may be detected by scrutinizing the patient's face for tone and symmetry. Facial weakness may be suspected by comparing the two sides of the face, looking for a difference

Table 4.3 Signs indicating probable diagnoses of lesions of the facial nerve at various topographic levels

Level	Signs	Probable diagnoses
Supranuclear cortex and internal capsule	Tone and upper face intact, loss of volitional movement with intact spontaneous expression, slurred speech (tongue weakness), hemiparesis (arm greater than leg) on side of facial involvement. Paresis of upper extremity begins with involvement of thumb, finger, and hand movement	Lesion of motor cortex or internal capsule on opposite side of facial involvement Paresis upper extremity usually middle cerebral artery; paresis lower extremity usually anterior cerebral artery
Opercular syndrome	Voluntary facial and lingual movements impaired, emotional and automatic movements preserved or exaggerated. Speech is dysarthric; laryngeal, sternocleidomastoid, and trapezius muscles involved. Weakness of the tongue, pharynx jaws, neck muscles, and upper extremity may occur. EEG may not be abnormal because of depth of lesion in operculum (insula or island of Reil complex). Upper face usually not spared as with other motor cortex lesions	Vascular, neoplastic, encephalitic, or traumatic lesion (operculum stippled)
Extrapyramidal	Increased salivary flow, spontaneous facial movement impaired, volitional facial movement intact. Masked face of Parkinsonism or dystonia, progressive hemifacial spasm	Tumor or vascular lesion of basal ganglia Parkinsonism. Meige's syndrome (cervical facial dystonia). Grimacing and choreiform movements
Midbrain	Involvement of face and oculomotor roots; loss of pupillary reflexes, external strabismus, and oculomotor paresis on opposite side of facial paresis	Unilateral Weber's syndrome (vascular lesion)
	Bilateral facial paresis with other cranial nerve deficits, emotional lability, hyperactive gag reflex, marked hyperreflexia associated with hypertension	Pseudobulbar palsy associated with multiple infarcts
Pontine nucleus	Involvement of cranial nerves VII and VI on side of lesion with gaze palsy on side of facial paresis Contralateral hemiparesis, ataxia, cerebellovestibular signs	Involvement of pons at level of VII and VI nuclei by pontine glioma, multiple sclerosis, encephalitis, infection, or polio
	Contralateral hemiplegia with ipsilateral facial palsy. Internal strabismus may be present on side of facial palsy	Possible lesion just above pontine facial nucleus, below decussation of corticobulbar tract. Millard–Gubler syndrome, Foville's syndrome
	Ipsilateral facial paresis, analgesia, Homer's cranial nerves VII and VI noted from time of birth with or without other congenital anomalies. Facial motor involvement usually incomplete sparing of comer of mouth or lower lip common. Another type of presentation is involvement of the lower lip with complete or partial sparing of upper face. Anomalies of the pinna, canal, or mandible associated with facial palsy indicate developmental defect of facial nerve	Developmental facial palsy (noted at birth). Oculofacial syndrome or Möbius syndrome. Thalidomide toxicity. Nondevelopmental facial palsy due to facial or abducens nerve anomalies is most often due to intranuclear lesions
Infranuclear, intracranial cerebellopontine angle	Impairment of hearing, especially discrimination out of proportion to pure tone scores. Possible ataxia, abnormalities of tearing or taste, stapes reflex decay, decreased corneal sensation. Facial motor deficit (late sign). Prolongation of the latency of waves III–V of auditory brainstem response. Anomalies on CT scan (usually not enhanced with contrast)	Vestibular schwannoma; see Chapter 18
	Abnormalities in trigeminal, acoustic–vestibular and facial nerve function, starting with facial pain or numbness. Lesion noted on CT (enhancement with contrast)	Meningioma

Table 4.3 continued

Level	Signs	Probable diagnoses
	Abnormalities of facial and acoustic–vestibular nerve function. May start with facial twitching. Erosion or arising in temporal bone. Lytic area evident on plane radiographs of temporal bone	Cholesteatoma or facial schwannoma; see Chapter 18
	Abnormalities of cranial nerves VII, VIII, IX, X, XI, and XII. Pulsatile tinnitus and purple-red pulsating mass bulging through the tympanic membrane	Glomus jugulare tumor
	Abnormalities of abducens nerve in addition to petrous apex to involve middle fossa	Glomus jugulare tumor extending to above
Skull base	Conductive or sensorineural hearing loss, acute or recurrent facial palsy. Positive family history, abnormalities of bone density on skull radiograph	Osteopetrosis
	Multiple cranial nerve involvement in rapid succession	Carcinomatous meningitis, leukemia, Landry–Guillain–Barré, mononucleosis, diphtheria, tuberculosis, sarcoidosis, malignant external otitis
Transtemporal bone, internal auditory canal, and labyrinthine segment of facial nerve	Ecchymosis around pinna and mastoid prominence (Battle's sign). Hemotympanum with sensorineural hearing loss (tuning fork lateralizes to normal side), vertigo, nystagmus (fast component away from involved side). Sudden complete facial paralysis following head trauma. Usually associated with basilar skull fracture, loss of consciousness, and cerebrospinal fluid leak. Transection of facial nerve more likely with this injury compared with longitudinal fracture	Temporal bone fracture (transverse, longitudinal, or combination)
Geniculate ganglion	Dry eye, and decreased taste and salivation. Erosion of geniculate ganglion area or middle fossa demonstrated by CT scan of temporal bone	Schwannoma, meningioma, cholesteatoma, cavernous hemangioma, arteriovenous malformation
	Ear pain, vesicles on pinna, dry eye, and decreased taste and salivary flow. Sensorineural hearing loss, nystagmus, vertigo, red chorda tympani nerve. Facial palsy may be complete, incomplete, or progress to complete over 14 days	Herpes zoster cephalicus (Ramsay Hunt syndrome)
	Same as above without vesicles, no other cause evident. Facial palsy may be complete, incomplete, or progress to complete over 10 days. Same as above but no recovery in 6 months	Idiopathic (Bell's) palsy, viral inflammatory immune disorder
	Ecchymoses around pinna and mastoid (Battle's sign), hemotympanum. Conductive hearing loss (tuning fork lateralizes to involved ear, bone air), no vestibular involvement unless stapes subluxed into vestibule (causes fluctuating sensorineural hearing loss and vertigo with nystagmus)	Longitudinal fracture of temporal bone. May be proximal or at the geniculate ganglion (dry eye), or distal to geniculate ganglion (tearing symmetrical). (Tear test valid only in acute injury)
Tympanomastoid	Decreased taste and salivation, loss of stapes reflex and symmetrical tearing. Sudden onset facial palsy VII that may be complete or incomplete or may progress to complete. Pain, vesicles, red chorda tympani	Herpes zoster cephalicus
	Pain without vesicles, red chorda tympani	Bell's palsy

Table 4.3 continued

Level	Signs	Probable diagnoses
	Red, bulging tympanic membrane, conductive hearing loss. Usually history of upper respiratory tract infection. Lower face may be involved more than upper face	Acute suppurative otitis media
	Foul drainage through perforated tympanic membrane. History of recurrent ear infection, drainage, and hearing loss	Chronic suppurative otitis media, most likely associated with cholesteatoma
	Pulsatile tinnitus, purple-red pulsatile mass noted through tympanic membrane	Glomus tympanicum or jugulare
	Recurrent facial paralysis, positive family history, facial edema, fissured tongue. May present with simultaneous bilateral facial paralysis	Melkersson–Rosenthal syndrome
Extracranial	Incomplete facial nerve paresis. Hearing, balance, tearing, stapes reflex, taste, and salivary flow spared	Penetrating wound of face; sequelae of parotid surgery; malignancy of parotid, tonsil, or oronasopharynx; rarely, with benign lesion of parotid gland compressing facial nerve
	Uveitis, salivary gland enlargement, fever	Sarcoidosis (Heerfordt's syndrome), lymphoma
Sites variable	Bilateral facial paralysis from birth	Möbius syndrome
	Bilateral facial paralysis, acquired	Landry–Guillain–Barré syndrome, sarcoidosis, mononucleosis, leukemia, idiopathic (Bell's) palsy
	Facial paralysis, especially simultaneous bilateral facial paralysis with symmetrical ascending paralysis, decreased deep tendon reflexes, minimal sensory changes. Abnormal spinal fluid (protein and few cells, albuminocytologic dissociation)	Landry–Guillain–Barré syndrome
	Deficits of cranial nerves VI and VII, or VII, VI, and III, possibly in association with other neurologic signs	Carcinoma of nasopharynx, metastatic carcinoma from breast, ovary, prostate, meningitis, leukemia, diabetes mellitus
Pseudobulbar palsy	Inappropriate or exaggerated laughing or crying. May be associated with marked increase in jaw jerk or gag reflex	Polyneuritis. Toxic, viral, or vascular lesion involving bilateral corticobulbar pathways

Source: Adapted with permission from Schaitkin et al 2000.[37]

or the presence of one or more of the following: forehead creases, eyebrow level, supratarsal fold sag, inclination of upper eye lashes (the facial nerve innervates pilomotor fibers to the eye lashes and paralysis may result in the lashes assuming a downward position), scleral show as a result of lower lid sagging, a blink lag, loss of the nasolabial crease, lower lip lag, lower teeth showing, and talking out of the side of the mouth. Patients with chronic facial palsy may show signs of synkinesis and twitching. Synkinesis is most obvious between the eye and mouth region, i.e., the eye is closed during mouth movements and eye closure causes twitching or sustained contracture of the zygomaticus muscles.

It is recommended to use a standard scheme to document the facial palsy with photographs (▶ Fig. 4.10) and if possible with a video for better dynamic accuracy. Furthermore, grading of the severity of the palsy is recommended to allow better comparison with other patients and for the follow-up. Several internationally validated grading systems are available and are presented in Chapter 7.

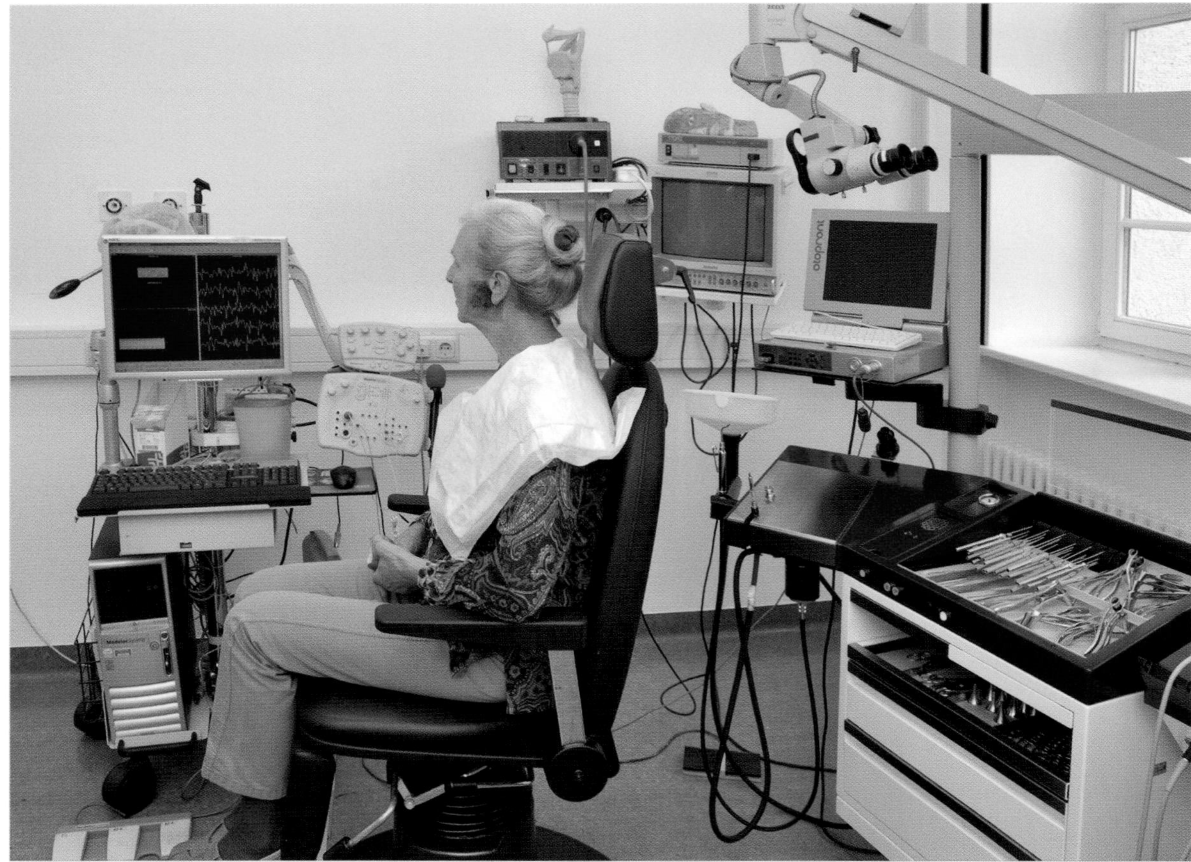

Fig. 4.5 Example of an examination room for patients with facial palsy, including a standard otorhinolaryngological unit and equipment for electrodiagnostic testing. The patient has a postoperative facial palsy after parotidectomy and also shows a positive iodine-starch test (Minor test) on the left side.

> !
>
> Examination of facial motor functions means testing the mimic function of the complete face. Otherwise a facial weakness or incomplete palsy can be overlooked.

4.3.2 Gross Neurological Examination

It is important to look for other neurologic signs as hints for a central palsy; see Chapter 27. Presence of simultaneous bilateral palsy, facial paralysis associated with other cranial nerve deficits, and slowly progressive facial weakness with or without hyperkinesis are such symptoms. Signs such as intact forehead movement, alterations in facial sensation, pupillary constrictions, corneal hypesthesia, and paresthesias of the extremities, although often associated with lesions in the cerebrocortex, cerebellopontine angle, or internal auditory canal, are nonspecific for a central palsy as they can also be found in patients with Bell's palsy.

4.3.3 Cranial Nerve Survey

As mentioned above, patients who present with facial paralysis require a complete otoneurological exam (► Fig. 4.5, ► Fig. 4.6, ► Fig. 4.7, ► Fig. 4.8, and ► Fig. 4.9). Many lesions causing a facial paralysis involve the nerve within the temporal bone. Also, it is of interest to note that 8 of the 12 cranial nerves pass through or by the temporal bone. Therefore a survey of cranial nerves V to XII should be studied in detail. Their function is most readily tested by one or more simple office tests.

4.3.4 Corneal Sensation

Testing for corneal sensation is part of the routine neurologic examination. A decreased or absent corneal sensation in association with a peripheral facial paralysis

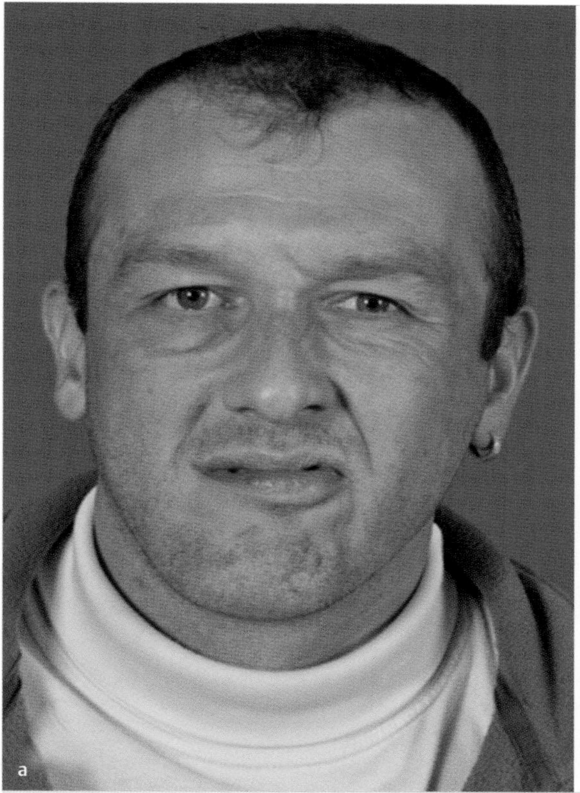

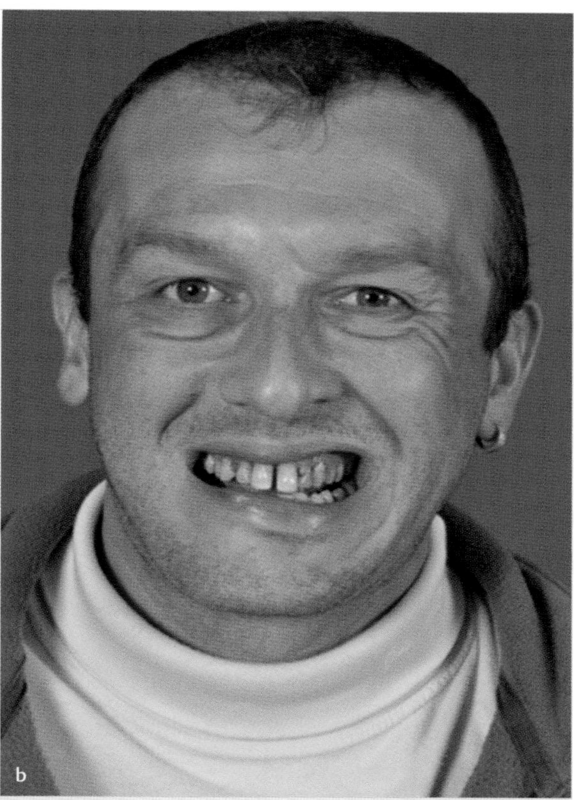

Fig. 4.6 Acute, incomplete facial palsy on the right side while (**a**) pursing the lips, and (**b**) showing the teeth. (Adapted with permission from Finkensieper M, Fabian Volk G, Guntinas-Lichius O. Facial nerve disorders [in German]. Laryngorhinootologie 2012;91(02):121–142.)

arouses suspicion of a cerebellopontine angle lesion and normally leads away from the diagnosis of Bell's palsy. However, it should be emphasized that loss of corneal sensation is entirely compatible with Bell's palsy. The frequency of diminished corneal sensation noticed with Bell's palsy is approximately 10%. Corneal sensation is determined by testing with a cotton wisp over the cornea on the paralyzed side. The apparent loss of sensation is most likely to represent a form of adaptation or exposure hypesthesia. Another possible explanation is involvement of the sensory fibers of the trigeminal nerve, which may be carried with the greater petrosal nerve to the cornea.

4.3.5 Keratitis

Detection and appropriate treatment of early corneal ulceration may prevent impairment of vision (corneal scarring) or loss of vision (corneal perforation). Eye pain, squinting, photophobia, pericorneal vascular flare, or hyperemia, suggest a keratitis, and positive fluorescein staining is diagnostic. Examination of the eye is described in more detail in Chapter 24. It is important during the initial examination as well as when considering reanimation surgery for the eye.

4.3.6 Palate Symmetry

The palate should be inspected for signs of asymmetry. If the involvement is at the level of the brainstem, skull base, or jugular foramen, not only will the palate be involved and pulled to the intact contralateral side, but there will also be weakness or paralysis of the vocal cord on the ipsilateral side. Involvement of the vagus will not only paralyze the ipsilateral vocal cord but will be associated with involvement of the superior laryngeal nerve as well. This leads to rotation of the posterior commissure to the abnormal side. Further, there will be paresis or paralysis of the superior and middle constrictor muscles, causing contraction of the pharynx on the uninvolved side only. This combination of deficits is responsible for hoarseness and aspiration; both symptoms are characteristically associated with a high vagal palsy.

4.3.7 Tongue Deviation

Palate asymmetry and sensory changes over the distribution of the trigeminal nerves suggest the presence of an interaxial lesion. Cranial nerve XII is evaluated by testing tongue movement. In some patients with flaccid

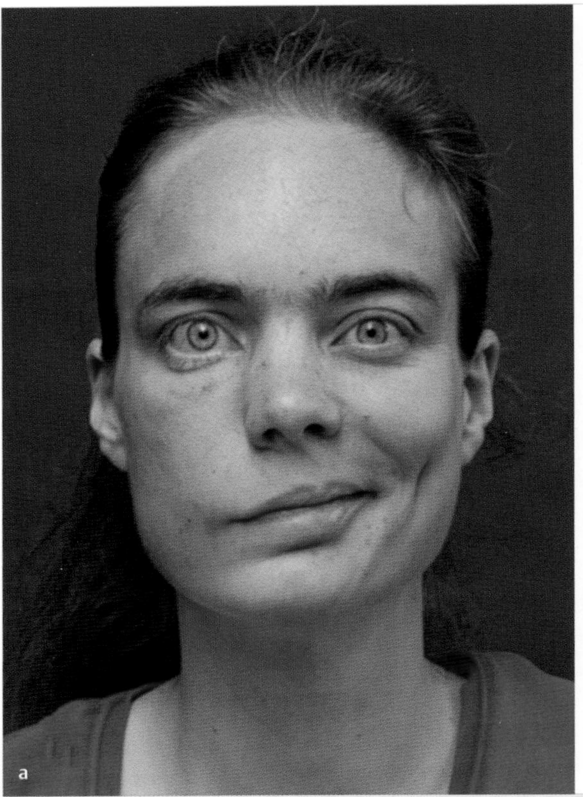

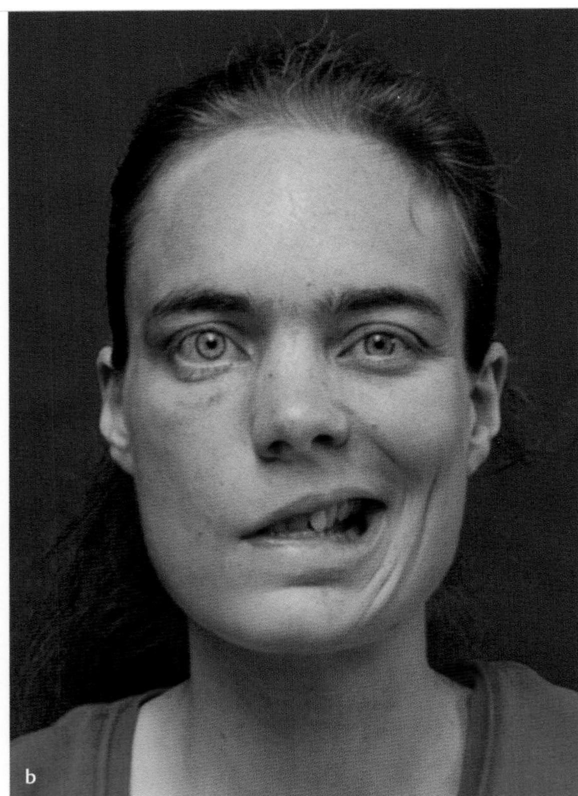

Fig. 4.7 Acute, complete facial palsy on the right side while (**a**) pursing the lips, and (**b**) showing the teeth. (Adapted with permission from Finkensieper M, Fabian Volk G, Guntinas-Lichius O. Facial nerve disorders [in German]. Laryngorhinootologie 2012;91(02):121–142.)

peripheral facial paralysis the tongue appears to be deviated upon protrusion, and it is usually pulled toward the normal side. Motor function of the tongue can be more accurately tested by having the patient push the tongue against the inside of the cheek while the examiner exerts counter pressure with the finger on the outside of the cheek. The absence of hemiatrophy of the tongue or fasciculations helps to rule out twelfth cranial nerve involvement. Examination of the hypoglossal nerve function is very important when considering facial nerve reanimation by a hypoglossal nerve transfer; see Chapter 20.

4.3.8 Loss of Taste and Taste Papillae

Loss of taste and taste papillae associated with facial nerve disorders has been reported. Although taste changes are commonly associated with Bell's palsy because of involvement of the chorda tympani nerve, altered taste has also been noted with lesions resulting from trauma, temporal bone surgery, inflammation, and neoplasms involving the middle ear, and temporal bone, and cerebellopontine angle.

4.3.9 Signs of Acquired Immunodeficiency Syndrome

Any of the head and neck manifestations of AIDS must be noted as these have been known to cause facial palsy on rare occasions. These physical findings include, but should not be limited to, adenoid hypertrophy in an adult, hairy leukoplakia, Kaposi's sarcoma, benign parotid cysts, molluscum contagiosum, and cervical lymphadenopathy.

4.3.10 Pain or Numbness

Pain associated with sudden onset of peripheral facial paralysis has been noted with Bell's palsy, herpetic neuropathy, and tumors. Therefore pain alone is not diagnostic. In addition, pain has not been found to have any prognostic significance. About 60% of patients complain of pain generally preceding the onset of Bell's palsy and this increases to 80 to 90% of patients with herpes zoster cephalicus. Bell's palsy patients most commonly complain of pain over the mastoid while patients with herpes zoster are more likely to complain of ear pain but this is not

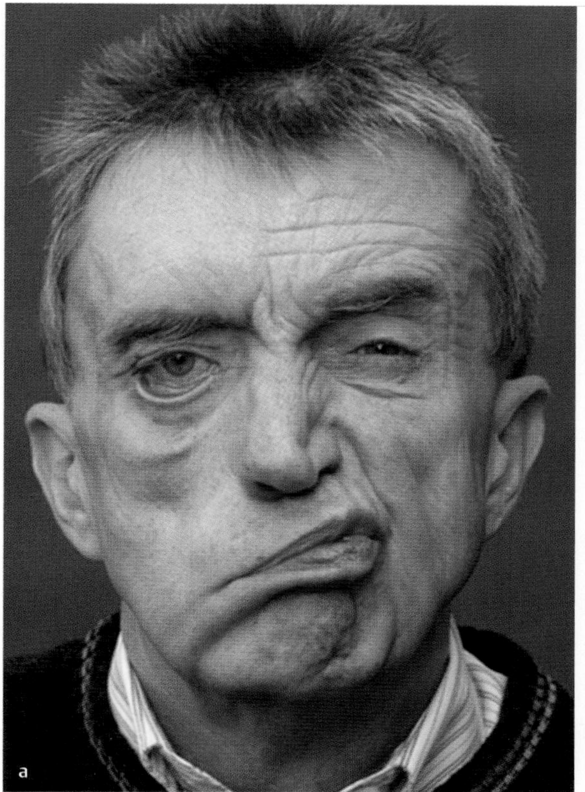

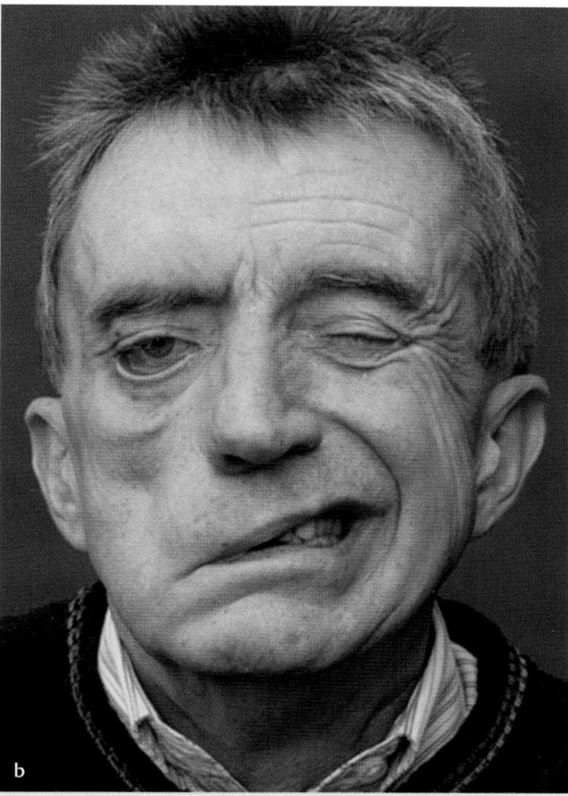

Fig. 4.8 Chronic facial palsy without regeneration on the right side while (**a**) pursing the lips, and (**b**) showing the teeth. (Adapted with permission from Finkensieper M, Fabian Volk G, Guntinas-Lichius O. Facial nerve disorders [in German]. Laryngorhinootologie 2012;91 (02):121–142.)

reliable enough to help in making a diagnosis. Involvement of cranial nerve VIII with hearing loss and dizziness is seen commonly with zoster and rarely with Bell's palsy.

4.3.11 Vesicles

The presence of vesicles is considered diagnostic of herpes varicella zoster cephalic neuropathy, Ramsay Hunt syndrome, as described in Chapter 10; however, it may be associated with herpes simplex type 1, and the two disorders may be clinically indistinguishable. Often vesicles will appear prior to the onset of facial paralysis or they may not appear until up to 10 days later. The distribution of the pain and vesicles maps out the ganglia and nerves involved. Involvement of cervical ganglia 2, 3, and 4 would be associated with pain and vesicles over the neck to the shoulder as well as across the lower posterior third of the face. Involvement of the lateral pinna would suggest involvement of the third division of the trigeminal nerve.

4.3.12 Ear

Evidence for involvement of the temporal bone is highly significant in establishing the cause of facial palsy. A history of acute or chronic ear infections, previous ear surgery, or any hearing and balance complaints must be thoroughly evaluated; see Chapter 17. A diagnosis of masked mastoiditis is suspected when there is a history of ear pain or hearing change on the side of the palsy in a patient who has taken antibiotics for recent symptoms of ear disease. Mastoid cell changes on computed tomography (CT) scan will help to support this diagnosis. Association of a facial paralysis with pulsatile tinnitus may suggest an arteriovenous malformation, a jugular or carotid anomaly compressing the facial nerve, or, more commonly, a glomus tumor; see Chapter 15. A sensorineural hearing loss together with involvement of the facial nerve suggests a lesion located in the internal auditory canal or cerebellopontine angle, as described in Chapter 18, while a conductive hearing loss and facial nerve involvement are in keeping with a lesion of the tympanic segment of the middle ear. The important point is that the presence of other temporal bone symptoms with a facial paralysis should prompt a search for a diagnosis.

4.3.13 Dizziness

Changes in balance with facial nerve involvement are most commonly seen with herpes zoster cephalicus but

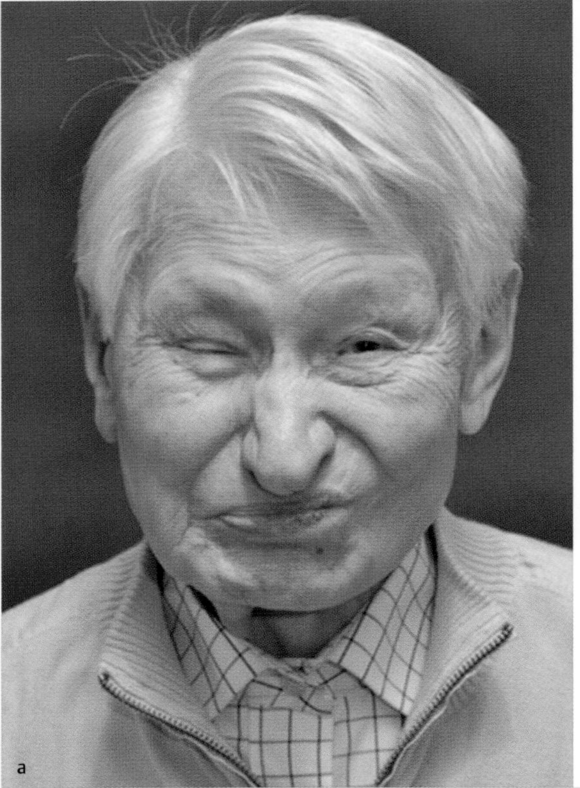

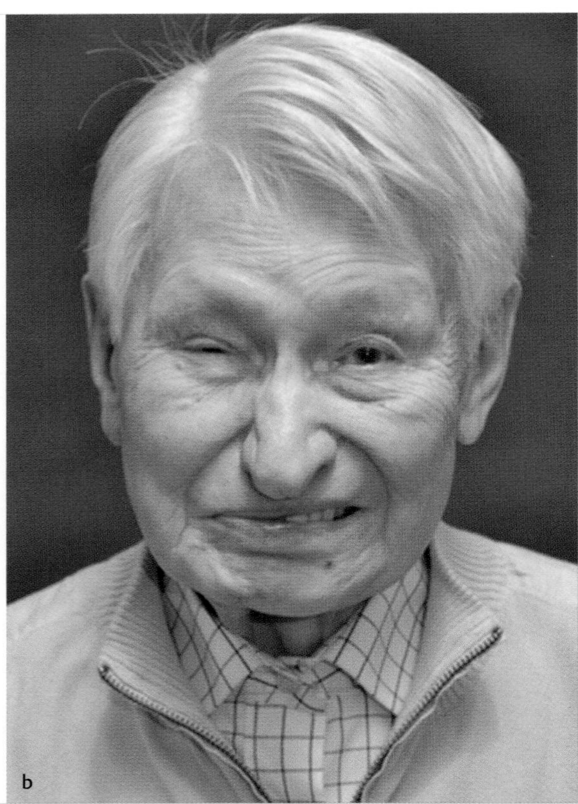

Fig. 4.9 Chronic facial palsy with defective healing on the left side while (**a**) pursing the lips, and (**b**) showing the teeth. Adapted with permission from Finkensieper M, Fabian Volk G, Guntinas-Lichius O. Facial nerve disorders [in German]. Laryngorhinootologie 2012;91 (02):121–142.)

also may be noted with a lesion in the cerebellopontine angle or internal auditory canal. The vestibular and facial nerves lie in close proximity in these areas and both structures may also be involved by a vestibular schwannoma; see Chapter 18. Dizziness and facial paralysis has also been noted with Bell's palsy, trauma, tumors, and multiple sclerosis. Dizziness from involvement of the peripheral vestibular system must be differentiated from true ataxia associated with a brainstem or cerebellar lesion; see Chapter 27.

4.4 Topodiagnostics

Topodiagnostic tests are nowadays mainly of historic interest. Surprisingly, they are still often used in clinical routine, although CT and magnetic resonance imaging (MRI) are available to detect a facial nerve lesion site much more precisely, as described in Imaging. In the pre-CT/MRI era, several topodiagnostic tests were developed to analyze the complex branching pattern of the facial nerve, with the idea of localizing the site of the lesion and possibly obtaining prognostic information. The most popular tests were gustometry, Schirmer's test for the evaluation of tear production, and the recording of the stapes reflex. Unfortunately, the results of all these and other tests show large intraindividual and interindividual variance.[28] All topodiagnostic tests have a very low positive predictive value for degeneration of the facial nerve. Topodiagnostic tests are worthless in patients with preoperative normal facial function.

> !
>
> The topodiagnostic accuracy of the so-called topodiagnostic tests is low.

4.4.1 Stapedial Reflex (Acoustic Reflex)

The stapedial reflex testing procedure involves presenting a suprathreshold stimulus to change the acoustic impedance of the ear. The reflex is normally activated

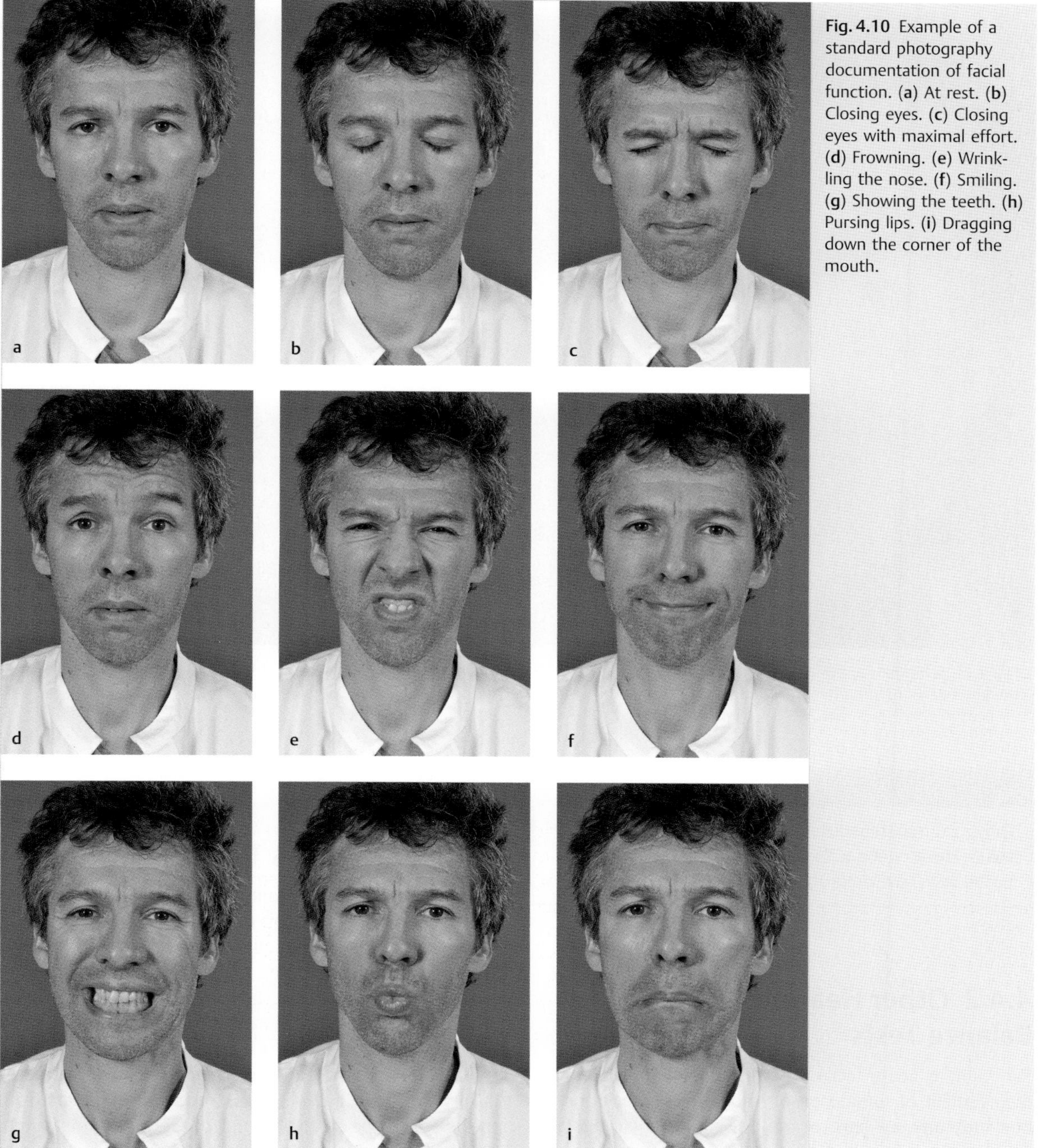

Fig. 4.10 Example of a standard photography documentation of facial function. (**a**) At rest. (**b**) Closing eyes. (**c**) Closing eyes with maximal effort. (**d**) Frowning. (**e**) Wrinkling the nose. (**f**) Smiling. (**g**) Showing the teeth. (**h**) Pursing lips. (**i**) Dragging down the corner of the mouth.

bilaterally. Normally, the ear's impedance increases when the reflex is activated. This change is caused by a contraction of the stapedius muscle and is measured in the ear containing the probe tip, i.e., the probe ear. The ear receiving the stimulus to activate the reflex is the stimulus ear. Dysfunction of the reflex can involve any part of the reflex arc, i.e., from the cochlea via the acoustic nerve to the brainstem, or from the brainstem via the facial nerve to the stapedius muscle. Therefore, the acoustic reflex test as a topodiagnostical test is useful only if an ear disease is ruled out. Topodiagnostically, the facial nerve is the first efferent branch. A normal acoustic reflex in a patient with acute facial palsy is prognostic for good recovery.[29] Unfortunately, the absence of the reflex at the onset of the palsy is of no prognostic significance.

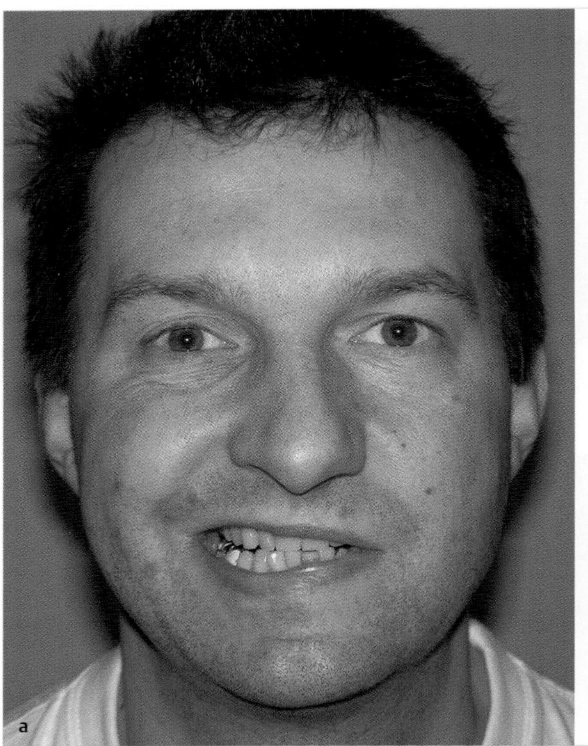

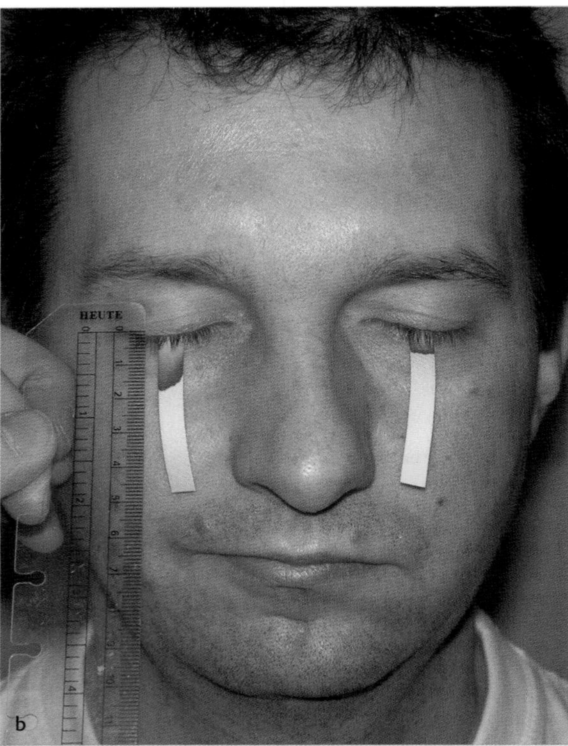

Fig. 4.11 Schirmer's test with pathological result. (**a**) Patient with incomplete facial palsy on the left side. (**b**) Decreased test function on the left side (< 15 mm after 5 min) indicating decreased tearing function.

> **!**
>
> Only a normal stapedial reflex is of (positive) prognostic value. The absence of the reflex and all other topodiagnostic tests have no prognostic value.

4.4.2 Other Hearing Tests and Balance Tests

Ear pain in acute facial palsy is mostly related to the involvement of somatosensory fibers of the facial nerve, but otoscopy as part of routine otorhinolaryngologic examination will help to rule out an otogenic cause of the facial palsy. The patient's history and symptoms will decide on the use of further hearing tests, and these may help to rule out a middle or inner ear disease when an abnormal stapedial reflex is found. Other hearing tests, such as brain stem evoked response audiometry, are of no topodiagnostic value but are part of the diagnostic work-up if a tumor, especially a vestibular schwannoma, has to be ruled out; see Chapter 18. Vestibular testing is indicated if the patient complains of dizziness. Vestibular tests including caloric testing have no topodiagnostic value but are standard in cases of vestibular schwannoma; see Chapter 18.

4.4.3 Schirmer's Test

Schirmer's test is carried out using 30 mm Schirmer's test strips, which are thin strips of filter paper with a notch to mark where the strip should be bent (▶ Fig. 4.11). The test is normally performed bilaterally. Before placement of the strips, excess tears should be dried gently with an absorbent tissue. The short end of the strip is placed between the eyelid and the eyeball, in the lateral third of the eyelid. The long end is placed hanging over the eyelashes. After 5 minutes, the distance in millimeters from the notch to the furthest point of wetting is measured. There are two variations in the test. First, it can be performed without local anesthetic drops, measuring both basal and reflex tearing: > 15 mm at 5 minutes is normal. Second, proxymetacaine eye drops can be instilled beforehand, measuring only basal tearing: > 10 mm at 5 minutes is normal.

Decreased tearing on the involved side may be due to lacrimal denervation. But Schirmer's test might be false positive if inflammation of the eye has led to massive tearing, if a paralytic ectropion with outward displacement of the inferior lacrimal puncta has led to collection of tears, or if the patient complains of excessive tearing because of defective healing with crocodile tears.

> !
>
> Schirmer's test can be false positive due to inflammation of the eye or dysfunction of the tear outflow.

4.4.4 Taste Test

The afferent fibers for taste function of the taste papillae of the anterior two-thirds of the tongue are carried through the chorda tympani nerve. Taste papillae atrophy can be seen using a binocular microscope within 5 to 10 days after a lesion of the chorda. Furthermore, the patient reports unilateral taste dysfunction or loss. Standard taste tests or electrogustometry can document the taste dysfunction but testing has no prognostic value. Furthermore, taste dysfunction can disappear in patients with chronic facial palsy, probably because of partial adaptation via the contralateral side.

4.5 Extended Diagnostics

4.5.1 Imaging

Due to their importance, imaging techniques for the facial nerve are described in detail in Chapter 5. Ultrasonography is the fastest, easiest, and cheapest method to complete the examination of the salivary glands to rule out a parotid tumor as reason for a facial palsy. CT and MRI are the preferential imaging modalities for examining the course of the facial nerve from the brainstem to the periphery.[30,31] CT is performed mainly for imaging of bony structures surrounding the facial nerve in the temporal bone, whereas MRI has a superior soft tissue contrast that enables imaging of the facial nerve itself. Replacement of the hyperintense fat tissue by hypointense soft tissue could be the first sign of perineural tumor spread on nonenhanced T1-weighted MRI. Even MRI has its limitations in evaluating very small perineural tumors causing facial palsy.[32] Notably, the facial plexus in the parotid gland is not imaged reliably with MRI, even after gadolinium administration.[33] MRI is optimal in detecting facial schwannomas, even those that are very small; see Chapter 18. Schwannomas show strong enhancement on T1-weighted images after gadolinium administration and are hypodense on T2-weighted images.[33] Three-dimensional T2-weighted fast spin-echo imaging allows identification of the facial nerve and its position relative to adjacent vestibular schwannomas larger than 25 mm.[34] MRI and CT can also show denervation changes such as muscle atrophy, leading to asymmetric facial muscles. Asymmetry on preoperative MRI might be a sensitive predictor of perineural invasion and could precede clinical facial palsy. Moreover, pronounced asymmetry on MRI is predictive of poor facial function after nerve grafting.[35] Recently, it has been shown that use of ultrasonography is feasible for very sensitive detection of facial muscle atrophy after a degenerative facial nerve lesion.[36] Furthermore, ultrasonography might help to discriminate between developmental and birth trauma facial palsy, as in the latter the images will show facial muscle whereas in congenital cases the muscles can be absent.

4.5.2 Electrodiagnostics

Various important electrophysiologic tests have been developed to classify the severity of nerve damage in patients with facial palsy. These methods are presented in detail in Chapter 6. Most important are electroneurography (ENoG) and electromyography (EMG). EMG with bipolar needle electrodes inserted directly into facial muscles is the mainstay for prognostic testing of facial nerve degeneration and regeneration. EMG is valuable in the assessment of signs of nerve degeneration beginning 14 days after onset of the nerve injury (such as the result of tumor infiltration), because Wallerian degeneration takes this long to reach the facial muscles. Typical spontaneous activities seen during needle EMG that indicate muscle denervation are positive sharp waves and fibrillation potentials. These abnormal spontaneous activities can sometimes be detected in patients with parotid cancer without any clinical sign of facial weakness. In such a case, the patient should be counseled about a higher probability that the facial nerve may be invaded and might require resection at least partially during surgery, although preoperative nerve function appears normal clinically. Vice versa, abnormal spontaneous activity for longer than 6 months in patients with facial palsy could be a sign of malignant tumor infiltration and the patient should undergo surgical exploration of the parotid gland and facial nerve, even if MRI or other imaging studies show no tumor lesion (▶ Fig. 4.12, ▶ Fig. 4.13, and ▶ Fig. 4.14).[32] EMG also assists in decision making concerning the optimal management of long-standing facial paralysis; see Chapter 19 and Chapter 20. First, the absence of insertional activity indicates massive muscle atrophy or could confirm the absence of any musculature, such as in patients with Möbius syndrome. Of course, nerve repair is not indicated in such cases. Second, the presence of muscle action potentials indicate that at least some axons are intact (i.e., nerve injury is incomplete). If the surgeon favors nerve repair, it has to be weighed against whether the result would be better than the actual status. Moreover, EMG should be used to monitor recovery after nerve repair because it anticipates clinical functions: depending on the type of nerve repair, regeneration potentials can be detected 4 to 6 months

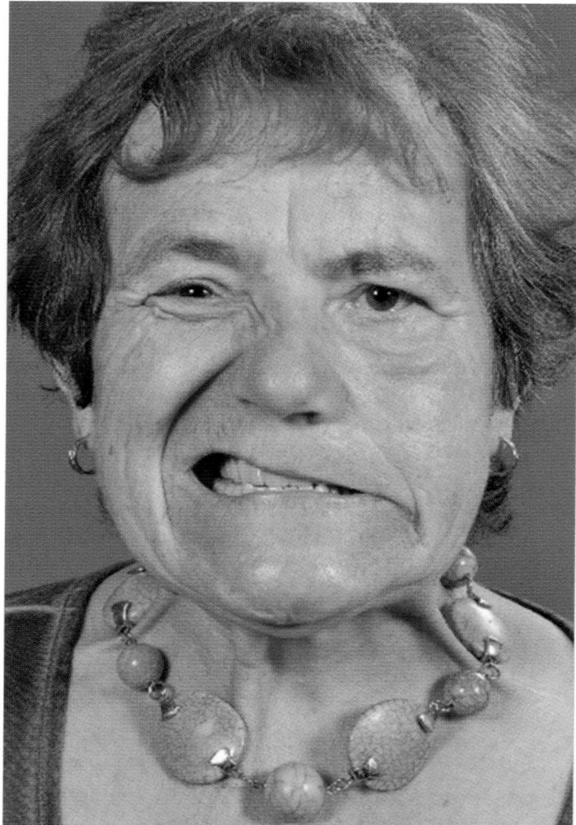

Fig. 4.12 Occult parotid adenoid cystic carcinoma with facial palsy. Persistent facial palsy on the left side without signs of regeneration over a year.

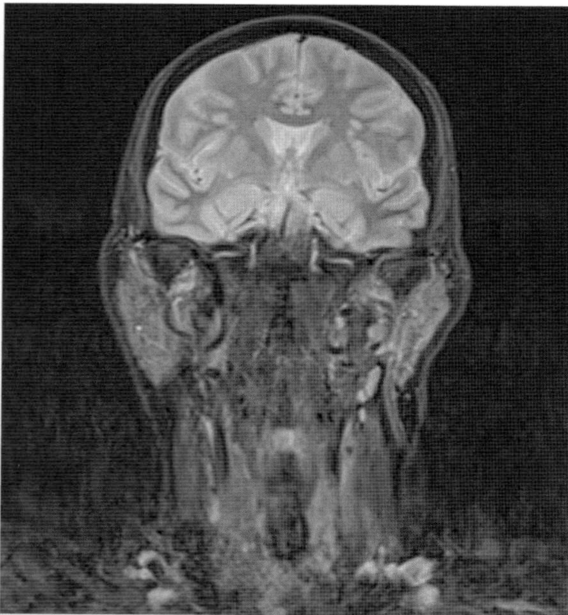

Fig. 4.13 Same patient as shown in ▶ Fig. 4.12. Repeated MRI without signs of a parotid tumor.

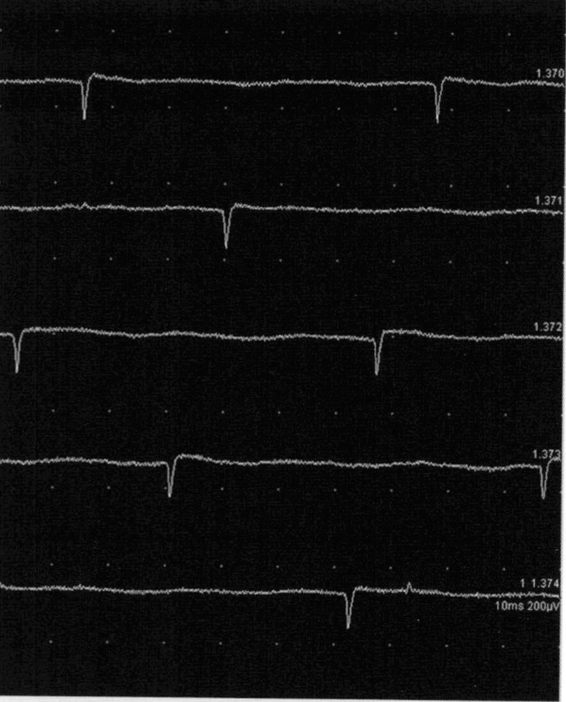

Fig. 4.14 Same patient as shown in ▶ Fig. 4.12 and ▶ Fig. 4.13. Needle EMG showed persistent pathologic fibrillation. Therefore, the extratemporal facial nerve was explored and a 0.5 cm adenoid cystic carcinoma was detected at the stylomastoid foramen with perineural infiltration of the facial nerve.

postoperatively. At this time, the patient will not show clinical movement. If no regeneration potentials are detected after 9 to 12 months postoperatively, the nerve repair has failed and a decision about other reanimation surgery has to be made.

4.5.3 Psychological Exploration

Acute and especially chronic facial palsy can have a major impact on the emotional and mental state of the patient. Patients with facial palsy might suffer from depression and increased anxiety. Their quality of life is reduced and they report social isolation and withdrawal. Social and emotional interactions are impeded. How such symptoms are detected and which patients might need a further exploration by a psychologist or a psychotherapist is described in Chapter 13.

4.6 Follow-up

Ideally, a special consultation hour is provided for new patients with facial palsy. This helps to bring in line follow-up visits with electrodiagnostic examinations, imaging, and other special diagnostics needed to follow-up patients with facial palsy (▶ Fig. 4.15). At the appropriate time, specialized physiotherapists can see the patient and treatment plans can be discussed. A patient with acute facial palsy should be monitored until full recovery or until recovery with defective healing stabilizes. An idiopathic palsy always shows nerve regeneration, whether with (in most cases) full recovery or not. If such a patient shows no signs of recovery, the diagnosis of idiopathic palsy has to be questioned. Furthermore, if a patient with acute palsy presents for evaluation within the first 2 weeks after onset, this might be too early to give a prognosis as to the probability of full recovery. Electrodiagnostics typically starts with ENoG during the first 10 days, as EMG will not give a reliable prognosis until 10 to 14 days after onset in many cases; see Chapter 6. Furthermore, repeat diagnostics, especially electrodiagnostics, during the follow-up help to confirm to initial diagnosis. After reconstructive surgery, particularly after facial nerve reconstruction surgery, regular follow-up visits help to support the patients during the phase until first signs of muscle recovery take place. For psychological reasons and to confirm the technical success of facial nerve surgery, electrodiagnostics normally show first signs of regeneration about 6 to 9 months after surgery, whereas clinical regeneration by muscle movement normally cannot be seen before 12 to 15 months after surgery; see Chapter 20.

!

A patient with acute facial palsy should be observed until full recovery or until recovery with defective healing shows no more changes.

4.7 Key Points

- Although idiopathic palsy is a common diagnosis, not all acute palsies are idiopathic (Bell's) palsies. An idiopathic palsy is still a diagnosis of exclusion.
- The clinical examination of the patient includes a physical, an otorhinolaryngologic, and a gross neurologic examination. Normally, electrodiagnostics are part of the standard examination. Depending on the initial results, extended diagnostic tests, including imaging studies and a variety of special diagnostics, might be necessary.

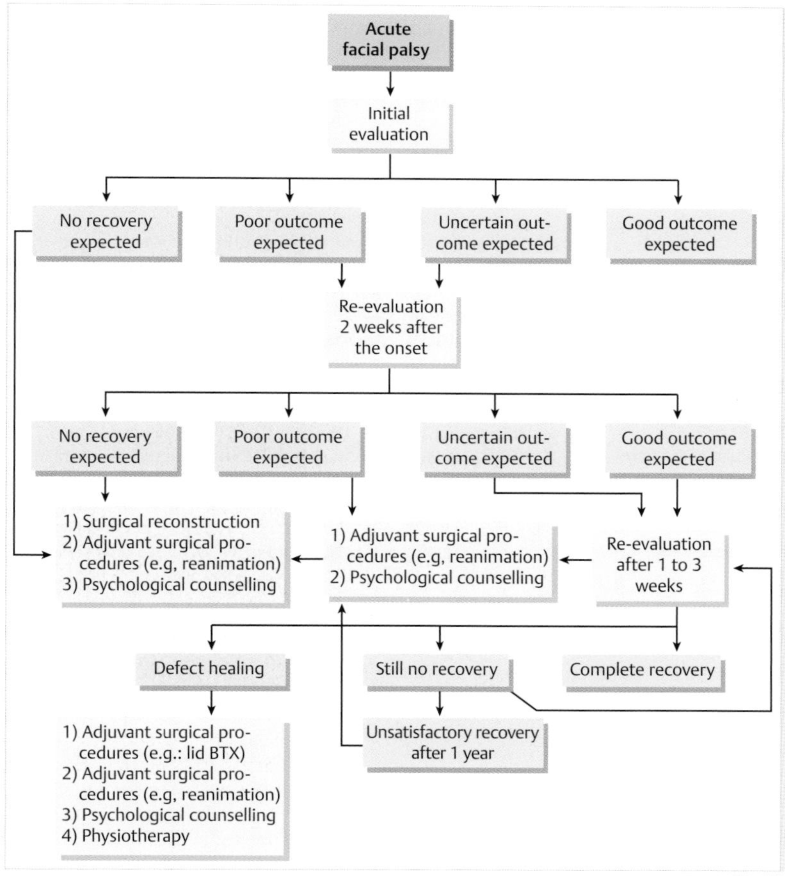

Fig. 4.15 Algorithm showing an idealized course of follow-up examinations for patients initially presenting with acute facial palsy. BTX, botulinum toxin.

- Now that we have computed tomography and magnetic resonance imaging diagnostics, the so-called topodiagnostic tests are more of historical interest.
- To treat patients with facial palsy requires observation of patients with acute palsy until a diagnosis is made, treatment is initiated, and recovery is complete. Patients with chronic facial palsy are often followed-up for life.

References

[1] Cawthorne T. Bell's palsies. Ann Otol Rhinol Laryngol 1963; 72: 774–779

[2] Critchlow WA, Chang D. Cheilitis granulomatosa: a review. Head Neck Pathol 2014; 8: 209–213

[3] Rivera-Serrano CM, Man LX, Klein S, Schaitkin BM. Melkersson-Rosenthal syndrome: a facial nerve center perspective. J Plast Reconstr Aesthet Surg 2014; 67: 1050–1054

[4] Pitts DB, Adour KK, Hilsinger RL, Jr. Recurrent Bell's palsy: analysis of 140 patients. Laryngoscope 1988; 98: 535–540

[5] May M, Hardin WB, Jr. Facial palsy: interpretation of neurologic findings. Trans Sect Otolaryngol Am Acad Ophthalmol Otolaryngol 1977; 84: ORL-710–ORL-722

[6] Desai SV, Law TJ, Needham DM. Long-term complications of critical care. Crit Care Med 2011; 39: 371–379

[7] D'Amore A, Viglianesi A, Cavallaro T et al. Guillain-Barré syndrome associated with acute onset bilateral facial nerve palsies. A case report and literature review. Neuroradiol J 2012; 25: 665–670

[8] Cornblath DR, Hughes RA. Treatment for Guillain-Barré syndrome. Ann Neurol 2009; 66: 569–570

[9] Kim YH, Choi IJ, Kim HM, Ban JH, Cho CH, Ahn JH. Bilateral simultaneous facial nerve palsy: clinical analysis in seven cases. Otol Neurotol 2008; 29: 397–400

[10] Kaygusuz I, Gödekmerdan A, Keleş E et al. The role of viruses in idiopathic peripheral facial palsy and cellular immune response. Am J Otolaryngol 2004; 25: 401–406

[11] Vargas DL, Stern BJ. Neurosarcoidosis: diagnosis and management. Semin Respir Crit Care Med 2010; 31: 419–427

[12] Tracy JA, Dyck PJ. Porphyria and its neurologic manifestations. Handb Clin Neurol 2014; 120: 839–849

[13] Lüttmann RJ, Teismann I, Husstedt IW, Ringelstein EB, Kuhlenbäumer G. Hereditary amyloidosis of the Finnish type in a German family: clinical and electrophysiological presentation. Muscle Nerve 2010; 41: 679–684

[14] Waterval JJ, Borra VM, Van Hul W et al. Sclerosing bone dysplasias with involvement of the craniofacial skeleton. Bone 2014; 60: 48–67

[15] Preuss SF, Veelken F, Galldiks N et al. A rare differential diagnosis in dysphagia: wound botulism. Laryngoscope 2006; 116: 831–832

[16] Ho K, Melanson M, Desai JA. Bell palsy in Lyme disease-endemic regions of Canada: a cautionary case of occult bilateral peripheral facial nerve palsy due to Lyme disease. CJEM 2012; 14: 321–324

[17] Krejcova H, Bojar M, Jerabek J, Tomas J, Jirous J. Otoneurological symptomatology in Lyme disease. Adv Otorhinolaryngol 1988; 42: 210–212

[18] Zaidi FH, Gregory-Evans K, Acheson JF, Ferguson V. Familial Bell's palsy in females: a phenotype with a predilection for eyelids and lacrimal gland. Orbit 2005; 24: 121–124

[19] Guntinas-Lichius O. Facial paralysis. In: Lang F, ed. Encyclopedia of Molecular Mechanisms of Disease. Stuttgart: Springer; 2009

[20] Michielse CB, Bhat M, Brady A et al. Refinement of the locus for hereditary congenital facial palsy on chromosome 3q21 in two unrelated families and screening of positional candidate genes. Eur J Hum Genet 2006; 14: 1306–1312

[21] Yanagihara N, Yumoto E, Shibahara T. Familial Bell's palsy: analysis of 25 families. Ann Otol Rhinol Laryngol Suppl 1988; 137: 8–10

[22] Couch RB. Nasal vaccination, Escherichia coli enterotoxin, and Bell's palsy. N Engl J Med 2004; 350: 860–861

[23] Vrabec JT, Isaacson B, Van Hook JW. Bell's palsy and pregnancy. Otolaryngol Head Neck Surg 2007; 137: 858–861

[24] Katz A, Sergienko R, Dior U, Wiznitzer A, Kaplan DM, Sheiner E. Bell's palsy during pregnancy: is it associated with adverse perinatal outcome? Laryngoscope 2011; 121: 1395–1398

[25] Jörg R, Milani GP, Simonetti GD, Bianchetti MG, Simonetti BG. Peripheral facial nerve palsy in severe systemic hypertension: a systematic review. Am J Hypertens 2013; 26: 351–356

[26] Vauzelle C, Beghin D, Cournot MP, Elefant E. Birth defects after exposure to misoprostol in the first trimester of pregnancy: prospective follow-up study. Reprod Toxicol 2013; 36: 98–103

[27] Rowhani-Rahbar A, Klein NP, Lewis N et al. Immunization and Bell's palsy in children: a case-centered analysis. Am J Epidemiol 2012; 175: 878–885

[28] Schaitkin BM, May M, Klein SR, et al. Topognostic, otovestibular, and electrical testing: diagnosis and prognosis. In: May M, Schaitkin BM, eds. The Facial Nerve. New York: Thieme; 2000:213–230

[29] Volk GF, Klingner C, Finkensieper M, Witte OW, Guntinas-Lichius O. Prognostication of recovery time after acute peripheral facial palsy: a prospective cohort study. BMJ Open 2013; 3: 3

[30] Phillips CD, Bubash LA. The facial nerve: anatomy and common pathology. Semin Ultrasound CT MR 2002; 23: 202–217

[31] Burmeister HP, Baltzer PA, Dietzel M et al. Identification of the nervus intermedius using 3 T MR imaging. AJNR Am J Neuroradiol 2011; 32: 460–464

[32] Jungehuelsing M, Sittel C, Fischbach R, Wagner M, Stennert E. Limitations of magnetic resonance imaging in the evaluation of perineural tumor spread causing facial nerve paralysis. Arch Otolaryngol Head Neck Surg 2000; 126: 506–510

[33] Jäger L, Reiser M. CT and MR imaging of the normal and pathologic conditions of the facial nerve. Eur J Radiol 2001; 40: 133–146

[34] Sartoretti-Schefer S, Kollias S, Valavanis A. Spatial relationship between vestibular schwannoma and facial nerve on three-dimensional T2-weighted fast spin-echo MR images. AJNR Am J Neuroradiol 2000; 21: 810–816

[35] Kaylie DM, Wax MK, Weissman JL. Preoperative facial muscle imaging predicts final facial function after facial nerve grafting. AJNR Am J Neuroradiol 2003; 24: 326–330

[36] Volk GF, Pohlmann M, Sauer M et al. Quantitative ultrasonography of facial muscles in patients with chronic facial palsy. Muscle Nerve 2014; 50: 358–365

[37] Schaitkin BM, May M, Klein SR. Office evaluation of the patient with facial paralysis. In: May M, Schaitkin BM, eds. The Facial Nerve. New York: Thieme; 2000

5 Imaging

Gerd Fabian Volk, Hartmut Peter Burmeister, and Orlando Guntinas-Lichius

5.1 Introduction

After the clinical examination, as described in Chapter 4, imaging is one of the most important diagnostic tools in patients with facial nerve diseases. The most important imaging methods are magnetic resonance imaging (MRI), computed tomography (CT), and ultrasonography (US).[1,2] The facial motor nerve has a very complex topographical course from its nucleus within the brainstem, through the temporal bone, and finally to its peripheral branches ending in the mimic muscles. Furthermore, the facial motor nerve is partly accompanied by parasympathetic, sensory, and taste nerve fibers; see Chapter 1. Ideally, imaging should detect the complete course of the facial nerve and should be able to differentiate the four nerve fiber qualities. In addition, imaging should, if possible, be able to differentiate congenital, infectious, traumatic, and neoplastic etiologies leading to facial nerve disorders. So far, there is no single imaging method fulfilling all these criteria.[3] MRI is the best method to identify soft tissue changes around and in the facial nerve. CT is performed mainly for imaging of bony structures surrounding the facial nerve in the temporal bone. Until recently, US was of interest only for the examination of the parotid gland to rule out a parotid tumor as reason for a peripheral facial nerve lesion. However, in 2013 it was shown that US is very sensitive at detecting facial muscle atrophy after a degenerative facial nerve lesion.[4] Hence, US might become an interesting tool to extend the diagnostic possibilities of facial nerve imaging. This new method is presented here in detail.

5.2 Indications for Imaging Studies

The facial nerve and the mimic muscles can be affected by a large number of different diseases all resulting in the same symptom: paresis, paralysis, and/or abnormal movement of the mimic muscles. The primary role of the clinical examination including patient's history is to set limits on the differential diagnosis. In many cases, the diagnosis can be made without any imaging studies; see Chapter 4. The etiology of the most frequent facial nerve disorders and comments on typical signs on imaging studies are presented in ▶ Table 5.1. As a rule of thumb, imaging planning can also be tailored to the suspected localization of the facial nerve lesion. The facial nerve nucleus and the cisternal and intracanalicular segments are best evaluated by contrast-enhanced MRI. All the intratemporal segments (the labyrinthine, tympanic, and mastoid segments) are evaluated by CT and MRI. The extratemporal course of the nerve is best examined by MRI. If the localization of the disease remains unclear, contrast-enhanced MRI is the first choice. Both MRI and CT are typically performed for malignant tumor staging related to the facial nerve. Evaluation of the facial muscles is performed by US or less frequently by MRI. A significant decrease in muscle size can be detected as soon as 1 to 2 months after complete facial muscle denervation induced by facial nerve lesion or by botulinum toxin injection.[5–7] MRI or US facial muscle studies can be used to monitor the facial muscle growth after reinnervation of the facial muscles, for instance after placement of a facial nerve graft.[6]

> **!**
>
> The most important imaging techniques are magnetic resonance imaging (MRI) and computed tomography (CT). MRI is the best method to identify soft tissue changes around and in the facial nerve. CT is performed mainly for imaging of bony structures surrounding the facial nerve in the temporal bone.

5.3 Magnetic Resonance Imaging

The method of choice to depict the typical course of the facial nerve within the brainstem with its first genu (medullary segment) is MRI. With MRI, the facial nerve is also identified in the cerebellopontine angle (CPA) anterior to the vestibulocochlear nerve within the CPA cistern. The intermediate nerve cannot always be separately resolved from the facial motor nerve with standard MRI at a field strength of 1.5 Tesla (T). Nowadays, high-resolution 3T-MRI of the skull base and the brainstem/CPA allows reliable depiction of the intermediate nerve in most cases (▶ Fig. 5.1).[8] MRI shows that both nerves, and the vestibulocochlear nerve, are covered by a common dural sheath.[9] The normal facial nerve appears as a hypointense linear structure in T2-weighted images or constructive interference in steady state (CISS) images, surrounded by T2-weighted hyperintense cerebrospinal fluid.

The labyrinthine, tympanic, and mastoid segments of the facial nerve are not well visualized in noncontrast T1-weighted images. The proximal extratemporal portion of the facial nerve in the parotid gland is best visualized with axial high-resolution T1-weighted images using a microscopic coil.[2] When performing MRI acquiring

Table 5.1 Frequent facial nerve disorders and indications for imaging studies

Category	Disease	Comment
Idiopathic; see Chapter 8	Bell's palsy	MRI of the brain and brainstem with gadolinium contrast demonstrates abnormal enhancement of the intracanalicular, labyrinthine, tympanic and mastoid segments and asymmetric enhancement of the tympanic and mastoid segments of the nerve. Reconsider MRI imaging if Bell's palsy does not show any signs of recovery or defective healing within 4 months, especially when initially (as it is the case in most cases of Bell's palsy) no MRI imaging was performed
Inflammatory; see Chapter 17	Sarcoidosis Guillain–Barré syndrome Multiple sclerosis	MRI with gadolinium enhancement shows abnormal enhancement of the facial nerve typically with involvement of other cranial nerves and parts of the brain
Infectious; see Chapter 10, Chapter 11, Chapter 12, Chapter 17	Acute or chronic otitis media	High-resolution CT is helpful to detect dehiscences of the fallopian canal related to acute or chronic otitis media. Extension of the infection into the brain can be depicted by enhanced CT or MRI with gadolinium enhancement
	Lyme disease[35]	MRI with gadolinium can be normal or may show bilateral enhancement of the facial nerves in Lyme disease
	Ramsey Hunt syndrome	MRI with gadolinium typically shows facial and trigeminal nerve enhancement
Traumatic; see Chapter 9	Temporal bone fracture	Fractures are best visualized on noncontrast high-resolution CT
Congenital; see Chapter 12	Congenital malformation/absence of the facial nerve/facial muscles[15] • Möbius syndrome • CHARGE syndrome • Aural atresia	Bony dehiscences and displacements of the bony facial canal are visualized with high-resolution CT. Hypoplasia or aplasia of the facial nerve is confirmed by MRI. Absence of facial muscles is best shown by US or by MRI
Vascular/central; see Chapter 27	Stroke, Brain tumor Multiple sclerosis[36]	Pathologies are best visualized on MRI
Neoplastic; see Chapter 16, Chapter 18, and Chapter 19	Vestibular schwannoma[37]	MRI is method of choice for initial diagnosis and follow-up. Treatment planning may benefit from additional CT images. US or MRI are helpful to estimate the degree of atrophy of facial muscle in patients with chronic palsy after vestibular schwannoma surgery
	Hemangioma[38]	Temporal bone CT shows mineralization of ossifying hemangiomas. MRI better reveals the number of involved facial nerve segments
	Paraganglioma	Treatment planning needs MRI and CT
	Malignant tumor	MRI is first method of choice. MRI with gadolinium is necessary for detecting perineural spread along the facial nerve. CT shows bony erosions of intratemporal tumors
Other	Hemifacial spasm	MRI can identify vessel loops compressing the facial nerve in the root exit zone of the cerebellopontine angle

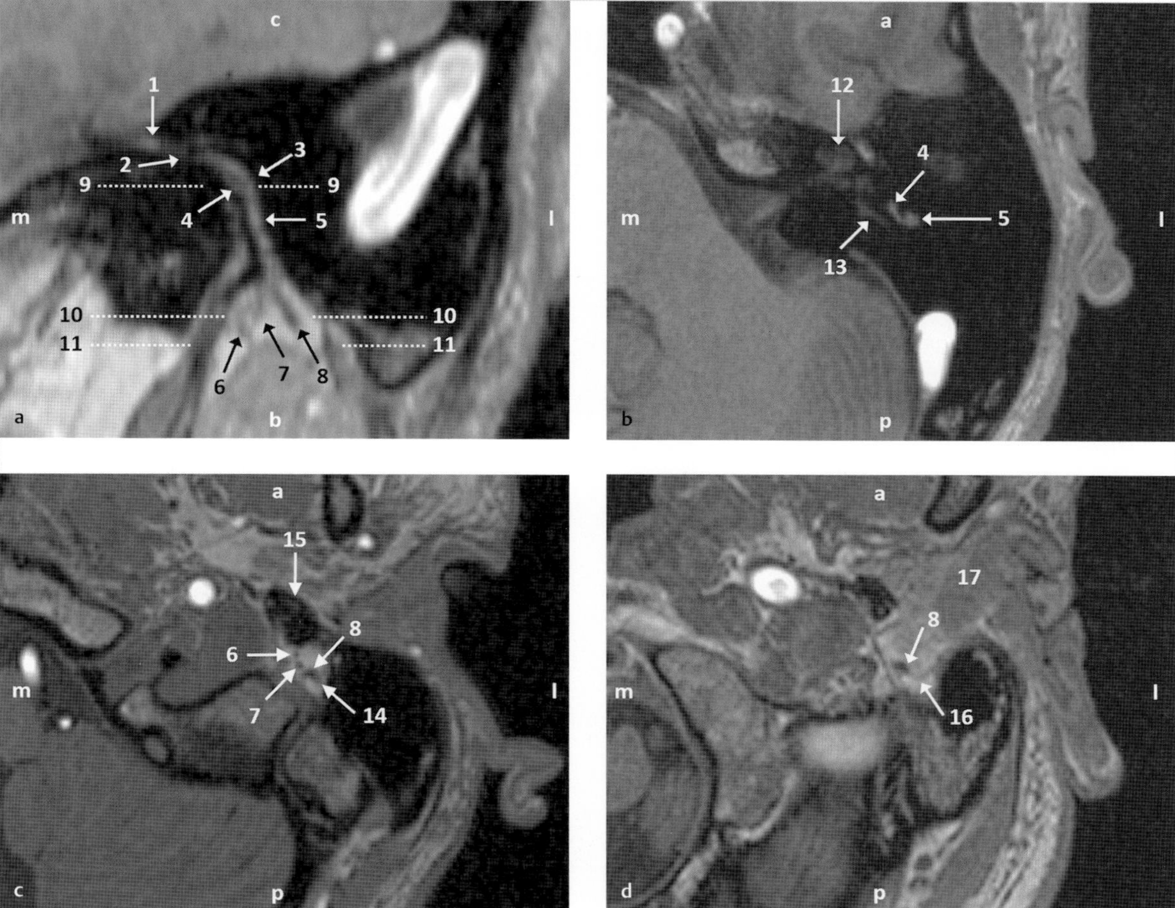

Fig. 5.1 High-resolution 3 Tesla MRI of small facial nerve branches using T1-weighted sequences. m, medial; l, lateral; c, cranial; b, basal; a, anterior; p, posterior.
(a) Parasagittal plane. 1, Geniculate ganglion; 2, tympanic segment 3, petrosal segment; 4, stapedial nerve; 5, mastoid segment; 6, stylohyoid branch; 7, digastric branch; 8, main trunk of the facial nerve; 9, sectional plane of axial image **(b)**; 10, sectional plane of axial image **(c)** in the stylomastoid foramen; 11, sectional plane of axial image **(d)** below the stylomastoid foramen. **(b)** Axial plane (sectional plane no. 9). 4, Stapedial nerve; 5, mastoid segment; 12, cochlea; 13, posterior semicircular canal. **(c)** Axial plane (sectional plane no. 10). 6, Stylohyoid branch; 7, digastric branch; 8, main trunk of the facial nerve; 14, stylomastoid foramen; 15, stylomastoid process. **(d)** Axial plane (sectional plane no. 11). 8, Main trunk of the facial nerve; 16, posterior auricular branch; 17, parotid gland.

gadolinium contrast-enhanced T1-weighted images, the normal facial nerve typically enhances slightly in the geniculate ganglion, tympanic, and mastoid segments.[10] In contrast, the cisternal, intracanalicular, and labyrinthine segments, and extratemporal portion of the facial nerve normally do not show such enhancement. Enhancement of the facial nerve in these segments and portions raises suspicion of inflammatory or neoplastic processes. Furthermore, asymmetric enhancement and/or thickening of the tympanic mastoid segments relative to the contralateral side should also be considered abnormal.[2] In Bell's palsy, such an enhancement of the intracanalicular, labyrinthine, geniculate ganglion, and tympanic and/or mastoid segments is often seen but has no prognostic value (▶ Fig. 5.2 and ▶ Fig. 5.3).[11] Not only CT but also MRI, especially high-resolution 3T-MRI with contrast enhancement, can depict the intratemporal segments of the facial nerve and even small branches such as the stapedial nerve, the posterior auricular branch, the digastric branch, and stylohyoid branch (see ▶ Fig. 5.1).[12]

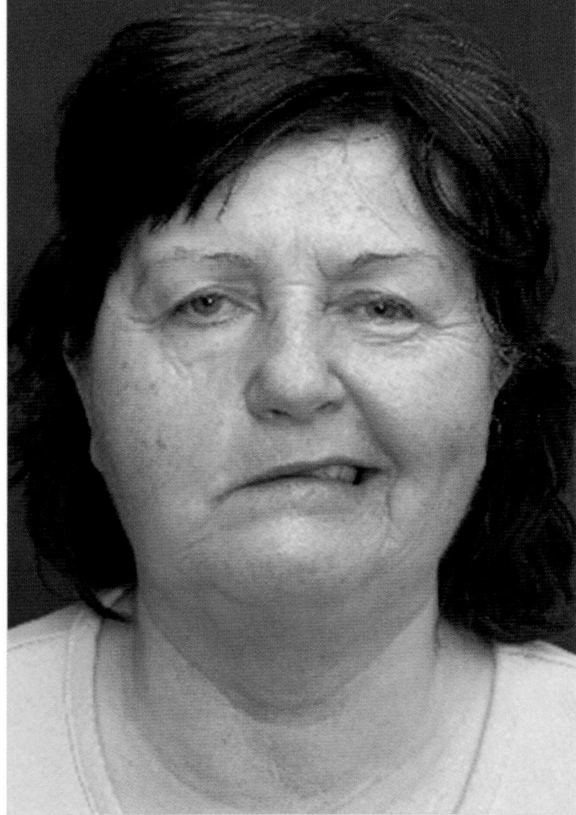

Fig. 5.2 A 66-year-old patient with incomplete Bell's palsy on the right side.

> **!**
>
> Magnetic resonance imaging (MRI) is the optimal method to distinguish the facial nerve from the other nerves in the cerebellopontine angle (CPA). Nevertheless, in large CPA tumors, for instance, a clear distinction is not always possible.

As in Bell's palsy, other inflammatory or infectious processes of or around the facial nerve can cause gadolinium enhancement in the affected nerve parts; these processes include sarcoidosis, multiple sclerosis, Lyme disease, and Ramsey Hunt syndrome. However, this enhancement is not specific for any disease and has, according to the current literature, no prognostic value.[13] It should be emphasized that it is the clinical presentation and eventually other diagnostic tools, and not normally the MRI, that establishes the correct diagnosis.

> **!**
>
> Any facial nerve enhancement on a magnetic resonance image with contrast (other than perineural invasion) is not diagnostic of any specific disease and has no prognostic value. It can help to localize a disease.

In contrast, in central facial palsy, as described in Chapter 27, MRI of the brain is the key diagnostic tool to define the affected brain region in patients with stroke or a brain tumor.[2] In patients with congenital facial palsy, MRI

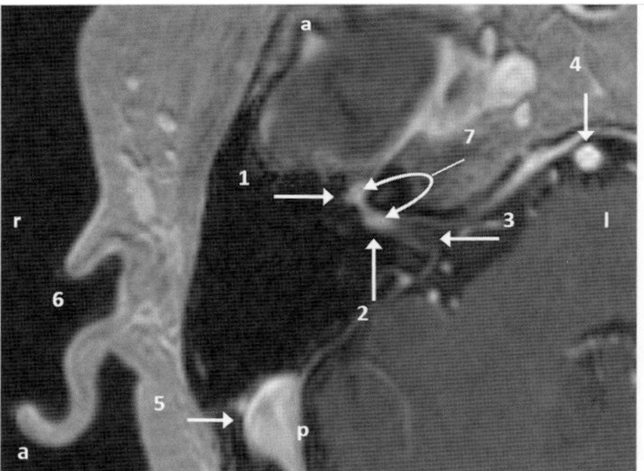

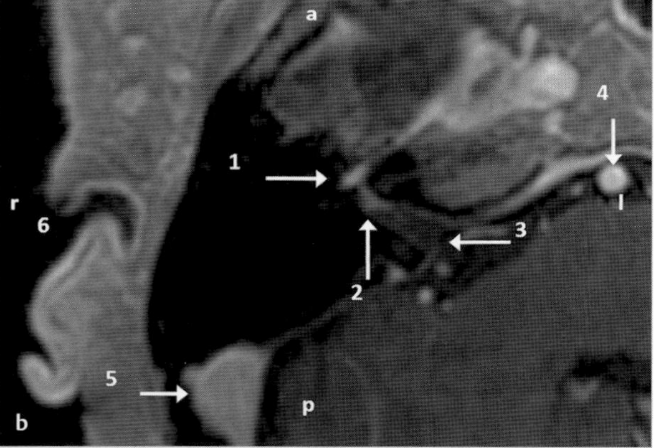

Fig. 5.3 High-resolution 3-Tesla MRI of the right petrous bone of the patient shown in ▶ Fig. 5.2; T1-weighted sequence after contrast media application, axial plane (slice thickness 0.6 mm). r, right; l, left; a, anterior; p, posterior. 1, Geniculate ganglion; 2, intrameatal segment; 3, inner auditory canal; 4, basilar artery; 5, sigmoid sinus; 6, auricle; 7, "bottleneck sign." **(a)** Initial MRI in the acute phase directly after symptom onset. The geniculate ganglion (1) and intrameatal segment (2) show strong enhancement. A typical "bottleneck sign" is visible in the acute phase. **(b)** Follow-up MRI 4 months later shows complete recovery. Geniculate ganglion (1) shows nearly complete physiologic enhancement and intrameatal segment (2) shows minimal residual pathologic enhancement.

can confirm hypoplasia, aplasia, or an abnormal course of the facial nerve (▶ Fig. 5.4, ▶ Fig. 5.5, and ▶ Fig. 5.6).[14,15] Therefore, a synopsis of MRI and CT is the standard imaging combination for defining extent of a vestibular schwannoma or neurofibroma (▶ Fig. 5.7, ▶ Fig. 5.8 and ▶ Fig. 5.9); see Chapter 18. If the vestibular schwannoma is very large, it might be difficult to distinguish the facial nerve from the schwannoma. In such a situation MRI three-dimensional (3D) modeling from diffusion tension tractography for 3D visualization of the facial nerve might

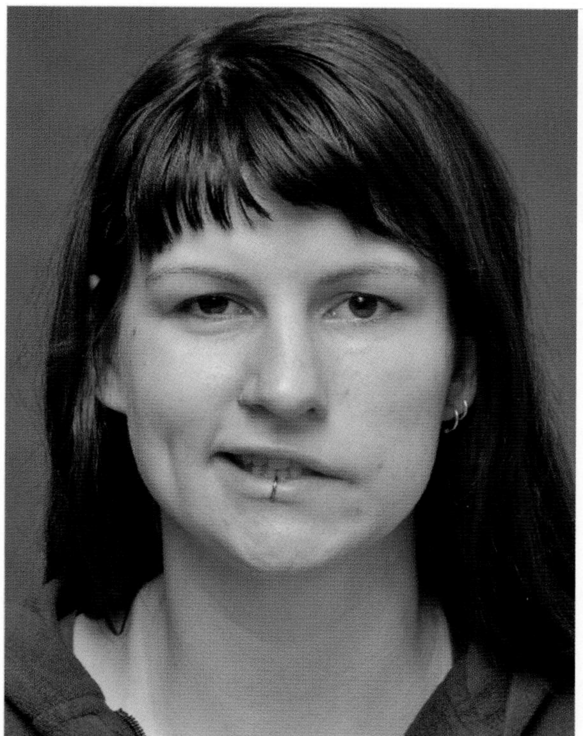

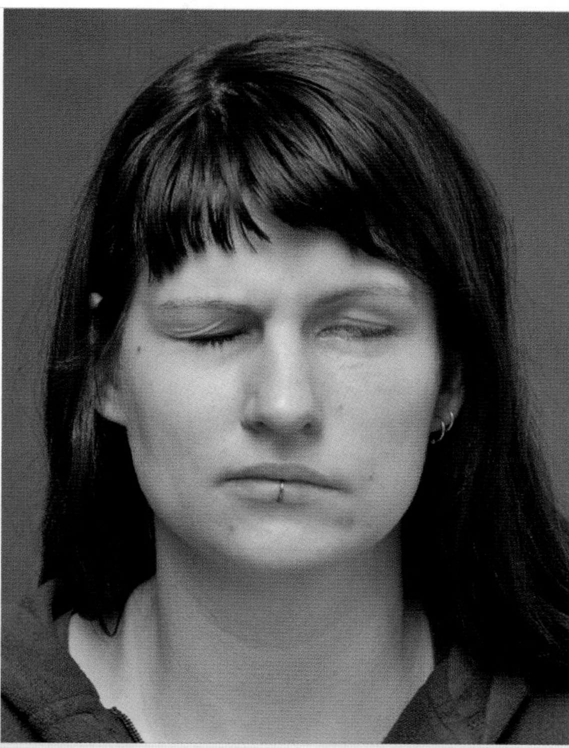

Fig. 5.4 A 29-year-old patient with congenital incomplete facial palsy on the left side and optic nerve atrophy on the left side. (**a**) Showing the teeth. (**b**) Closing the eyes.

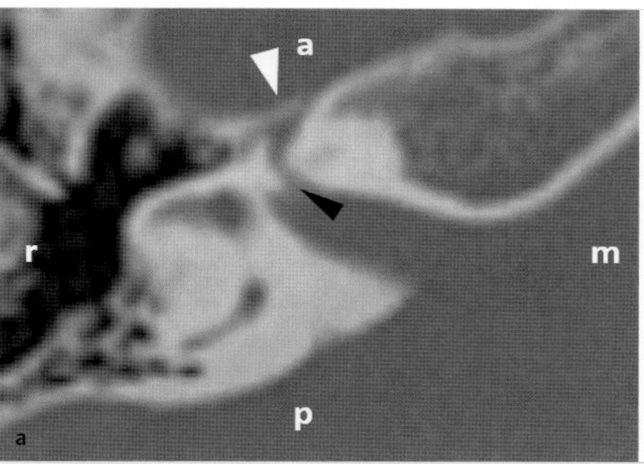

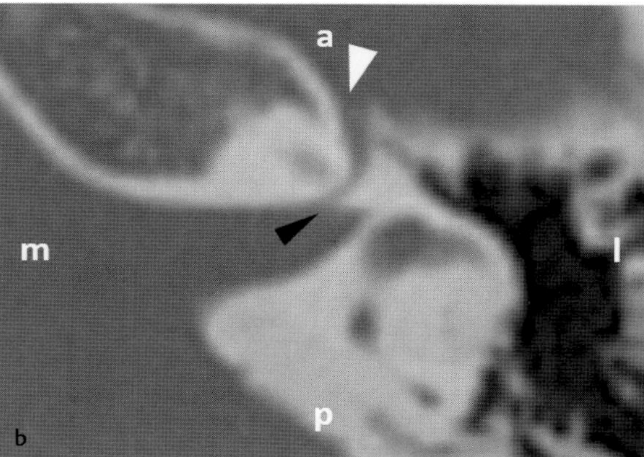

Fig. 5.5 (a,b) High-resolution CT of the petrous bone of the patient shown in ▶ Fig. 5.4, axial plane (slice thickness 1.0 mm). The caliber of both the right and the left internal auditory canal is regular. The caliber of the labyrinthine segment of the facial nerve canal on the left side seems hypoplastic compared with the right side (*black arrowheads*), whereas the fossa of the geniculate ganglion (*white arrowheads*) and the canal of the greater petrosal nerve on the left side appear larger compared with the right side. r, right; l, left; a, anterior; p, posterior; m, medial.

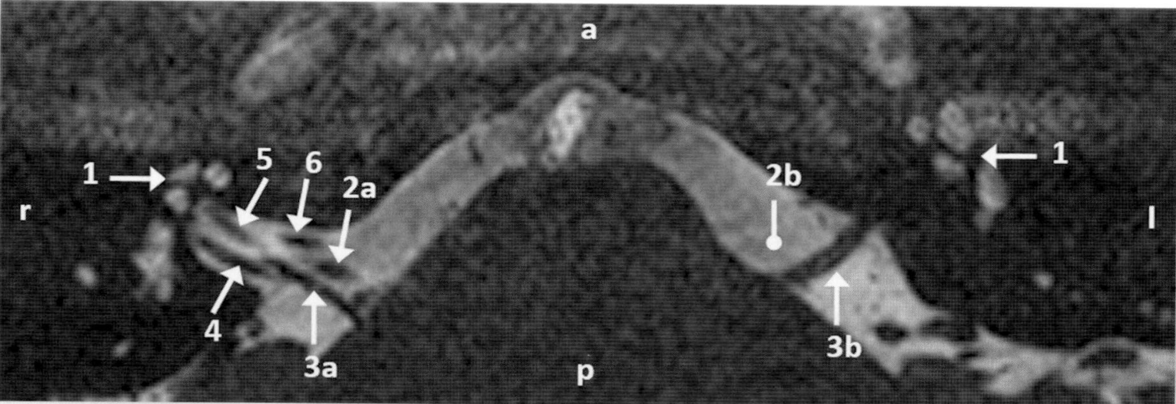

Fig. 5.6 A 3-Tesla MRI of the right petrous bone of the patient shown in ▶ Fig. 5.4, CISS, axial plane (slice thickness 0.4 mm). 1, Cochlea; 2, facial nerve with normal course and caliber on the right side (2a), missing facial nerve (2b) on the left side; 3, vestibulocochlear nerve on the right side (3a), the vestibulocochlear nerve (3b) on the left side appears to be a bit thickened; 4, vestibular nerve; 5, cochlear nerve; 6, branch of the anterior inferior cerebellar artery. r, right; l, left; a, anterior; p, posterior; m, medial.

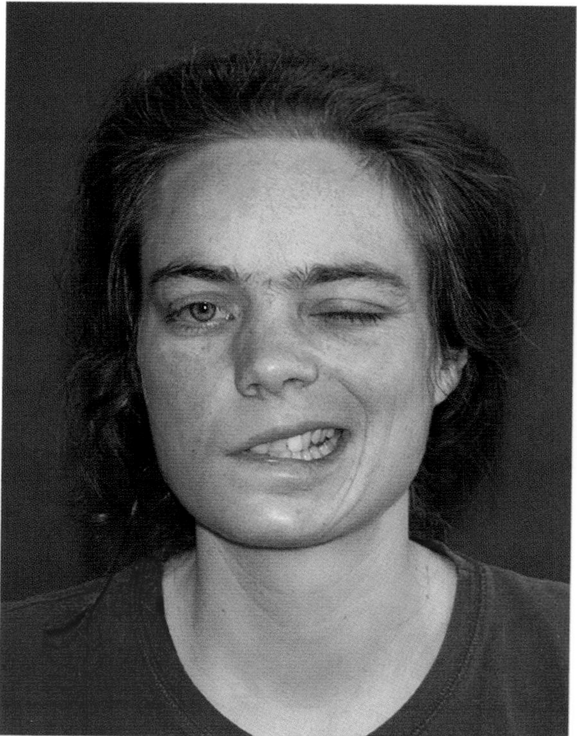

Fig. 5.7 A 36-year-old patient with neurofibroma of the greater petrosal nerve on the right side presenting with facial palsy as first clinical sign of the tumor.

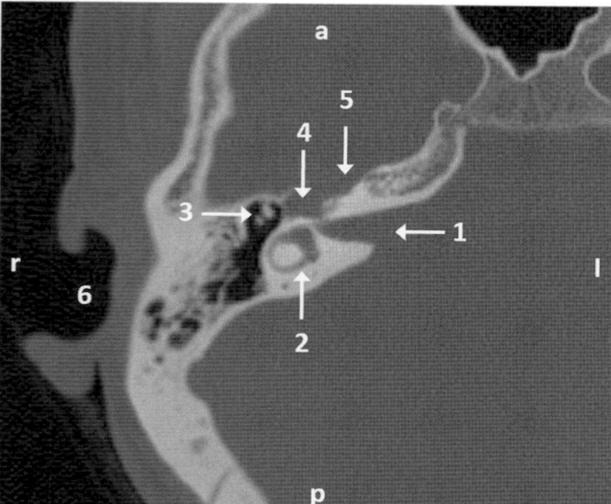

Fig. 5.8 High-resolution CT of the right petrous bone of the patient shown in ▶ Fig. 5.7, bone algorithm, axial plane (slice thickness 0.6 mm). 1, Internal auditory canal; 2, lateral semicircular canal; 3, cavum tympani/incudomalleolar joint; 4, dilatation of the fossa of the geniculate ganglion due to the expanding neurofibroma of the greater petrosal nerve; 5, erosion of the anterior surface of the petrous bone along the course of the greater petrosal nerve; 6, auricle. r, right; l, left; a, anterior; p, posterior; m, medial.

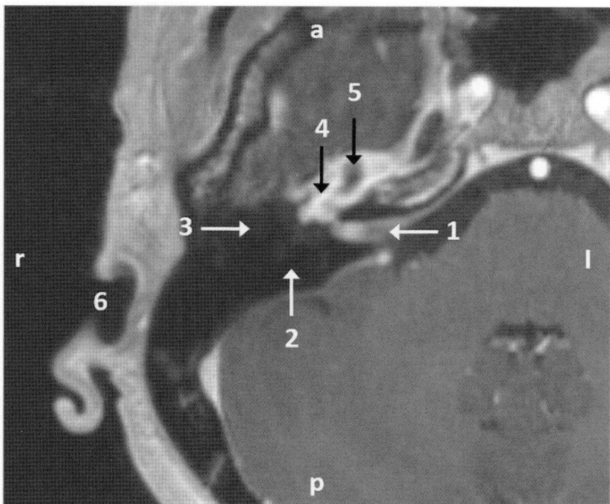

Fig. 5.9 A 3-Tesla MRI of the right petrous bone of the patient shown in ▶ Fig. 5.7, T1-weighted sequence after contrast media application, axial plane (slice thickness 0.6 mm). 1, Inner auditory canal with congestion-based enhancement of the venous plexus; 2, lateral semicircular canal; 3, cavum tympani; 4, dilatation of the fossa of the geniculate ganglion due to the expanding neurofibroma of the greater petrosal nerve with congestion-based venous enhancement and a small slightly enhancing neurofibroma mass; 5, erosion of the anterior surface of the petrous bone along the course of the greater petrosal nerve, with enhancing rim around the central non-enhancing neurofibroma mass; 6, auricle. r, right; l, left; a, anterior; p, posterior; m, medial.

be helpful.[16] Facial nerve schwannomas are much rarer but can be best detected by MRI and can occur anywhere along the facial nerve. MRI is also the first choice for malignant tumor diagnosis related to facial palsy. Nevertheless, a very small tumor presenting with facial palsy as first clinical sign can be undetectable by MRI and become obvious only by exploration (▶ Fig. 5.10 and ▶ Fig. 5.11). The most frequent site for a malignant tumor to affect the facial nerve is the extratemporal portion of the nerve affected by parotid neoplasms. MRI with gadolinium is also helpful to detect perineural spread along facial nerve branches.

Only a few studies have been published showing that the degree of mimic muscle atrophy can also be detected by MRI.[5,17–19] MRI also can be used for the monitoring of structural changes of the facial muscles after reconstructive surgery.[7,20]

5.4 Computed Tomography

CT is frequently used to image the course of the facial nerve canal within the temporal bone to the point of the stylomastoid foramen. CT does not allow imaging of the healthy facial nerve in the CPA and of the extratemporal course. If the intratemporal course of the facial nerve is of main interest, high-resolution temporal bone CT is recommended.[9,21] Temporal bone CT is a standard tool to evaluate the caliber in vestibular schwannomas in the CPA, in the porus acusticus, and in the internal auditory canal, and might be helpful to make a rough estimate of the course of the facial nerve (see ▶ Fig. 5.8); see Chapter 18. The intratemporal course of the facial nerve and the bony facial canal can be depicted in high-resolution CT. Here, CT allows an evaluation of the facial nerve and facial nerve canal erosion or destruction in patients with inflammation, trauma, or a tumor. CT shows the relation of the facial nerve canal to the ossicles and the oval window. This is also of interest in patients with chronic otitis media with cholesteatoma, or in those with congenital anomalies with facial palsy.[22]

In patients with a temporal bone fracture, CT is of great interest in planning treatment, and for forecasting prognosis of patients with facial palsy a classification of the type of fracture is of importance (▶ Fig. 5.12, ▶ Fig. 5.13, and ▶ Fig. 5.14).[23] Nowadays, most surgeons and radiologists prefer a classification that considers insults to the otic capsule instead of the petrous bone; see Chapter 9.[23,24] However, the fracture lines often do not appear in only one slice of the axial or coronal view, but take diverse directions through multiple CT slides. In such cases multiplanar reconstructive imaging of temporal bone CT is very helpful.[23] Three-dimensional CT reconstructions of the temporal bone also allow one to measure the diameters of the different intratemporal facial nerve segments with high precision. CT reconstructions show us that the narrowest point in the fallopian canal occurs in the transition from the internal auditory canal to the geniculate ganglion and it is this vulnerable spot that is felt to be most susceptible to the insult from Bell's palsy.[25]

!

High-resolution computed tomography (CT) is the first choice to detect intratemporal facial nerve canal erosion or destruction from inflammation, trauma or tumors. CT depicts well the relation of the facial nerve canal to any disease in the temporal bone.

CT is not the preferential method for an evaluation of the mimic muscles. There has been only one small case series published focusing on some exemplary facial muscles demonstrating that CT can show qualitatively the consequences of end-stage appearance of denervation, such as severe atrophy, asymmetrical facial muscle size, or fatty infiltration.[26] CT, like MRI, has the drawback that sectional

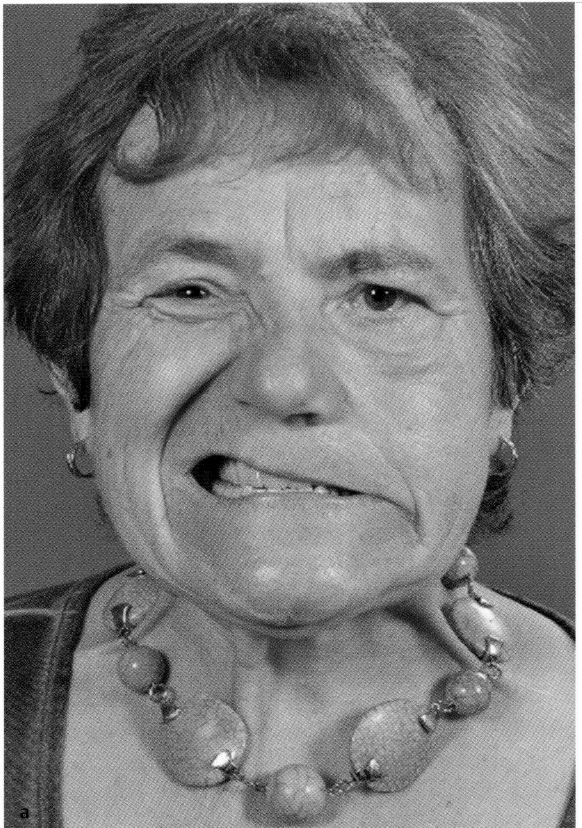

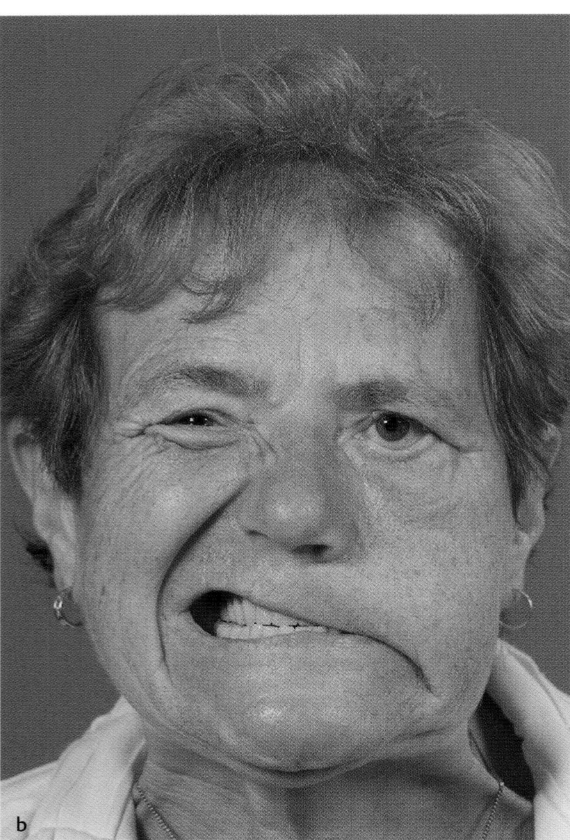

Fig. 5.10 A 67-year-old patient with facial palsy on the left side for 2 years. She was initially diagnosed with Bell's palsy and inconspicuous MRI. (**a**) Initial facial palsy. (**b**) Two years later prior to surgery, with no clinical signs of recovery. See MRI in Fig 5.11.

planes often do not correspond to the axial symmetry of the face. Furthermore, when repeated investigations of the facial muscles in a single patient is planned, the radiation exposure and the high organizational and financial effort are important drawbacks in comparison with facial US.

5.5 Ultrasonography

A first report on visualization of the muscles of facial expression with US in 15 volunteers was published in 1988.[27] Interestingly, although currently possible, applications of US have not been explored further in detail. Due to technical developments resulting in better image quality and higher resolution in recent years, some of the perioral mimic muscles, mainly with an orthodontic focus, have been analyzed by US investigations.[28–30] Protocols have been established for a standardized quantitative US investigation of most of the important facial muscles.[4,31] Furthermore, age and gender-specific reference data for dynamic facial muscle US in adults have been published.[32] Finally, the usefulness of the clinical application of US in patients with chronic facial palsy or defective healing of facial palsy has been shown.[6,33]

!

It is relatively new to use ultrasonography for facial nerve and facial muscle diagnostics. It is a fast and easy method to depict the status of the facial muscles.

The application of US as a diagnostic tool for facial nerve diagnostics is not yet well disseminated. Therefore, the application is explained here in more detail. The ultrasound images in this chapter were obtained with a

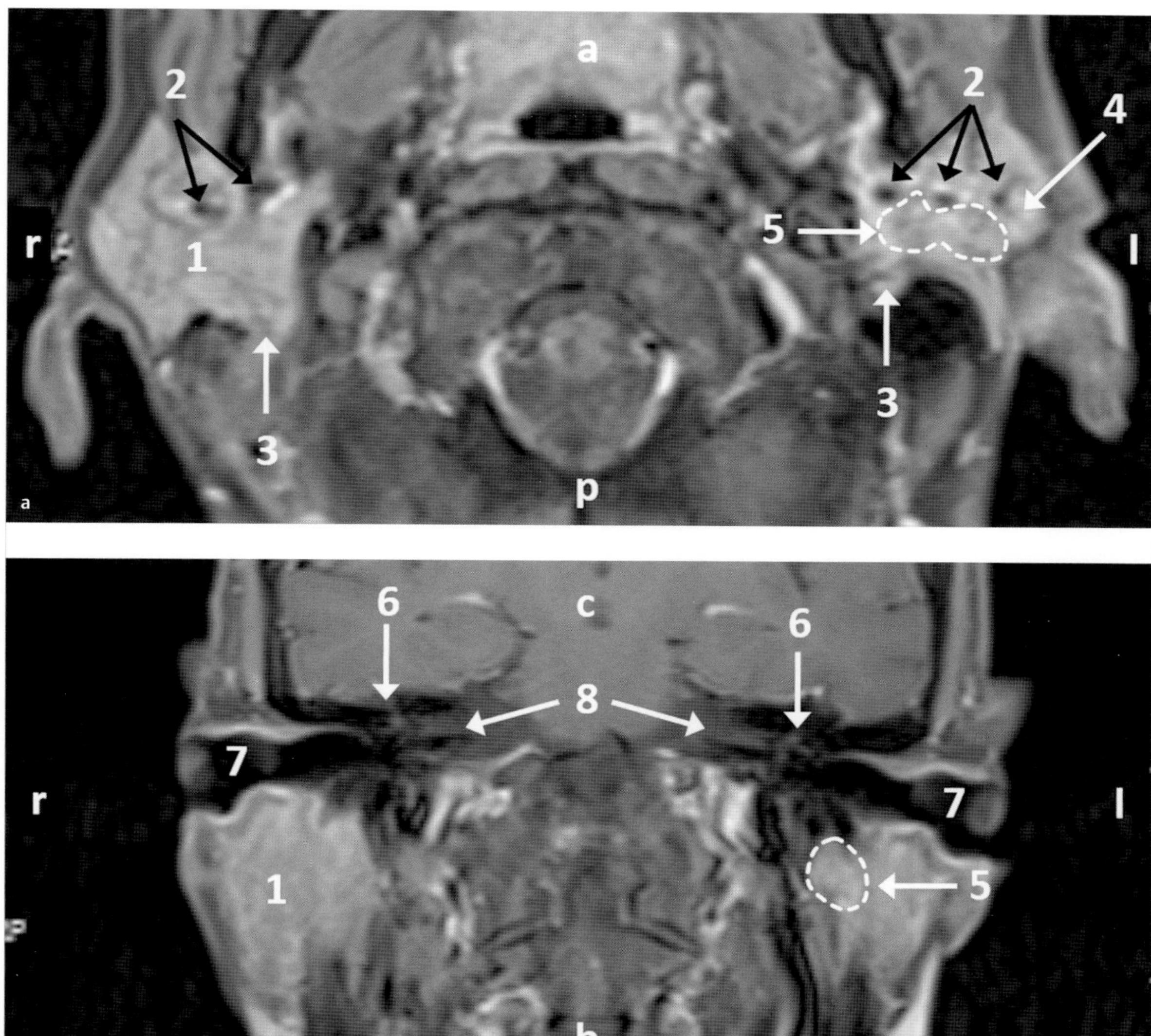

Fig. 5.11 A 1.5-Tesla MRI of the skull base and parotid gland, fat-saturated T1-weighted sequences after contrast media application. **(a)** Axial plane, and **(b)** coronal plane (slice thickness 5 mm). The MRI was repeated because of persistent pathologic spontaneous fibrillation potentials in facial EMG MRI. The images are of the latest MRI, which again did not show a parotid tumor or perineural enhancement of the facial nerve. Nevertheless, because of the EMG result, the parotid and the extratemporal facial nerve were explored. Surgery detected a 5 mm adenoid cystic carcinoma with facial nerve infiltration. 1, Normal right parotid gland; 2, retromandibular veins; 3, facial nerve exiting the stylomastoid foramen; 4, atrophic left parotid gland due to diffuse tumor infiltration; 5, location of the adenoid cystic carcinoma (histologically verified) showing an atypical appearance with only very small cysts and nearly no contrast enhancement (initially overlooked in MRI but detected with ultrasound; white dashed line); 6, vestibulocochlear system; 7, external auditory canal; 8, inner auditory canal. r, right; l, left; a, anterior; p, posterior; m, medial.

standard diagnostic ultrasound system (HD11 XE, Philips). Our protocol used two different linear-array transducers: one transducer with 3 to 12 MHz (L12–3, Philips) and the other with 7 to 15 MHz (L15–7io, Philips). The orbicularis oculi and the orbicularis oris muscle were analyzed with the 7 to 15 MHz transducer due to better visualization of the muscles with this transducer. All other facial muscles and the muscles of mastication (temporalis and master muscle as control muscles in some special situations) were analyzed with the 3 to 12 MHz probe (▸ Fig. 5.15 and ▸ Fig. 5.16). The mechanical index was set to 1.5 for the L12–3 transducer and to 1.4 for the L15–7io transducer. The thermal index for both transducers was 0.6 and the gain was set to 75 dB, i.e., using constant time gain compensation. The resulting pictures have a resolution of 1,280 × 1,040 pixels

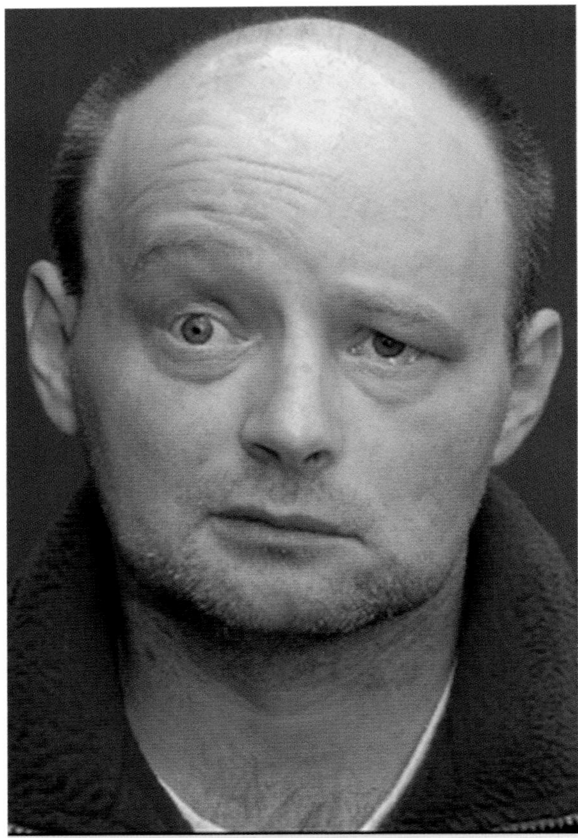

Fig. 5.12 A 45-year-old patient 5 days after temporal bone fracture with facial palsy on the left side.

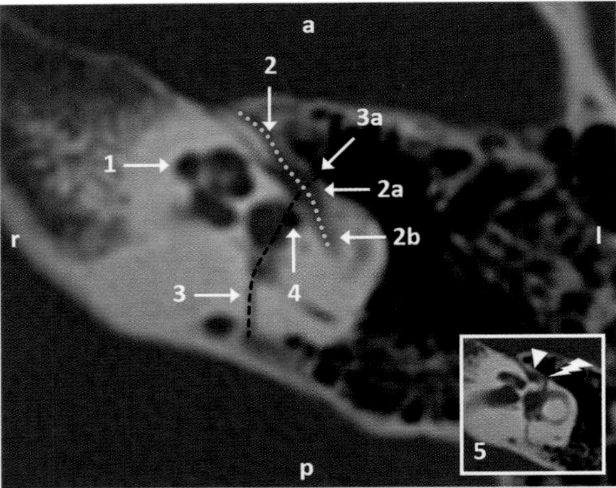

Fig. 5.13 High-resolution CT of the left petrous bone of the patient shown in ▶ Fig. 5.12, bone algorithm, para-axial plane (slice thickness 1.25 mm). 1, Cochlea; 2, course of the nerve (*yellow dotted line*): the greater petrosal nerve (2), tympanic segment (2a), and the proximal mastoid segment (2b); 3, fracture (*black dashed line*),including the broken lateral bony wall of the tympanic segment (3a); 4, small hypodense intravestibular air-bubble indicating that the fracture involves the vestibular system and the transvestibular course of the fracture; 5, (inset) details of the slice depicting the fracture's transtympanic course just lateral to the geniculate ganglion (*white arrowhead*). r, right; l, left; a, anterior; p, posterior; m, medial.

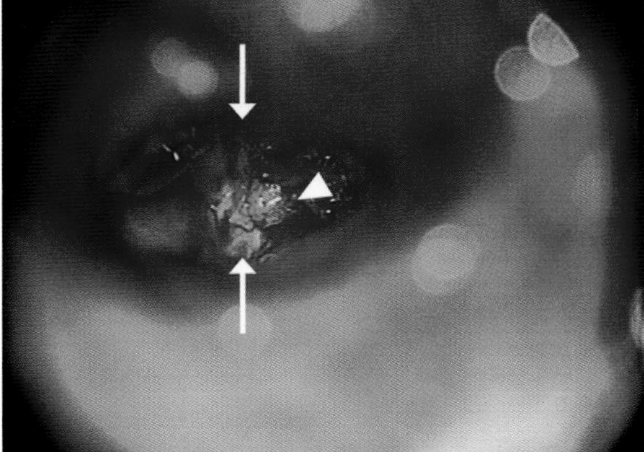

Fig. 5.14 Transmastoid exploration of the patient shown in ▶ Fig. 5.12, showing the fracture line (*arrows*) in the tympanic segment of the facial nerve and bony debris of the facial canal (*arrowhead*).

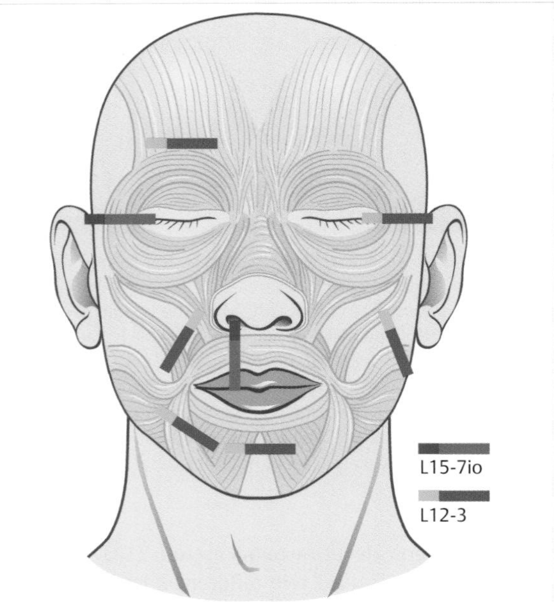

Fig. 5.15 Optimal positions of the ultrasound probe to detect the facial muscles. In the following examples two different transducers are used: L12–3 (blue) and L15–7io (green; both from Philips). The orientation of the markers of the probes is indicated in yellow and red, respectively.

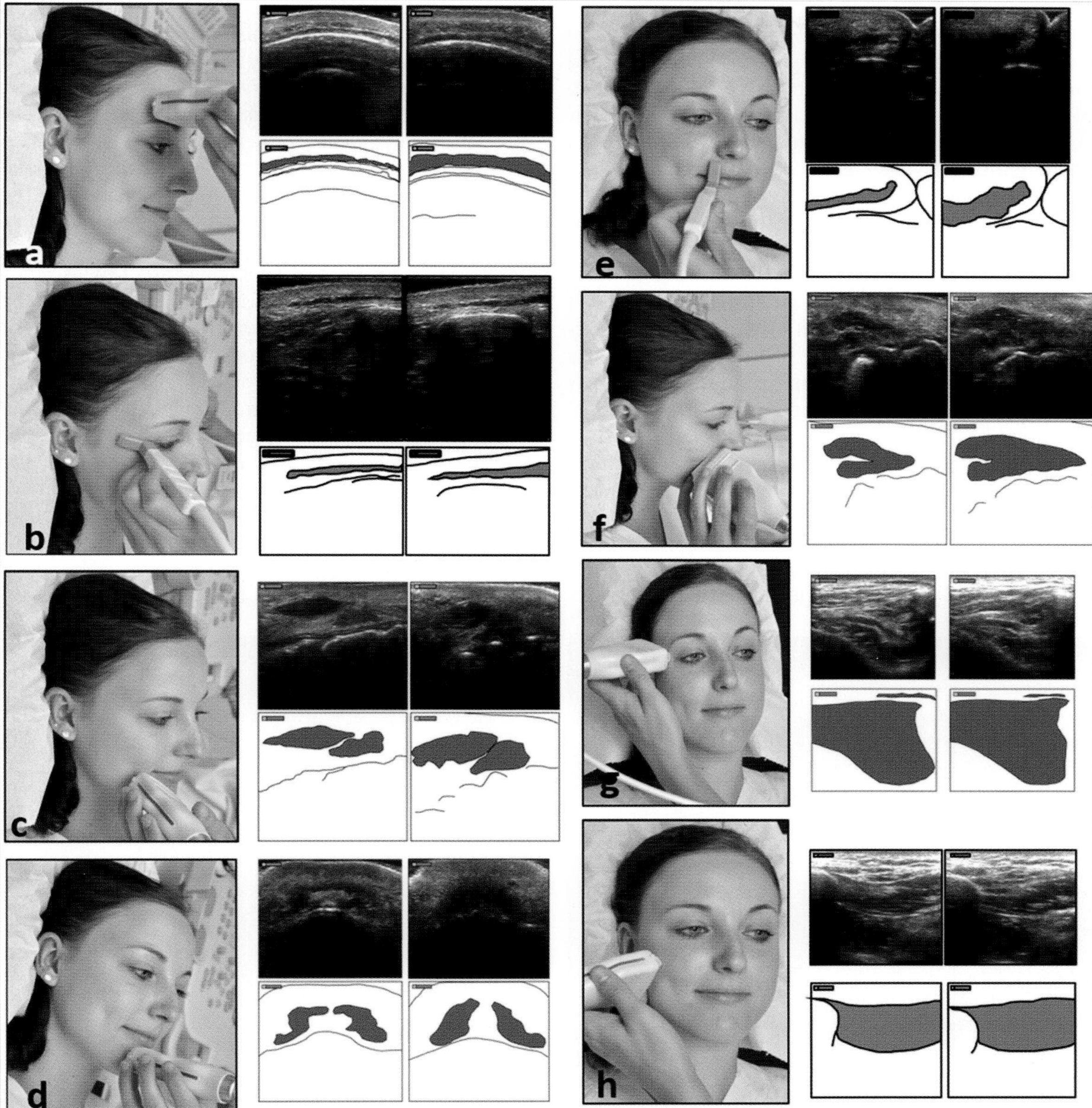

Fig. 5.16 (a–f) Landmarks and optimal visualization of six important facial muscles. **(g,h)** The chewing muscles are shown as references. Clinical images showing the optimal positions of the ultrasound probe (left), ultrasound images of the optimal plane (top right), and illustration of the optimal visualization of the target muscle (bottom right). Left column: at rest; right column: during contraction. **(a)** Frontal muscle. **(b)** Orbicularis oculi muscle. **(c)** Depressor anguli oris/labii inferioris muscle. **(d)** Mentalis muscle. **(e)** Orbicularis oris muscle. **(f)** Zygomaticus major muscle. **(g)** Temporalis muscle. **(h)** Masseter muscle.

(60 Hz, 256 gray-scale levels [8 bit]). All equipment settings were kept constant during the measurements of the facial muscles. All measurements were performed with transmission gel but without any other coupling media. The transducer was always placed perpendicular to the skin surface. Special importance was taken to position the transducer gently and without pressure against the facial skin. It was possible to maintain the same position of the transducer relative to the examined muscle during contraction. All subjects were examined in the supine position while completely relaxed. Directed activation of facial muscles was used to confirm the correct position of the transducer. Furthermore, the patients were instructed to precisely maintain a maximal contraction for 2 seconds to allow an analysis of each muscle during maximal contraction, if of interest.

In most cases US scans are feasible of seven mimic muscle pairs: the frontalis, orbicularis oculi, zygomaticus major, depressor anguli oris, depressor labii inferioris, orbicularis oris, and mentalis muscles. These facial muscles can be identified in a reliable manner. All other facial muscles cannot be identified in all subjects or with sufficient reliability. Separation of the zygomatic major muscle from the zygomatic minor muscle is not possible in all patients using US, partly due to image quality, and partly to anatomic variability. Additionally, a distinct delineation of the nasalis muscle and other small facial muscles is not possible. Furthermore, reproducible separation of the nasalis muscle from parts of the levator labii superioris muscle is not achievable. In addition to the mimic muscles innervated by the facial nerve, in most cases two other muscles are analyzed as control muscles: the temporalis and masseter muscles. This is done because these neighboring muscles are not innervated by the facial nerve. In patients with facial palsy, when the motor trigeminal nerve is not affected, these muscles should not show any relevant side difference. The identification of relevant anatomical landmarks that allow facial muscle identification and standardized planes for transducer positioning for optimal imaging at each site are described in detail in ▶ Table 5.2.

In patients with facial palsy and chronic denervation, the facial muscles typically are atrophied, i.e., they appear thinner during sonographical examination (▶ Fig. 5.17, ▶ Fig. 5.18, and ▶ Fig. 5.19). After facial nerve

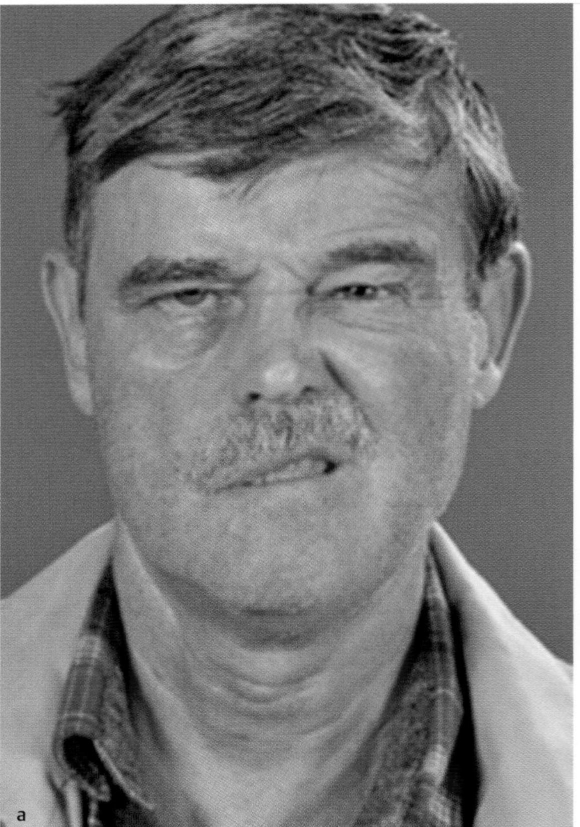

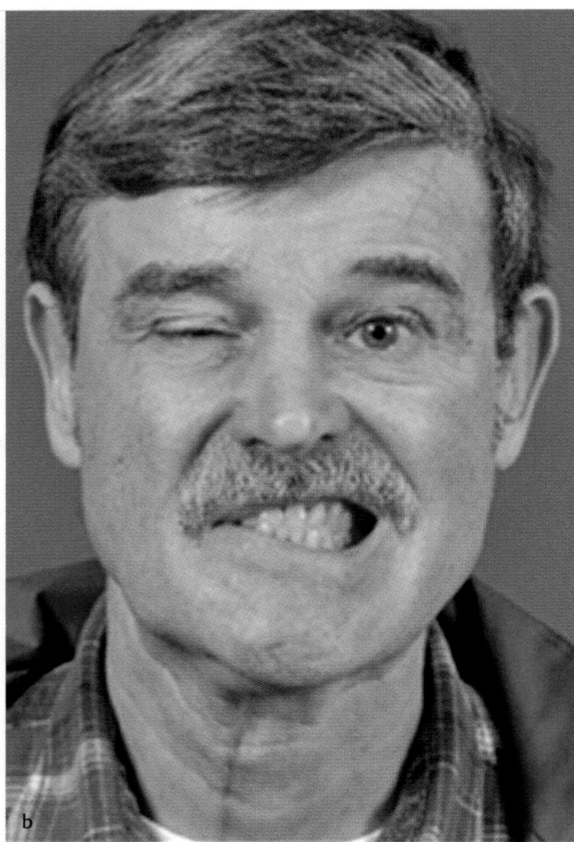

Fig. 5.17 A 59-year-old patient with facial palsy on right side after vestibular schwannoma surgery. **(a)** Four months after surgery with severe muscle atrophy on the paralyzed side. **(b)** Two years later with defective healing and regrowth of the facial muscles on the paralyzed side.

Table 5.2 Identification of the facial muscles during ultrasonography

Muscle	Transducer (MHz)	Landmarks	Imaging plane	Maneuver for muscle activation
Mimic muscles innervated by the facial nerve				
Occipitofrontalis, frontal belly (frontal muscle)	L12–3	Frontal bone, eye brow	Transverse position 1–2 cm cranial eye brow	Frowning
Corrugator supercilii	L12–3	Midline, eyebrows, superciliary arch	Transverse position, between eyebrows	Squinting
Procerus	L15–7io	Bridge of the nose, frontal bone, nasal bone	Sagittal position, midline, between frontal bone and nasal bone	Wrinkling the nose
Orbicularis oculi	L15–7io	Frontal process of zygomatic bone, lateral margin of the orbit	Transverse position perpendicular on the frontal process	Twinkling
Nasalis	L15–7io	Nasal bone, frontal process of maxilla, minor alar cartilage of both sides	Along nasal bone and frontal process of maxilla lateral of both sides to wing of the nose	Wrinkling the nose
Zygomaticus major	L12–3	Nasolabial fold, maxilla, upper row of teeth	Cranial and parallel to nasolabial fold	Smiling, pulling the corner of the mouth upwards
Zygomaticus minor	L12–3	Lateral inferior orbital rim, orbicularis oris muscle	Orthogonal to lateral orbital rim	Smiling, pulling the upper lip superiorly
Levator labii superioris	L12–3	Midpoint of lower orbital rim, pupil, orbicularis oris muscle, zygomatic minor muscle	Nearly sagittal position, parallel to zygomatic minor muscle	Elevating upper lip, showing the upper incisors
Levator labii superioris alaeque nasi	L12–3	Medial lower orbital rim, upper incisors	Between commissura medialis palpebralis and angle of the mouth	Elevating upper lip, flaring nostrils
Buccinator	L12–3	Upper and lower molar teeth	Nearly sagittal, level of second molar teeth	Sucking, pressing cheeks against molar teeth
Orbicularis oris	L15–7io	Columella, philtrum, upper lip	Sagittal position within the philtrum	Pressing the lips together
Depressor anguli oris	L12–3	Infralabial fossa, mandibular premolar teeth, supra-angular mandible	Positioning parallel to lower angular mandible, movement in craniocaudal direction along supra-angular mandible	Pulling the corners of the mouth downward
Depressor labii inferiors	L12–3	Infralabial fossa, mandibular premolar teeth, supra-angular mandible, facial artery	Positioning parallel to lower angular mandible, movement in craniocaudal direction along supra-angular mandible	Pulling the corners of the mouth downward
Risorius	L12–3	Lower row of teeth, relation to orbicularis oris, depressor anguli oris and depressor anguli oris	Lateral to angle of the mouth, parallel to body of the mandible	Smiling
Mentalis	L12–3	Mandible, protuberantia mentalis, contralateral muscle	Horizontal position, movement form point of the chin to lower lip	Pressing the lips together
Superficial muscles of mastication innervated by the trigeminal nerve				
Temporalis	L12–3	Lateral orbital rim, infratemporal fossa, greater wing of sphenoid bone, squama ossis of temporal bone	Transverse position, level of pupil, on the temple	Clenching the teeth
Masseter	L12–3	Facies lateralis of zygomatic bone, zygomatic arc	Between middle third of zygomatic arc and angle of the mandible	Clenching the teeth

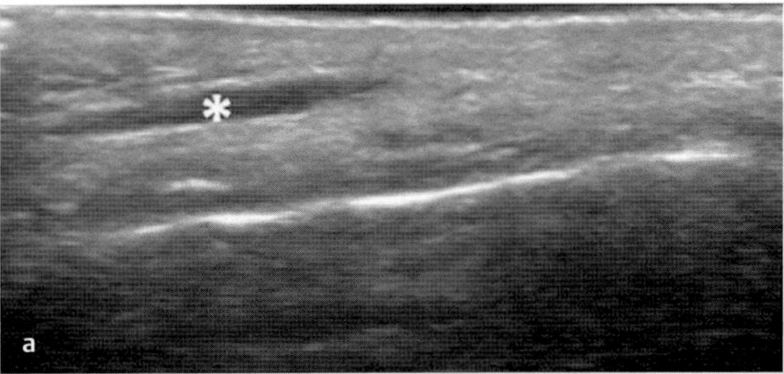

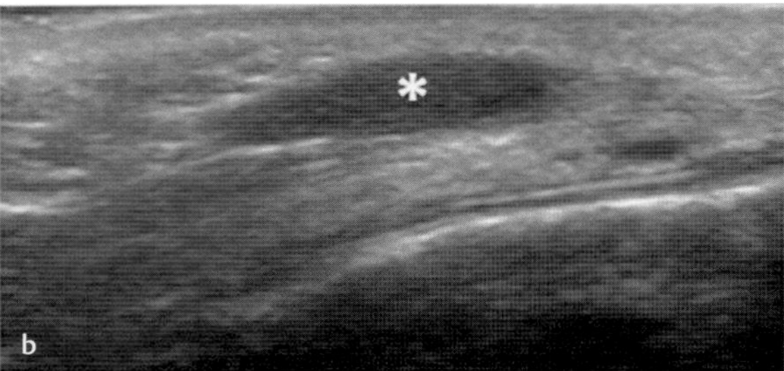

Fig. 5.18 Ultrasound of depressor anguli oris (*asterisk*) muscle of the right paralyzed side of the patient shown in ▶ Fig. 5.17, showing an increase in muscle area over time. **(a)** Four months after surgery. **(b)** Two years later.

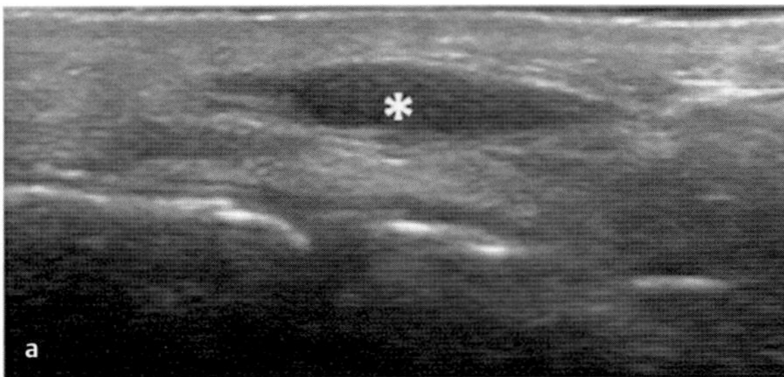

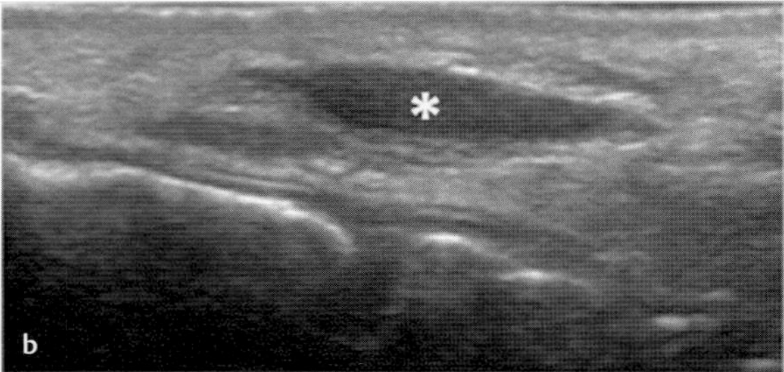

Fig. 5.19 Ultrasound of the depressor anguli oris muscle (*asterisk*) of the contralateral left normal side of the patient shown in ▶ Fig. 5.17, without a change in muscle area. **(a)** Four months after surgery. **(b)** Two years later.

reconstruction, US can be used to monitor the regeneration by repeated US of the facial muscles, typically showing a progressive facial muscle regrowth.

A single study has measured the facial nerve diameter at the stylomastoid foramen in 37 patients with Bell's palsy.[34] A larger diameter at onset was associated with a worse outcome. It should be emphasized that these results should be considered as preliminary as no other group has confirmed these data.

5.6 Key Points

- Diagnosis starts with clinical investigations. Imaging studies in patients with facial nerve disorders follow from these clinical findings.
- Magnetic resonance imaging is the best method to identify soft tissue changes around and in the facial nerve.
- Computed tomography is performed mainly for imaging of bony structures surrounding the facial nerve in the temporal bone.
- Ultrasonography offers very sensitive detection of facial muscle atrophy and subsequent regeneration.

References

[1] Veillon F, Taboada LR, Eid MA et al. Pathology of the facial nerve. Neuroimaging Clin N Am 2008; 18: 309–320

[2] Gupta S, Mends F, Hagiwara M, Fatterpekar G, Roehm PC. Imaging the facial nerve: a contemporary review. Radiol Res Pract 2013; 2013: 248039

[3] Singh AK, Bathla G, Altmeyer W et al. Imaging Spectrum of facial nerve lesions. Curr Probl Diagn Radiol 2015; 44: 60–75

[4] Volk GF, Wystub N, Pohlmann M, Finkensieper M, Chalmers HJ, Guntinas-Lichius O. Quantitative ultrasonography of facial muscles. Muscle Nerve 2013; 47: 878–883

[5] Koerte IK, Schroeder AS, Fietzek UM et al. Muscle atrophy beyond the clinical effect after a single dose of OnabotulinumtoxinA injected in the procerus muscle: a study with magnetic resonance imaging. Dermatol Surg 2013; 39: 761–765

[6] Volk GF, Pohlmann M, Sauer M, Finkensieper M, Guntinas-Lichius O. Quantitative ultrasonography of facial muscles in patients with chronic facial palsy. Muscle Nerve 2014; 50: 358–365

[7] Volk GF, Karamyan I, Klingner CM, Reichenbach JR, Guntinas-Lichius O. Quantitative magnetic resonance imaging volumetry of facial muscles in healthy patients with facial palsy. Plast Reconstr Surg Glob Open 2014; 2: e173

[8] Burmeister HP, Baltzer PA, Dietzel M et al. Identification of the nervus intermedius using 3 T MR imaging. AJNR Am J Neuroradiol 2011; 32: 460–464

[9] Phillips CD, Bubash LA. The facial nerve: anatomy and common pathology. Semin Ultrasound CT MR 2002; 23: 202–217

[10] Al-Noury K, Lotfy A. Normal and pathological findings for the facial nerve on magnetic resonance imaging. Clin Radiol 2011; 66: 701–707

[11] Burmeister HP, Baltzer PA, Volk GF et al. Evaluation of the early phase of Bell's palsy using 3 T MRI. Eur Arch Otorhinolaryngol 2011; 268: 1493–1500

[12] Burmeister HP, Hause F, Baltzer PA et al. Improvement of visualization of the intermediofacial nerve in the temporal bone using 3 T magnetic resonance imaging: part 1: the facial nerve. J Comput Assist Tomogr 2009; 33: 782–788

[13] Burmeister HP, Baltzer PA, Klingner CM, Pantel M, Kaiser WA. CT and MR imaging of the facial nerve [in German] HNO 2010; 58: 433–442

[14] Giesemann AM, Neuburger J, Lanfermann H, Goetz F. Aberrant course of the intracranial facial nerve in cases of atresia of the internal auditory canal (IAC). Neuroradiology 2011; 53: 681–687

[15] Keraliya AR, Naphade PS. Congenital unilateral facial nerve agenesis. Neurology 2014; 82: 2252–2253

[16] Chen DQ, Quan J, Guha A, Tymianski M, Mikulis D, Hodaie M. Three-dimensional in vivo modeling of vestibular schwannomas and surrounding cranial nerves with diffusion imaging tractography. Neurosurgery 2011; 68: 1077–1083

[17] Kaylie DM, Wax MK, Weissman JL. Preoperative facial muscle imaging predicts final facial function after facial nerve grafting. AJNR Am J Neuroradiol 2003; 24: 326–330

[18] Kaylie DM, Jackson CG, Aulino JM, Gardner EK, Weissman JL. Preoperative appearance of facial muscles on magnetic resonance predicts final facial function after acoustic neuroma surgery. Otol Neurotol 2004; 25: 622–626

[19] Farrugia ME, Kennett RP, Hilton-Jones D, Newsom-Davis J, Vincent A. Quantitative EMG of facial muscles in myasthenia patients with MuSK antibodies. Clin Neurophysiol 2007; 118: 269–277

[20] Gargiulo P, Klingner CM, Friogeirsson EA, Burmeister HP, Volk GF, Guntinas Lichius O. Side differences im MRI-scans in facial palsy: 3-D modelling, segmentation and grey value analysis. 23rd European Modeling and Simulation Symposium (Simulation in Industry). Rome, 2011

[21] Tüccar E, Tekdemir I, Aslan A, Elhan A, Deda H. Radiological anatomy of the intratemporal course of facial nerve. Clin Anat 2000; 13: 83–87

[22] Fu Y, Dai P, Zhang T. The location of the mastoid portion of the facial nerve in patients with congenital aural atresia. Eur Arch Otorhinolaryngol 2014; 271: 1451–1455

[23] Lim JH, Jun BC, Song SW. Clinical feasibility of multiplanar reconstruction images of temporal bone CT in the diagnosis of temporal bone fracture with otic-capsule-sparing facial nerve paralysis. Indian J Otolaryngol Head Neck Surg 2013; 65: 219–224

[24] Dahiya R, Keller JD, Litofsky NS, Bankey PE, Bonassar LJ, Megerian CA. Temporal bone fractures: otic capsule sparing versus otic capsule violating clinical and radiographic considerations. J Trauma 1999; 47: 1079–1083

[25] Vianna M, Adams M, Schachern P, Lazarini PR, Paparella MM, Cureoglu S. Differences in the diameter of facial nerve and facial canal in bell's palsy—a 3-dimensional temporal bone study. Otol Neurotol 2014; 35: 514–518

[26] Harnsberger HR, Dillon WP. Major motor atrophic patterns in the face and neck: CT evaluation. Radiology 1985; 155: 665–670

[27] Balogh B, Frühwald F, Millesi W, Millesi H, Firbas W. Sonoanatomy of the muscles of facial expression. Surg Radiol Anat 1988; 10: 101–106

[28] McAlister RW, Harkness EM, Nicoll JJ. An ultrasound investigation of the lip levator musculature. Eur J Orthod 1998; 20: 713–720

[29] Satiroğlu F, Arun T, Işik F. Comparative data on facial morphology and muscle thickness using ultrasonography. Eur J Orthod 2005; 27: 562–567

[30] de Korte CL, van Hees N, Lopata RG, Weijers G, Katsaros C, Thijssen JM. Quantitative assessment of oral orbicular muscle deformation after cleft lip reconstruction: an ultrasound elastography study. IEEE Trans Med Imaging 2009; 28: 1217–1222

[31] Alfen NV, Gilhuis HJ, Keijzers JP, Pillen S, Van Dijk JP. Quantitative facial muscle ultrasound: feasibility and reproducibility. Muscle Nerve 2013; 48: 375–380

[32] Volk GF, Sauer M, Pohlmann M, Guntinas-Lichius O. Reference values for dynamic facial muscle ultrasonography in adults. Muscle Nerve 2014; 50: 348–357

[33] Volk GF, Pohlmann M, Finkensieper M, Chalmers HJ, Guntinas-Lichius O. 3D-Ultrasonography for evaluation of facial muscles in patients with chronic facial palsy or defective healing: a pilot study. BMC Ear Nose Throat Disord 2014; 14: 4

[34] Lo YL, Fook-Chong S, Leoh TH et al. High-resolution ultrasound in the evaluation and prognosis of Bell's palsy. Eur J Neurol 2010; 17: 885–889

[35] Campbell J, McNamee J, Flynn P, McDonnell G. Teaching NeuroImages: facial diplegia due to neuroborreliosis. Neurology 2014; 82: e16–e17

[36] Uzawa A, Mori M, Ito S, Kuwabara S. Neurological picture. Isolated abducens and facial nerve palsies due to a facial collicular plaque in multiple sclerosis. J Neurol Neurosurg Psychiatry 2011; 82: 85–86

[37] Copeland WR, Hoover JM, Morris JM, Driscoll CL, Link MJ. Use of preoperative MRI to predict vestibular schwannoma intraoperative consistency and facial nerve outcome. J Neurol Surg B Skull Base 2013; 74: 347–350

[38] Yue Y, Jin Y, Yang B, Yuan H, Li J, Wang Z. Retrospective case series of the imaging findings of facial nerve hemangioma. Eur Arch Otorhinolaryngol

6 Electrophysiology

Hans-Christoph Scholle, Nikolaus-Peter Schumann, and Gerd Fabian Volk

6.1 Introduction

The etiology and pathogenesis of facial nerve paresis is multifactorial.[1] Therefore, in most cases the clinical decision-making for the optimal treatment of a patient with facial nerve paresis is often based on a so-called diagnosis of exclusion. After a sophisticated anamnesis, including a complete otorhinolaryngologic and neurologic examination as well as appropriate laboratory and imaging investigations, electrophysiologic analyses can complete the determination of diagnosis and improve the prognostic conclusions.[2]

This chapter encompasses electrophysiologic basics, the pathophysiology of facial nerve disorders, and the methods used for their evaluation.

6.2 Definition

Facial nerve dysfunction can provoke different degrees of one-sided flaccid paresis of facial muscles with corresponding disturbances of their coordination and activation patterns. The patient may have an enlarged palpebral fissure with Bell's phenomenon, reduced nasolabial and possibly forehead contours (see section 6.4), as well as changed sensory functions such as hyperacusis or disturbances of gustatory sense or salivation. The etiology can be idiopathic (Bell's palsy) or a wide variety of inflammatory, congenital, or neoplastic sources; more details are given in Chapter 4. Bell's palsy is more common than other types of facial paresis.[3] In later phases of disease muscle synkinesis, the involuntary contractions of muscles that are not involved in the primary programmed movement, is possible.[4]

6.3 Physiology behind Electrophysiologic Diagnostics

To better understand the electrophysiologic methods presented in this chapter, the practitioner must understand the physiology of the facial motor system. This chapter will focus on the facial motor system (for more details on the physiology of the facial nerve; see also Chapter 2.

After a sufficient depolarization of the facial nerve by different kinds of stimuli, sequences of action potentials are evoked that activate a variable number of motor units to be adequate to the required muscle contraction during a certain motor task. A motor unit consists of a motoneuron and its innervated muscle fibers. The number of innervated muscle fibers is variable and depends on muscle size. In small muscles, such as those of the facial region, the number of muscle fibers per motor unit is low,[5] which correlates with the precise motor control adjustment function of these muscles. The action potentials are transmitted to the muscles via motor end plates. Normally, the amplitude and duration of motor unit action potentials (MUAPs) are characteristic of the number of innervated muscle fibers and can be recorded by needle electromyography (N-EMG). In contrast, surface electromyography (S-EMG) usually permits only a registration of compound muscle action potentials, which is a summation of motor unit action potentials. The higher the number of activated motor units the denser is the motor unit activation pattern that can be recorded during voluntary muscle contraction (EMG interference pattern). N-EMG and S-EMG are explained in detail later in this chapter.

> **!**
>
> A motor unit consists of a facial motoneuron and all muscle fibers innervated by this motoneuron. If a motoneuron is activating its related muscle fibers by an action potential, a motor unit action potential (MUAP) can be recorded by a needle inserted in the muscle. This method is called needle electromyography. A recording on the surface of the muscle, called surface electromyography, allows the registration of the sum of MUAPs in the range of the surface electrode.

6.4 Pathology and its Electrophysiologic Correlates

Disturbances of facial muscle function can be provoked by central and peripheral sources. The central causes are localized in the region of corticonuclear tract, which encompasses the relevant pathways between the cortex and the facial nucleus (▶ Fig. 6.1). The corticonuclear tract can be interfered by either functional or morphological alterations (lesions). Dysfunction of the peripheral facial nerve occurs along the pathway from the facial nerve nucleus to the facial muscles (▶ Fig. 6.1). These peripheral lesions are more frequent than central lesions.[6] Peripheral facial nerve dysfunction can be classified into three different subtypes of severity: neurapraxia, axonotmesis, and neurotmesis. Neurapraxia is characterized by functional nerve deficits, not by morphological nerve failure; more details on the classification are given in Chapter 9. Axonotmesis is defined as a disturbance of axonal nerve fibers, but the covering myelin sheath is kept. Neurotmesis is distinguished as complete disconnection of the facial nerve.[7]

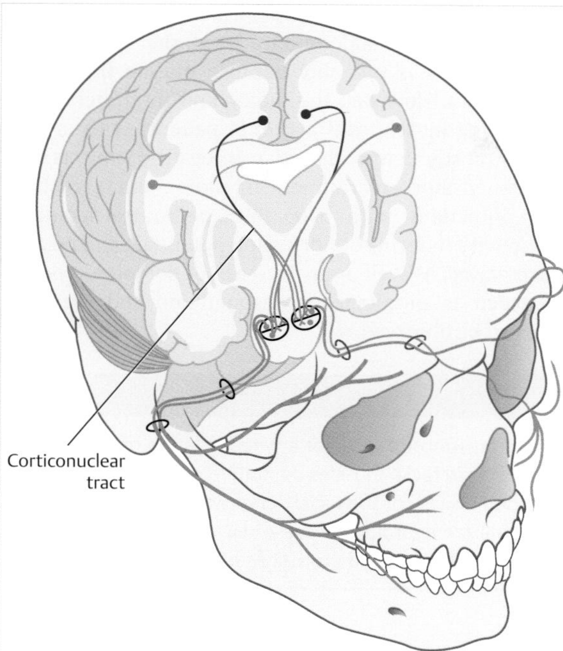

Fig. 6.1 Facial muscle function influenced by neuroanatomical characteristics. The light green and red points indicate the right and left motor cortex. These points mark the beginning of corticonuclear tracts to facial nuclei. Most of these motor pathways cross to the contralateral side of brainstem. However, the upper part of facial nuclei receives ipsilateral fibers of corticonuclear tracts supplying the muscles in the upper facial region. The dark green and brown points mark areas of caudal cingulum appropriated for involuntary (emotional) facial movements.

!

An important task of electrodiagnostics is to differentiate between neurapraxia, axonotmesis, and neurotmesis. Depending on the point in time after a facial nerve lesion, electrodiagnostics cannot always differentiate between the three types of nerve injury. The significance of electrodiagnostics can be increased when repeated several times during the time course of a facial nerve lesion, and may be enhanced when using several electrodiagnostics methods.

In the acute phase of facial paresis (during the first 3 days), the diagnostic differentiation of central and peripheral causes by using electrophysiologic methods can be problematic. If the history and clinical examination suggest a stroke, the usual recommendations, including brain imaging, have to be considered (note: time is brain); there is more information on central lesions of the facial nerve in Chapter 27. If an acute stroke has been excluded, transcranial magnetic stimulation can be helpful to differentiate between a central and peripheral facial paresis; see Transcranial Magnetic Stimulation and Magnetic Evoked Potentials.

During the first days after a facial nerve lesion, electrodiagnostics cannot differentiate between central and peripheral facial nerve lesion. Other diagnostic methods are needed; see Chapter 27. They can be helpful to look at peripheral lesions for nerve continuity.

The greater the number of facial nerve axons that are functionally or morphologically impaired, the more distinct the rarefication of EMG interference pattern in N-EMG and S-EMG. This rule is valid for neurapraxia, axonotmesis, and neurotmesis. In the case of neurapraxia, normally the electrophysiologic configuration of motor units is not changed. However, in axonotmesis or neurotmesis the duration of motor units and the number of their potential phases can increase. About 2 to 4 weeks postlesion, the appearance of pathologic spontaneous activity is possible (fibrillation potentials, positive sharp waves; see ▶ Fig. 6.5). The instability of the muscle membrane and an enhanced response of muscle fibers to acetylcholine have been described.[8] Pathologic spontaneous activity is a negative prognosticator, i.e., the probability of full recovery decreases with the appearance of pathologic spontaneous activity. If the facial nerve regenerates, i.e., axons sprout out of the lesion site and regrow to the target muscles (spontaneously or after nerve suture), regeneration potentials can occur, which have a positive prognostic meaning and often a polyphasic structure. Furthermore, as a consequence of neurotmesis, a defective healing with synkinesis is inevitable; for further details see Transcranial Magnetic Stimulation and Magnetic Evoked Potentials.

!

The number of functionally or morphologically lesioned facial nerve axons normally correlates with the rarefication of the electromyographic (EMG) interference pattern during activation of the related facial muscles.

!

Pathologic spontaneous activity during EMG recording at rest is always a sign of axon degeneration in the facial nerve.

6.4.1 Supranuclear Lesions

Between the cortex and the facial nucleus, pathways are situated that belong to the supranuclear structures. Most of these fibers cross the midline to the contralateral facial nucleus region.[9] Therefore, a disturbance of the left-sided corticonuclear tract could appear as a contralateral, right-sided paresis. In contrast, the portion of the facial nucleus that innervates the upper facial muscles (forehead and palpebral muscles) receives fibers from both sides of the corticonuclear tract (see ▶ Fig. 6.1). It is for this reason that supranuclear lesions do not cause symptoms in the upper facial muscle areas; see also Chapter 27. The corticonuclear tract can be disturbed by a variety of neoplasms, trauma, metabolic causes, and circulatory issues, as well as nonspecific inflammatory disorders.

6.4.2 Infranuclear Lesions

All nerve dysfunctions distal to the facial nucleus are termed infranuclear (▶ Fig. 6.1). Infranuclear disorders can manifest as variable degrees of unilateral flaccid paresis, as well as changes in taste, lacrimation, and salivation. Pathologic processes affecting the facial nerve in the fallopian canal, distal to the geniculate ganglion, also produce one-sided flaccid paresis of facial muscles. They can be accompanied by changes of gustatory sense and salivation (from the chorda tympani), but spare lacrimation. Disturbances of the facial nerve in the region of the stylomastoid foramen and further distally are purely motor disturbances.[6]

6.4.3 Synaptic Lesions

Disturbed neuromuscular transmission can also be assessed in facial muscles (e.g., ocular form of myasthenia gravis). Patients with this disorder may have a reduced duration of MUAPs and an increase of polyphasic potentials of N-EMG. In this condition, there is a decrease of S-EMG amplitudes, especially of proximal body muscles, evoked by repetitive nerve stimulation; for further details see Transcranial Magnetic Stimulation and Magnetic Evoked Potentials.[10]

6.4.4 Muscular Lesions

This group of dysfunctions is subdivided into specific muscular diseases, which are named myopathies (muscle dystrophy, myotonia, and myositis), and disturbances of muscle function, which have many etiologies, for example on the basis of neoplastic, metabolic, and endocrine disorders.

Electrophysiologic diagnostics of the several kinds of myopathies is difficult. As myopathies do not play a major role in facial nerve disorders, only some general aspects of EMG for myopathy will be presented here. Overall, the motor unit pattern in myopathies is characterized by reduced duration and amplitude of the single motor units.[11,12] This is probably because muscle fibers have dropped out. However, the motor unit interference pattern during muscle contraction in patients with myopathies is mostly denser than that in healthy subjects (due to compensatory recruitment of motor units). Furthermore, in patients with myopathies, pathologic spontaneous activity in terms of fibrillation potentials and positive sharp waves, as well as an increase of polyphasic potentials such as simultaneous degeneration and regeneration, can be observed.

!

Electrodiagnostic signs for a synaptic lesion or a muscular lesion in facial muscles do not indicate a circumscribed disease of the facial nerve system but a more generalized neurologic disease also affecting the face. These findings should prompt referral to a neurologist.

6.5 Electrophysiologic Diagnostic Work-Up

Promising higher objectivity and reliability than, for example, classic topognostic testing, electrical testing has become the mainstay for prognostic testing of the facial nerve. Adour credits Duchenne in the 1800s as one of the earliest electrodiagnostic practitioners. In discussing "rheumatismal" facial palsy, Duchenne noted that the palsies that persisted had absent muscular contractility on nerve stimulation. He claimed his tests could reliably predict prognosis.[13] In 2013, the American Academy of Otolaryngology—Head and Neck Surgery Foundation published a clinical practice guideline for the treatment of Bell's palsy. This guideline recommended offering electrodiagnostic testing primarily in cases of complete paralysis, as patients with incomplete paralysis already, by and large, have a good prognosis.[14] However, clinicians should refer patients to a facial nerve specialist when new or worsening neurologic findings occur at any point, ocular symptoms develop, or when, after 3 months, there is still an incomplete facial recovery. Also in these cases, use of electrodiagnostic tests is justified. In the following sections it will be shown that in the hands of a facial nerve specialist, specialist electrodiagnostics support the diagnostics in most cases of complete facial palsy.

6.5.1 Needle Electromyography

The first part of the electrophysiologic investigation of patients is usually N-EMG. Using a small EMG needle, all the facial muscles can easily be investigated. There are several types of indwelling electrodes, of which needle electrodes are the most versatile: they occur as monopolar, concentric, bipolar concentric, and single-fiber needle electrodes.

The *monopolar needle electrode* is a stainless steel needle fully insulated with a thin insulating coating, except for the tip. Solid needles are used for diagnostic purposes; for EMG-guided injection of botulinum toxin, the needle is hollow (▶ Fig. 6.2). The recording area of this electrode is spherical. The reference electrode is placed at a myoelectric inactive location of the body and may be a surface electrode. For facial EMG, a suitable place for the reference electrode is the skin over the manubrium sterni because of a lack of interfering muscles close by and the symmetric position in the midline of the patient.

The *concentric needle electrode* (▶ Fig. 6.3) consists of a hollow steel needle with a steel, silver, or platinum wire running through the needle, which is fully insulated except for the tip. The potential difference between the outer shaft of the needle and the tip of the wire is measured by connecting each of these to one port of the differential amplifier. Since the electrode cannula acts as a shield, the electrode has directional recording characteristics controlled by the angle and position of the bevel. Therefore, a simple axial rotation of the electrode may significantly alter the individual motor units recorded.

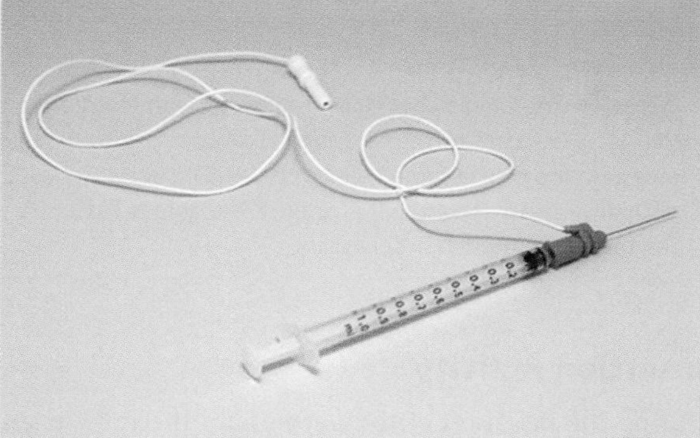

Fig. 6.2 Monopolar EMG cannula for EMG-guided application of botulinum toxin.

Comparing monopolar with concentric needle electrodes, potentials recorded by *monopolar needle electrodes* tend to be larger and longer with more phases than those recorded with concentric needle electrodes. This difference is based on the existence of more muscle fibers within the zone of detection, as well as on fewer cancellations due to potentials being recorded from the cannula of the electrode.

The *bipolar concentric electrode* is sometimes called *bifilar* or *double concentric*. It is a hollow needle containing two platinum wires, each of which is insulated except for its tip. The outer shaft is grounded, and the two internal wires are each connected to one side of the differential amplifier, so that the potential difference between the two wires is measured. The recording range of the bipolar concentric electrode is restricted to the area between the two tips of the wires within the shaft, which makes it unsatisfactory for many clinical routine purposes. Such bipolar electrodes may be useful primarily for experimental studies. The potentials are shorter and lower in the voltage than those recorded with concentric needle electrodes. For *single-fiber EMG*, a fine wire capable of recording a single muscle fiber action potential is embedded at the tip of the needle shaft acting as reference.[15]

Selection of Electrode Type

For comparative or quantitative evaluation, the same electrode type must be used when obtaining reference

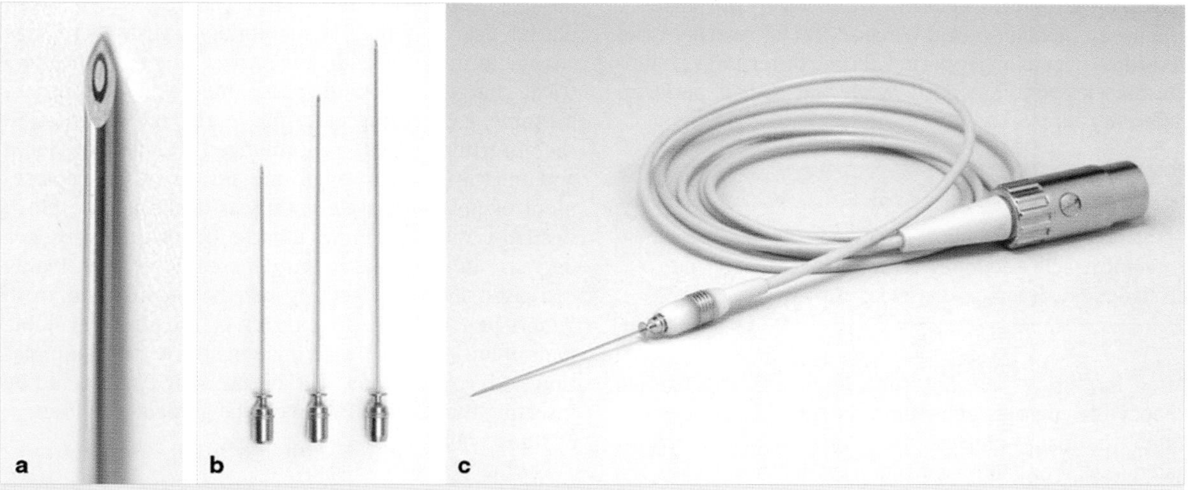

Fig. 6.3 Concentric EMG needles. **(a)** Tip of a concentric needle electrode. **(b)** Concentric needle electrodes of different sizes: 0.50 × 60 mm, 0.45 × 50 mm, and 0.45 × 38 mm. **(c)** Concentric needle electrode 0.45 × 38 mm with cable and DIN plug.

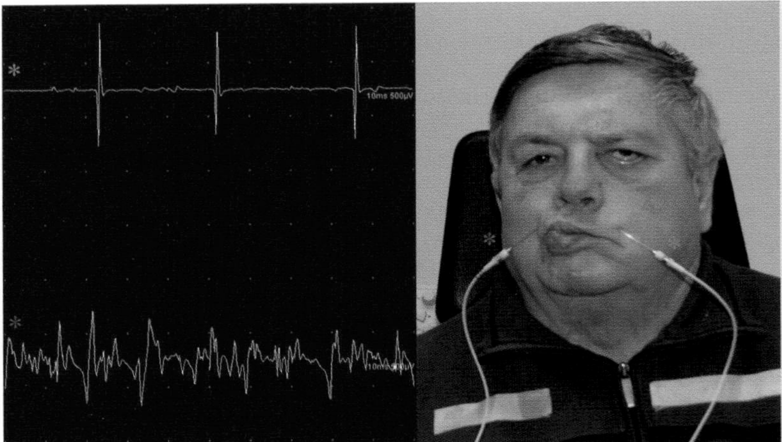

Fig. 6.4 Two-channel N-EMG recording of the orbicularis oris muscle during voluntary muscle movement. The left paretic side (*green asterisk*) shows only a single motor unit firing, while on the healthy right side (*red asterisk*) a normal dense recruitment pattern is recorded.

values, because of the previously mentioned differences between electrode types. Filter settings must also be consistent. In general, monopolar electrodes pick up potentials from a larger spherical region than concentric electrodes. Unfortunately, bipolar concentric electrodes are not commercially available at the moment. Studies comparing different needle types for facial EMG are not available. In the past, a major part of the laryngeal EMG reports on MUAP characteristics in the thyroarytenoid and cricothyroid muscles have used concentric electrodes, which has resulted in their preferred use despite weaker selectivity. One study used commercially available single-fiber EMG electrodes and provided normative data on 10 adults. Measures of jitter and fiber density may have clinical significance.[16] Single-fiber EMG is preferred for the diagnosis of neuromuscular junction abnormalities.[17,18]

For the transcutaneous approach to the facial muscles, it is recommended to use concentric needle electrodes, providing a uniform field for MUAP waveform analysis. The use of bipolar hooked wires allows for selected cases recording over a longer period of time or recording multiple muscles simultaneously while the patient performs different tasks.

!

The standard for needle electromyography is to use concentric needle electrodes. Be aware that other needles offer other advantages for selected cases.

After having chosen the suitable needle, one should choose the muscles depending on the clinical question. Often, the main branches of the facial nerve are investigated (e.g., if one looks for reinnervation in the case of a complete facial nerve/axonotmesis). In this case the frontalis, orbicularis oculi, oris, and zygomaticus muscle may be chosen. Of course, such a scheme is not fixed and can be adapted (▶ Fig. 6.4).

!

It is recommended to perform needle electromyography (N-EMG) in accordance to a standard protocol for routine investigation of the same facial muscles. Of course, in facial palsies restricted to parts of the face, only N-EMG of the region of interest is necessary.

Insertion Activity

During the insertion of the needle into the muscle, an insertion activity response should occur. Typically, the insertion of the needle causes bursts of electrical activity. These should last no longer than several hundred milliseconds. They are caused by the fact that the needle itself contains some electrical energy, which, when placed near the muscle membrane, causes a relative change in the surrounding electrical energy. If the electrical charges surrounding the muscle membrane are unstable, e.g., during early nerve and muscle injuries, the insertion activity is prolonged. Healing of nerve and muscle injuries sometimes results in the replacement of normal muscle with scar tissue or fat, which insulates the remaining muscle fibers and causes a decrease in insertion activity. Increased or even highly increased insertion activity can be recorded in fresh denervated muscles as a result of the more unstable membrane potential reacting sensitively on manipulation with contractions. The muscle activity triggered by inserting the needles into it can be graded as follows:

1. No activity.
2. Normal activity (< 300 ms).
3. Increased activity.
4. Highly increased activity.

!

During needle electromyography (N-EMG) examinations these three activities should be evaluated:

- Insertion activity
- Spontaneous activity during rest
- Activity during voluntary activity

Spontaneous Activity at Rest

In a resting muscle and a nonmoving electrode, the examiner should check the N-EMG for pathologic spontaneous activity. Under normal conditions, no spontaneous electrical activity should be present during rest. However, a severely denervated muscle can show some such activity in the form of unstable electrical charges. Such spontaneous activity implies that the muscle is degenerating or that the nerve has been injured and that the injury is ongoing. Spontaneous activity can include fibrillation potentials, increased insertion fibrillations (insertion activity), complex repetitive discharges, and sharp positive waves. Specifically, fibrillation potentials are defined as low-amplitude, short-duration units generated by a single muscle fiber, indicating axonal degeneration (see ▶ Fig. 6.5e). However, this symptom may occur only 10 to 14 days after the injury or later, since it takes some time for the nerve to degenerate to such a degree that the release of the neurotransmitter acetylcholine into the neuromuscular junction is completely fatigued and no more depolarization of the muscle will occur. This degree of denervation occurs only in severe nerve injury. Spontaneous activity indicates a poor prognosis for recovery. Once regeneration begins, the muscle receives electrical impulses from the regenerated nerve and the spontaneous activity ceases.

!

Pathologic spontaneous activity is an important finding on electromyography (EMG), but occurs only after 14 days or later. Repeat examinations may be necessary if the first EMG was done before this.

Spontaneous activity should be recorded and classified as:

1. No reproducible pathologic spontaneous activity.
2. Little pathologic spontaneous activity.
3. Moderate pathologic spontaneous activity.
4. Dense pathologic spontaneous activity.

Activity during Voluntary Muscle Movement

Neural lesions may result in a reduced number of normal motor unit potentials and reduced recruitment during voluntary activity. Recruitment is defined as the activation of motor units with increasing strength of voluntary muscle contraction. It reflects the number of MUAPs identifiable during increasing activation when performing tasks such as voicing or smiling; see also Physiology behind Electrophysiologic Diagnostics. Preferentially, individual action potentials are evaluated in correspondence with minimal activation. Maximal activation (interference pattern = dense recruitment pattern) of the muscle should be recorded and graded as follows (▶ Fig. 6.5):

1. No activity.
2. Single-fiber pattern.
3. Severe decreased recruitment pattern.
4. Mildly decreased recruitment pattern.
5. Normal/dense recruitment pattern.

Synkinetic Activity

In order to reveal synkinesis, the patient is asked to perform agonistic and antagonistic maneuvers to provoke physiologic and synkinetic activity while recording EMG; details on background of synkinesis are given in Chapter 3.

Evaluation of the EMG Results

For clinical routine use, it is convenient to classify electrophysiologic findings according to Seddon[7] into neurapraxia, axonotmesis, or neurotmesis; see also Pathology and its Electrophysiologic Correlates. For neurapraxia, the diagnostic criterion on EMG is the detection of a rarefied recruitment pattern or of single action potentials during voluntary contraction without pathologic spontaneous activity (e.g., positive sharp waves or fibrillation activity). Axonotmesis should be suspected if spontaneous activity, indicating neural degeneration, is detected. This may be the case 10 to 14 days or later after the onset of paralysis. This classification includes a certain level of prognosis on recovery, since neurapraxia is most likely to recover completely within 8 to 12 weeks, whereas axonotmesis is thought to have only a poor chance of recovery to a perfect level. If reinnervation occurs following axonotmesis, it is usually associated with sequelae, such as synkinesis, due to neuronal misdirection. The result is a simultaneous activation of several facial muscles. This kind of dysfunction following reinnervation is called "autoparalytic syndrome" when antagonistic muscles are coactivated, outbalancing their force so little to no movement is visible when looking on the skin. The motionless wrinkle-free forehead after reinnervation is a typical example of the autoparalytic syndrome. Neurotmesis, i.e., the complete destruction of the whole nerve structure across its entire diameter, is assumed to never recover unless the damaged nerve endings have direct contact.

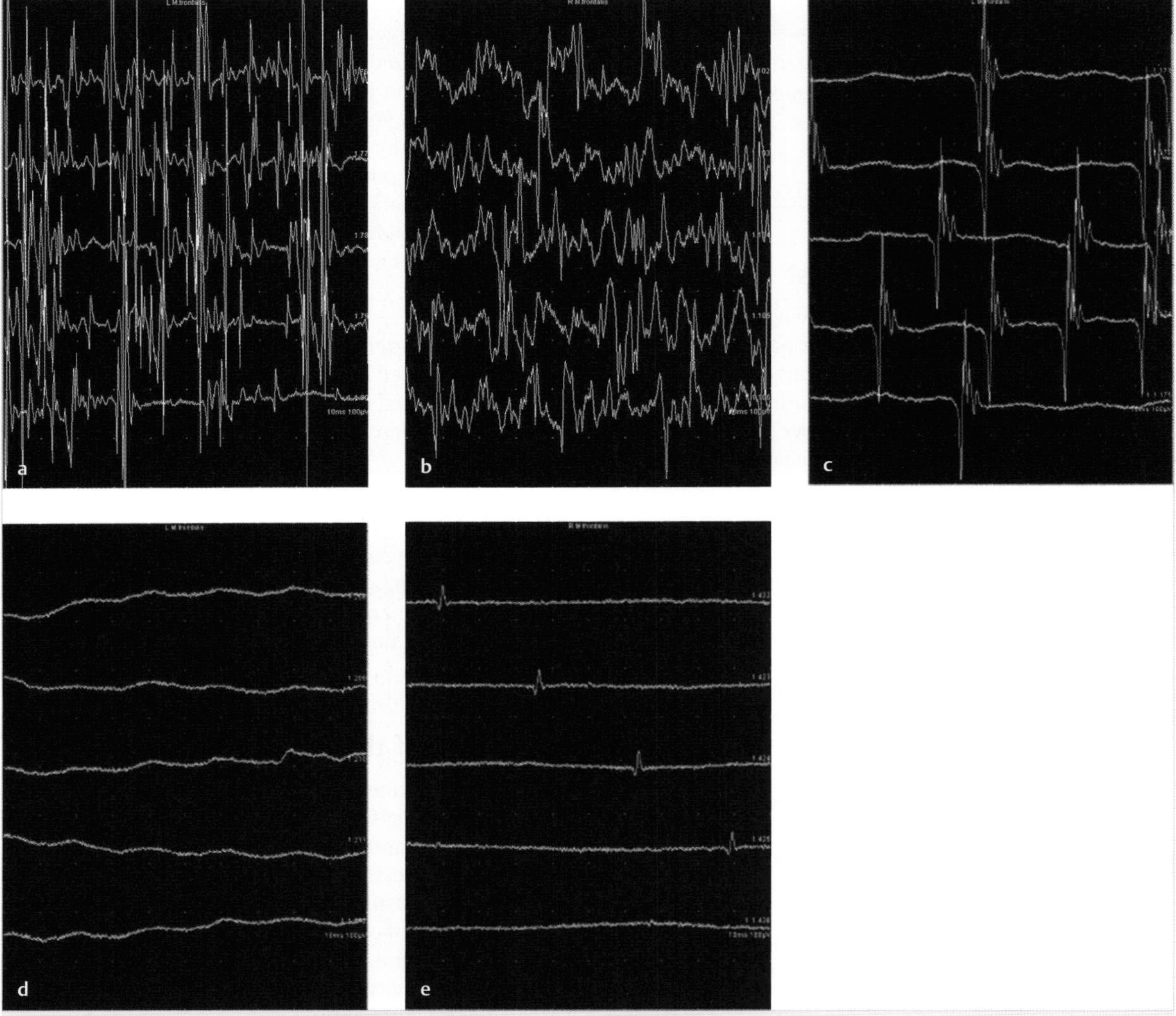

Fig. 6.5 Examples of activation (interference patterns) of the frontalis muscle recorded with a concentric needle electrode 0.45 × 38 mm during contraction. (a) Normal/dense recruitment pattern. (b) Mildly decreased recruitment pattern with some polyphasic reinnervation potentials. (c) Single-fiber pattern with polyphasic reinnervation potentials. (d) No activity. (e) Pathologic spontaneous activity as a sign for denervation.

Waveform Morphology

Waveform morphology refers to the shape, amplitude, and duration of the MUAPs, which are the electrical signals captured by the EMG. The normal facial motor unit potential is biphasic or triphasic, with a downward positive spike and an upward negative spike. Although it is strongly dependent on the needle used for recording, it usually has an amplitude of 200 to 500 mV and lasts about 5 to 7 milliseconds. The amplitude of the MUAP reflects the number and the strength of the muscle fibers innervated by one axon, while the duration of the MUAP depends on the velocity and synchrony of the neural input, which in turn is influenced by the insulation of the nerve. Nerves that are well insulated and have an intact and functioning sheath are able to transmit electrical impulses faster, because electrical impulses are transmitted from one node of Ranvier to another, the so-called saltatory conduction. The shape of the MUAP reflects changes in the electrical activity of the muscle membrane; normally measured in a certain distance to the motor end plates, it has a biphasic pattern. MUAPs recorded close to motor end plates often appear with more than three phases and are called polyphasic. These are physiologic and normal polyphasic MUAPs with no pathologic value. In the small facial muscles such recordings are hard to avoid. The investigator should not confuse these physiologic polyphasic MUAPS with pathologic polyphasic MUAPs. In case of doubt, the investigator should repeat the investigation after shifting the needle to a different place in the muscle.

> ⚠
>
> Polyphasic potentials recorded close to motor end plates are normal and not a sign of axonal regeneration of a nerve lesion.

The MUAPs of the facial muscles are smaller and shorter as compared with the skeletal muscles of the limbs. Of course, this is related to the small and short character of the mimic muscles as compared with other muscles. Nevertheless the waveform morphology of the MUAP provides, along with other information, aspects of the phase of recovery. After injury, the nerve goes through a process of degeneration, followed by regeneration. During degeneration, there is no neural input into the muscle, and in the first days before pathologic spontaneous activity occurs, no motor unit potential waveforms are produced. Abnormal MUAP morphologies are produced during the period of regeneration. During the early phases of regeneration, tiny nerves return to the muscles, which are atrophied during the time of denervation. Early in the regrowth process, the insulation of the nerve is decreased. The combination of the tiny, minimally insulated nerves and the weak muscle fibers produces electrical signals on the EMG that are seen as MUAPs with small amplitudes, long durations, and polyphasic shapes. These waveforms are sometimes referred to as nascent units and imply the presence of a recent nerve injury. At this time, the clinical picture is still one of complete paralysis.

> !
>
> During early regeneration, electromyography will show small amplitude, long duration polyphasic shapes referred to as nascent units. These electrical findings precede clinical improvement.

Regeneration Potentials

During regeneration, the nerve functions become more regular and the nerves become better insulated through regrowth of their sheaths. The muscle fibers become stronger and gain mass. However, not all nerve fibers regenerate. Fibers that do regenerate usually branch more extensively than they did before the injury, and they spread to innervate as many denervated muscle fibers as possible. The MUAPs that are produced as a result of this ongoing regeneration have greater amplitudes than normal. These MUAPs have a prolonged duration and are often described as giant polyphasic potentials (▶ Fig. 6.6).

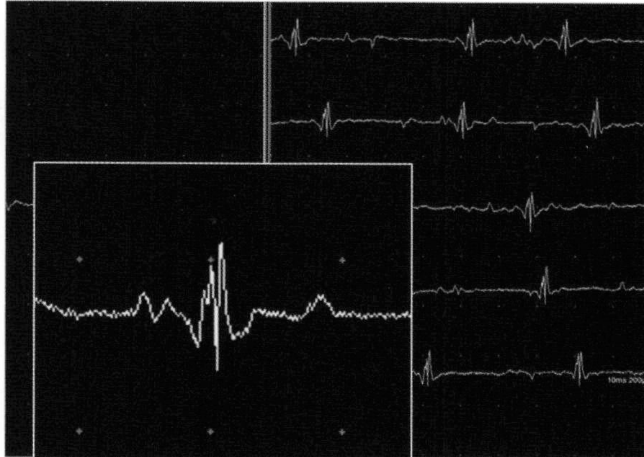

Fig. 6.6 Reinnervation action potentials with typical polyphasic waveform configuration.

Previous nerve injury can be inferred from their presence. Such a recovery is clinically accompanied by mass movements and synkinesis. The ingrowing axon branches off different twigs can reach widely separated muscles. Early signs of synkinesis can be found with EMG by having the patient contract muscles other than the one in which the needle is placed. Often, one finds the presence of MUAPs that can only be recruited by contracting another muscle. Alternatively, one can also use a two-channel recording and position two EMG needles in different muscles. In the case of synkinesis, an exact synchronous firing of one MUAP in the two different muscles is recorded during contraction.

> !
>
> Detection of giant polyphasic potentials during voluntary facial muscle movements in the time course after facial nerve lesion is a sign of facial nerve regeneration.

If the nerve is not injured but the muscle is damaged, the morphology of the motor unit potential is different; see also Muscular Lesions. The intact nerve functions well, i. e., the duration of the MUAP is normal. Instead, the electrical charges in the muscle membrane are abnormal, resulting in a polyphasic shape. The amplitude, which reflects the decreased muscle mass and force of contraction, is decreased. The different waveform morphology can be classified as described in detail in ▶ Table 6.1. The important waveforms are:

- Normal biphasic motor unit potential.
- Early (sometimes polyphasic) reinnervation potentials with low amplitude and long duration.
- Giant polyphasic reinnervation potentials with high amplitude and long duration.
- Myogenic polyphasic potentials with low amplitude but in many cases normal duration.

Table 6.1 Documentation of electromyography

Side of examination	Frontalis	Oculi	Oris	Zygomaticus	Right	Left
Insertion activity						
No activity						
Normal activity (< 300 ms)						
Increased activity						
Highly increased activity						
Spontaneous activity						
No reproducible pathologic spontaneous activity						
Little pathologic spontaneous activity						
Moderate pathologic spontaneous activity						
Dense pathologic spontaneous activity						
Volitional activity						
No activity						
Single-fiber pattern						
Strongly decreased recruitment pattern						
Mildly decreased recruitment pattern						
Normal/dense recruitment pattern						
Morphology of waveform						
Normal biphasic motor unit potential						
Early polyphasic reinnervation potentials with low amplitude and long duration						
Giant polyphasic reinnervation potentials with high amplitude and long duration						
Myogenic polyphasic potentials with low amplitude but normal duration						

6.5.2 Electroneurography

Electroneurography and Needle Electromyography in the First Days of Onset of the Facial Nerve Lesion

In the first few days after the onset of an acute palsy, EMG may detect the presence of voluntary motor unit action potentials (VMUAPs). This indicates that the lesion has not yet become complete. Detection of such potentials is of particular value when the paralysis follows a traumatic insult because it means that the nerve has not been completely transected. Because the only absolute indication for exploring a facial nerve that has been compromised by trauma is transection, this may obviate the need for surgery in some cases.

There is general agreement that nerve degeneration is a sign of major neural damage leading to poor outcome in most cases. However, it is subject to debate which test is most appropriate to detect neural degeneration. Electroneurography (ENoG) has been discredited for this purpose by several authors.[19,20] Numerous investigators have had cases in which an evoked compound facial muscle action potential could not be obtained, while at the same time N-EMG detected voluntary muscle contraction. Fisch postulated that this phenomenon was due to early deblocking of nerve fibers.[21] However, a convincing pathophysiologic explanation for this puzzling finding is still lacking.

A patient who has a severed facial nerve may maintain a normal latency and normal muscle action potential for 48 to 72 hours on ENoG. Over a course of 5 to 6 days, the response to ENoG will be very quickly lost. N-EMG would reveal absent voluntary muscle action potentials at the moment of injury, but this could be true even if the nerve were only in a neurapraxic state, meaning that the presence of VMUAP is proof that the nerve is intact, but the absence does NOT mean that the nerve has been transected. Fibrillation potentials, indicating degeneration, may not appear on the N-EMG for 2 weeks after the injury. The tip of the needle should be relocated repeatedly within the muscle examined in order to search for fibrillation activity. Nevertheless, the detection of pathologic spontaneous activity by N-EMG is a much more reliable tool to identify nerve degeneration than a decreased amplitude in ENoG.[22,23] With prognostication based mainly on N-EMG, a high positive predicative value of 92.4% for favorable outcome has been shown; defective recovery was the correct prognosis in 80.8% of cases in the series. It can be summarized that N-EMG is the most appropriate tool to identify nerve degeneration as the most reliable sign predicting unfavorable outcome when detecting pathologic spontaneous activity. However, reliable prognostic information is not obtainable earlier than 10 to 14 days after onset of palsy. When N-EMG results show reduced voluntary activity but no clear sighs of denervation, ENoG, especially when repeated during the time course of the facial palsy, might be helpful.

Electroneurography in Later Phases of Facial Nerve Lesion

In the 1960s, the first attempts at clinical facial nerve testing based on electrophysiologic principles were made. The nerve excitability test stimulated the facial nerve over its main trunk while the examiner watched the patient's face for the first sign of muscle contraction (▶ Fig. 6.7). By definition, prognosis was poor if the electric current for stimulating the paretic side was more than 2.0 mA higher than in the healthy side. The maximum stimulation test followed the same setup, but supramaximal stimulation well over the level of excitation was used before comparing both sides of the face. Both the nerve excitability test and the maximum stimulation test were soon found to be seriously flawed, with subjective interpretation of results being the most obvious drawback.[24] In 1977 Esslen[25] introduced ENoG for prognostication of facial palsies. In this test, which was also called neuronography, electroneuronography, or neuromyography, the nerve is stimulated supramaximally next to the stylomastoid foramen in the retromandibular area. Using surface electrodes in the nasolabial groove, the evoked muscle contraction is recorded (▶ Fig. 6.8 and ▶ Fig. 6.9). In short Esslen's conclusions were:

- In healthy persons with no facial palsy, the left/right difference is less than 3% on average.
- In patients with facial palsy, the ratio of amplitudes between the paretic and the normal side reflects the proportion of the surviving neurons.
- If the amplitude of the paretic side is less than 10% on the 4th day of palsy, the prognosis must be considered poor.

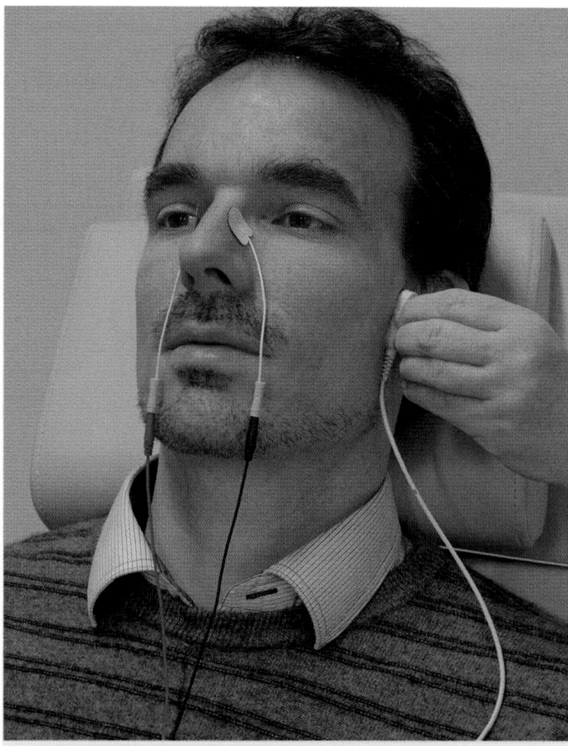

Fig. 6.7 For facial ENoG, electrodes are placed on each side of the nose. In order to test the facial nerve an electrical stimulator is used. The stimulator is placed along the side of the face just in front of the ear, and varying levels of electrical current up to 50 mA are applied. The test can be uncomfortable but is performed as quickly as possible to minimize patient discomfort. Results obtained can indicate how well the facial nerve is working and can provide information regarding the likelihood that the nerve will recover.

Esslen recommended monitoring of the facial nerve conduction by repeated ENoG over several days. A progressive decay of evoked potential amplitude is assumed to reflect ongoing neuronal degeneration. Fisch[26] further promoted ENoG and established 90% axonal degeneration as the critical value for poor prognosis depending on the rate of degeneration and the cause of paralysis. Since knowledge about physiologic side differences is a prerequisite for assessing pathologic cases, other authors have tried to reproduce Esslen's results. Until the early 1980s there were studies supporting Esslen's data; but there was also skepticism. In 1980 Adour[27] compared ENoG with maximal nerve excitability testing and discredited ENoG for high test–retest fluctuation of 16%. Unfortunately, in Adour's paper, only absolute data were given on left/right differences and information on statistical analysis that could help interpretation of the data were not supplied.

There is increasing evidence that either the intrasubject left/right differences are not as constant as initially postulated or that the recording technique is not

Nerve / point of stimulation	point of recording	Distance cm	Latency ms	Amp.2-4 mV	Duration %	Stim.
Left N facialis						
Infraauricular	M. orb. ocul.	12	3.60	2.9	100	49mA
Infraauricular	M. orb. ocul.	12	3.65	2.8	97,5	49mA
Right N facialis						
Infraauricular	M. orb. ocul.	12	3.75	0.6	100	49mA
Infraauricular	M. orb. ocul.	12	3.85	0.7	91.6	49mA

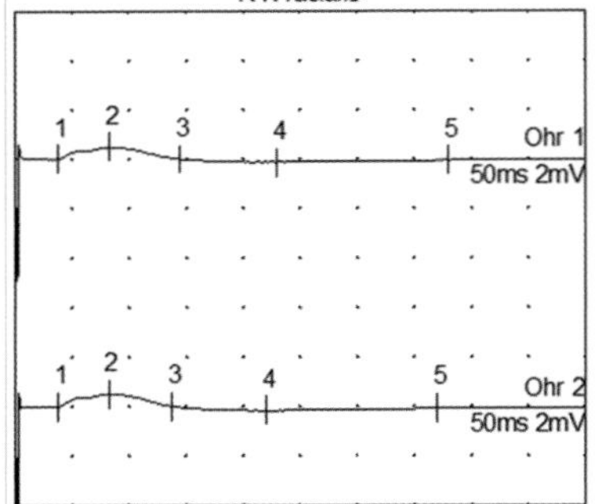

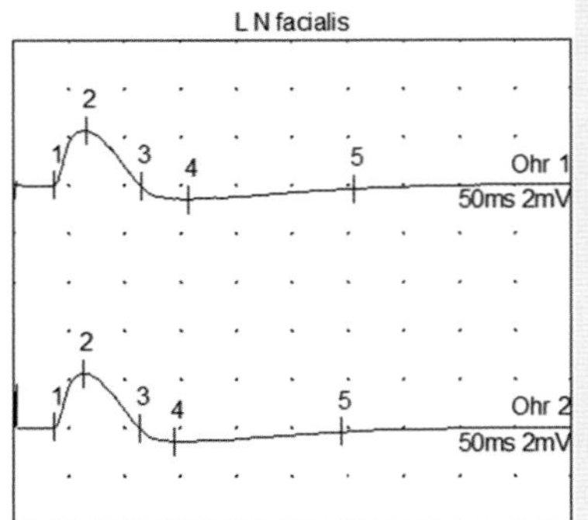

Fig. 6.8 ENoG: complete peripheral facial paresis. ENoG result:

- Right facial nerve (M. orb. ocul.): motor amplitude decreased (0.6 mV, threshold 0.8), normal latency.
- Left facial nerve (M. orb. ocul.): normal motor response.

Nerve / point of stimulation	Point of recording	Distance cm	Latency ms	Amp.2-4 mV	Duration %	Stim.
Right N facialis						
Ohr	M. orb. ocul.	12	3.70	2.1	100	58mA
Ohr	M. orb. ocul.	12	3.75	2.1	100	58mA
Left N facialis						
Ohr	M. orb. ocul.	12	4.25	1.5	100	100mA
Ohr	M. orb. ocul.	12	4.20	1.6	105	100mA

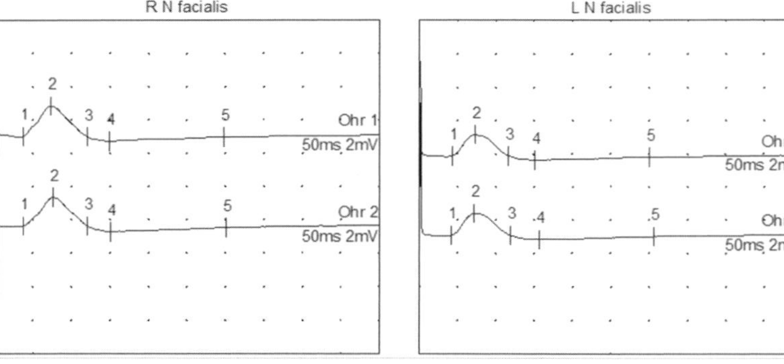

Fig. 6.9 ENoG: incomplete peripheral facial paresis. ENoG result:

- Right facial nerve (M. orb. ocul.): normal motor response, normal latency.
- Left facial nerve (M. orb. ocul.): normal motor response.

yet optimal. In 1992 Coker examined three different techniques of ENoG in normal subjects and in patients with advanced paralysis.[28] In normal subjects, side-to-side differences varied greatly depending on the recording technique applied. The mean percentages and standard deviations (SDs) ranged from 11.8 ± 9.48% SD for an optimized recording technique developed by Coker, up to 31.6 ± 32.1% SD for a standardized recording technique. However, only 10 subjects underwent a second examination in this study. Thus, this investigation is of limited value in determining the influence of time on the constancy of the evoked compound action potential. Nevertheless, Coker generally concluded that ENoG is a reliable and valid system of measurement. Conversely, there is one remarkable statement in that study alluding to Esslen's results: "In this study the only means of reducing the intrasubject side-to-side compound action potential (CAP) amplitude differences to 3% or less was to 'match' the amplitudes on the monitor during the test procedure and alter the fixed positions of electrode on both sides of the face until similar results were obtained." Neuwirth-Riedl conducted a similar study with the goal of optimizing ENoG of the facial nerve.[29] In that investigation, even under most favorable test conditions, an average side difference of 22% for the bilaterally recorded electroneurograms was found in normal test persons.

In 1998 a study was published that not only reinvestigated side-to-side differences in healthy subjects, but also for the first time evaluated retest reliability within the same subjects at four 1-week intervals.[30] It showed a mean amplitude ratio of 32.5%. Repeated measurements on the same individual differed substantially from 0 to 80%. These data did not support the hypothesis of symmetrical facial evoked compound potentials postulated by Esslen and Fisch. Furthermore, the study was able to show that the amplitude ratio is not even constant in repeated measurements of the same individual. First, variables inherent in the recording techniques were blamed, such as type of electrode, interelectrode distance, impedance, or electrode location. Stimulation technique may also be responsible, since the applied current might dissipate differently in different test persons and there might be intersubject variation in the current required to ensure supramaximal stimulation. Furthermore, there may be individual patient factors of influence such as skin resistance, different distribution of muscle mass, or different tolerance levels to the intensity of stimulation.

Nevertheless, even with high test–retest variability across time, ENoG is a tool that is widely used for monitoring facial nerve function. Patients with Bell's palsy showing greater than 90% compound action potential reduction in the affected side may be submitted to surgical decompression of the facial nerve in some centers, even in recent years.[31] However, there is evidence that predictability of recovery from Bell's palsy using ENoG is poor. Sinha was able to show that outcome was equal in 15 patients who met surgical criteria based on ENoG, but who did not undergo surgery.[20] In summary, due to intrinsic flaws in the test concept, with physiologic variability of the individual evoked compound action potential being the most important factor, results of ENoG should be interpreted with caution. ENoG does not yield a reliable prognosis and it cannot be recommended as a single source of data on which treatment decisions could be based.[23]

However, when EMG results show no clear signs of denervation, ENoG can be helpful, especially when repeated during the time course of the facial palsy (see ▶ Fig. 6.8 and ▶ Fig. 6.9).[19,22]

> **!**
>
> Electroneurography (ENoG) is a widely used tool for monitoring facial nerve function. Nevertheless, results of ENoG should be interpreted with caution. It cannot be recommended as a single source of data on which treatment decisions could be based. At best, ENoG should be used in combination with EMG.

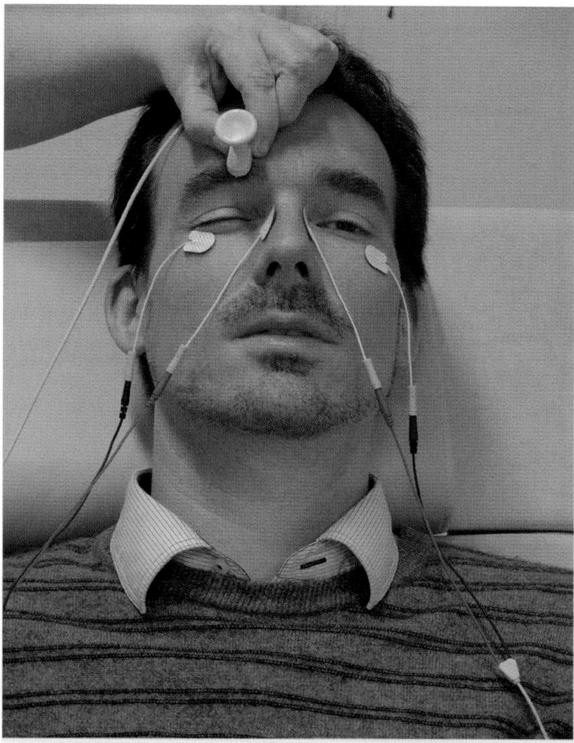

Fig. 6.10 Blink reflex. The trigeminal nerve is electrostimulated via the supraorbital nerve (V1) for studying the blink reflexes recorded from orbicularis oculi muscle.

6.5.3 Blink Reflex

The blink reflex electrical test uses an electrical stimulus for initiating a reflexive closure of the eyelids (▶ Fig. 6.10, ▶ Fig. 6.11 and ▶ Fig. 6.12), which can be detected via EMG. Often this reflex is measured with two channels and recorded with surface electrodes over the orbicularis oculi muscle (e.g., with an electrode at the lateral canthus and one below the eye).[32,33] In clinical practice, the electrical stimulus is delivered mainly above the exit of the supraorbital nerve (which can easily be located by palpating the rim of the orbit: the supraorbital foramen) with 10 to 20 mA and 0.2 millisecond duration. By rotating the stimulator, the stimulus artifact can be often lowered. The response consists of a fast, ipsilateral response in the orbicularis oculi muscle (R1) with a latency of around 10 milliseconds and a second bilateral response with a latency of about 30 milliseconds. The first response is a monosynaptic or bisynaptic response travelling from the trigeminal nerve nucleus with only one or two synapses (excitatory) on the facial nucleus and facial axons only to the muscles around the eye. Due to its monosynaptic or bisynaptic character, the response has a very fixed latency and little variability. In contrast, the R2 response is very variable and dependent

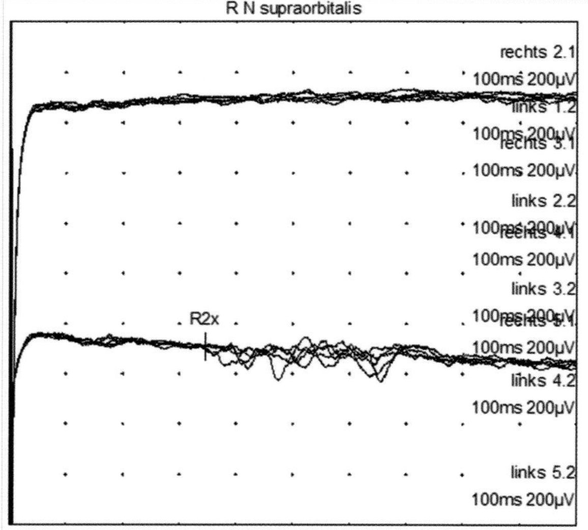

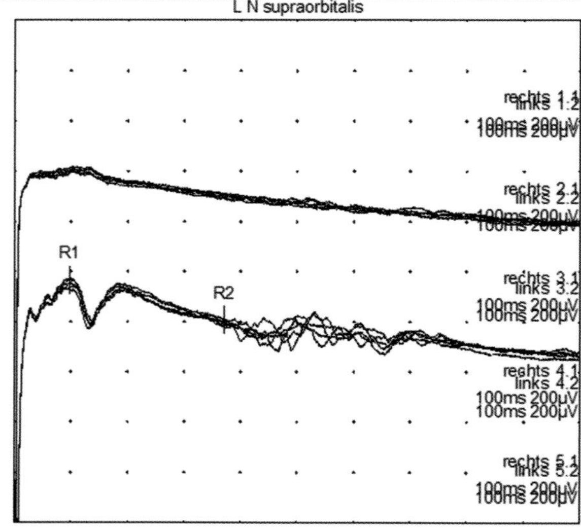

Nerve / point of stimulation	R1 ms	R2 ms	R2x ms
Right N supraorbitalis			
Left			34.50
Left N supraorbitalis			
Left	9.75	37.05	

Fig. 6.11 Blink reflexes of a complete peripheral facial paresis. Results for blink reflex:
- Right: no R1component, no R2 component.
- Left: no R2x component.

on arousal, attention, and other influences. For clinical use, the following thresholds can be used: R1 latency less than 13 milliseconds, ipsilateral R2 latency less than 41 milliseconds, and contralateral R2 latency less than 44 milliseconds. The relative latency differences between sides should be no more than 1.2 milliseconds between each R1 and no more than 8 milliseconds between each R2.[34]

Normal Values for the Blink Reflex

Stimulation of the supraorbital nerve with 10 to 20 mA and 0.2 millisecond duration, recording at the orbicularis oculi muscle:

R1 latency less than 13 milliseconds, ipsilateral R2 latency less than 41 milliseconds, and contralateral R2 latency less than 44 milliseconds. The relative latency differences between sides should be no more than 1.2 milliseconds between each R1 and no more than 8 milliseconds between each R2.

The course of the reflex is via the trigeminal nucleus, descending to the trigeminal spinal nucleus, and consequently with a bilateral projection on the facial nucleus ending again in the eyelid-closing muscles. In contrast to the electrical stimulation at the ear for standard ENoG as described above, this reflex has the advantage of measuring the facial nerve along its entire course, including its proximal part. Furthermore, a detailed analysis of the different reflex parts can point to afferent (trigeminal nerve), brainstem, or efferent lesions of the reflex arc. For example, a slowing in the trigeminal nerve results in an even slowing of all responses, including the contralateral R2, while an affliction of the facial nerve does not disturb the contralateral R2.[35]

!

The blink reflex might help to differentiate a peripheral facial nerve lesion from a trigeminal nerve lesion or a brainstem lesion.

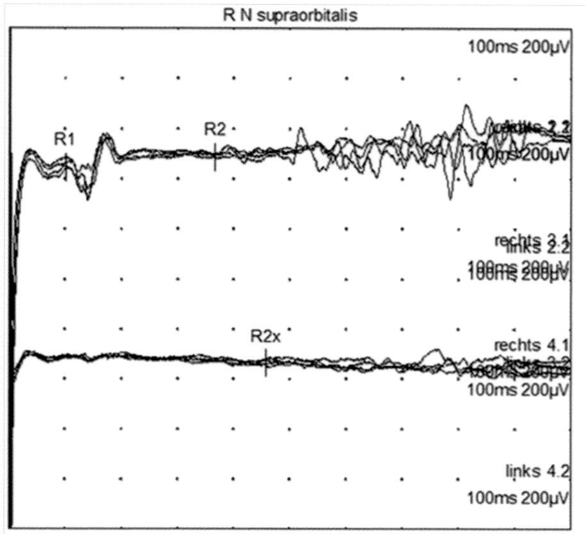

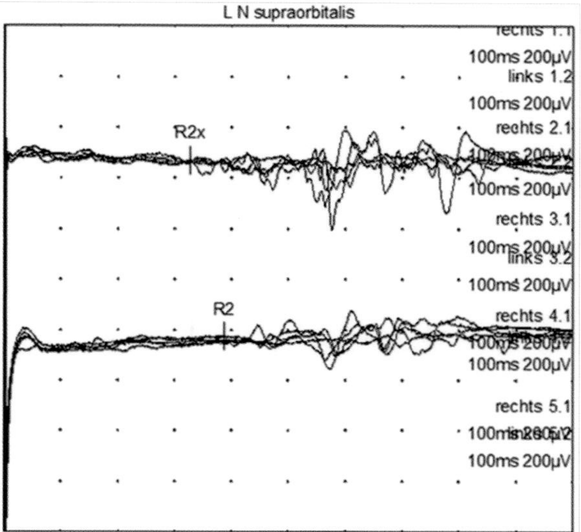

Nerve / point of stimulation	R1 ms	R2 ms	R2x ms
Left N supraorbitalis			
Right			32.75
Left		38.75	
Right N supraorbitalis			
Right	10.05		
Left			45.75
Right		36.75	

Fig. 6.12 Blink reflexes of an incomplete peripheral facial paresis. Results for blink reflex:

- Right: R2x component with increased latency (45.8 ms, threshold 39.2). Latency between R2 and R2x increased (9 ms, threshold 8).
- Left: No R1component, R2 shows increased latency (38.8 ms, threshold 38).

Another interesting aspect of the blink reflex is its change when stimulated twice in succession. Due to a form of habituation, the second response is of lower amplitude. This habituation can be diminished because of, among other things, a lack of inhibition of interneurons at the level of the brainstem. Blepharospasm, a focal dystonia affecting an involuntary closure of the eyelids, is an example of such a disease. Typically, the habituation of the blink reflex is strongly diminished in blepharospasm.[36]

6.5.4 Transcranial Magnetic Stimulation and Magnetic Evoked Potentials

Magnetic stimulation is a technique that uses fast changing magnetic fields to stimulate excitable structures. For magnetic stimulation, a magnetic field of up to 2 Tesla, but short duration of only 2 to 3 milliseconds, is generated. This magnetic field passes through tissues, including bone, without losing almost any power.[37] In conducting media such as fluids, the magnetic field is changed into an electric field, which can evoke a nerve depolarization. So, basically, the nerve is stimulated as in ENoG, with the magnetic field serving as mediator (▶ Fig. 6.13, ▶ Fig. 6.14 and ▶ Fig. 6.15). However, in contrast to electrostimulation, no direct access to the stimulated structure is necessary, and so nerve segments hidden in bony structures can be stimulated. In theory, it should be possible to magnetically stimulate the facial nerve proximal to an intratemporal lesion. It is very easy and almost painless to stimulate the facial nerve with the coil of the magnetic stimulator situated over the parieto-occipital region. At low stimulus levels (around 30–40% of the maximal output), supramaximal responses can be obtained. The technique seemed to be ideal for electrophysiologic examinations of the facial nerve, and expectations were high when it was first used. An altered response to stimulation distal to the lesion requires a

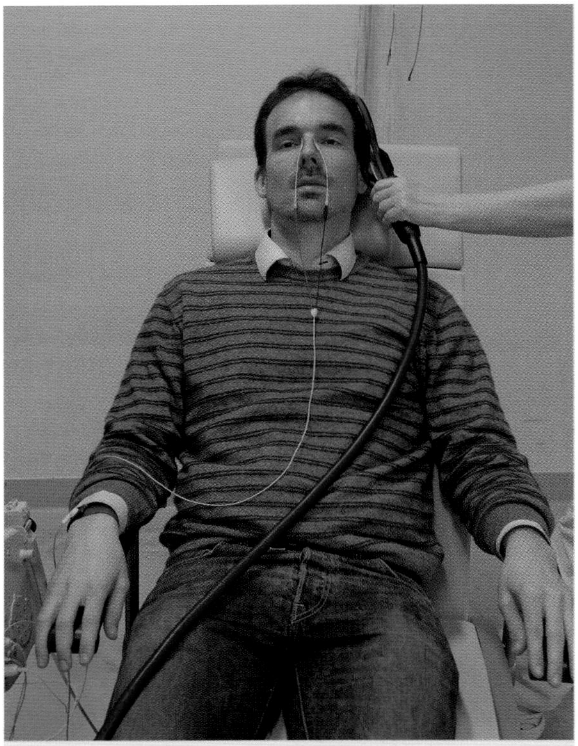

Fig. 6.13 Magnetic stimulation. For magnetic evoked potentials of the facial muscles, electrodes are placed in the same manner as for ENoG on each side of the nose to record compound action potentials. The facial nerve is stimulated with a coil inducing an electric current by a magnetic pulse in the ipsilateral inner ear canal. The correct placement of the coil is very important. If the coil is placed in a position that is too cranial, there can be a contralateral reaction by stimulation of the motor cortex.

period of 2 to 5 days before Wallerian degeneration reaches the site of stimulation (see ▶ Fig. 6.5). In contrast, magnetic stimulation can provide information regarding the severity of the injury earlier than classic electrical tests and allows for earlier estimation of prognosis in cases of Bell's palsy or trauma.

However, clinical routine use revealed several disadvantages limiting the value of magnetic stimulation. Since focusing a magnetic field is almost impossible, the location of the actual site of excitation remained unclear for quite a while. The hypothesis of stimulating the facial nerve at its nuclear origin was proven wrong; today most authors agree that the site of depolarization is the entry of the nerve into the fallopian canal.[36] Consequently, stimulation proximal to the lesion is not possible when there are pathologic changes in the cerebellopontine angle. As an alternative, stimulating the contralateral cortex is possible; however, the recorded pattern of excitation is complex and reliable interpretation of peripheral neural damage is almost impossible.[38,39]

!

Transcranial magnetic stimulation (TMS) can be used to stimulate the motor cortex to induce a facial muscle response on the contralateral side. More frequently, TMS is used to stimulate the parieto-occipital region to release a facial muscle response on the ipsilateral side; however, when TMS is used in this way, it is still unknown where exactly the facial nerve is stimulated.

The prognostic value of TMS in facial nerve palsies is low: a complete loss of excitability using magnetic stimulation has been found even in nerves that are only minimally affected.[40] In contrast to ENoG, where the progressive amplitude decay is presumed to reflect the status of the nerve, no scalable answer is recorded following magnetic stimulation. This "yes-or-no" pattern of results makes any differentiated interpretation almost impossible. As a consequence, magnetic stimulation is not used routinely, but maybe an additional option for selected cases, e.g., in unconscious patients or if a stimulation of the facial nerve proximal to the temporal bone is required.

!

Transcranial magnetic stimulation (TMS) does not allow a graduated evaluation of a facial nerve lesion. Furthermore, the prognostic value of TMS is at least doubtful. Therefore, TMS has not so far made its way into routine settings of facial electrodiagnostics.

6.5.5 Surface Electromyography

Facial movements are based upon sensitive graduated interactions of facial and masticatory muscles. Such intermuscular coordination is based on complex motor control processes, including hierarchically different levels of the central nervous system. In addition, it requires normal function of the peripheral motor nerves. Functional deficits, as appear in facial paresis, may be assessed qualitatively by clinical exploration using facial movements, but objective quantitative characterization is only possible by EMG techniques; see Physiology Behind Electrophysiologic Diagnostics. The method delivers insight into neuromuscular excitation patterns and their changes. The N-EMG allows the investigation of superficial and deep muscle layers. It is spatially highly selective because of the very small conductive surface of the needle electrode. However, N-EMG is an invasive technique and it can be painful. A single needle EMG registration is poorly reproducible and not representative for a muscle as a whole. For a neurologic diagnosis the needle electrode has to be moved into several regions of the muscle in order to

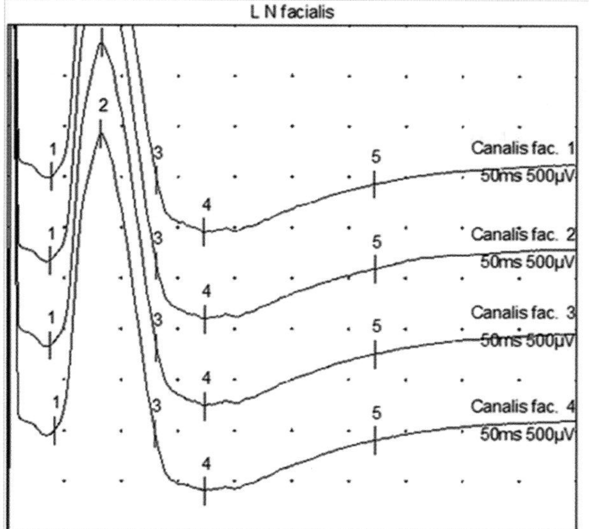

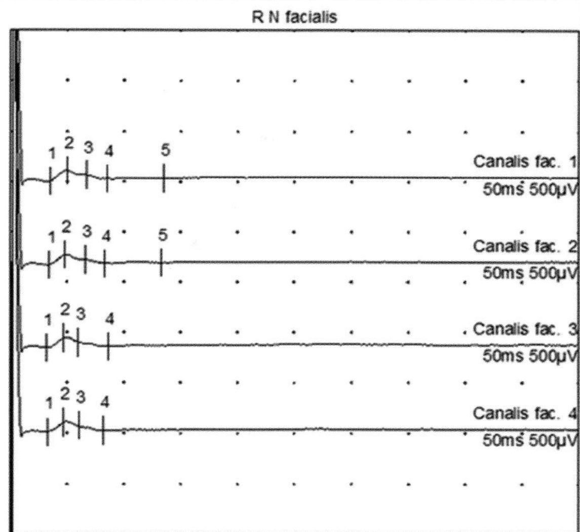

Nerve / point of stimulation	Latency ms	Ampl. mV
Right N facialis		
Canalis fac.	3.50	0.1
Canalis fac.	3.45	0.1
Canalis fac.	3.15	0.1
Canalis fac.	3.25	0.1
Left N facialis		
Canalis fac.	3.85	3.6
Canalis fac.	3.75	3.5
Canalis fac.	3.80	3.6
Canalis fac.	4.15	3.5

Fig. 6.14 Magnetic evoked potentials of a complete peripheral facial paresis.
Results:
- Right: decreased amplitude (Ampl.).
- Left: normal amplitude.

assess changes of MUAPs statistically. The spatial selectivity of the needle EMG also limits the characterization of muscle function as well as the evaluation of intermuscular coordination. The N-EMG amplitude is not suited to quantify how much different muscles are involved in a facial movement. Conversely, the multichannel S-EMG[18,41–43] enables a functional characterization of complex activity and coordination patterns of the facial muscles.

The technique for S-EMG is noninvasive. The myoelectrical activities are recorded by surface electrodes placed on the skin above the facial muscles and hence the method is free of pain. If surface electrodes are fixed, no further manipulation is necessary. Because there are no painful sensations during S-EMG examination, it does not cause stress to the patient. Therefore, S-EMG does not influence muscle contraction and coordination patterns during facial movements. Surface electrodes are not highly selective spatially. Instead, they integrate the myoelectrical activity of several motor units over a larger area as opposed to needle electrodes. In this way they include myoelectrical activity from more distant and deeper sources. Nevertheless, the more distant the source the smaller is the contribution to the measured S-EMG activity. A further advantage of S-EMG is the chance of simultaneous EMG registration from different facial muscles as well as muscle regions via multichannel application (e.g., the electrode scheme in ▶ Fig. 6.16). Such simultaneous examinations are needed because more than one muscle is generally involved in facial movements. In addition to the

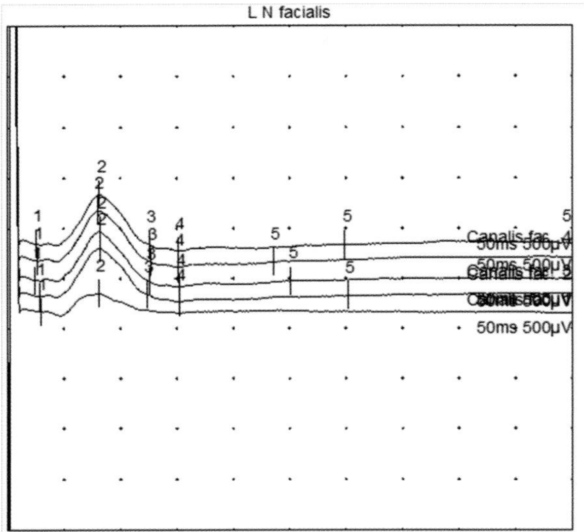

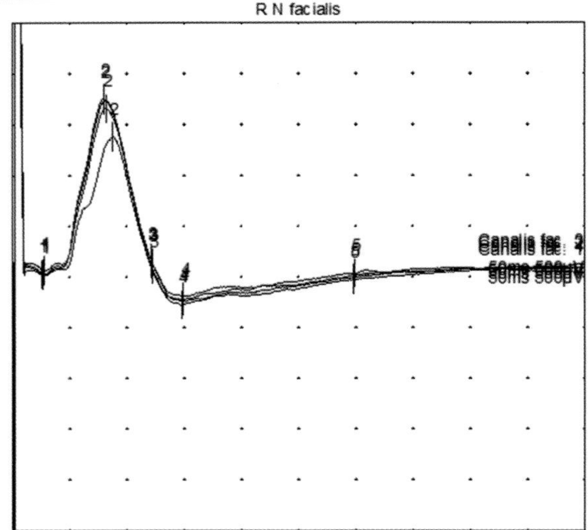

Nerve / point of stimulation	Latency ms	Ampl. mV
Left N facialis		
Canalis fac.	3.00	0.2
Canalis fac.	2.85	0.6
Canalis fac.	2.50	0.6
Canalis fac.	2.70	0.6
Canalis fac.	2.55	0.6
Right N facialis		
Canalis fac.	2.55	1.7
Canalis fac.	2.75	1.9
Canalis fac.	2.70	2.0
Canalis fac.	2.70	2.0

Fig. 6.15 Magnetic evoked potentials of an incomplete peripheral facial paresis.
Results:
- Right: normal amplitude (Ampl.).
- Left: decreased amplitude.

agonist whose origin and insertion defines the main force direction, there are also synergists actively supporting modulation of the soft tissue of the face, as well as antagonists. These antagonists always work in addition to the agonist and its synergists. Antagonistic muscle forces limit the movement of the facial soft tissue from the opposite direction. The varying force vectors of the facial muscles involved create the actual facial expression, i.e., the modeling of the soft tissue. Neuronal recruiting processes control the muscle force. Muscle forces are enhanced if the motoneuron firing rates of already working motor units increase, or additional motor units, especially greater motor units, start working. Therefore facial movements are the result of the differentiated activation of motor units and their associated muscle fibers located in different facial muscles.

> **!**
>
> Surface electromyography is the method of choice for detailed muscle analysis of the interaction of different facial muscles during distinct movements or emotional expressions.

S-EMG registers the action potentials of these motor units. The myoelectrical activity is not equal in each region of facial muscles.[44] Therefore, surface electrode positioning on the muscle is not arbitrary. It has to be specified in order to qualify the variability of the mean EMG amplitude.

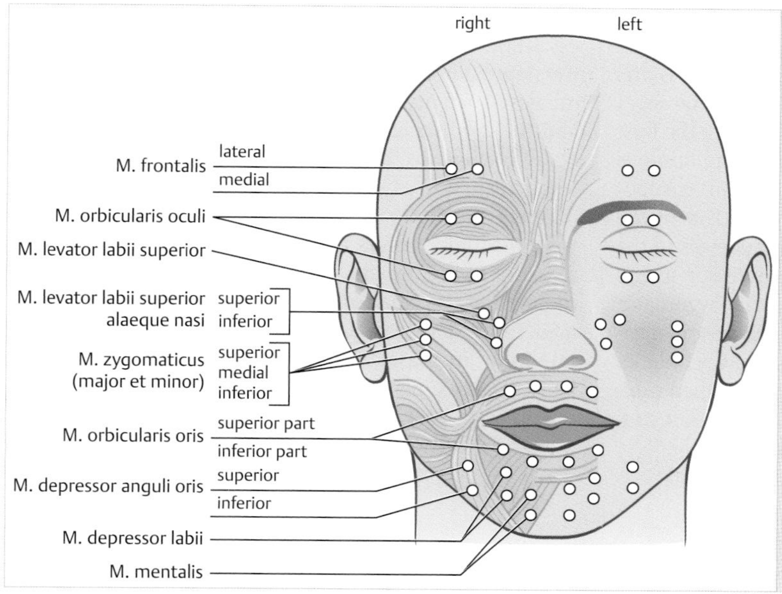

Fig. 6.16 Electrode scheme. Circles represent electrodes. (Adapted from Schumann et al 2010.[44])

Surface electromyograms may be recorded monopolarly or bipolarly. The bipolar registration is less prone to artificial interference. However, it represents only the superficial part of myoelectrical sources. To enable comparability between muscles and test series, interelectrode distance needs to be held constant and electrode pairs needs to be placed on a parallel axis to the muscle fibers.

In the following examples, a monopolar (unipolar) electrode arrangement is used (▶ Fig. 6.16). The S-EMG measurement is performed between the different electrodes above the muscles and the indifferent common reference electrode placed in a muscle-free area (e.g., earlobe). In this way, deeper muscle layers are more represented than in a bipolar electrode placement. More than one electrode can be placed on the same muscle. Therefore, it is also possible to search for intramuscular differences of myoelectrical activity distribution.

Because of their superficial position the following facial muscles are sufficiently detectable for S-EMG: frontalis, orbicularis oculi, zygomatic, levator labii superioris/levator labii superioris alaeque nasi, orbicularis oris, depressor anguli oris, depressor labii, and mentalis muscles.

These muscles are quite small. Hence, the surface electrodes used in EMG registration should have a small diameter (e.g., 4 mm). Moreover, low-weight cables between electrodes and amplifiers are needed to avoid distortion of the facial soft tissues. With respect to the reproducibility of S-EMG mean amplitude, the examiner must pay attention to the positioning of surface electrodes (▶ Fig. 6.16). The localization of electrode positions is carried out using anatomical topographic landmarks.

S-EMG is recorded while subjects perform facial movements for test purposes, including: pressing the lips together, pulling the corners of the mouth downwards, smiling (pulling the corners of the mouth upwards and backwards), depressing the lower lip, protruding the lower lip, pulling the upper lip upwards, pulling the upper lip upwards and depressing the lower lip simultaneously, pursing the lips, blowing out the cheeks, whistling with a similar tone pitch, exhaling forcefully with moderately closed lips (a more diffuse whistling), opening the lips as wide as possible while the jaw is closed, wrinkling the nose, raising the eyebrows up and wrinkling the forehead, contracting the eyebrows, closing the eyelids forcefully, squinting the eyes, closing the right eyelid, and closing the left eyelid. However, subjects who carry out instructions do not always do the same movement. Therefore, facial movements have to be defined with respect to extent, duration, and correctness of the performance. This is especially important if S-EMG is to characterize the course of disease.

After obtaining the EMG recording, the interference pattern of the electromyograms needs to be checked for artifacts. The next step of EMG analysis is quantification by calculating characteristic values of the mean EMG activity, e.g., the mean rectified EMG amplitude, root mean square, and square root of the spectral EMG power. An S-EMG registration of a single facial muscle is not very meaningful. However, simultaneous S-EMG registrations of many facial muscles allow the creation of S-EMG activity profiles of facial movements. They express the coordination between the participating facial muscles. There are facial movements showing important different coordination patterns, and others with similar muscle participation but different activation levels. Facial muscles that are not directly involved in the actual facial movement show higher mean S-EMG amplitude than at rest. Facial test movements, as commonly performed during a clinical examination of facial nerve function, show typical EMG activity profiles. For example, in both facial movements, pursing lips and whistling with a similar tone pitch, the highest mean EMG activity is found in the orbicularis oris muscle (▶ Fig. 6.17). There are intramuscular differences within the orbicularis oris muscle during pursing the lips: within the orbicularis oris the mean S-EMG amplitude is higher in the inferior part of the muscle than in its superior part, and also higher in the lateral part than in the medial part. In comparison, the EMG activity levels of the mentalis, the depressor labii, and the depressor anguli oris muscles are lower. The EMG levels of the zygomatic, levator labii superioris, and levator labii superioris alaeque nasi muscles are still lower again, but always higher than at rest. This demonstrates that the ring-shaped orbicularis oris muscle—while pursing the lips—does not contract alone, but together with other facial muscles.

During pressing the lips together (▶ Fig. 6.17), the highest S-EMG activity is found above the orbicularis oris and the depressor anguli oris muscles and there is a little less increased activity above the mentalis, the depressor labii, and the zygomatic muscles. The frontalis, the orbicularis oculi, and, in part, the levator labii superioris muscles are less activated.

Doing voluntary smiling (▶ Fig. 6.17), the maximum S-EMG activity occurs above the zygomatic muscles. The mean S-EMG amplitudes of the muscles around the mouth and the chin (orbicularis oris, mentalis, depressor labii, and depressor anguli oris muscles) also show important increases. The levator labii superioris, and the levator labii superioris alaeque nasi muscles, as well as the inferior part of the orbicularis oculi muscle, show moderate S-EMG activity.

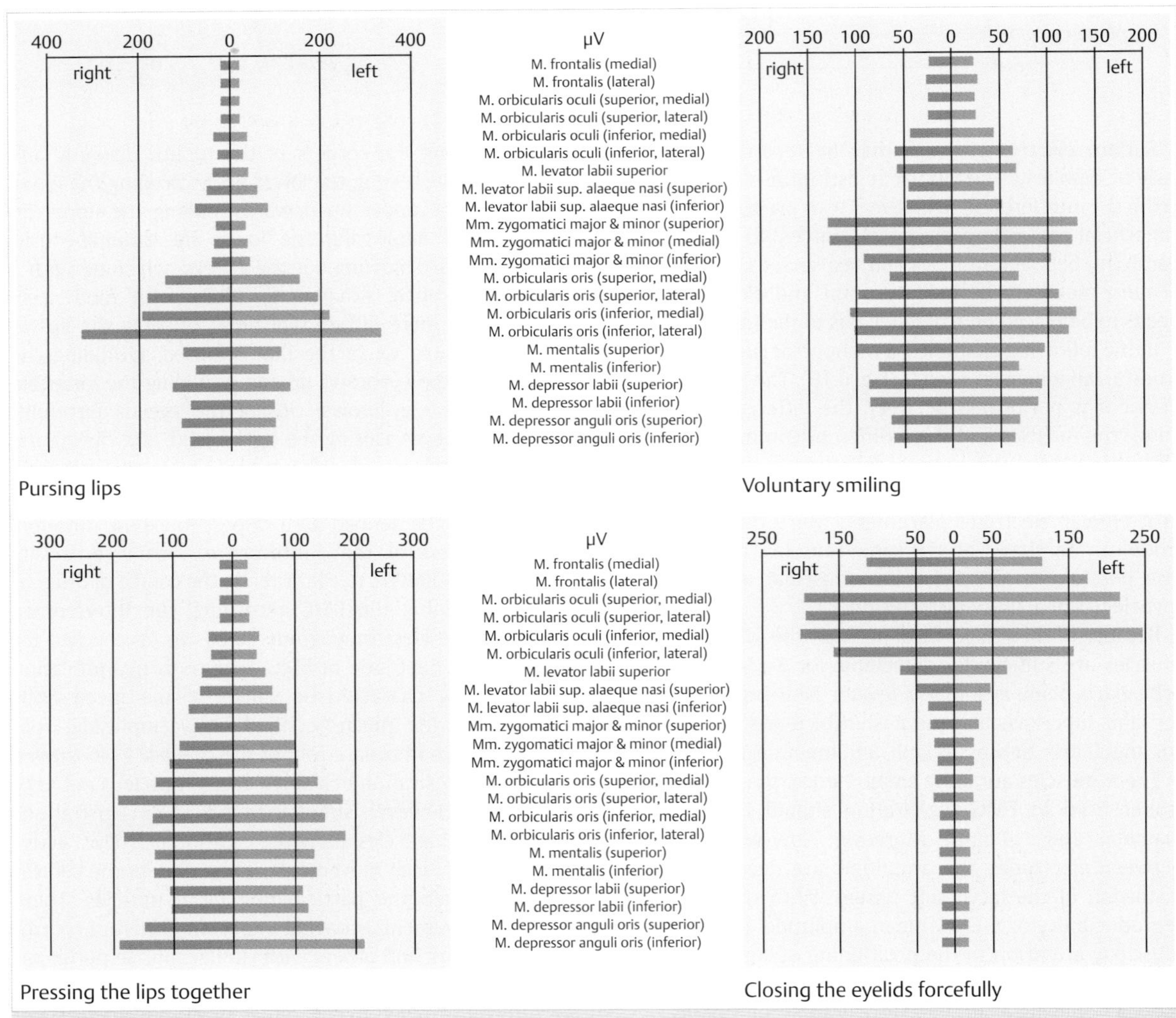

Fig. 6.17 S-EMG profiles of the 30 healthy young males while performing facial movements. Displayed is the normalized mean S-EMG amplitude (square root of spectral S-EMG power, median in microvolts [µV]) recorded monopolarly, corresponding to the electrode scheme demonstrated in ▶ Fig. 6.16. Red bars, right side; blue bars, left side.

When closing the eyelids forcefully (▶ Fig. 6.17), the S-EMG activity increases, especially above the orbicularis oculi muscle and to a lesser extent above the frontalis muscle. The other recorded facial muscles show S-EMG activity at a lower level.

Between the right and the left side of the face, no statistical differences in muscle activation were found within a sample of young healthy men (▶ Fig. 6.17). On the other hand, the individuals of this sample showed between-side differences of up to 30%. Therefore side differences in mean S-EMG amplitudes up to 30% do not indicate a disturbance of the facial muscle activation process.

When analyzing EMG activity profiles, one first notices the location of maximum EMG activity (▶ Fig. 6.17). This area signifies the muscle area most involved with a particular facial movement. As noted above, this will be the orbicularis oris muscle while pursing the lips and the zygomatic muscles while smiling voluntarily, or the orbicularis oculi muscle while closing the eyelids (▶ Fig. 6.17). In addition to these leading muscles of facial movement, further muscles can be identified that provide more fine-tuning. Based on the increase and decrease of the mean S-EMG amplitude one can see how much a muscle is involved and what significance it has for a facial movement. In addition to the orbicularis oris muscle, the mentalis, depressor labii, and depressor anguli oris muscles are also active when pursing lips or whistling, and the zygomatic, levator labii superioris, and levator labii superioris alaeque nasi contract less strongly (▶ Fig. 6.17). The mentalis muscles pull the soft tissues of the chin upwards. This process unloads the inferior part of the orbicularis oris muscle during pursing the lips.

The other muscles—considering origin and insertion—counteract the orbicularis oris muscle. Actually, they pull the lips apart. Apparently, antagonistic muscle forces are necessary in order to center the pursed lips. The depressor labii, depressor anguli oris, zygomatic, levator labii superioris, and levator labii superioris alaeque nasi muscles brace the ring-shaped contracted orbicularis oris muscle from different directions. They regulate and control the position of the pursed lips. This also means that a unilateral reduction of muscle forces caused by facial paresis leads to a change in position of the pursed lips.

!

Surface electromyography can give detailed information on compensatory mechanisms of facial movements in patients with chronic facial palsy or defective healing after facial nerve regeneration as a result of severe nerve trauma or nerve repair. This information is very useful for the treating physician to use in designing surgical or medical (botulinum toxin) therapy, and as much or more so for creating physical therapy routines.

In a patient with facial paresis (acute idiopathic peripheral paresis of the left side) (▶ Fig. 6.18) the surface EMG profiles show significant differences between the sides. The mean EMG amplitudes are smaller on the affected than on the nonaffected side.

These examples demonstrate how the S-EMG activity profiles reflect the coordination between facial muscles. Cross-talk potentially complicates the interpretation, and should be taken into account. MUAPs from facial muscles immediately below the surface are especially represented in the surface electromyogram. These muscles are not always clearly separated from a morphological point of view. To some extent they overlap each other, such as, for example, the depressor anguli oris, depressor labii, and mentalis muscles. Moreover, there are regions where the fibers of different muscles are interwoven, for example in the corner region of the mouth, the modiolus anguli oris. Due to the topographical proximity of myoelectrical sources and the propagation of MUAPs via volume conduction, cross-talk of myoelectrical activities between the closely neighboring muscles cannot be ruled out. This is a general problem of the S-EMG.[45] However, the effects of cross-talk can be narrowed down. For testing purposes, isolated contraction of a single facial muscle is hardly possible. Nevertheless, the extent of cross-talk can be estimated by varying the facial test movement, so that one or other facial muscle activates preferentially. The difference can be seen in the mean EMG amplitude of neighboring electrodes. In a monopolar (unipolar) electrode arrangement, cross-talk is also possible via the common indifferent reference electrode, even if it is placed on a muscle-free region such as the ear lobe. Muscles in close vicinity to the ear lobes can create electrical potentials there. These interferences affect all monopolar EMG channels to the same extent. They can slightly raise the base level of the mean EMG amplitude. However, the differences between the monopolar EMG channels, i.e., the differences between the facial muscles, do not change.

6.6 Key Points

- Modern techniques of electrophysiologic investigation, such as electroneurography and needle electromyography, and also multichannel surface electromyography, are important tools that allow objective assessments of facial nerve function at a comparatively early stage of palsy.
- Prognosis concerning return of facial function is possible with remarkable accuracy.
- However, at the present time, within the first days of paralysis it is impossible to identify patients developing complete degeneration with reasonable certainty.

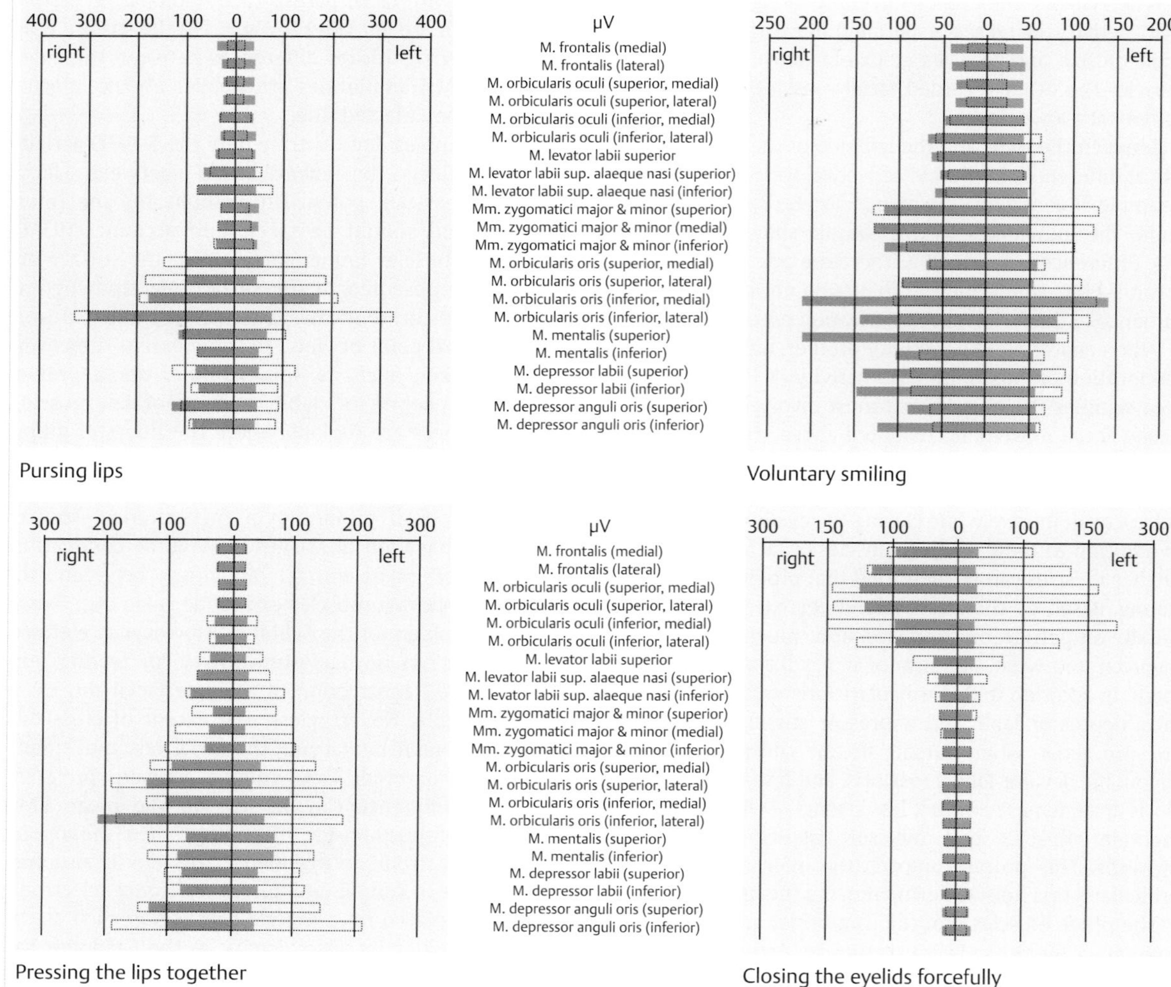

Fig. 6.18 S-EMG profiles of a patient with acute idiopathic peripheral facial paresis on the left side (31-year-old man) in comparison with the healthy control group data. The S-EMG was recorded monopolarly on the 4th day after the beginning of the paresis, corresponding to the electrode scheme in ▶ Fig. 6.16. Displayed is the mean S-EMG amplitude (square root of spectral S-EMG power, median in microvolts [µV]). Red bars, right side of the patient; blue bars, left side of the patient; white bars, healthy control group data shown in ▶ Fig. 6.17. Note the differences between the sides in the S-EMG amplitudes in the patient and the deficits in comparison with healthy control group data.

References

[1] Brackmann DE, Fetterman BL. Cranial nerve VII: facial nerve. In: Goetz GC, ed. Textbook of Clinical Neurology. Philadelphia: Saunders Elsevier; 2007:185–98

[2] Valls-Solé J. Electrodiagnostic studies of the facial nerve in peripheral facial palsy and hemifacial spasm. Muscle Nerve 2007; 36: 14–20

[3] Rowlands S, Hooper R, Hughes R, Burney P. The epidemiology and treatment of Bell's palsy in the UK. Eur J Neurol 2002; 9: 63–67

[4] Peitersen E. The natural history of Bell's palsy. Am J Otol 1982; 4: 107–111

[5] Feinstein B, Lindegard B, Nyman E, Wohlfart G. Morphologic studies of motor units in normal human muscles. Acta Anat (Basel) 1955; 23: 127–142

[6] Gilden DH. Clinical practice. Bell's palsy. N Engl J Med 2004; 351: 1323–1331

[7] Seddon HJ. Three types of nerve injury. Brain 1943; 66: 237–288

[8] Tackmann W. Disorders affecting the peripheral motor and sensory neurons. Electromyography. In: Ludin HP, ed. Handbook of EEG and Clinical Neurophysiology (revised series, volume 5). Amsterdam: Elsevier Science; 1995:321–433

[9] Urban PP, Wicht S, Vucorevic G et al. The course of corticofacial projections in the human brainstem. Brain 2001; 124: 1866–1876

[10] Özdemir C, Young RR. The results to be expected from electrical testing in the diagnosis of myasthenia gravis. Ann N Y Acad Sci 1976; 274: 203–222

[11] Kugelberg E. Electromyograms in muscular disorders. J Neurol Neurosurg Psychiatry 1947; 10: 122–133

[12] Kugelberg E. Electromyography in muscular dystrophies: differentiation between dystrophies and chronic lower motor neurone lesions. J Neurol Neurosurg Psychiatry 1949; 12: 129–136

[13] Adour KK. Facial nerve electrical testing. In Jackler RK, Brackmann DE, eds. Neurotology. St Louis: Mosby; 1994:1283

[14] Baugh RF, Basura GJ, Ishii LE et al. Clinical practice guideline: Bell's palsy. Otolaryngol Head Neck Surg 2013; 149 Suppl: S1–S27
[15] Date K, Nishimura Y, Minatogawa T, Iritani H, Satomi F, Kumoi T. The utility of single-fiber electromyography in facial nerve paralysis. Eur Arch Otorhinolaryngol 1994: S205–S207
[16] Koufman JA, Postma GN, Whang CS et al. Diagnostic laryngeal electromyography: The Wake Forest experience 1995–1999. Otolaryngol Head Neck Surg 2001; 124: 603–606
[17] Guld C, Rosenfalck A, Willison RG. Technical factors in recording electrical activity of muscle and nerve in man. Electroencephalogr Clin Neurophysiol 1970; 28: 399–413
[18] Basmajian JV, Stecko G. A new bipolar electrode for electromyography. J Appl Physiol 1962; 17: 849
[19] May M, Blumenthal F, Klein SR. Acute Bell's palsy: prognostic value of evoked electromyography, maximal stimulation, and other electrical tests. Am J Otol 1983; 5: 1–7
[20] Sinha PK, Keith RW, Pensak ML. Predictability of recovery from Bell's palsy using evoked electromyography. Am J Otol 1994; 15: 769–771
[21] Fisch U. Prognostic value of electrical tests in acute facial paralysis. Am J Otol 1984; 5: 494–498
[22] Volk GF, Klingner C, Finkensieper M, Witte OW, Guntinas-Lichius O. Prognostication of recovery time after acute peripheral facial palsy: a prospective cohort study. BMJ Open 2013; 3: e003007
[23] Grosheva M, Wittekindt C, Guntinas-Lichius O. Prognostic value of electroneurography and electromyography in facial palsy. Laryngoscope 2008; 118: 394–397
[24] May M, Harvey JE, Marovitz WF, Stroud M. The prognostic accuracy of the maximal stimulation test compared with that of the nerve excitability test in Bell's palsy. Laryngoscope 1971; 81: 931–938
[25] Esslen E. The acute facial palsies: investigations on the localization and pathogenesis of meato-labyrinthine facial palsies. Schriftenr Neurol 1977; 18: 1–164
[26] Fisch U. Maximal nerve excitability testing vs electroneuronography. Arch Otolaryngol 1980; 106: 352–357
[27] Adour KK, Sheldon MI, Kahn ZM. Maximal nerve excitability testing versus neuromyography: prognostic value in patients with facial paralysis. Laryngoscope 1980; 90: 1540–1547
[28] Coker NJ. Facial electroneurography: analysis of techniques and correlation with degenerating motoneurons. Laryngoscope 1992; 102: 747–759
[29] Neuwirth-Riedl K, Burian M, Nekahm D, Gstöttner W. Optimizing of electroneuronography of the facial nerve. ORL J Otorhinolaryngol Relat Spec 1990; 52: 360–367
[30] Sittel C, Guntinas-Lichius O, Streppel M, Stennert E. Variability of repeated facial nerve electroneurography in healthy subjects. Laryngoscope 1998; 108: 1177–1180
[31] Gantz BJ, Rubinstein JT, Gidley P, Woodworth GG. Surgical management of Bell's palsy. Laryngoscope 1999; 109: 1177–1188
[32] Trontelj MA, Trontelj JV. Reflex arc of the first component of the human blink reflex: a single motoneurone study. J Neurol Neurosurg Psychiatry 1978; 41: 538–547
[33] Ongerboer de Visser BW. Afferent limb of the human jaw reflex: electrophysiologic and anatomic study. Neurology 1982; 32: 563–566
[34] Kennelly KD. Electrodiagnostic approach to cranial neuropathies. Neurol Clin 2012; 30: 661–684
[35] Kimura J, Powers JM, Van Allen MW. Reflex response of orbicularis oculi muscle to supraorbital nerve stimulation. Study in normal subjects and in peripheral facial paresis. Arch Neurol 1969; 21: 193–199
[36] Zwarts MJ, van Weerden TW. Electrodiagnostics of the facial nerve. In: Beurskens CHG, eds. The Facial Palsies: Complementary Approaches. Utrecht: Lemma; 2005
[37] Benecke R, Meyer BU, Schönle P, Conrad B. Transcranial magnetic stimulation of the human brain: responses in muscles supplied by cranial nerves. Exp Brain Res 1988; 71: 623–632
[38] Rimpiläinen I, Karma P, Eskola H, Häkkinen V. Magnetic facial nerve stimulation in normal subjects. Three groups of responses. Acta Otolaryngol Suppl 1992; 492: 99–102
[39] Rösler KM, Hess CW, Schmid UD. Investigation of facial motor pathways by electrical and magnetic stimulation: sites and mechanisms of excitation. J Neurol Neurosurg Psychiatry 1989; 52: 1149–1156
[40] Schriefer TN, Mills KR, Murray NM, Hess CW. Evaluation of proximal facial nerve conduction by transcranial magnetic stimulation. J Neurol Neurosurg Psychiatry 1988; 51: 60–66
[41] Ohyama M, Obata E, Furuta S, Sakamoto K, Ohbori Y, Iwabuchi Y. Face EMG Topographic analysis of mimetic movements in patients with Bell's palsy. Acta Otolaryngol Suppl 1988; 446: 47–56
[42] Cacou C, Greenfield BE, Hunt NP, McGrouther DA. Patterns of coordinated lower facial muscle function and their importance in facial reanimation. Br J Plast Surg 1996; 49: 274–280
[43] Lapatki BG, Stegeman DF, Jonas IE. A surface EMG electrode for the simultaneous observation of multiple facial muscles. J Neurosci Methods 2003; 123: 117–128
[44] Schumann NP, Bongers K, Guntinas-Lichius O, Scholle HC. Facial muscle activation patterns in healthy male humans: a multi-channel surface EMG study. J Neurosci Methods 2010; 187: 120–128
[45] Dimitrov GV, Disselhorst-Klug C, Dimitrova NA, Schulte E, Rau G. Simulation analysis of the ability of different types of multi-electrodes to increase selectivity of detection and to reduce cross-talk. J Electromyogr Kinesiol 2003; 13: 125–138

7 Grading

Orlando Guntinas-Lichius and Mira Finkensieper

7.1 Introduction

There is still no international agreement or even any national consensus for reporting the facial malfunction at onset of a facial palsy or for reporting the recovery and long-term sequelae.[1,2] Clinicians need a uniform, objective, accurate, reliable, easy, and sensitive facial grading system to determine facial function that requires little time at low cost. This ideal method has yet to be found. The current most frequently used grading system to describe the motor deficits of mimic function, the nonmotor malfunctions, and also to assess the communicative and emotional impact are summarized in this chapter. The advantages and disadvantages of the different facial grading systems are presented.

7.2 Definition

Facial nerve grading covers all methods of formally assessing the functions related to the facial nerve. Grading should be able to evaluate the consequences of an acute or chronic facial palsy. Primarily, a facial nerve grading system describes the motor function or dysfunction of the mimic muscles that serve as the most important component of nonverbal communication and emotional expression. The assessment of the motor function can be performed at rest (static function) and during voluntary facial movements (dynamic function). Facial nerve grading can also cover the assessment of the nonmotor functions of the facial nerve, especially of the visceroefferent nerve fibers (to the parotid and lacrimal gland), and visceroafferent nerve fibers (for taste sensation). Facial nerve grading should also describe the defective healing after aberrant regeneration of the facial nerve including motor and nonmotor dysfunction. Finally, facial nerve grading is divided into subjective grading and objective grading. Subjective grading is performed by a professional rater or by the patient himself. In contrast, objective grading is performed using mathematical measurements and computer-based analysis.

!

Facial nerve grading can include the assessment of facial function at rest and during voluntary facial movements, defective healing, nonmotor function, nonverbal communication, and emotional expression.

7.3 Subjective Grading

Most evaluation systems used today are subjective depending on the judgment of a trained observer. Most subjective systems are easy to apply, but all these methods have issues with the lack of a sensitive, reproducible, and quantitative analysis. Patients' examples for subjective grading with several actually applied systems are presented in ▶ Fig. 7.1, ▶ Fig. 7.2, and ▶ Fig. 7.3. The reliability of a grading system is determined by the sum of errors made by each examiner in a test–retest situation (intraobserver reliability). A reliable method also implies a low interobserver variability defined as a minimal difference in the score obtained by different examiners. Systematic grading started in the 1960s with the gross five-point scales by Botman and Jongkees,[3] and another by Peitersen.[4] Adour and Swanson in the early 1980s were the first to develop a weighted system giving the eye and mouth region more weight than the forehead region.[5] All these and some other less well-known systems are no longer popular, but they prepared the ground for the subsequent systems that are used nowadays.

Most subjective systems lack reliable and quantitative data on facial muscle function, and often have an insufficient intraobserver and interobserver reliability.

7.3.1 House–Brackmann Facial Grading System

House improved the Botman and Jongkees system subclassifying the moderate degrees of facial palsy.[6] At the same time Brackmann developed the first objective method to evaluate facial function.[7] In his system movements of eye and mouth are measured using a 0.25 mm scale. The affected and the healthy side are compared. Both systems were the basis for the House–Brackmann facial grading system.[8] It is a well-accepted grading system. It was adopted by the American Academy of Otolaryngology—Head and Neck Surgery (AAOHNS) in 1985 and recommended as the American standard for the assessment of facial nerve function by the Facial Nerve Disorders Committee (of the AAOHNS) (▶ Table 7.1). The retest reliability is reported to have 77% correlation. In contrast, the interobserver variability is reported to be lower than 10% in some studies, but in other studies it is significantly higher.[9] Using the House–Brackmann facial grading system, the most difficult area for grading is

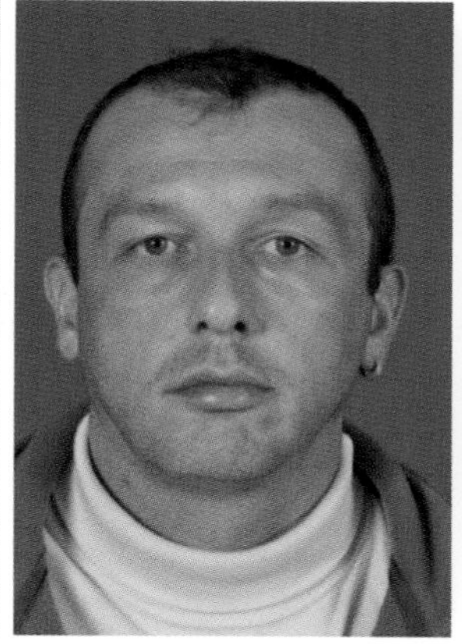

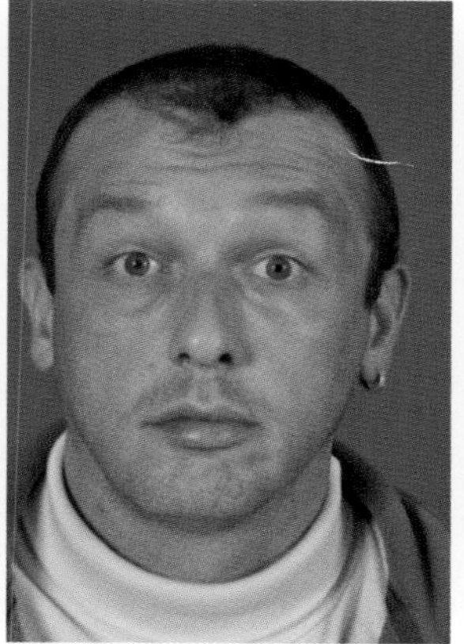

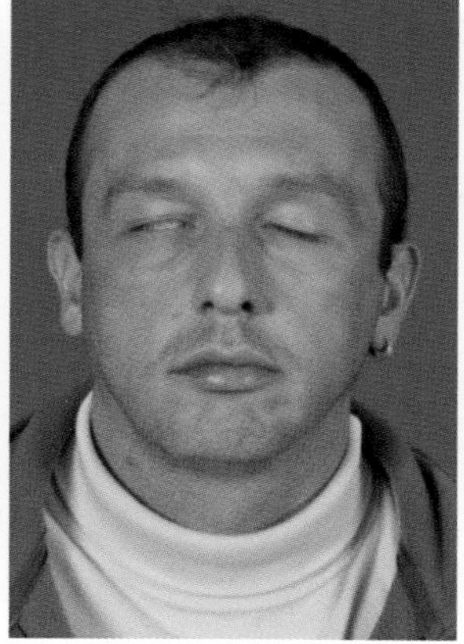

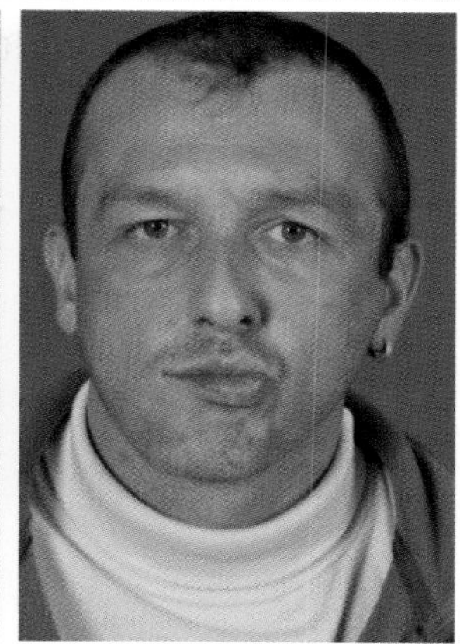

House–Brackmann Facial Grading System

Grade	Description	Characteristics
I	Normal	Normal facial function in all areas
II	Slight dysfunction	Gross: slight weakness noticeable on close inspection; may have very slight synkinesis. At rest: normal symmetry and tone. Motion: forehead-moderate to good function; eye-complete closure with minimum effort: mouth-slight asymmetry.
(III)	Moderate dysfunction	Gross: obvious but not disfiguring difference between two sides; noticeable but not severe synkinesis, contracture, and/or hemifacial spasm. At rest: normal symmetry and tone. Motion: forehead-slight to moderate movement; eye-complete closure with effort; mouth-slightly week with maximum effort.
IV	Moderately severe dysfunction	Gross: obvious weakness and/or disfiguring asymmetry. At rest: normal symmetry and tone. Motion: forehead-none; eye-incomplete closure; mouth-asymmetric with maximum effort.
V	Severe dysfunction	Gross: only barely perceptible motion. At rest: asymmetry. Motion: forehead-none; eye-incomplete closure; mouth-slight movement.
VI	Total paralysis	No movement

Stennert´s Facial Paralysis Index

Characteristics	No	Yes
At rest:		
Difference between palpebral fissures ≥ 3mm	✕	
Ectropion	✕	
Loss of nasolabial sulcus (if present on normal side)	✕	
Drop of angle of the mouth ≥ 3mm	✕	
Motion:		
Frowning: Less than 50% of normal side	✕	
Incomplete lid closure: by slight innervation (as in sleep)		✕
Incomplete lid closure: by maximal innervation	✕	
By exposure of teeth: Upper and lower canine teeth not visible	✕	
By exposure of teeth: 2nd upper incisor not visible in full width	✕	
Whistling: Less than 50% decrease in distance between filtrum and angulus oris compared to normal side	✕	
Paralysis index (maximal 10 points):		0/1

Sunnybrook (Toronto) Facial Grading System Part A

Resting symmetry compared to normal side (choose one description only)		
Eye	Normal	⓪
	Narrow	1
	Wide	1
	Eyelid surgery	1
Cheek (Nasolabial fold)	Normal	⓪
	Absent	2
	Less pronounced	1
	More pronounced	1
Mouth	Normal	⓪
	Corner dropped	1
	Corner pulled up/out	1
	Resting symmetry score = Total x 5 =	0

Part B

Standard expressions	Symmetry of voluntary movement (degree of muscle excursion compared to normal side): Unable to initiate movement/ no movement -Gross asymmetry	Initiate slight movement -Severe asymmetry	Initiate movement with mild excursion -Moderate asymmetry	Movement almost complete -Mild asymmetry	Movement complete -Symmetry	Synkinesis (degree of involuntary muscle contraction): None: No synkinesis or mass movement	Mild: Slight synkinesis	Moderate: Obvious but not disfiguring synkinesis	Severe: Disfiguring synkinesis/ Gross mass movements
Forehead wrinkle	1	2	3	④	5	⓪	1	2	3
Gentle eye closure	1	2	③	4	5	⓪	1	2	3
Open mouth smile	1	2	3	④	5	⓪	1	2	3
Snari	1	2	3	④	5	⓪	1	2	3
Lid pucker	1	2	③	4	5	⓪	1	2	3
	Voluntary movement score = Total x 4 = 72					Synkinesis score = Total = 0			
Composite score = Voluntary movement score-Resting symmetry score-Synkinesis score = 72									

Fig. 7.1 Grading of acute incomplete facial palsy. Grading of an acute palsy might be difficult or even impossible when using a grading system which includes an evaluation of facial synkinesis. Because of the absence of time to develop synkinesis, grading of synkinesis in cases of acute facial palsy is impossible.

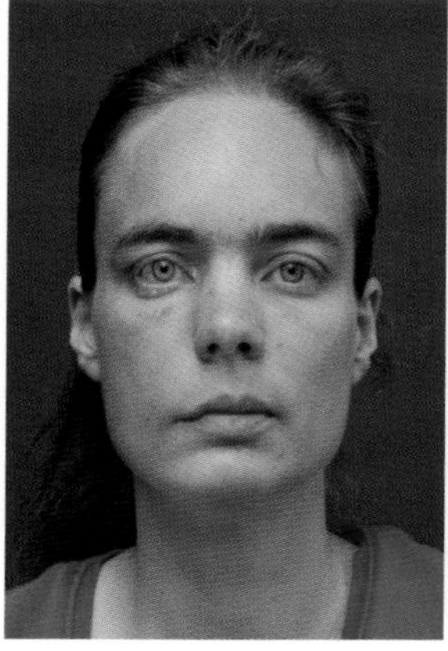
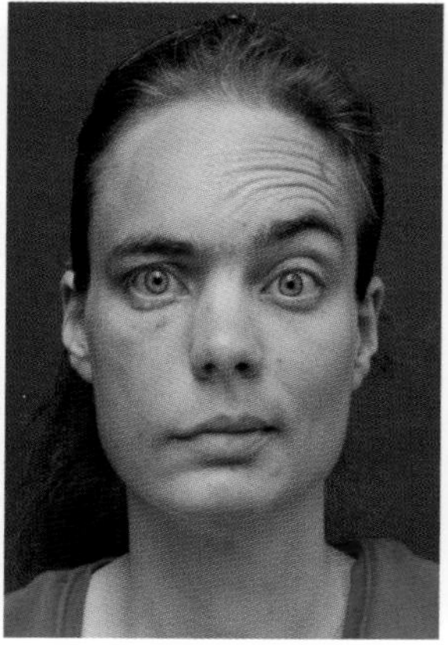
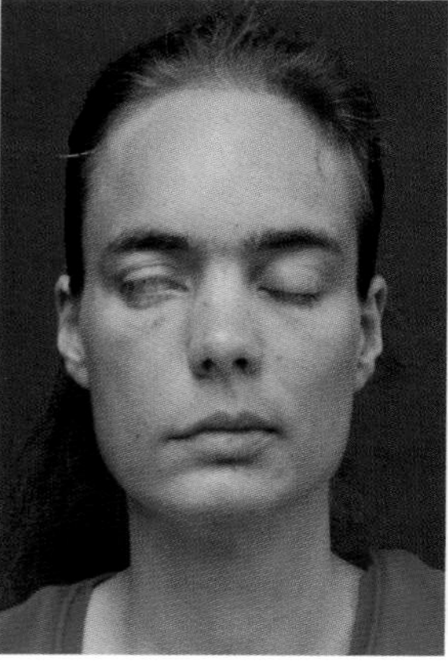
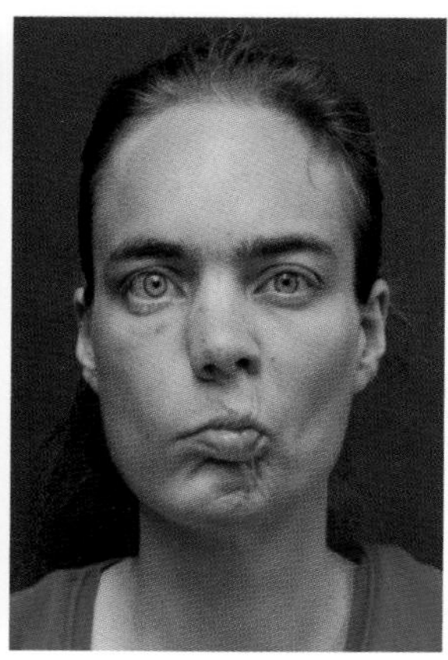

House–Brackmann Facial Grading System

Grade	Description	Characteristics
I	Normal	Normal facial function in all areas
II	Slight dysfunction	Gross: slight weakness noticeable on close inspection; may have very slight synkinesis. At rest: normal symmetry and tone. Motion: forehead-moderate to good function; eye-complete closure with minimum effort: mouth-slight asymmetry.
III	Moderate dysfunction	Gross: obvious but not disfiguring difference between two sides; noticeable but not severe synkinesis, contracture, and/or hemifacial spasm. At rest: normal symmetry and tone. Motion: forehead-slight to moderate movement; eye-complete closure with effort; mouth-slightly week with maximum effort.
IV	Moderately severe dysfunction	Gross: obvious weakness and/or disfiguring asymmetry. At rest: normal symmetry and tone. Motion: forehead-none; eye-incomplete closure; mouth-asymmetric with maximum effort.
(V)	Severe dysfunction	Gross: only barely perceptible motion. At rest: asymmetry. Motion: forehead-none; eye-incomplete closure; mouth-slight movement.
VI	Total paralysis	No movement

Stennert´s Facial Paralysis Index

Characteristics	No	Yes
At rest:		
Difference between palpebral fissures ≥ 3mm		X
Ectropion	X	
Loss of nasolabial sulcus (if present on normal side)		X
Drop of angle of the mouth ≥ 3mm		X
Motion:		
Frowning: Less than 50% of normal side		X
Incomplete lid closure: by slight innervation (as in sleep)		X
Incomplete lid closure: by maximal innervation		X
By exposure of teeth: Upper and lower canine teeth not visible		X
By exposure of teeth: 2nd upper incisor not visible in full width		X
Whistling: Less than 50% decrease in distance between filtrum and angulus oris compared to normal side		X
Paralysis index (maximal 10 points):		3/6

Sunnybrook (Toronto) Facial Grading System Part A

Resting symmetry compared to normal side (choose one description only)		
Eye	Normal	0
	Narrow	1
	Wide	(1)
	Eyelid surgery	1
Cheek (Nasolabial fold)	Normal	0
	Absent	2
	Less pronounced	(1)
	More pronounced	1
Mouth	Normal	0
	Corner dropped	(1)
	Corner pulled up/out	1
	Resting symmetry score = Total x 5 =	15

Part B

Standard expressions	Symmetry of voluntary movement (degree of muscle excursion compared to normal side): Unable to initiate movement/ no movement -Gross asymmetry	Initiate slight movement -Severe asymmetry	Initiate movement with mild excursion -Moderate asymmetry	Movement almost complete -Mild asymmetry	Movement complete -Symmetry	Synkinesis (degree of involuntary muscle contraction): None: No synkinesis or mass movement	Mild: Slight synkinesis	Moderate: Obvious but not disfiguring synkinesis	Severe: Disfiguring synkinesis/ Gross mass movements
Forehead wrinkle	(1)	2	3	4	5	(0)	1	2	3
Gentle eye closure	1	2	(3)	4	5	(0)	1	2	3
Open mouth smile	1	(2)	3	4	5	(0)	1	2	3
Snari	1	(2)	3	4	5	(0)	1	2	3
Lid pucker	1	(2)	3	4	5	(0)	1	2	3
	Voluntary movement score = Total x 4 = 40					Synkinesis score = Total = 0			
Composite score = Voluntary movement score-Resting symmetry score-Synkinesis score = 25									

Fig. 7.2 Grading of acute complete facial palsy.

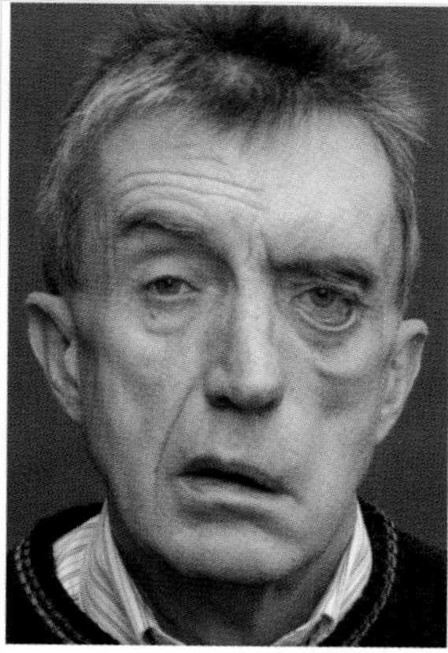
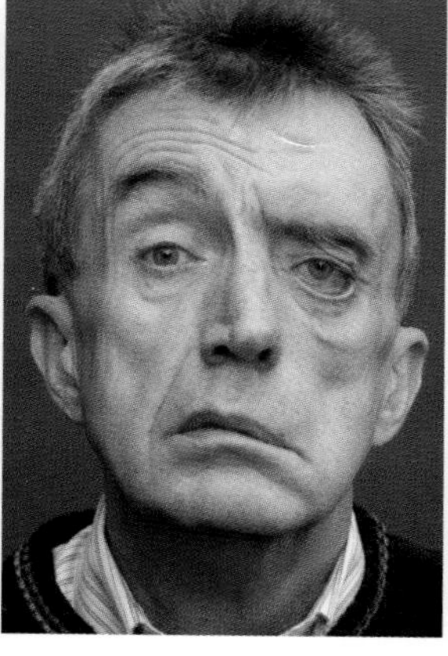
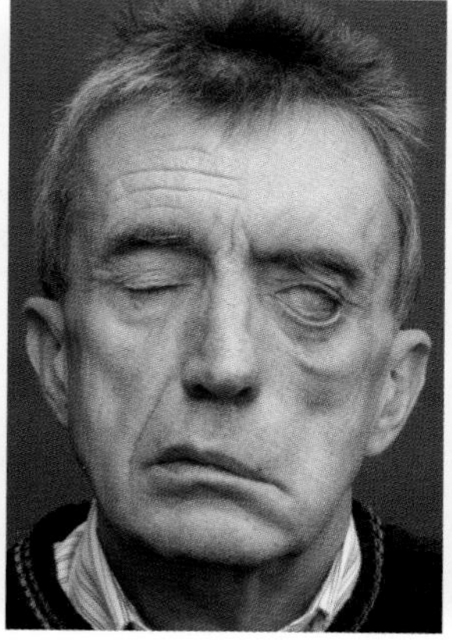
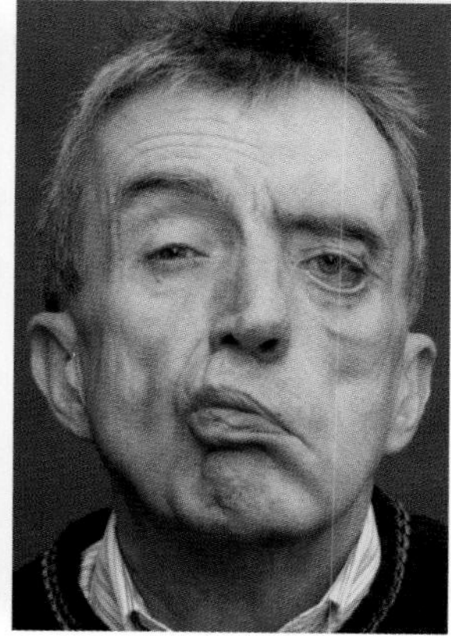

House–Brackmann Facial Grading System

Grade	Description	Characteristics
I	Normal	Normal facial function in all areas
II	Slight dysfunction	Gross: slight weakness noticeable on close inspection; may have very slight synkinesis. At rest: normal symmetry and tone. Motion: forehead-moderate to good function; eye-complete closure with minimum effort: mouth-slight asymmetry.
III	Moderate dysfunction	Gross: obvious but not disfiguring difference between two sides; noticeable but not severe synkinesis, contracture, and/or hemifacial spasm. At rest: normal symmetry and tone. Motion: forehead-slight to moderate movement; eye-complete closure with effort; mouth-slightly week with maximum effort.
IV	Moderately severe dysfunction	Gross: obvious weakness and/or disfiguring asymmetry. At rest: normal symmetry and tone. Motion: forehead-none; eye-incomplete closure; mouth-asymmetric with maximum effort.
V	Severe dysfunction	Gross: only barely perceptible motion. At rest: asymmetry. Motion: forehead-none; eye-incomplete closure; mouth-slight movement.
(VI)	Total paralysis	No movement

Stennert´s Facial Paralysis Index

Characteristics	No	Yes
At rest:		
Difference between palpebral fissures ≥ 3mm		✕
Ectropion		✕
Loss of nasolabial sulcus (if present on normal side)		✕
Drop of angle of the mouth ≥ 3mm		✕
Motion:		
Frowning: Less than 50% of normal side		✕
Incomplete lid closure: by slight innervation (as in sleep)		✕
Incomplete lid closure: by maximal innervation		✕
By exposure of teeth: Upper and lower canine teeth not visible		✕
By exposure of teeth: 2nd upper incisor not visible in full width		✕
Whistling: Less than 50% decrease in distance between filtrum and angulus oris compared to normal side		✕
Paralysis index (maximal 10 points):		4/6

Sunnybrook (Toronto) Facial Grading System Part A

Resting symmetry compared to normal side (choose one description only)		
Eye	Normal	0
	Narrow	1
	Wide	(1)
	Eyelid surgery	1
Cheek (Nasolabial fold)	Normal	0
	Absent	(2)
	Less pronounced	1
	More pronounced	1
Mouth	Normal	0
	Corner dropped	(1)
	Corner pulled up/out	1
	Resting symmetry score = Total x 5 =	20

Part B

Standard expressions	Symmetry of voluntary movement (degree of muscle excursion compared to normal side): Unable to initiate movement/ no movement -Gross asymmetry	Initiate slight movement -Severe asymmetry	Initiate movement with mild excursion -Moderate asymmetry	Movement almost complete -Mild asymmetry	Movement complete -Symmetry	Synkinesis (degree of involuntary muscle contraction): None: No synkinesis or mass movement	Mild: Slight synkinesis	Moderate: Obvious but not disfiguring synkinesis	Severe: Disfiguring synkinesis/ Gross mass movements
Forehead wrinkle	(1)	2	3	4	5	(0)	1	2	3
Gentle eye closure	1	(2)	3	4	5	(0)	1	2	3
Open mouth smile	(1)	2	3	4	5	(0)	1	2	3
Snari	(1)	2	3	4	5	(0)	1	2	3
Lid pucker	(1)	2	3	4	5	(0)	1	2	3
	Voluntary movement score = Total x 4 = 24					Synkinesis score = Total = 0			
Composite score = Voluntary movement score-Resting symmetry score-Synkinesis score = 4									

Fig. 7.3 Grading of chronic complete facial palsy.

Table 7.1 House–Brackmann Facial Grading System

Grade	Description	Characteristics
I	Normal	Normal facial function in all areas
II	Slight dysfunction	Gross: slight weakness noticeable on close inspection; may have very slight synkinesis At rest: normal symmetry and tone Motion: forehead—moderate to good function; eye—complete closure with minimum effort; mouth—slight asymmetry
III	Moderate dysfunction	Gross: obvious but not disfiguring difference between two sides; noticeable but not severe synkinesis, contracture, and/or hemifacial spasm At rest: normal symmetry and tone Motion: forehead—slight to moderate movement; eye—complete closure with effort; mouth—slightly weak with maximum effort
IV	Moderately severe dysfunction	Gross: obvious weakness and/or disfiguring asymmetry At rest: normal symmetry and tone Motion: forehead—none; eye—incomplete closure; mouth—asymmetric with maximum effort
V	Severe dysfunction	Gross: only barely perceptible motion At rest: asymmetry Motion: forehead—none; eye—incomplete closure; mouth—slight movement
VI	Total paralysis	No movement

Source: House and Brackmann 1985.[8]

generally the separation between grades 3 and 4.[10] The House–Brackmann facial grading system and almost all other subjective grading scales were not designed to assess facial nerve function after nerve reconstruction or facial reanimation. They were also not designed to be used acutely because they rely on changes over time (such as synkinesia). As with other systems the House–Brackmann system is hard to use it when parts of the face have varying degrees of recovery.

Although the House–Brackmann facial grading system is the most popular facial nerve grading system, be aware of its limitations.

7.3.2 Yanagihara's Facial Grading Scale

In the 1980s Yanagihara developed a simple unweighted system assessing the face at rest and by nine movements, first with a five-point scale, and in a later version with a three-point scale (▶ Table 7.2).[11] In his hands, the three-point scale was as effective as the five-point scale. Symptoms of defective healing are not considered. This grading system continues to be a standard method in Japan. Evaluations by physicians using this system correlate well with self-evaluations by patients.

7.3.3 Stennert's Index

Stennert's grading system was also developed in the 1980s and is still popular in Europe.[12] It describes facial function in more detail. It is a double-weighted system that places a value on the face at rest that is lower than the value for motion (40% versus 60%). Moreover, the movement of the mouth is weighted higher than the other facial regions (▶ Table 7.3). Secondary defects are assessed separately (▶ Table 7.4). Hence, it is designed to scale either acute or chronic facial paralyses. As yet there are no data regarding test–retest reliability and interobserver variability. Stennert's index is used primarily in Europe.

7.3.4 May Facial Nerve Grading Scale

The May facial nerve grading scale was specially developed to describe the facial function after reconstructive surgery (▶ Table 7.5)[13]; however, it is limited by its subjectivity and has not yet found general acceptance.

7.3.5 Sunnybrook (Toronto) Facial Grading System

The Sunnybrook (Toronto) facial grading system was published in 1996 and is also a subjective grading system.[14] It is very popular nowadays and has been used in several recent studies on facial palsy and facial nerve recovery.

Table 7.2 Yanagihara's Facial Grading Scale

Characteristic	Scale of five rating						Scale of three rating		
At rest	0	1	2	3	4	5	0	2	4
Wrinkle forehead	0	1	2	3	4	5	0	2	4
Blink	0	1	2	3	4	5	0	2	4
Closure of eye lightly	0	1	2	3	4	5	0	2	4
Closure of eye tightly	0	1	2	3	4	5	0	2	4
Closure of eye on involved side only	0	1	2	3	4	5	0	2	4
Wrinkle nose	0	1	2	3	4	5	0	2	4
Whistle	0	1	2	3	4	5	0	2	4
Grin	0	1	2	3	4	5	0	2	4
Depress lower lip	0	1	2	3	4	5	0	2	4

Source: Yanagihara 1977.[11]

Table 7.3 Stennert's Facial Paralysis Index

Characteristics	No	Yes (1 point)
At rest:		
Difference between palpebral fissures ≥ 3 mm		
Ectropion		
Loss of nasolabial sulcus (if present on normal side)		
Droop of angle of the mouth ≥ 3 mm		
Motion:		
Frowning: less than 50% of normal side		
Incomplete lid closure: by slight innervation (as in sleep)		
Incomplete lid closure: by maximal innervation		
By exposure of teeth: upper and lower canine teeth not visible		
By exposure of teeth: 2nd upper incisor not visible in full width		
Whistling: less than 50% decrease in distance between philtrum and angle of the mouth compared with normal side		
Paralysis index (maximal 10 points):		

Source: Stennert et al 1977.[12]

Table 7.4 Stennert's Secondary Defect Facial Paralysis Index

Characteristic	No	Yes
Hyperacusis		
Taste impaired		
Synkinesia between forehead/eye/nasolabial sulcus/corner of mouth/chin		
Synkinesia between more than three areas		
Generalized secondary spasms		
Contractures		
Lacrimation less than 70%		
Lacrimation less than 70% and incomplete lid closure		
Lacrimation 0%		
Crocodile tears		
Defect healing index		

Source: Stennert et al 1977.[12]

The system explicitly considers facial function at rest and in voluntary motion. Moreover, degrees of synkinesia are assessed for different regions of the face, and severity is graded (▶ Table 7.6 and ▶ Table 7.7). It has been reported to be more sensitive than the House–Brackmann facial grading system in discriminating changes in facial nerve

Table 7.5 May's Facial Grading System (designed as post reanimation grading system)

Grade	Description	Characteristics
I	Superb	Minimal mass movements with separation of expressions
II	Excellent	Can smile and close eye, but only at the same time; obvious mass movement without separation of expressions
III	Good	Smile but cannot close eye/eye closed but cannot smile
IV	Fair	Incomplete eye closure and/or weak mouth movement
V	Poor	Tone intact, symmetry at rest, but no movement, 2 years after surgery without change
VI	Failure	Flaccid, tone lost

Source: May 1980.[13]

Table 7.6 Sunnybrook (Toronto) Facial Grading System Part A

Resting symmetry compared with normal side (choose one description only)		
Eye	Normal	0
	Narrow	1
	Wide	1
	Eyelid surgery	1
Cheek (nasolabial fold)	Normal	0
	Absent	2
	Less pronounced	1
	More pronounced	1
Mouth	Normal	0
	Corner dropped	1
	Corner pulled up/out	1
	Resting symmetry score = total × 5	

Source: Ross et al 1996.[14]

Table 7.7 Sunnybrook (Toronto) Facial Grading System Part B

	Symmetry of voluntary movement (degree of muscle excursion compared with normal side)					Synkinesis (degree of involuntary muscle contraction)			
Standard expressions	Unable to initiate movement/no movement	Initiate slight movement	Initiate movement with mild excursion	Movement almost complete mild symmetry	Movement complete symmetry	None: no synkinesis or mass movement	Mild: slight synkinesis	Moderate: obvious but not disfiguring synkinesis	Severe: disfiguring synkinesis/gross mass movements
Forehead wrinkle	1	2	3	4	5	0	1	2	3
Gentle eye closure	1	2	3	4	5	0	1	2	3
Open mouth smile	1	2	3	4	5	0	1	2	3
Snarl	1	2	3	4	5	0	1	2	3
Lip pucker	1	2	3	4	5	0	1	2	3
	Voluntary movement score = total × 4					Synkinesis score = total			
Composite score = voluntary movement score – resting symmetry score – synkinesis score									

Source: Ross et al 1996.[14]

regeneration. Although a subjective scale, it has good interobserver reliability between 69 and 85%.[15] One shortcoming is that only synkinesia and no other secondary defects such as contractures, spasms, and crocodile tears are covered.

> !
>
> When looking for a subjective facial nerve grading system, the Sunnybrook (Toronto) facial grading system is a good choice. It is relatively easy to remember and use. It analyzes sections of the face independently for movement and synkinesia, and this further enables one to document longitudinal changes.

7.3.6 Facial Nerve Grading System 2.0

Recently an updated version of the House–Brackmann facial grading system was presented by the Facial Nerve Disorders Committee of the AAOHNS and was called the Facial Nerve Grading System 2.0 (FNGS 2.0; ▶ Table 7.8).[16] To overcome disadvantages of the House–Brackmann facial grading system, it incorporates regional scoring of facial movement and additional information. The intraobserver and interobserver agreements have been shown to be high. When using FNGS 2.0, nominal improvement is seen in percentage of exact agreement of grade, and there is a reduction of instances of examiners differing by more than one grade. It also offers improved agreement in differentiating between House–Brackmann grades 3 and 4.

7.4 Objective Grading Systems

7.4.1 Burres–Fisch Linear Measurement Index and the Nottingham System

A grading system based on objective measurements has the benefit of eliminating observer bias and subjectivity. In the 1990s, Burres and Fisch introduced an objective grading system based on five facial expressions.[17,18] The shortening

Table 7.8 Facial Nerve Grading System 2.0

	Region			
Score	**Brow**	**Eye**	**Nasolabial fold**	**Oral**
1	Normal	Normal	Normal	Normal
2	Slight weakness	Slight weakness	Slight weakness	Slight weakness
3	Obvious weakness	Obvious weakness	Obvious weakness	Obvious weakness
4	Asymmetry at rest	Asymmetry at rest	Asymmetry at rest	Asymmetry at rest
5	Trace movement	Trace movement	Trace movement	Trace movement
6	No movement	No movement	No movement	No movement
Secondary movement (global assessment across the entire face)				
Score	**Degree of movement**			
0	None			
1	Slight synkinesia			
Reporting: sum scores for each region and secondary movement				
Grade	**Total score**			
I	4			
II	5–9			
III	10–14			
IV	15–19			
V	20–23			
VI	24			

Source: Vrabec et al 2009.[16]

of several distances is defined regarding nine anatomic landmarks that are compared on both sides of the face. The Burres-Fisch Linear Measurement Index is calculated by deploying a sequence of seven algorithms (▸ Table 7.9). In distinction to the House–Brackmann facial grading system, the index represents a continuously graded scale, thereby allowing finer distinction of facial function. Measures for secondary defects are not incorporated. Most importantly, the system is time consuming. This might be the reason why it has never found wide distribution and acceptance. Nevertheless, it is worthwhile to look at the Burres-Fisch Linear Measurement Index and also its simplification, the Nottingham system (▸ Table 7.10),[19] because elements of such metric measurements can be analyzed using computer-assisted image systems.

7.4.2 Neely's Facial Analysis Computerized Evaluation system

Neely and colleagues were the first at the end of the last century to use digital images to perform computer evaluation of facial function.[20–22] Image sets of the eyebrow, eye, and mouth areas of the face are evaluated by a computer algorithm that measures the degree of facial deformation during facial expression to compose an index. Briefly, the program was later termed the Facial Analysis Computerized Evaluation (FACE) system. When validated against the House–Brackmann facial grading scale, FACE was clearly valid and far more sensitive to small degrees of facial change. FACE is a computerized image subtraction program. Standard video image sets are imported into the

Table 7.9 Burres-Fisch Linear Measurement Index

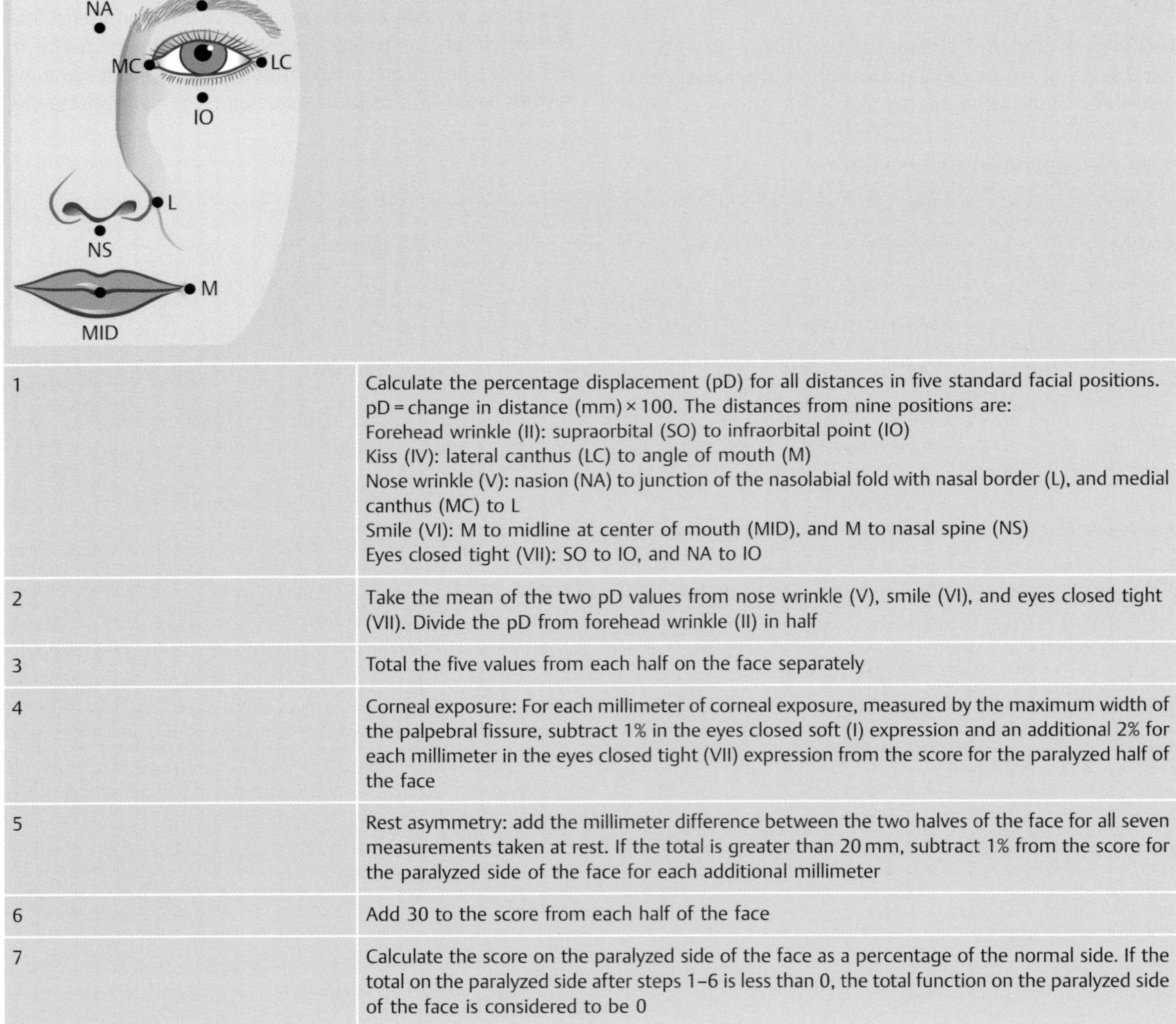

1	Calculate the percentage displacement (pD) for all distances in five standard facial positions. pD = change in distance (mm) × 100. The distances from nine positions are: Forehead wrinkle (II): supraorbital (SO) to infraorbital point (IO) Kiss (IV): lateral canthus (LC) to angle of mouth (M) Nose wrinkle (V): nasion (NA) to junction of the nasolabial fold with nasal border (L), and medial canthus (MC) to L Smile (VI): M to midline at center of mouth (MID), and M to nasal spine (NS) Eyes closed tight (VII): SO to IO, and NA to IO
2	Take the mean of the two pD values from nose wrinkle (V), smile (VI), and eyes closed tight (VII). Divide the pD from forehead wrinkle (II) in half
3	Total the five values from each half on the face separately
4	Corneal exposure: For each millimeter of corneal exposure, measured by the maximum width of the palpebral fissure, subtract 1% in the eyes closed soft (I) expression and an additional 2% for each millimeter in the eyes closed tight (VII) expression from the score for the paralyzed half of the face
5	Rest asymmetry: add the millimeter difference between the two halves of the face for all seven measurements taken at rest. If the total is greater than 20 mm, subtract 1% from the score for the paralyzed side of the face for each additional millimeter
6	Add 30 to the score from each half of the face
7	Calculate the score on the paralyzed side of the face as a percentage of the normal side. If the total on the paralyzed side after steps 1–6 is less than 0, the total function on the paralyzed side of the face is considered to be 0

Source: Burres and Fisch 1986.[17]

Table 7.10 The Nottingham System

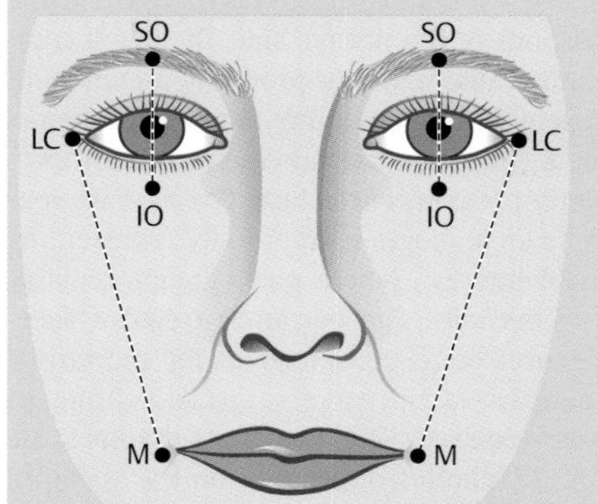

Part 1	Differences to face at rest (mm)	Healthy side	Paralyzed side
	Raise eyebrows: distance supra-orbital (SO) to infraorbital point (IO)		
	Close eyes tightly: distance SO to IO		
	Smile: distance lateral canthus (LC) to corner of mouth (M)		
	Calculate (sum on paralyzed side − sum on healthy side) × 100		
Part 2	Presence (P) or absence (A) of hemifacial spasm, contractures, synkinesia		
Part 3	Presence (Y) or absence (N) of crocodile tears, decreased lacrimation, dysgeusia		
Score	Expressed in a term such as 65AY, i.e., 65% of facial function, A = absence of secondary defects, and Y = presence of other effects		

Source: Murty et al 1994.[19]

FACE program. All of the pixels of the facial image at rest are subtracted from the pixels in each sequential image frame in motion during the prescribed expression. This process results in a new gray-scale image set composed of only changed pixel values. If an area of the face does not move, the subtracted pixel value in that area is zero or black; when an area moves, the subtracted absolute pixel value is greater than zero and turns varying degrees of gray or white. The intensity of facial movement is congruent with the intensity of whiteness seen on the subtracted image. All pixel changes are summed and can be plotted over the time during defined expressions.

7.4.3 Facial Landmark-Based Computer Systems and Programs

In 2002, Linstrom from New York presented a videocomputer interactive system using preselected facial landmarks to study linear displacements of the face during defined facial expressions.[23] The asymmetry of facial displacement between both sides is calculated and expressed in percentages. This system seems to be appropriate to detect changes in the face and the test–retest reliability is about 73 to 99%. Moreover, it allows for a quantification of synkinesia. A similar system called videomimicography was introduced by Dulguerov and colleagues from Geneva. As a result of the fast technical developments in the recent years none of these computer systems have been widely employed; alternatively it is possible to use standard software such as Adobe Photoshop. The patient's face is marked and digitally photographed in standardized expressions such as at rest, forehead wrinkling, snarl, and smiling (showing their teeth). Pictures are transferred to a computer and vertical axes of resting photos (as the reference pictures) are determined using the software. Three points are marked on the picture including the midpoint between the inside corners of the eyes, the midpoint of the upper lip, and the midpoint of the chin to draw the vertical axis. The vertical line divides the face into two parts. Then, the shortest distance from the vertical line to each marker (corners of lips) is measured in the normal and impaired sides in the resting photos. To measure the differences between the marker positions at rest and when posing various facial expressions, the prepared photos showing dynamic movements (such as wrinkling, smiling, or snarling) are put on the photos prepared at rest, i.e., the unchanged parts of the face were placed exactly on their counterparts. Finally, alteration of the marker positions is measured in millimeters by the software.

> ⚠
>
> Although it might look easy to use Adobe Photoshop or equivalent software programs for (semi)automatic image analysis, international standards still need to be defined to allow comparison of the data of different centers.

7.4.4 Three-Dimensional Video Analysis and Surface Analysis

In 1999, Frey and coworkers from Vienna introduced a quantitative and three-dimensional (3D) video analysis system to measure facial function on both sides.[24] It is a marker-based system. The patient's head is positioned between a mirror system to get three different views of the face simultaneously. Standardized static and dynamic points are marked on the face. Within only a few minutes a digital video is taken from standardized facial movements. Analysis and visualization are performed later offline, with an image analyzing program. Alterations of specific distances between static and dynamic points are measured over time. The degree of pathologic facial asymmetry is quantified by comparison of the healthy and paralytic sides. The power of this system to quantify results of dynamic facial reconstruction in patients with facial palsy has been demonstrated in several studies from the Vienna group. It would be worthwhile to test the system in other departments also. There are now several commercial 3D/4D surface-imaging systems on the market. Such systems are primarily used in plastic and aesthetic surgery. To date, there are no publications on using such commercial applications explicitly for patients with facial palsy.

7.4.5 Glasgow Facial Palsy Scale

The Glasgow Facial Palsy Scale (GFPS) software is an open source for computer facial video analysis website (http://www.GFPS.org.uk).[25] GFPS works with videos recorded with standard video cameras of the subject against a plain background performing five standard movements. Briefly, GFPS uses facial recognition techniques, the boundaries of different regions of both sides of the face at rest and then in every frame during each movement. The software records the pixel changes per frame in each separate region of the face and compares them to the resting frame by a subtraction algorithm. The pixel changes on the palsied side of the face are then compared with those in the corresponding regions of the normal side. By digital computing, the program automatically produces a consistent objective measurement of the House–Brackmann overall grading and also a consistent measurement of the movement in the different regions of the face. The data are represented similar to an audiogram graphically representing the five regions of interest, where pixel change replaces measurements of decibels. The output is called a *Facogram*. Data are expressed as percentage of the movement of the healthy side. No facial markers, special lighting, or head fixation are required. The Facogram graphics are produced in 7 to 15 minutes depending on the speed of hardware and amount of information recorded.

7.4.6 Facial Assessment by Computer Evaluation

In response to the need for development of a diagnostic assessment tool that could rapidly provide quantitative data regarding resting position and dynamic excursion of key facial structures, the Massachusetts Eye and Ear Infirmary developed a Java-based software program, Facial Assessment by Computer Evaluation (also abbreviated FACE), which provides this information quickly and easily from standard patient photographs (▶ Fig. 7.4).[26] Pictures of five standard movements important in human facial function and communication receive attention by facial reanimation specialists: brow elevation with attempted brow raising, palpebral fissure narrowing with attempted eye closure, midupper lip excursion with attempted smiling, oral commissure excursion with attempted smiling, and midlower lip excursion with articulation of the sound "ee". The program evaluates seven facial distances relevant in the paralyzed face at rest: brow ptosis, superior eyelid malposition, inferior eyelid malposition, nasal base ptosis, midupper lip malposition, oral commissure malposition, and philtral deviation toward the healthy side. The FACE program needs a mean time of about 1.3 minutes to complete a full set of measurements. Recently, the system was reported as also being capable of providing a comprehensive measure of ocular synkinesia.

> !
>
> The Facial Assessment by Computer Evaluation (FACE) should be definitively tested and validated in more facial nerve centers, because it might have the potential to define a new standard for an objective facial grading system.

7.4.7 Facial Action Coding System

Facial expression is widely used to evaluate emotional impairment in psychological and neuropsychiatric

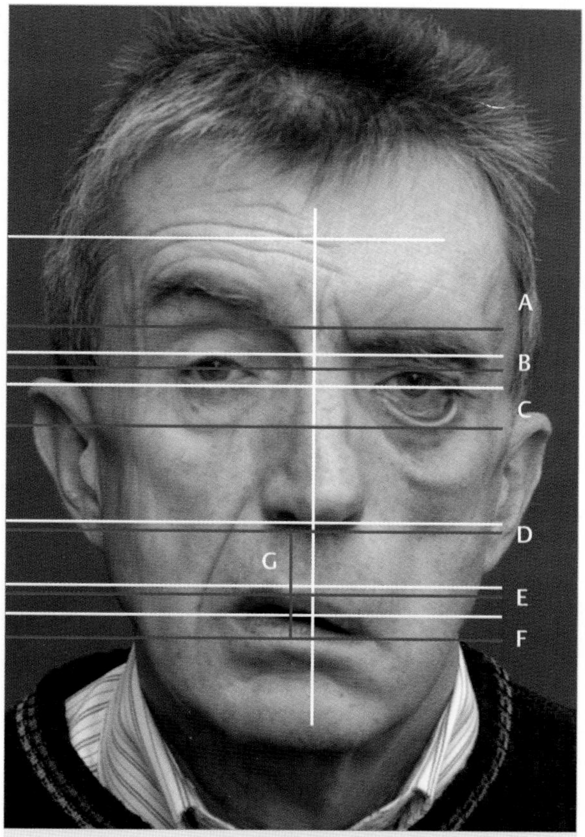

Fig. 7.4 The seven relevant distances in facial paralysis at rest. Horizontal lines (white, healthy side; red, paralyzed side) represent brow ptosis (A), superior eyelid malposition (B), inferior eyelid malposition (C), nasal base ptosis (D), midupper eyelid ptosis (E), and oral commissure malposition (F). (G) represents philtral deviation.

disorders. Ekman and Friesen's Facial Action Coding System (FACS) encodes movements of individual facial muscles from distinct momentary changes in facial appearance. FACS is popular in psychological research on emotional behavior. FACS encodes the movement of specific facial muscles called action units, which reflect distinct momentary changes in facial appearance. It is suitable for analyzing the small differences in facial affect. FACS rating requires that the human rater is extensively trained and it is time consuming. To overcome these limitations, automated FACS computer-based systems have been developed. The technology automatically tracks faces in a video, extracts geometric and texture features, and produces temporal profiles of each facial muscle movement. These profiles are quantified to compute frequencies of single and combined action units in videos. Recently, automated FACS analysis was introduced to assess patients with facial palsy.[27] Such an analysis is of special value when deficits in emotional expression need to be characterized in patients with facial palsy.

!

Computer-based Facial Action Coding System analysis might allow objective assessment of facial motor function and emotional function.

7.5 Assessment of Nonmimic Motor Function and Nonmotor Facial Nerve Functions

The facial nerve also directs motor fibers for the stapedial muscle and the posterior belly of the digastric muscle. Testing of the latter muscle is not included in any facial grading. Stapedial reflex testing is part of the traditional topognostic tests, as the reflex should still be functional when facial nerve injury takes place distal to the stapedial nerve. Stapedial reflex testing is typically not used for grading facial nerve injury although it has been used as a prognostic predictor for functional outcome by some groups. Gustatory tests, Schirmer's test, and the measurement of the salivary flow rate are other traditional topognostic tests involving nonmotor functions of the facial nerve, but also typically not included in facial nerve grading. Stennert's Secondary Defect Facial Paralysis Index (▶ Table 7.4) includes nonmotor functions by the assessment of lacrimation and crocodile tears.

7.6 Assessment of the Communicative and Emotional Function

Patients with peripheral facial paralysis often suffer from problems with eating and drinking. These problems are not covered by any of the previously mentioned facial nerve grading systems. Moreover, the patients are affected not only by physical dysfunction but also by psychological disturbances. Emotional problems may exist longer than the paralysis, and there is no correlation between extent of recovery and persisting psychological problems. Therefore, it is recommended to include scores for the social and emotional disabilities of these patients. This can be done with generic instruments to measure health-related quality of life, for instance with an internationally validated tool such as the Short Form-36 (SF-36) questionnaire. This tool allows patients with facial dysfunction to be compared with patients with other diseases. Disease-specific instruments that are more sensitive for patients with facial dysfunction are also available. The two most commonly used and best validated questionnaires are presented here.

7.6.1 Facial Disability Index

The Facial Disability Index (FDI) was developed during the 1990s in the Facial Nerve Center at the University of Pittsburgh. It is a 10-question self-reporting questionnaire that compares two domains: the physical disabilities with the social and emotional disabilities of the patient (▶ Table 7.11). The FDI includes aspects of the mouth, eye, and entire face, and the influence of the palsy on emotions and everyday activities.

7.6.2 Facial Clinimetric Evaluation Scale Instrument

The Facial Clinimetric Evaluation (FaCE) scale was developed in 2001 at the Baylor College of Medicine, Houston (▶ Table 7.12 and ▶ Table 7.13). It also measures facial impairment and disability. The 15-item scale includes six domains: facial movement, facial comfort, oral function, eye comfort, lacrimal control, and social function.

!

To measure general health-related quality of life, use Short Form-36 or a comparable tool. To measure facial palsy–specific quality of life, use the Facial Disability Index (FDI) or the Facial Clinimetric Evaluation (FaCE) Scale Instrument.

Table 7.11 Facial Disability Index (FDI)

Please choose the most appropriate response. Each question considers the function during the past month						
Physical function subscale	**Score[a]**					
1 How much difficulty did you have keeping food in your mouth, moving food around in your mouth, or getting food stuck in your cheek while eating?	5	4	3	2	1	0
2 How much difficulty did you have drinking from a cup?	5	4	3	2	1	0
3 How much difficulty did you have saying specific sounds while speaking?	5	4	3	2	1	0
4 How much difficulty did you have with your eye tearing excessively or becoming dry?	5	4	3	2	1	0
5 How much difficulty did you have with brushing your teeth or rinsing your mouth?	5	4	3	2	1	0
[c]Physical function score = [[sum (questions 1–5) − N] ÷ N] × (100 ÷ 4), where N is the number of questions answered						
Social/wellbeing function subscale	**Score[b]**					
6 How much of the time have you felt calm and peaceful?	6	5	4	3	2	1
7 How much of the time did you isolate yourself from people around you?	6	5	4	3	2	1
8 How much of the time did you get irritable toward those around you?	6	5	4	3	2	1
9 How often did you wake up early or wake up several times during your night-time sleep?	6	5	4	3	2	1
10 How often has your facial function kept you from going out to eat, shop, or participate in family or social activities?	6	5	4	3	2	1
[c]Social score = [[sum (questions 6–10) − N] ÷ N] × (100 ÷ 5), where N is the number of questions answered						

Source: VanSwearingen and Brach 1996.[28]
[a]Physical subscale: usually did with no difficulty (5), a little difficulty (4), some difficulty (3), much difficulty (2); or usually did not do because of health (1), or other reasons (0).
[b]Social/wellbeing subscale: all of the time (6), most of the time (5), a good bit of the time (4), some of the time (3), a little bit of the time (2), none of the time (1). For items 7–10, the scoring is reversed.
[c]The calculation instructions are not part of the questionnaire for the patient. [AU: Please check the changes to the calculations of the scores in the table]

Table 7.12 Facial Clinimetric Evaluation (FaCE) Scale Instrument

You may already have answered these or similar questions before. Please answer all questions as best as you can. The following statements are about how you think your face is moving:					
Circle only one number	**One side**	**Both sides**	**I have no difficulty**		
When I try to move my face, I have difficulties on	1	2	0		
If you have problems on both sides, answer the questions in the remainder of the survey with regard to the more affected side, or with regard to both sides if they are equally affected in the past week:					
Circle only one number on each line	**Not at all**	**Only if I concentrate**	**A little**	**Almost normally**	**Normally**
1. When I smile, the affected side of my mouth goes up	1	2	3	4	5
2. I can raise my eyebrow on the affected side	1	2	3	4	5
3. When I pucker my lips, the affected side of my mouth moves	1	2	3	4	5
The following are statements about how you might feel because of your face or the problems. Please rate how often each of the following statements applied to you during the past week:					
Please circle only one number on each line	**All of the time**	**Most of the time**	**Some of the time**	**A little of the time**	**None of the time**
4. Parts of my face feel tight, worn out, or uncomfortable	1	2	3	4	5
5. My affected eye feels dry, irritated, or scratchy	1	2	3	4	5
6. When I try to move my face, I feel tension, pain or spasm	1	2	3	4	5
7. I use eye drops or ointment in the affected eye	1	2	3	4	5
8. My affected eye is wet or has tears in it	1	2	3	4	5
9. I act differently around people because of my face or facial problem	1	2	3	4	5
10. People treat me differently because of my face or facial problem	1	2	3	4	5
11. I have problems moving food around in my mouth	1	2	3	4	5
12. I have problems with drooling or keeping food in my mouth or off my chin and clothes	1	2	3	4	5

Source: Kahn et al 2001.[29]

7.6.3 Assessment of Psychological Distress, Anxiety, and Depression

Patients with chronic facial palsy (and also patients with acute palsy) can develop severe psychological complaints that go hand in hand with disturbances of interpersonal communication and stigmatization. These problems are explored in detail in Chapter 13 and Chapter 14. The most common problems reported by patient are distress, anxiety, and depression. These complaints are normally not addressed by the otolaryngologist. The severity of psychological disturbances does not necessarily correlate with the severity of the motor function disturbance. Major depression is a frequent finding in patients with chronic facial palsy. Appropriate tools to assess such problems include the Hospital Anxiety and Depression Scale (HADS) or the Beck Depression Inventory (BDI, BDI-II).

7.7 Key Points

- There is no international agreement on a simple, sensitive, reproducible facial nerve grading system. Such a system should combine the assessment of the face as a

Table 7.13 Facial Clinimetric Evaluation (FaCE) Scale Instrument (continuation)

The next statements refer to how you felt in the past week or how you got along with your facial nerve paralysis. Please estimate how well you concur with each statement:					
Please circle only one number per line	**Strongly agree**	**Agree**	**Don't know**	**Disagree**	**Strongly disagree**
13. My face feels tired, I feel tension, pain or cramp	1	2	3	4	5
14. My appearance has changed my willingness to take part in social activities or to meet my family and friends	1	2	3	4	5
15. Because of the difficulties with eating, I have avoided going to a restaurant or in other people's homes	1	2	3	4	5
Additional comments: Thank you!					
Calculation (not part of the questionnaire for the patient) Facial Movement Score = ((Items 1 + 2 + 3) – #valid)/4 × (#valid) × 100 Facial Comfort Score = ((Items 4 + 6 + 16) – #valid)/4 × (#valid) × 100 Oral Function Score = ((Items 11 + 12) – #valid)/4 × (#valid) × 100 Eye Comfort Score = ((Items 5 + 7) – #valid)/4 × (#valid) × 100 Lacrimal Control Score = ((Items 8) – #valid)/4 × (#valid) × 100 Social Function Score = ((Items 9 + 10 + 14 + 15) – #valid)/4 × (#valid) × 100 Total Score = ((Sum of all 15 items) – #valid)/4 × (#valid) × 100 #valid = number of items within the domain for which an adequate response was given.					

Source: Kahn et al 2001.[29]

whole, but also discriminate regional differences in the face, and accurately detect signs of defective healing. It should have high test–retest reliability and a low interobserver variability, including subjective and objective criteria, and ideally be inexpensive. It should be sufficiently sensitive to measure whether treatments are improving outcome.

- Due to the advances in computer technology, especially faster data acquisition, digital image analysis systems provide the optimal basis for an ideal internationally accepted facial nerve grading system. Commercialized 3D/4D surface-imaging systems offer the optimal platform for the development of the optimal facial grading system. Such systems should be tested in patients with facial palsy and for monitoring patients after facial nerve reconstruction.
- New software tools such as the Facial Assessment by Computer Evaluation (FACE) program can be used for evaluation of photographs. It needs to be tested on a large scale in international trials, optimally using a web-based approach.
- The otolaryngologist often lacks the expertise and time to deal in detail with the communicative and emotional dysfunction of the patient. Therefore, qualified personnel should use tests such as the Facial Disability Index (FDI) or the Facial Clinimetric Evaluation (FaCE) Scale Instrument and work with the patient on the significant health problems related to their facial nerve disorder. In the near future, affordable and easy-to-use automated image analysis tools will also be available for objective measurement of such psychological components of facial nerve disorders.

References

[1] Kang TS, Vrabec JT, Giddings N, Terris DJ. Facial nerve grading systems (1985–2002): beyond the House-Brackmann scale. Otol Neurotol 2002; 23: 767–771

[2] Guntinas-Lichius O, Beurskens CH, van Gelder RS, Heymans PG, Manni JJ, Nicolai SPA. The facial nerve grading systems. In: Beurskens CHG, van Gelder RS, Heymans PG, Manni JJ, Nicolai JPA, eds. The Facial Palsies. Utrecht: Lemma Publishers; 2005:51–68

[3] Botman JW, Jongkees LB. The result of intratemporal treatment of facial palsy. Pract Otorhinolaryngol (Basel) 1955; 17: 80–100

[4] Peitersen E, Andersen P. Spontaneous course of 220 peripheral nontraumatic facial palsies. Acta Otolaryngol 1966; 224–296

[5] Adour KK, Swanson PJ, Jr. Facial paralysis in 403 consecutive patients: emphasis on treatment response in patients with Bell's palsy. Trans Am Acad Ophthalmol Otolaryngol 1971; 75: 1284–1301

[6] House JW. Facial nerve grading systems. Laryngoscope 1983; 93: 1056–1069

[7] Brackmann DE, Barrs DM. Assessing recovery of facial function following acoustic neuroma surgery. Otolaryngol Head Neck Surg 1984; 92: 88–93

[8] House JW, Brackmann DE. Facial nerve grading system. Otolaryngol Head Neck Surg 1985; 93: 146–147

[9] Evans RA, Harries ML, Baguley DM, Moffat DA. Reliability of the House and Brackmann grading system for facial palsy. J Laryngol Otol 1989; 103: 1045–1046

[10] Yen TL, Driscoll CL, Lalwani AK. Significance of House-Brackmann facial nerve grading global score in the setting of differential facial nerve function. Otol Neurotol 2003; 24: 118–122

[11] Yanagihara N. Grading of facial palsy. In: Fisch U, ed. Facial Nerve Surgery. Birmingham, Alabama: Aesculapius Publishing Co; 1977

[12] Stennert E, Limberg CH, Frentrup KP. An index for paresis and defective healing—an easily applied method for objectively determining therapeutic results in facial paresis [in German] HNO 1977; 25: 238–245

[13] May M. Management of cranial nerves I through VII following skull base surgery. Otolaryngol Head Neck Surg (1979) 1980; 88: 560–575

[14] Ross BG, Fradet G, Nedzelski JM. Development of a sensitive clinical facial grading system. Otolaryngol Head Neck Surg 1996; 114: 380–386

[15] Kayhan FT, Zurakowski D, Rauch SD. Toronto Facial Grading System: interobserver reliability. Otolaryngol Head Neck Surg 2000; 122: 212–215

[16] Vrabec JT, Backous DD, Djalilian HR et al. Facial Nerve Disorders Committee. Facial Nerve Grading System 2.0. Otolaryngol Head Neck Surg 2009; 140: 445–450

[17] Burres S, Fisch U. The comparison of facial grading systems. Arch Otolaryngol Head Neck Surg 1986; 112: 755–758

[18] Rickenmann J, Jaquenod C, Cerenko D, Fisch U. Comparative value of facial nerve grading systems. Otolaryngol Head Neck Surg 1997; 117: 322–325

[19] Murty GE, Diver JP, Kelly PJ, O'Donoghue GM, Bradley PJ. The Nottingham System: objective assessment of facial nerve function in the clinic. Otolaryngol Head Neck Surg 1994; 110: 156–161

[20] Neely JG, Cheung JY, Wood M, Byers J, Rogerson A. Computerized quantitative dynamic analysis of facial motion in the paralyzed and synkinetic face. Am J Otol 1992; 13: 97–107

[21] Moran CJ, Neely JG. Patterns of facial nerve synkinesis. Laryngoscope 1996; 106: 1491–1496

[22] Neely JG, Wang KX, Shapland CA, Sehizadeh A, Wang A. Computerized objective measurement of facial motion: normal variation and test-retest reliability. Otol Neurotol 2010; 31: 1488–1492

[23] Linstrom CJ. Objective facial motion analysis in patients with facial nerve dysfunction. Laryngoscope 2002; 112: 1129–1147

[24] Frey M, Giovanoli P, Gerber H, Slameczka M, Stüssi E. Three-dimensional video analysis of facial movements: a new method to assess the quantity and quality of the smile. Plast Reconstr Surg 1999; 104: 2032–2039

[25] Romeo M, O'Reilly B, Robertson BF, Morley S. Validation of the Glasgow Facial Palsy Scale for the assessment of smile reanimation surgery in facial paralysis. Clin Otolaryngol 2012; 37: 181–187

[26] Hadlock TA, Urban LS. Toward a universal, automated facial measurement tool in facial reanimation. Arch Facial Plast Surg 2012; 14: 277–282

[27] Haase D, Kemmler M, Guntinas-Lichius O, Denzler J. Measuring Facial Action Unit Activation Intensities using Active Appearance Models. German Association for Pattern Recognition (DAGM) Conference, August, 28–31, 2012, Graz, Austria

[28] Van Swearingen JM, Brach JS. The Facial Disability Index: reliability and validity of a disability assessment instrument for disorders of the facial neuromuscular system. Phys Ther 1996; 76: 1288–1298, discussion 1298–1300

[29] Kahn JB, Gliklich RE, Boyev KP, Stewart MG, Metson RB, McKenna MJ. Validation of a patient-graded instrument for facial nerve paralysis: the FaCE scale. Laryngoscope 2001; 111: 387–398

Part III

Management of Acute Peripheral Facial Palsy

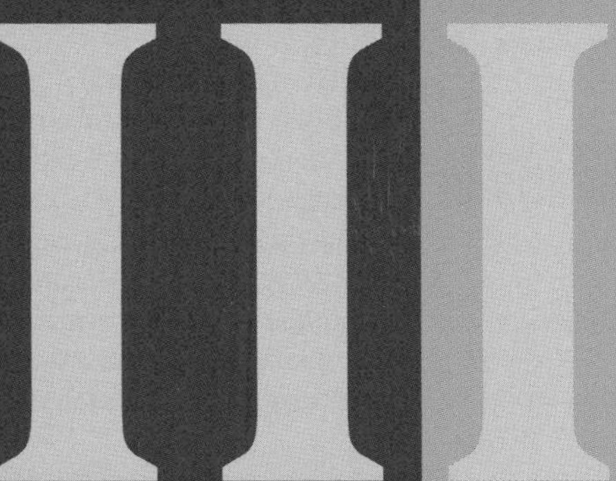

8 Bell's Palsy

Eric Smouha and Elizabeth Toh

8.1 Introduction

Bell's palsy is a common and distressing condition. It is the most common cause of acute unilateral facial nerve palsy, and may be accompanied by retroauricular pain, hyperacusis, and excessive lacrimation. The cause is not known, but the prevailing thinking is that it is caused at least in some patients by reactivated herpes simplex virus (HSV).[1–4] It is very important to differentiate idiopathic Bell's palsy from secondary causes with known treatments, such as ear infections, Lyme disease, and parotid tumors. The recommended treatment of Bell's palsy is corticosteroids, administered as early as possible after onset, and 70% will achieve a completely normal recovery with or without treatment.[5] Many other treatments have been proposed and will be discussed further in this chapter.

8.2 Definition

Bell's palsy, first described in 1924 by Charles Bell,[6] is defined as acute unilateral facial nerve paresis or paralysis with onset in less than 72 hours and without an identifiable cause. It is considered a diagnosis of exclusion, after all other potential causes have been ruled out.

8.3 Epidemiology and Etiology

Bell's palsy is relatively common, affecting between 15 and 40 out of 100,000 people per year.[7] It can occur at any age and may involve children as well. It affects males and females in roughly equal proportions. It may be more common during the third trimester of pregnancy. It is usually unilateral but may be bilateral in between 4 and 12% of cases. Bilateral alternating facial palsy is almost always due to idiopathic Bell's palsy; simultaneous bilateral palsy should lead to a suspicion of Guillain–Barré syndrome, sarcoidosis, Lyme disease, HIV infection, or other systemic disorder. Recurrent unilateral facial nerve palsy is also usually due to idiopathic Bell's palsy, but on occasion may be due to Melkersson–Rosenthal syndrome, a tumor, such as facial nerve hemangioma, or to anatomic compression of the facial nerve, and should always be evaluated by imaging.

> **!**
>
> Contralateral recurrence is more common than ipsilateral recurrence in Bell's palsy (2:1).
>
> Ipsilateral recurrence of facial paralysis should always be evaluated radiologically.

Bell's palsy is the most common cause of facial nerve palsy, representing over 60% of cases.[5,8] In a study of 2,570 cases of acute facial nerve paresis in Denmark over a 25-year period, 66% of the cases were classified as idiopathic Bell's palsy, with the remainder caused by tumors, infections, trauma, diabetes, or systemic diseases.[5] A similar percentage was observed in a study of 1,000 patients by Adour at al.[8] Bell's palsy is believed to be of viral etiology. Despite this, there is no diagnostic test that proves the cause, and therefore the diagnosis of Bell's palsy remains a diagnosis of exclusion, after all other neoplastic, inflammatory, and traumatic causes have been ruled out.

Bell's palsy can occur at any age, but is less common below the age of 15 years and above the age of 60. Bell's palsy affects the right and left side equally, and male and female gender in equal distribution, and there is no seasonal variability. Six percent of cases are recurrent, and 4% are familial. Seventy percent of cases will show complete paralysis at presentation.[5]

> **!**
>
> At presentation, 70% of cases of Bell's palsy are complete and 30% are incomplete.

The best available evidence suggests that etiology of Bell's palsy is now believed to be due to reactivated HSV.[1] This relationship was originally hypothesized by McCormick in 1972 based on the fact that the virus is sequestered in neural ganglia.[2] A classical study by Murakami et al showed that the HSV genome was present within facial nerve endoneurial fluid and muscle in 79% (9 of 14) patients with Bell's palsy but not in patients with varicella zoster (VSV) or normal controls.[3] The samples were derived from live patients who underwent surgical decompression of the facial nerve, and the viral genome was detected using polymerase chain reaction followed by hybridization with Southern blot analysis. HSV genome was also isolated from oral secretions of Bell's palsy patients. However, the presence of HSV genome has not been detected in cerebrospinal fluid or tear samples of Bell's palsy patients,[4,9] and HSV and VSV were found in relatively high incidence in the geniculate and other cranial nerve ganglia of cadaver specimens from patients without Bell's palsy.[10,11] The presence of the viral genome in the facial nerve therefore does not constitute proof of causality, because HSV infection is prevalent in the general population and dormant viral particles may reside in the neural ganglia of asymptomatic subjects.[12] Features that raise doubt about HSV as the etiologic agent include its much more frequent expression and re-expression in its mucocutaneous form (cold sores are much more prevalent than facial palsy and often recur, while 90% of cases of Bell's palsy occur only once), and the relative rarity of palsies of other cranial nerves that may harbor HSV.[13]

The pathology of the facial nerve in Bell's palsy has been studied by several authors.[14–20] In acute cases, the entire nerve is infiltrated by inflammatory cells. Myelin breakdown, axonal changes, and edema are present, and Wallerian degeneration of various degrees has been demonstrated. Liston believed the observed changes suggested viral neuritis,[17] but Matsumoto concluded the pathological findings were multiple and could include vascular, inflammatory, or degenerative causes.[18] Michaels observed congestion and infiltration of the nerve by lymphocytes in the internal auditory meatus and proximal fallopian canal, features indicating compression of the nerve in the proximal fallopian canal.[19] May and Schlaepfer studied chorda tympani specimens and found varying degrees of inflammation, which were not well correlated with clinical symptoms, salivary flow, or overall prognosis.[20]

8.4 Clinical Features

Bell's palsy begins acutely, with facial motor weakness developing over the course of one to three days (▸ Fig. 8.1 and ▸ Fig. 8.2). Sixty percent of patients will have pain in external auditory meatus or in the postauricular area, i.e., in the distribution of the common sensory fibers of the facial nerve. Pain precedes the onset of motor weakness

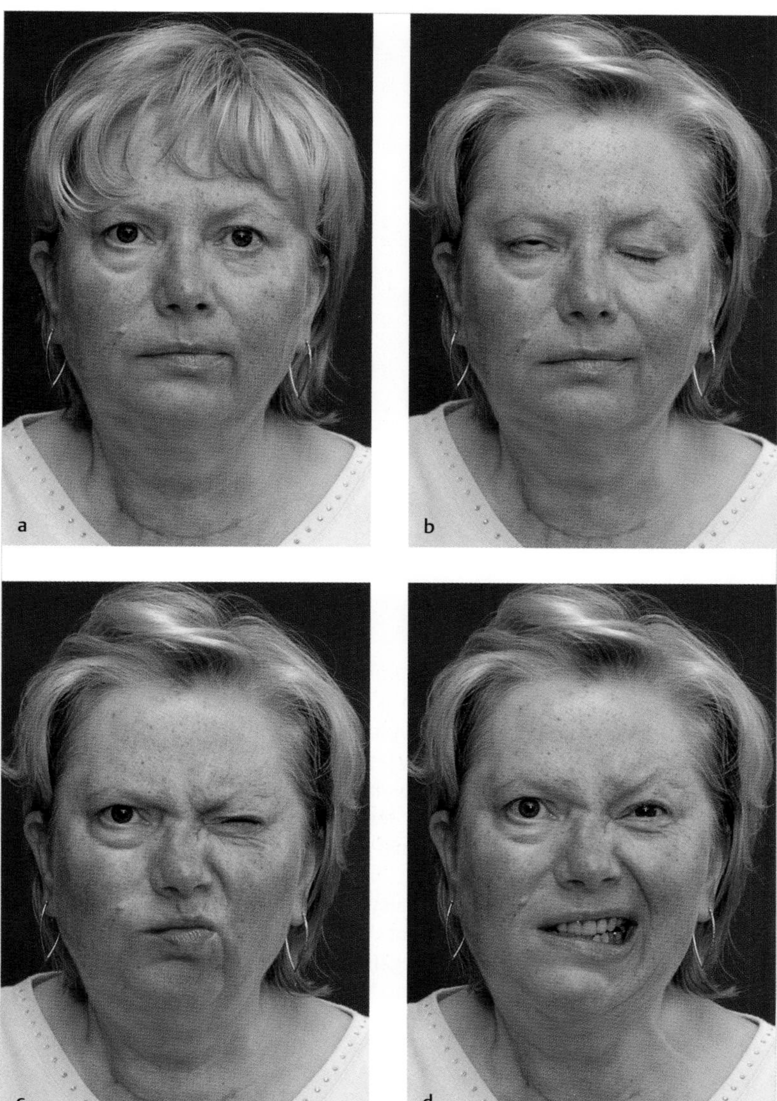

Fig. 8.1 Patient with Bell's palsy treated with tapered corticosteroids, pictured 3 days after onset: **(a)** at rest, **(b)** closing the eyes, **(c)** wrinkling the nose, **(d)** showing the teeth.

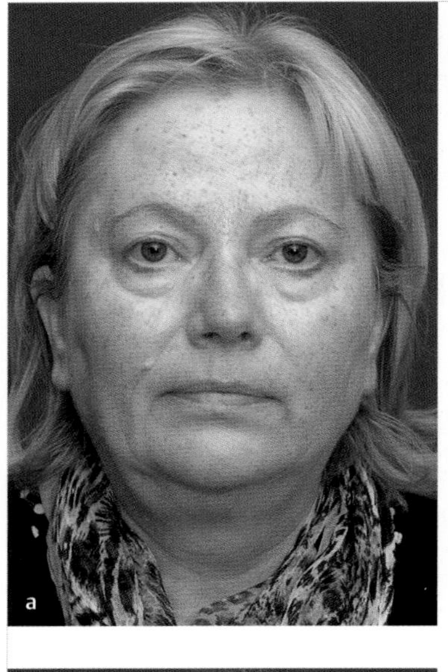

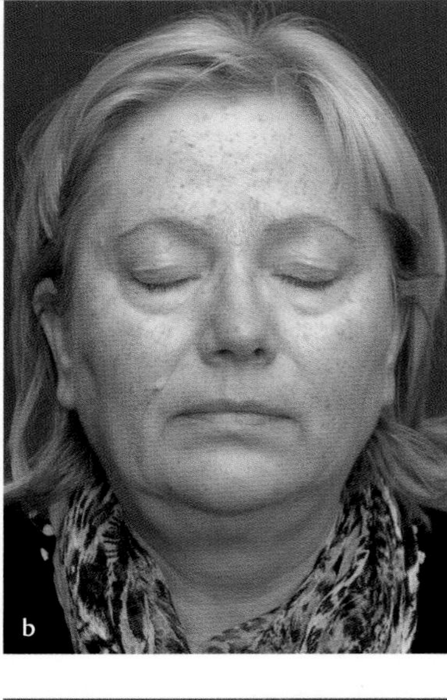

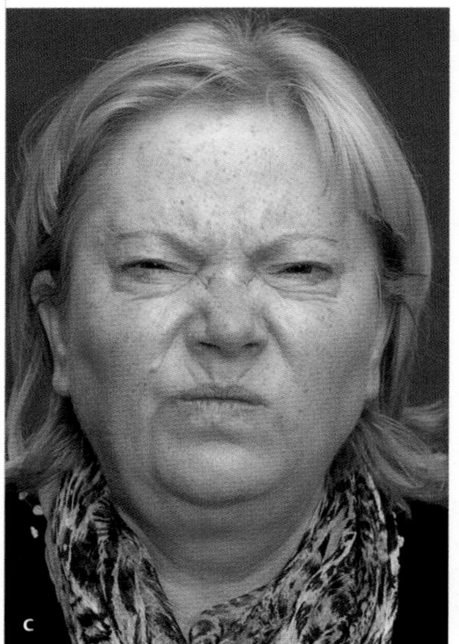

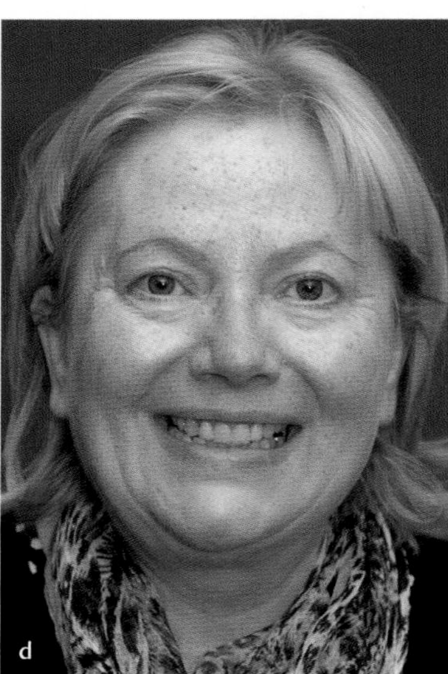

Fig. 8.2 The patient shown in ▶ Fig. 8.1, 3 months later: **(a)** at rest, **(b)** closing the eyes, **(c)** wrinkling the nose, **(d)** showing the teeth.

in about 25% of cases. The other functions of the facial nerve are also affected. There may be hyperacusis, dry mouth, dysgeusia, dry eye, and dry nose. Some patients also report facial "numbness."

The Clinical Practice Guidelines of the American Academy of Otolaryngology—Head and Neck Surgery[21] have listed the following clinical features of Bell's palsy:

- Bell's palsy is rapid in onset (< 72 hours).
- Bell's palsy is diagnosed when no other medical etiology is identified as a cause of the facial weakness.
- Bilateral Bell's palsy is rare.
- Currently, no cause for Bell's palsy has been identified.
- Other conditions may cause facial paralysis, including stroke, brain tumors, tumors of the parotid gland or infratemporal fossa, metastatic cancer involving the facial nerve, and systemic and infectious diseases, including zoster, sarcoidosis, and Lyme disease.
- Bell's palsy is typically self-limited.
- Bell's palsy may occur in men, women, and children but is more common in those 15 to 45 years old; those with diabetes, upper respiratory ailments, or compromised immune systems; or during pregnancy.

Once the facial palsy begins, it may take days to weeks to resolve. All patients will experience at least partial recovery; failure to regain any function at all after 4 months should elicit a search for another etiology for facial weakness. The majority of patients (approximately 70%) will recover function fully, while a few will have permanent partial palsy.

> !
>
> All patients will experience at least partial recovery. If the patient does not show any recovery, the initial diagnosis of Bell's palsy should be questioned and the diagnostic work-up should be repeated.

8.5 Diagnostic Work-Up

Bell's palsy is a diagnosis of exclusion, so the evaluation of the patient with acute facial nerve paresis depends principally on a thorough history and physical examination. If the symptoms and signs are consistent with Bell's palsy, no other laboratory or radiologic examinations are routinely required.[21] The history should confirm the elements listed in Clinical Features, namely rapid onset progressing to maximal weakness within 72 hours, presence of postauricular pain (common), hyperacusis, excessive tearing, and occasionally subjective "numbness." The history should also verify the absence of other neurologic symptoms such as hearing loss, dizziness, dysphagia, or diplopia. The physical examination should confirm the presence of a unilateral peripheral facial nerve palsy, along with absence of additional neural deficits and absence of pathology in the ears, head and neck, parotid gland, and skull base. Peripheral facial nerve palsy involves the upper and lower facial branches; lower facial weakness with sparing of the brow and mimetic function signifies a central nervous system lesion. This is a fundamental aspect of the physical examination.[22] The presence of other cranial nerve deficits should initiate a search for central nervous system etiologies, such as Guillain–Barré syndrome, sarcoidosis, or a skull base tumor (Adour and colleagues have asserted that Bell's palsy is a polycranial neuropathy,[23] as they attribute sensory symptoms to fifth nerve involvement and dysacusis to eighth nerve involvement, but this is controversial).

The differential diagnosis of facial paralysis is extensive, and includes all forms of infectious, inflammatory, neoplastic, traumatic, and congenital lesions that can affect the facial nerve; for differential diagnoses see Chapter 4.[21] Herpes zoster oticus (Ramsay Hunt syndrome) is characterized by painful vesicles in the distribution of the mandibular nerve (V3 dermatome); this is caused by a reactivated varicella zoster virus ("shingles") and has a worse prognosis than idiopathic Bell's palsy; more details are given in Chapter 10. Zoster can occasionally occur without vesicular rash and may be confused with idiopathic Bell's palsy; the presence of severe pain in the V3 distribution should suggest this diagnosis.[16] Eighth nerve complaints are common with Ramsay Hunt and do not occur with Bell's palsy. The distinction is important because zoster has a worse prognosis than idiopathic Bell's palsy and should be treated with antiviral drugs.

In endemic areas, evidence of Lyme disease should be sought; for more information on Lyme disease see Chapter 11.[24,25] Lyme disease is a tick-borne borreliosis characterized by a pathognomonic rash (erythema migrans), although the rash may have resolved and gone unnoticed before the facial palsy begins. Because of this, diagnostic serology should be obtained on patients with Bell's palsy who live in Lyme-endemic areas and present between the months of June and November.[26] The enzyme-linked immunosorbent assay (ELISA) is a serologic test that identifies antibodies in the bloodstream of patients who have been exposed to Lyme disease, and should serve as the initial diagnostic test. The ELISA has high sensitivity but imperfect specificity, and a positive result should be confirmed by western blot assay. The prognosis for recovery is excellent (99%) but patients with Lyme disease should be treated with a month-long course of an appropriate antibiotic, such as doxycycline, because they may continue to harbor the infectious agent despite recovery.[24] Certain cases of facial palsy will be associated with central nervous system manifestations of Lyme disease, and, in these cases, spinal fluid serology and treatment with intravenous ceftriaxone should be considered.[27]

Certain clinical features that are not characteristic of Bell's palsy deserve mention, because these should trigger a search for another etiology (See Box 8.1 (p. 116)). Palsy that is gradual in onset (greater than 72 hours) should raise the suspicion of a lesion causing extrinsic compression of the nerve, such as a cholesteatoma or neoplasm of the facial nerve, skull base, or parotid. Palsy that spares the brow and mimetic function is central in origin, and should raise the possibility of stroke; likewise facial paresis accompanied by somatic hemiparesis should suggest pathology in the motor cortex of the brain. Polycranial neuropathies could be associated with central nervous system pathology or skull base tumors. Segmental facial palsy (i.e., sparing of certain branches) should raise the suspicion of a lesion distal to the stylomastoid foramen, such as a parotid tumor. Facial paralysis that fails to show any sign of recovery after 4 months is also suspicious, as all cases of Bell's palsy will show at least partial return of function within that time frame.[5,7] Patients who have a history of a previous malignancy should undergo work-up for the possibility of metastatic disease.

The risk of Bell's palsy is increased in patients with diabetes.[27] Diabetes is more common among patients with Bell's palsy than among persons who have never had that disease. According to Adour et al, the diabetic patient is more prone than the nondiabetic to nerve degeneration, and to having recurrent or bilateral facial palsy, and it is suggested that patients over 40 years old be screened for diabetes.[27] Peitersen regards facial palsy in diabetes as a neuropathy distinct from idiopathic Bell's palsy,[5] but in the absence of a conclusive etiologic test, it is not clear that this is a separate disease.

Box 8.1 Clinical features that are not typical of Bell's palsy

- Gradual onset
- Slow progression beyond 2 weeks
- Hyperkinesis
- Segmental paresis/paralysis
- Bilateral simultaneous palsy
- Presence of other cranial neuropathies
- Associated neurologic symptoms
- Absence of onset of recovery by 4 months
- History of malignancy

A segmental facial palsy, with sparing of certain facial nerve branches, should raise the suspicion of a lesion distal to the stylomastoid foramen, such as a parotid tumor.

Bell's palsy appears to occur more commonly in pregnancy. Hilsinger et al found a threefold increase in incidence versus nonpregnant women.[28] Most cases occurred in the third trimester and immediately postpartum. Although Hilsinger felt the prognosis was similar for Bell's palsy of pregnancy, some authors believe it to have a worse prognosis.[29,30]

Box 8.2 Causes of recurrent alternating facial palsy

- Bell's palsy
- Melkersson–Rosenthal syndrome

Box 8.3 Causes of bilateral facial palsy

- Guillain–Barré syndrome
- Sarcoidosis
- Lyme disease
- Skull base trauma
- Infectious mononucleosis
- HIV infection

Bell's palsy usually occurs on only one side of the face and only once during the patient's life; however, occasionally it occurs bilaterally or more than once.[31] Recurrent Bell's palsy occurs in between 3 and 15% of cases (the differences in incidence between studies might be regional). Some authors have found the prognosis for recurrent forms to be identical for single episodes,[32–34] while others have found it to be worse.[35] Recurrent palsy may be ipsilateral or contralateral, and simultaneous or sequential. Recurrent alternating palsy is almost always idiopathic Bell's. Simultaneous bilateral palsy and recurrent ipsilateral palsy should initiate a search for an underlying cause.

Causes of recurrent alternating and bilateral facial palsy are listed in Box 8.2 (p. 116) and Box 8.3 (p. 116).

Understandably, Bell's palsy causes psychological distress that might need treatment; see Chapter 13 and Chapter 14. Patients often believe that they are having a stroke, and they need to be reassured about the cause of their condition as well as the statistical likelihood of satisfactory recovery. For patients with complete facial nerve paralysis, the timing of the recovery cannot be predicted, and so these patients should be followed closely for the first few weeks to detect signs of early improvement. Improvement of function that is detected within 3 weeks of onset is associated with a favorable prognosis.

!

Patients with Bell's palsy who have complete facial paralysis should be followed at least until they show signs of recovery.

Ancillary tests that can be obtained in the work-up of Bell's palsy include: imaging studies that may reveal a structural lesion such as tumor, fracture, or stroke; electrodiagnostic tests that may evaluate the integrity of peripheral motor function; and "topognostic" tests that evaluate nonmotor function of the nerve (stapedial function, gustation, salivation, and tearing) as well as the site of lesion of the nerve palsy; more details are given in Chapter 4. Audiometry and electronystagmography can also be used, to evaluate the adjacent eighth cranial nerve.

Imaging studies can demonstrate the anatomy of the nerve from the brainstem to the periphery, although they are only indicated in selected patients; details of facial nerve imaging are given in Chapter 5. Magnetic resonance imaging (MRI) is the most sensitive imaging modality, and will demonstrate a tumor, plaque, or cerebrovascular lesion affecting the facial nerve. MRI should be performed with gadolinium enhancement unless medically contraindicated. Segmental enhancement of the nerve is commonly seen in Bell's palsy (▶ Fig. 8.3).[36] The degree of facial nerve enhancement is not correlated with severity or outcome.[37] Computed tomography (CT) scanning demonstrates the bony fallopian canal, and is useful if trauma had occurred, or as a supplement to MRI when the need exists to visualize the temporal bone or to look for bony erosion, e.g., in the presence of tumor or infections. The Clinical Practice Guidelines recommend that imaging should not be routinely performed in Bell's palsy, but reserved for atypical cases that are suspicious for other etiologies, such as recurrent palsy, paresis of isolated nerve branches, additional cranial nerve deficits, or palsy that fails to recover after 4 months.[21]

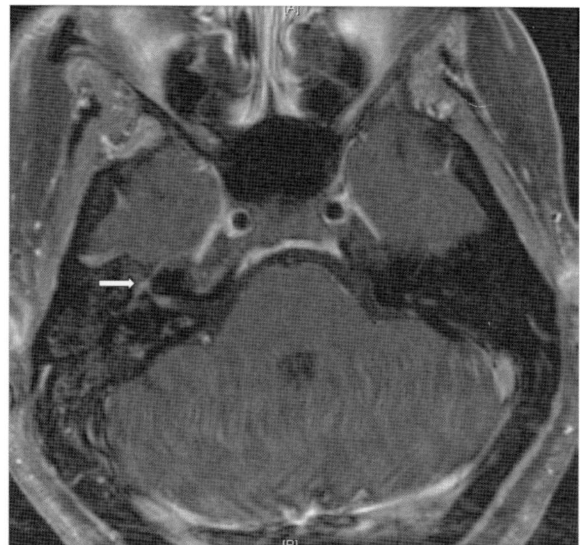

Fig. 8.3 T1-weighted axial MRI scan of the brain with gadolinium enhancement showing diffuse enhancement of the geniculate ganglion (*arrow*) and tympanic and labyrinthine segments of the facial nerve in a patient with right Bell's palsy.

!

Enhancement of the facial nerve is due to hypervascularity, and is not prognostically significant in Bell's palsy. Compare both sides on magnetic resonance imaging scans. Enhancement may persist after recovery and may sometimes occur in a normal nerve.

Electrodiagnostic testing may have prognostic value in cases of complete facial paralysis; details are given in Chapter 6. Electrical testing has also been used in selecting patients for surgical decompression of the facial nerve, although the value of this treatment has come into question. Topognostic tests, which examine lacrimation, gustatory function, stapedial contraction, and salivation, have been used historically to determine the site of lesion of the nerve.

Historically, the minimal nerve excitability (Hilger) test was the first test used to assess function. The nerve is stimulated using a device capable of delivering a fixed current through a bipolar ball-type electrode placed on the face near the stylomastoid foramen. The minimal stimulus setting capable of evoking a visible facial contraction is determined on the affected side and compared with that on the normal side. The test is simple to conceptualize and perform, but does not yield accurate prognostic information. The maximal nerve excitability test (MNET) uses a suprathreshold stimulus level to evoke a facial contraction on the affected and normal sides, and compares the degree of contraction, as determined by visual estimation. The test may have prognostic value by determining the number of remaining functional axons, but the result is not quantitative and therefore clinically unreliable.

Electroneuronography (ENoG) is a better test. ENoG is similar in principle to MNET in using a suprathreshold current to stimulate the nerve, but improves on MNET by measuring facial contraction quantitatively. ENoG utilizes a bipolar stimulating electrode to deliver a constant-current stimulus to the face, and a pair of surface electrodes placed in a standard location on the nasolabial crease record the electrical depolarization of facial muscles. A suprathreshold stimulation is delivered to the facial nerve near the stylomastoid foramen, which recruits all the functioning axons. Alternatively, stimulation of the buccal branch produces a reliable response with less current, and therefore less patient discomfort. The amplitude of the resulting facial contraction is measured on the normal and affected sides, and the amplitude ratio is calculated. The test is initially performed at least 3 days following the onset of facial palsy (before 3 days, axonal degeneration has not yet occurred). The test is repeated at intervals, and the amplitude ratio plotted as a function of time. The prognostic value of ENoG has been studied by Fisch.[38] If the response on the affected side declines to less than 10% of the normal side within 14 days of onset of complete paralysis, there is severe axonal degeneration and this implies a poor prognosis. ENoG is only useful in cases of complete facial palsy; incomplete facial paresis has a good prognosis and electrical testing provides no additional prognostic information.[39,40] ENoG requires synchronous firing and is therefore not as reliable in recurrent cases of a slow paralysis where there has been degeneration and regeneration.

!

Electroneurography is valuable prognostically when used between day 3 and day 14 after onset of complete paralysis.

Electromyography (EMG) uses needle electrodes inserted into the facial muscles to measure spontaneous depolarizations and the responses to voluntary or evoked muscle contraction. EMG is more sensitive than ENoG because it is not affected by the loss of neural synchrony during neural regeneration and is less dependent on electrode placement (when performing ENoG, some centers use a standard surface electrode placement and some move to find the optimal placement for maximal recording).[41] Evoked electromyography (EEMG), in which the nerve is electrically stimulated near its main trunk, gives equivalent information to EnoG.[42] The response amplitude of the normal and affected sides can be measured and compared as a ratio, and the prognosis determined by the degree of degeneration of time.

EMG also allows the determination of muscle end plate potentials, and this helps reveal the functional status of the nerve. The presence of motor unit action potentials during voluntary facial contraction implies functioning motor end plates, a favorable finding.[43] If the clinical examination of the patient shows a complete palsy but EMG reveals voluntary facial contraction s, the palsy is electrophysiologically incomplete and shows a better outcome than a clinically and electrophysiologically complete palsy.[44] Absence of action potentials implies axonal loss. Fibrillation potentials at rest are a sign of random muscle activity and indicate muscle denervation. Sharp waves, asynchronous bursts of electrical activity, and fibrillation potentials are the earliest manifestation of axonal denervation. These are typically identified between 1 and 4 weeks after nerve injury. EMG may not show spontaneous activity up to 2 weeks after a severe neuronal injury, and therefore is not informative during this early time period.

!

Electromyography has high prognostic value beyond 14 days after onset of the palsy: detection of pathologic spontaneous activity is prognostic of incomplete recovery.

Topognostic tests of facial nerve function examine the nonmotor functions of the nerve and can give information about the site of lesion; see also Chapter 4. These include tests of tearing, stapedial contraction, salivation, and gustation. Tearing can be evaluated using Schirmer's test, in which a strip of filter paper is placed in the inferior conjunctival fornix, without anesthesia, and tears are wicked away from the normal and affected sides for a prescribed amount of time, 5 minutes. The affected side is compared with the normal side. Less than 25% tearing is considered significant.

Stapedial function is measured by immittance audiometry. During tympanometry, a sound is applied to the sealed ear canal at a level 60 to 80 dB SL, and deflection of the tracer tone is sought. The acoustic reflex can be tested with the probe tone presented in the ipsilateral and contralateral ear. The facial nerve is the efferent limb of the stapedial reflex, therefore the muscle contraction will be absent on the affected side with the probe tone presented to either ear. The stapedial reflex is absent in over two-thirds of patients with Bell's palsy initially and usually returns 1 to 2 weeks before clinical recovery of facial function is evident.[5] A normal acoustic reflex is a good predictor of complete recovery; however the lack of an acoustic reflex is not a poor prognostic sign.[44]

Salivary flow can be measured quantitatively by cannulating the Wharton's duct on both sides. Gustation can be measured by electrogustometry.

The results of topognostic tests are, in general, poorly correlated with prognosis in Bell's palsy, and therefore are not routinely indicated. In other forms of acquired facial paralysis, they may provide information about the site of lesion. For example, lacrimal fibers exit the facial nerve at the geniculate ganglion, therefore a positive Schirmer's test implies a lesion proximal to the first genu, in the meatal or labyrinthine segment of the nerve.

8.6 Treatment

8.6.1 Eye Care

Incomplete eye closure, reduced blink frequency, and decreased tearing, which may occur in Bell's palsy, predispose to corneal desiccation and exposure keratopathy. Untreated, this may lead to permanent visual impairment. Eye lubrication and protection therefore remain a top priority in management of patients with moderate-to-severe facial paralysis. Aggressive eye lubrication and use of a moisture chamber are recommended if incomplete eye closure is observed. Caution should be exercised with use of eye patches and eye taping, especially in individuals with reduced corneal sensation since corneal abrasions may occur if the upper lid inadvertently retracts under the eye patch/tape. Complaints of eye pain, burning, visual changes, and visible signs of eye irritation should prompt an emergent consultation with ophthalmology for further evaluation. In individuals who continue to have bothersome eye symptoms or who are unable to cooperate with aggressive eye care, a temporary tarsorrhaphy, external reversible lid loading or upper eyelid gold weight placement may occasionally be indicated; details on surgery of the eye are given in Chapter 24.

!

Eye lubrication and protection therefore remain a top priority in management of patients with moderate-to-severe facial paralysis.

8.6.2 Medical Treatment of Bell's Palsy

Bell's palsy patients are fortunate in two ways. They have a very high spontaneous recovery rate without treatment (70% House–Brackmann I and 15% House–Brackmann II) and the natural history has been more robustly studied than for most diseases.[5] However, trying to show that the remaining 15% can be improved with medical therapy has led to some confusion and controversy as to the ideal medical regimen.

Oral Steroids

Since neural edema and entrapment neuropathy are thought to be the primary pathologic processes resulting in facial nerve dysfunction in Bell's palsy, treatment with oral steroids has been extensively investigated and is well supported by several randomized controlled trials. The anti-inflammatory effects of steroids are aimed at reducing nerve swelling and therefore improving functional recovery.

Both Sullivan and Engstrom report large randomized, double-blind, placebo-controlled studies comparing outcomes of patients with Bell's palsy treated with prednisolone, antiviral therapy, combination therapy, and placebo agents.[45,46] Both trials report administration of treatment within 72 hours of onset of symptoms and treatment duration of 10 days. Sullivan reported a significantly larger proportion of patients with complete recovery of facial function at 3 months (83% prednisolone versus 63.6% placebo) and 9 months (94.4% prednisolone versus 81.6% placebo) in the prednisolone group compared with the placebo group.[45] Prednisolone was also found to shorten the time to complete recovery of function in Bell's palsy.[46] Oral steroid therapy may also significantly reduce unwanted long-term sequelae of Bell's palsy, such as synkinesis.[47,48]

> **!**
>
> Oral corticosteroids are the standard treatment for Bell's palsy; they are most effective when initiated within 72 hours of onset of symptoms and with treatment duration of 10 days.

The administration of oral steroids early in the course of Bell's palsy is now strongly supported by both the American Academy of Neurology and the American Academy of Otolaryngology—Head and Neck Surgery.[21,49] The recommendations of the American Academy of Otolaryngology—Head and Neck Surgery for the diagnostic work-up and treatment of Bell's palsy are summarized in ▶ Fig. 8.4 and ▶ Fig. 8.5. The large placebo-controlled trials and the guidelines seem to be clearly associated with change in management of patients with Bell's palsy, i.e., there are rising trends in prednisolone therapy in the recent years. Nevertheless and unfortunately, some patients still do not receive any medical treatment.[50] The exact dosing of prednisone varies but generally starts with 60 mg/day for 5 to 10 days with a slow taper over the subsequent 5 to 7 days. Peptic ulcer prophylaxis may be used as needed. All patients should be carefully counseled on the potential side effects and risks associated with oral steroid therapy, including mood changes, acute psychosis, gastrointestinal irritation and bleeding, altered glucose metabolism,

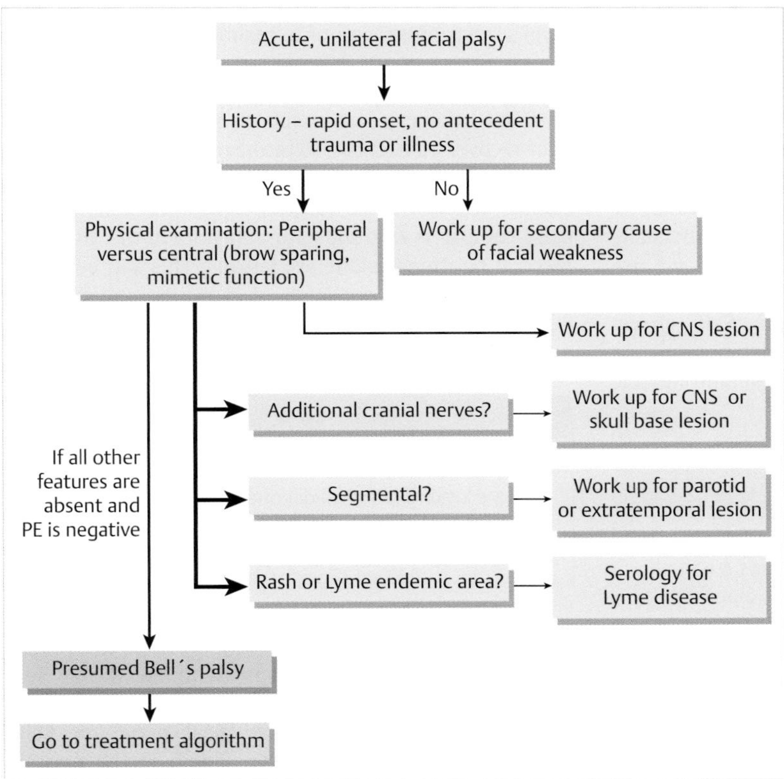

Fig. 8.4 Algorithm summarizing the most important steps of the diagnostic work-up of Bell's palsy. CNS, central nervous system; PE, physical examination.

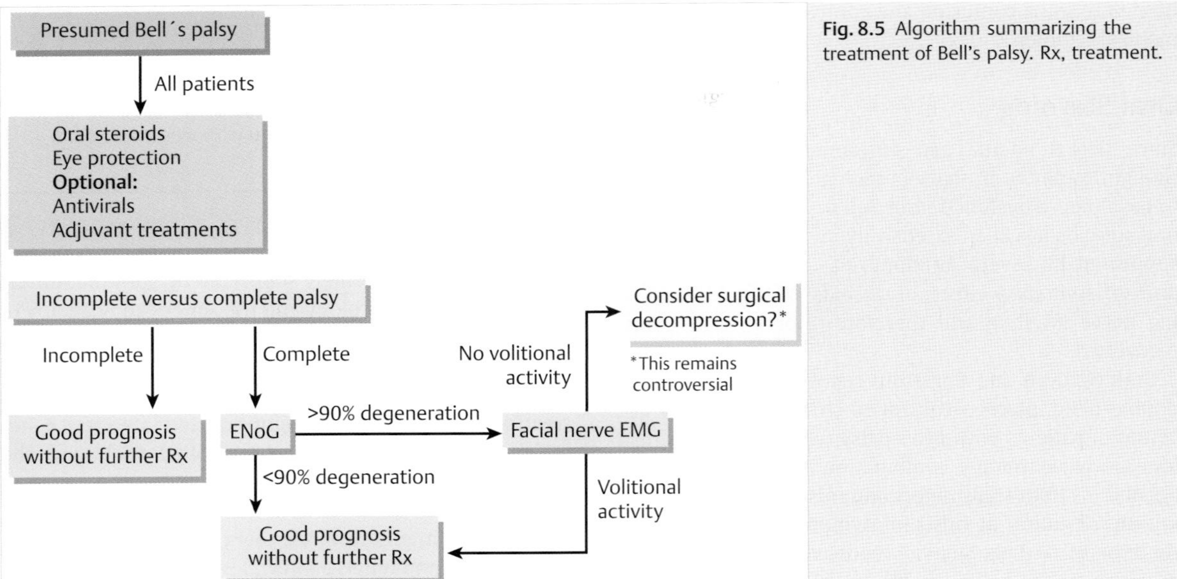

Fig. 8.5 Algorithm summarizing the treatment of Bell's palsy. Rx, treatment.

glaucoma, and avascular necrosis of the femoral head. In pregnant and diabetic patients, steroids should be used with caution.

Antiviral Therapy

In large reviews, antiviral monotherapy has not been found to offer any additional therapeutic benefit in Bell's palsy even though herpes simplex virus reactivation is thought to play a role in the disease. Patients treated with acyclovir or valacyclovir alone demonstrated no better functional recovery when compared with patients treated with placebo agents, and did worse than patients treated with oral steroids.[45,46] However, when combined with prednisolone administered within 72 hours of onset, there may be a small yet not statistically significant benefit.[49] Valacyclovir and famciclovir are preferred both for easier dosing schedules and higher bioavailability compared with acyclovir. Side effects related to antiviral therapy are infrequent but include nausea, vomiting, diarrhea, and rarely renal and hepatic insufficiency.

> Although these recent studies suggest use of prednisone alone, they are not without flaws. The groups are small and patients continue to be able to achieve a perfect 100%, House–Brackmann grade I result after 3 months. These studies may not be the final word on the medical treatment of Bell's palsy.

8.6.3 Surgical Decompression

Surgical decompression of the facial nerve for Bell's palsy remains controversial. The proposed pathophysiologic mechanism in Bell's palsy is thought to be entrapment neuropathy. Decompression of the entrapped nerve would logically offer some theoretic benefit. Improved neural regeneration has been demonstrated in cats after surgical decompression of experimentally induced facial nerve compression.[51] Proponents of surgical decompression for Bell's palsy endeavor to improve the odds of favorable recovery in the subset of patients at risk for poor recovery based on electrodiagnostic testing. To date, large randomized controlled studies demonstrating the clinical superiority of surgical decompression in Bell's palsy compared with the natural history of the disease or medical treatment alone are lacking. This can be attributed largely to the challenge of capturing patients with Bell's palsy within the first 2 weeks of onset of complete paralysis.

> Controlled studies on facial nerve decompression surgery are lacking. Surgical decompression in Bell's palsy has not yet been shown to be superior to the natural history of the disease or medical treatment alone.

The site of pathology in Bell's palsy has evolved over the decades from the mastoid segment to the meatal segment of the facial nerve. Ballance was the first to report surgical decompression of the facial nerve for Bell's palsy with slitting of the nerve sheath in the mastoid segment.[52] The benefit of decompression of the mastoid segment has since been refuted after meta-analyses of pooled data from available randomized studies.[53] Adour randomized 40 patients to surgical and nonsurgical treatment and reported no benefit of early or late decompression of the mastoid segment in which nerve excitability testing showed evidence of impending or actual nerve degeneration.[54] Similarly, a small randomized study by Mechelse in 1971 reported no benefit with surgical decompression compared with nonsurgical treatment.[55] Transmastoid decompression of the vertical facial nerve is no longer recommended for Bell's palsy.

The fallopian canal is narrowest in the labyrinthine segment, starting from the meatal foramen. In 1972, Fisch reported intraoperative findings of nerve edema proximal to the geniculate ganglion in 94% of patients who underwent combined transmastoid and middle fossa facial nerve decompression.[39] He subsequently reported improved functional recovery in patients with Bell's palsy who underwent surgical decompression of the labyrinthine facial nerve via a middle fossa approach compared with control patients treated nonsurgically.[56] This segment of the facial nerve has become the focus of surgical decompression for Bell's palsy. In 1999, Gantz reported on a prospective multi-institutional case–control study supporting middle fossa decompression of the facial nerve and reported improved functional outcomes in surgically treated patients with poor prognostic indicators for recovery.[57] Patients with greater than 90% degeneration on ENoG and no spontaneous EMG activity within 14 days of onset of paralysis, were offered surgical decompression. Ninety-one percent of 34 surgically treated patients achieved House–Brackmann grades I to II function. Of the 36 control subjects with similar electrical test results who elected not to undergo surgery, 58% had persistent weakness at 7 months (House–Brackmann grades III to IV). Several other case series have also reported good functional outcomes with middle fossa decompression of the facial nerve with more variable time treatment time frames.[58,59]

Based on the available literature, middle fossa decompression of the meatal foramen and labyrinthine facial nerve may be offered to Bell's palsy patients who have 90% or more degeneration on ENoG testing within the first 14 days of onset of complete paralysis and absence of motor unit action potentials on voluntary EMG testing. In those with poor or no hearing in the affected ear, a translabyrinthine approach is used. The risk of iatrogenic facial nerve injury, sensorineural hearing loss, dizziness, cerebrospinal fluid leak, meningitis, and cerebrovascular events related to craniotomy surgery and facial nerve decompression must be weighed heavily against the potential benefit of improved long-term functional outcomes. A Cochrane review failed to show any benefit of surgical decompression for Bell's palsy.[53] There remains a lack of consensus on the role of surgical decompression for Bell's palsy, mostly attributable to multiple factors including the paucity of high-quality evidence supporting this treatment and the challenging logistics of evaluating Bell's palsy patients within the recommended surgical window. Only half of neurotologists surveyed believe that surgical decompression should be the standard of care, and one-third had not performed a surgical decompression for Bell's palsy in the last 10 years.[60]

> **!**
>
> Surgical decompression of the meatal segment of the facial nerve for patients with appropriate electrodiagnostic testing remains controversial.

8.6.4 Adjunctive Therapies

Massage therapy, facial exercises, acupuncture, and electrical stimulation have been used as adjunctive modalities for managing patients with facial paralysis. The true benefit of these therapies has yet to be proven; see the discussion in Chapter 26.[61] However, given the concomitant lack of evidence demonstrating harm with these treatment modalities, any of these may be offered to the patient with Bell's palsy if skilled therapists are available for these therapies.

8.7 Outcomes and Prognosis

All patients with acute facial palsy should be followed closely within the first couple weeks of onset. During the first 2 weeks after onset of complete paralysis, close attention should be directed at following the time course of progression in electrodiagnostic test results. Surgical decompression of the facial nerve may be offered to those who meet electrical criteria for this treatment within the initial 2-week time frame. Any patient with an acute unilateral facial palsy who fails to demonstrate any sign of recovery at 4 months should be worked-up further to rule out other etiologies.

Most patients with Bell's palsy demonstrate some recovery within 2 to 3 weeks after onset of symptoms and complete recovery within 4 to 6 months. Incomplete paresis and early onset of recovery are good prognostic factors. Patients with incomplete nerve palsy will generally recover all or most of their function. In Peitersen's study, 94% of patients with incomplete palsy achieved normal function, whereas 61% of patients with complete paralysis returned to normal function.[5] Also, greater degrees of recovery were observed in patients who began to recover earlier, in younger patients, and in patients who did not have postauricular pain. Recovery of mimetic function began within 3 weeks in 85% of patients with Bell's palsy, and over 80% of these patients achieved normal function. The remaining 15% of the patients did not see any onset of recovery until 3 to 5 months after onset, and very few of those achieved complete recovery of function. These patients all had complete paralysis, and the late onset of recovery implies a severe conduction block of the nerve with muscle denervation. Age is certainly a factor that influences degree of recovery. Bell's palsy in children under 14 recovers 90% of the time, whereas in adults over age 60, only one-third will recover fully.

Bell's palsy patients with incomplete recovery and long-term sequelae may require additional treatment, including facial reanimation surgery. This topic is covered in detail in Section VI of this textbook. The emotional and psychological impact of facial dysfunction cannot be underestimated. Appropriate counseling and support must be offered to these patients.

8.8 Key Points

- Clinical features that are not characteristic of Bell's palsy and that should trigger a search for another etiology:
  - Palsy that is gradual in onset (greater than 72 hours) —this should raise the suspicion of a cholesteatoma or neoplasm of the facial nerve, skull base, or parotid.
  - Palsy that spares the brow and mimetic function—this is central nervous system in origin.
  - Polycranial neuropathies—these could be associated with central nervous system pathology or skull base tumors.
  - Segmental facial palsy (i.e., sparing of certain branches)—this suggests a lesion distal to the stylomastoid foramen, such as a parotid tumor.
  - Facial paralysis that fails to show any sign of recovery after 4 months.
- Recurrent Bell's palsy occurs in between 3 and 15% of cases, ipsilateral (one-third) or contralateral (two-thirds), and simultaneous or sequential:
  - Recurrent alternating palsy is either Melkersson–Rosenthal syndrome or from Bell's palsy.
  - Simultaneous bilateral palsy and recurrent ipsilateral palsy should initiate a search for an underlying cause.
- Early recovery of function is the most important prognostic sign in Bell's palsy:
  - Patients who show some degree of recovery within 3 weeks will go on to have normal function > 80% of the time.
  - Patients who show no recovery before 3 months will not achieve normal function.
- Electrodiagnostic testing is helpful in prognosticating recovery when facial paralysis becomes complete.
- Imaging of the facial nerve is not routinely recommended for Bell's palsy.
- Oral steroids with or without antiviral therapy have been demonstrated to improve functional recovery in Bell's palsy when administered within 72 hours of onset.
- Surgical decompression of the facial nerve for Bell's palsy remains controversial.

References

[1] Adour KK, Byl FM, Hilsinger RL, Jr, Kahn ZM, Sheldon MI. The true nature of Bell's palsy: analysis of 1,000 consecutive patients. Laryngoscope 1978; 88: 787–801

[2] McCormick DP. Herpes-simplex virus as a cause of Bell's palsy. Lancet 1972; 1: 937–939

[3] Murakami S, Mizobuchi M, Nakashiro Y, Doi T, Hato N, Yanagihara N. Bell palsy and herpes simplex virus: identification of viral DNA in endoneurial fluid and muscle. Ann Intern Med 1996; 124: 27–30

[4] Lazarini PR, Vianna MF, Alcantara MP, Scalia RA, Caiaffa Filho HH. Herpes simplex virus in the saliva of peripheral Bell's palsy patients. Braz J Otorhinolaryngol 2006; 72: 7–11

[5] Peitersen E. Bell's palsy: the spontaneous course of 2,500 peripheral facial nerve palsies of different etiologies. Acta Otolaryngol Suppl 2002: 4–30

[6] Bell C. On the nerves; giving an account of some experiments on their structure and functions, which lead to a new arrangement of the system. Phil Trans R Soc Lond 1821; 111: 398–424

[7] Peitersen E. The natural history of Bell's palsy. Am J Otol 1982; 4: 107–111

[8] Adour KK, Bell DN, Hilsinger RL, Jr. Herpes simplex virus in idiopathic facial paralysis (Bell palsy). JAMA 1975; 233: 527–530

[9] Pitkäranta A, Piiparinen H, Mannonen L, Vesaluoma M, Vaheri A. Detection of human herpesvirus 6 and varicella-zoster virus in tear fluid of patients with Bell's palsy by PCR. J Clin Microbiol 2000; 38: 2753–2755

[10] Stjernquist-Desatnik A, Skoog E, Aurelius E. Detection of herpes simplex and varicella-zoster viruses in patients with Bell's palsy by the polymerase chain reaction technique. Ann Otol Rhinol Laryngol 2006; 115: 306–311

[11] Steiner I, Spivack JG, O'Boyle DR, II, Lavi E, Fraser NW. Latent herpes simplex virus type 1 transcription in human trigeminal ganglia. J Virol 1988; 62: 3493–3496

[12] Linder T, Bossart W, Bodmer D. Bell's palsy and Herpes simplex virus: fact or mystery? Otol Neurotol 2005; 26: 109–113

[13] Steiner I, Mattan Y. Bell's palsy and herpes viruses: to (acyclo)vir or not to (acyclo)vir? J Neurol Sci 1999; 170: 19–23

[14] Sadé J. Pathology of Bell's palsy. Arch Otolaryngol 1972; 95: 406–414

[15] Proctor B, Corgill DA, Proud G. The pathology of Bell's palsy. Trans Sect Otolaryngol Am Acad Ophthalmol Otolaryngol 1976; 82: ORL70–ORL80

[16] May M, Podvinec M, Ulrich J, et al. Idiopathic Bell's palsy, Herpes zoster cephalicus, and other facial nerve disorders of viral etiology. In: May M, ed. The Facial Nerve, Thieme, New York, 1986

[17] Liston SL, Kleid MS. Histopathology of Bell's palsy. Laryngoscope 1989; 99: 23–26

[18] Matsumoto Y, Pulec JL, Patterson MJ, Yanagihara N. Facial nerve biopsy for etiologic clarification of Bell's palsy. Ann Otol Rhinol Laryngol Suppl 1988; 137: 22–27

[19] Michaels L. Histopathological changes in the temporal bone in Bell's palsy. Acta Otolaryngol Suppl 1990; 470: 114–117, discussion 118

[20] May M, Schlaepfer WM. Bell's palsy and the chorda tympani nerve: a clinical and electron microscopic study. Laryngoscope 1975; 85: 1957–1975

[21] Baugh RF, Basura GJ, Ishii LE et al. Clinical practice guideline: Bell's palsy. Otolaryngol Head Neck Surg 2013; 149 Suppl: S1–S27

[22] Gilden DH. Clinical practice. Bell's palsy. N Engl J Med 2004; 351: 1323–1331

[23] Adour KK, Hilsinger RL, Jr, Callan EJ. Facial paralysis and Bell's palsy: a protocol for differential diagnosis. Am J Otol 1985 Suppl: 68–73

[24] Clark JR, Carlson RD, Sasaki CT, Pachner AR, Steere AC. Facial paralysis in Lyme disease. Laryngoscope 1985; 95: 1341–1345
[25] Smouha EE, Coyle PK, Shukri S. Facial nerve palsy in Lyme disease: evaluation of clinical diagnostic criteria. Am J Otol 1997; 18: 257–261
[26] Halperin JJ, Golightly M Long Island Neuroborreliosis Collaborative Study Group. Lyme borreliosis in Bell's palsy. Neurology 1992; 42: 1268–1270
[27] Luft BJ, Steinman CR, Neimark HC et al. Invasion of the central nervous system by Borrelia burgdorferi in acute disseminated infection. JAMA 1992; 267: 1364–1367Erratum in: JAMA 1992;19:268:872
[28] Adour K, Wingerd J, Doty HE. Prevalence of concurrent diabetes mellitus and idiopathic facial paralysis (Bell's palsy). Diabetes 1975; 24: 449–451
[29] Gillman GS, Schaitkin BM, May M, Klein SR. Bell's palsy in pregnancy: a study of recovery outcomes. Otolaryngol Head Neck Surg 2002; 126: 26–30
[30] Hilsinger RL, Jr, Adour KK, Doty HE. Idiopathic facial paralysis, pregnancy, and the menstrual cycle. Ann Otol Rhinol Laryngol 1975; 84: 433–442
[31] Yanagihara N, Mori H, Kozawa T, Nakamura K, Kita M. Bell's palsy. Nonrecurrent v recurrent and unilateral v bilateral. Arch Otolaryngol 1984; 110: 374–377
[32] Pitts DB, Adour KK, Hilsinger RL, Jr. Recurrent Bell's palsy: analysis of 140 patients. Laryngoscope 1988; 98: 535–540
[33] Boddie HG. Recurrent Bell's palsy. J Laryngol Otol 1972; 86: 117–120
[34] Devriese PP, Pelz PG. Recurrent and alternating Bell's palsy. Ann Otol Rhinol Laryngol 1969; 78: 1091–1104
[35] Chung DH, Park DC, Byun JY, Park MS, Lee SY, Yeo SG. Prognosis of patients with recurrent facial palsy. Eur Arch Otorhinolaryngol 2012; 269: 61–66
[36] Schwaber MK, Larson TC, III, Zealear DL, Creasy J. Gadolinium-enhanced magnetic resonance imaging in Bell's palsy. Laryngoscope 1990; 100: 1264–1269
[37] Sartoretti-Schefer S, Brändle P, Wichmann W, Valavanis A. Intensity of MR contrast enhancement does not correspond to clinical and electroneurographic findings in acute inflammatory facial nerve palsy. AJNR Am J Neuroradiol 1996; 17: 1229–1236
[38] Fisch U. Prognostic value of electrical tests in acute facial paralysis. Am J Otol 1984; 5: 494–498
[39] Fisch U, Esslen E. Total intratemporal exposure of the facial nerve. Pathologic findings in Bell's palsy. Arch Otolaryngol 1972; 95: 335–341
[40] Tojima H, Aoyagi M, Inamura H, Koike Y. Clinical advantages of electroneurography in patients with Bell's palsy within two weeks after onset. Acta Otolaryngol Suppl 1994; 511: 147–149
[41] Adour KK, Sheldon MI, Kahn ZM. Maximal nerve excitability testing versus neuromyography: prognostic value in patients with facial paralysis. Laryngoscope 1980; 90: 1540–1547
[42] Sinha PK, Keith RW, Pensak ML. Predictability of recovery from Bell's palsy using evoked electromyography. Am J Otol 1994; 15: 769–771
[43] Sillman JS, Niparko JK, Lee SS, Kileny PR. Prognostic value of evoked and standard electromyography in acute facial paralysis. Otolaryngol Head Neck Surg 1992; 107: 377–381
[44] Volk GF, Klingner C, Finkensieper M, Witte OW, Guntinas-Lichius O. Prognostication of recovery time after acute peripheral facial palsy: a prospective cohort study. BMJ Open 2013; 3: e003007
[45] Sullivan FM, Swan IRC, Donnan PT et al. Early treatment with prednisolone or acyclovir in Bell's palsy. N Engl J Med 2007; 357: 1598–1607
[46] Engström M, Berg T, Stjernquist-Desatnik A et al. Prednisolone and valaciclovir in Bell's palsy: a randomised, double-blind, placebo-controlled, multicentre trial. Lancet Neurol 2008; 7: 993–1000
[47] Berg T, Bylund N, Marsk E et al. The effect of prednisolone on sequelae in Bell's palsy. Arch Otolaryngol Head Neck Surg 2012; 138: 445–449
[48] Axelsson S, Berg T, Jonsson L, Engström M, Kanerva M, Stjernquist-Desatnik A. Bell's palsy - the effect of prednisolone and/or valaciclovir versus placebo in relation to baseline severity in a randomised controlled trial. Clin Otolaryngol 2012; 37: 283–290
[49] Gronseth GS, Paduga R American Academy of Neurology. Evidence-based guideline update: steroids and antivirals for Bell palsy: report of the Guideline Development Subcommittee of the American Academy of Neurology. Neurology 2012; 79: 2209–2213
[50] Morales DR, Donnan PT, Daly F, Staa TV, Sullivan FM. Impact of clinical trial findings on Bell's palsy management in general practice in the UK 2001–2012: interrupted time series regression analysis. BMJ Open 2013; 3: e003121
[51] Yamamoto E, Fisch U. Experimentally induced facial nerve compression in cats. Acta Otolaryngol 1975; 79: 390–395
[52] Ballance C, Duel AB. The operative treatment of facial palsy: by the introduction of nerve grafts into the fallopian canal and by other intratemporal methods. Arch Otolaryngol 1932; 15: 1–70
[53] McAllister K, Walker D, Donnan PT, Swan I. Surgical interventions for the early management of Bell's palsy. Cochrane Database Syst Rev 2011: CD007468
[54] Adour KK, Swanson PJ, Jr. Facial paralysis in 403 consecutive patients: emphasis on treatment response in patients with Bell's palsy. Trans Am Acad Ophthalmol Otolaryngol 1971; 75: 1284–1301
[55] Mechelse K, Goor G, Huizing EH et al. Bell's palsy: prognostic criteria and evaluation of surgical decompression. Lancet 1971; 2: 57–59
[56] Fisch U. Surgery for Bell's palsy. Arch Otolaryngol 1981; 107: 1–11
[57] Gantz BJ, Rubinstein JT, Gidley P, Woodworth GG. Surgical management of Bell's palsy. Laryngoscope 1999; 109: 1177–1188
[58] Kim IS, Shin SH, Kim J, Lee WS, Lee HK. Correlation between MRI and operative findings in Bell's palsy and Ramsay Hunt syndrome. Yonsei Med J 2007; 48: 963–968
[59] Bodénez C, Bernat I, Willer JC, Barré P, Lamas G, Tankéré F. Facial nerve decompression for idiopathic Bell's palsy: report of 13 cases and literature review. J Laryngol Otol 2010; 124: 272–278
[60] Smouha E, Toh E, Schaitkin BM. Surgical treatment of Bell's palsy: current attitudes. Laryngoscope 2011; 121: 1965–1970
[61] Teixeira LJ, Valbuza JS, Prado GF. Physical therapy for Bell's palsy (idiopathic facial paralysis). Cochrane Database Syst Rev 2011; 7: CD006283

9 Facial Nerve Trauma

Peter L. Santa Maria, Mira Finkensieper, Orlando Guntinas-Lichius, and Robert K. Jackler

9.1 Introduction

After idiopathic facial palsy, trauma of the facial nerve is the most common cause of facial palsy.[1] The exact lesion site has to be localized and a detailed assessment of type and extent of the injury is mandatory. Important tools are imaging and electrophysiologic tests. Treatment varies according to type of injury, severity, location, onset of the lesion, and wishes of the patient.

9.2 Definition

Facial nerve trauma is an acute trauma of the peripheral facial nerve. It can have an external origin or be the result of an iatrogenic injury. Facial nerve trauma can affect all six segments of the facial nerve from its exit from the facial nucleus (intracranial segment), the cerebellopontine angle up to the internal auditory canal (meatal segment), the three intratemporal segments (labyrinthine, tympanic, and mastoid segment), and the extratemporal segment from the stylomastoid foramen to the division into the branches in the face.

> **!**
>
> Decision making in facial nerve trauma depends heavily on the precise localization of the trauma to the intracranial, intratemporal, or extratemporal segment of the facial nerve.

The facial nerve is composed of neuronal axons surrounded by non-neuronal cells and connective tissues providing a complex stromal connective tissue scaffold. This complex is important to understanding the classification of facial nerve injuries (▶ Table 9.1, ▶ Fig. 9.1).[2] The classification into three categories by Seddon is important as it is frequently used to describe the results of electromyographic examinations of the facial nerve; see also Chapter 6. Seddon's classification is based on the presence of demyelination and the extent of damage to the axons and the connective tissues of the nerve.[3] The mildest form of injury is called neurapraxia, defined by focal demyelination without damage to the axons or the connective tissues. Neurapraxia typically occurs from mild compression or traction of the nerve. The next level is axonotmesis, which involves direct damage to the axons in addition to focal demyelination while maintaining continuity of the nerve's connective tissues. The most severe form of injury is called neurotmesis, which is a full transection of the axons and connective tissue layers, resulting in complete discontinuity of the nerve. The classification of Sunderland is more accurate in distinguishing the extent of damage in the connective tissues.[4] Sunderland's grade I and grade V correspond with Seddon's neurapraxia and neurotmesis, respectively. Grades II to IV, however, are all forms of axonotmesis with increasing amounts of connective tissue damage. In grade II, axon damage is observed with no damage present in the connective tissue. Grade III involves damage to the endoneurium and grade IV includes damage to the perineurium. A grade VI lesion was later introduced by Mackinnon and Dellon to denote combinations of grade III to V injuries along a damaged nerve.[5] Although Sunderland's classification determines more correctly the different types of nerve injury, there is no current diagnostic tool available to allow such an exact classification in the individual patient with traumatic facial palsy. The timing of onset of facial palsy is an important factor for treatment planning. An immediate onset of facial palsy is defined by start of the symptoms coincident with the injury. Late-onset (delayed) paresis is defined as a palsy occurring any time after the trauma and is common after temporal bone trauma.

Table 9.1 Classification of nerve injuries

Seddon	Sunderland	Type of injury	Comment
Neurapraxia	Grade I	Focal segmental demyelination	Due to mild compression or traction of the nerve
Axonotmesis	Grade II	Axon damaged with intact endoneurium	Moderate compression or blunt trauma, viral infection
Axonotmesis	Grade III	Axon and endoneurium damaged with intact perineurium	Moderate compression or blunt trauma
Axonotmesis	Grade IV	Axon, endoneurium, and perineurium damaged with intact epineurium	Moderate compression or blunt trauma
Neurotmesis	Grade V	Complete nerve transection	Typical iatrogenic lesion or fire arm/knife injury
Neurotmesis	Grade VI (MacKinnon and Dellon)	Mixed levels of injury along the nerve	Severe and complex facial trauma

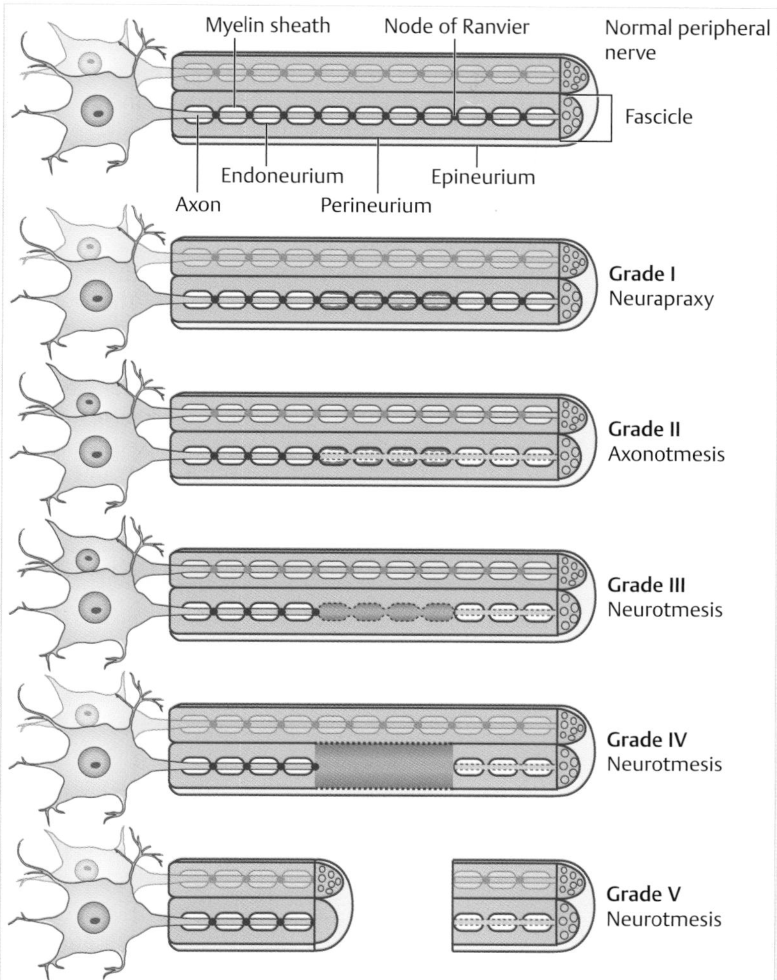

Fig. 9.1 Classification of facial nerve trauma according to Sunderland's classification (see ▶ Table 9.1).

> **!**
>
> It is very important for further treatment planning to define whether the patient has an immediate- or delayed-onset traumatic facial palsy.

9.3 Epidemiology and Etiology

Due to the long and complicated course of the facial nerve, the cause of facial nerve trauma and the site of the lesion can be manifold (▶ Table 9.2). In general terms, the causes of injury are categorized as accidental (external) trauma or surgical (unavoidable or iatrogenic) trauma.[6] The prevalence of traumatic lesions in series of patients with facial palsy has been described to be between 5 and 25%,[7–9] depending mainly on the frequency of severe traffic accidents and violent conflicts.

Table 9.2 Most frequent causes and lesion sites of facial nerve trauma

Site of facial nerve trauma	Most frequents causes
Intracranial	• Brain injury • Avulsion at brainstem • Surgical lesion
Intratemporal	• Temporal bone fracture • Fire arm injury • Blunt injury • Thermal burn • Chemical burn • Surgical lesion
Extratemporal	• Facial fracture • Fire arm injury • Facial contusion and laceration • Puncture injury • Blast injury • Birth canal trauma • Surgical lesion

In large series, depending on the reference being used, surgical trauma (three-fourth of cases) is much more frequent than accidental trauma in the western world (one-fourth of cases). According to the lesion site, facial nerve trauma is divided into intracranial, intratemporal, and extratemporal lesions. The leading causes for surgical trauma are vestibular schwannoma surgery (two-thirds of cases), parotid surgery (one-fourth of cases), and otologic surgery for chronic otitis media and temporal bone tumors. The importance of the facial nerve in parotid and vestibular schwannoma surgery is explored in more detail in Chapter 18 and Chapter 19.

Half of the accidental causes of facial paralysis are localized in the temporal bone,[10] mainly in combination with temporal bone fracture. Blunt head trauma is the most frequent (30–70%) reason for facial palsy in cases of temporal bone fracture.

Temporal bone fractures in the past have been classified into longitudinal and transverse fractures according to their plane with the long axis of the petrous ridge of the temporal bone. Longitudinal fractures generally pass in a plane anterior to the otic capsule and are usually secondary to temporoparietal impact (▶ Fig. 9.2), compared with transverse fractures, which are perpendicular to the long axis of the petrous ridge and usually secondary to fronto-occipital impact (▶ Fig. 9.3 and ▶ Fig. 9.4). When there is a combination of these they are termed mixed fractures.[11] The fracture patterns follow predictable paths of least resistance (▶ Fig. 9.5 and ▶ Fig. 9.6).

A newer classification describes the fractures as either otic capsule sparing or otic capsule violating. Otic capsule sparing fractures usually involve the squamous part, superior external auditory canal, tympanic membrane, or mastoid. Otic capsule violating fractures usually spare the external auditory canal and more often involve the jugular foramen or foramen magnum (▶ Fig. 9.7, ▶ Fig. 9.8 and ▶ Fig. 9.9).[12]

Traditionally, using the older classification, it was taught that longitudinal fractures occurred in 80% of patients and transverse fractures in 20%. The reality is that true longitudinal fractures are rare with most being considered oblique.[11] The highest proportion is mixed, being a combination of longitudinal and transverse. In one large cohort the frequency of occurrence was 29% longitudinal, 26% transverse, and 45% mixed. Using the new classification they were described as 93% otic capsule sparing compared with 7% otic capsule violating.

> **!**
>
> The newer classification of otic capsule sparing and otic capsule violating fractures provides a clinically relevant classification that relates to the likelihood of facial nerve injury.

Facial nerve injury occurs in 7 to 10% of temporal bone fractures,[13] including up to 30% in otic capsule violating

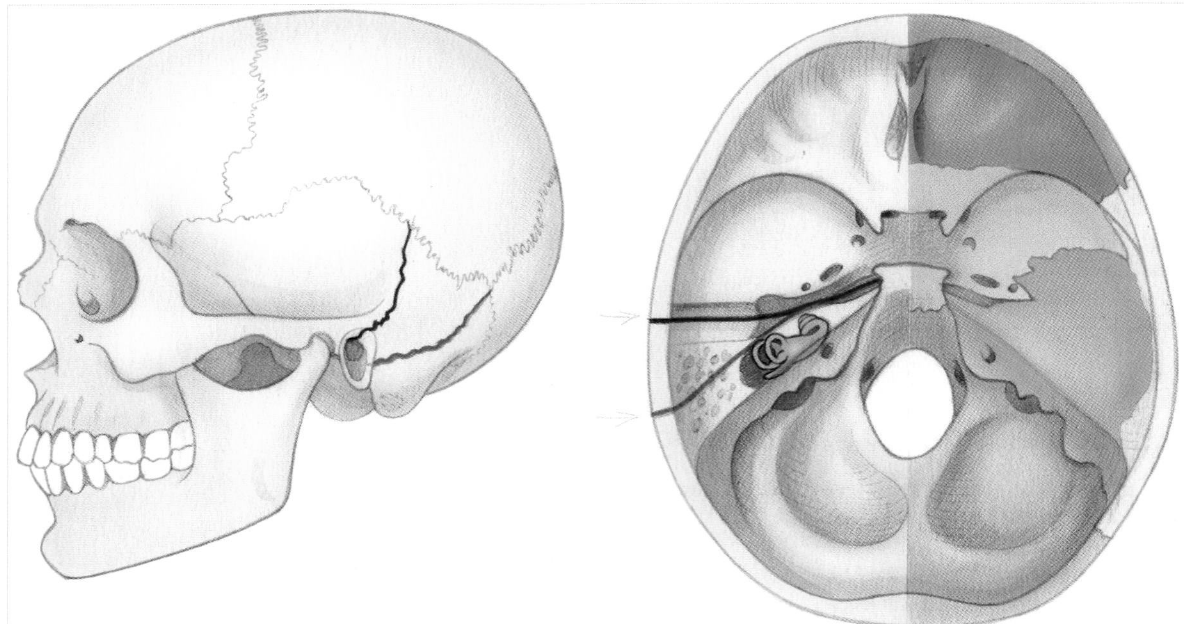

Fig. 9.2 The more common pathways of longitudinal fractures. (Image provided courtesy of Chris Gralapp and Robert Jackler, Department of Otolaryngology–Head and Neck Surgery, Stanford School of Medicine, California, USA)

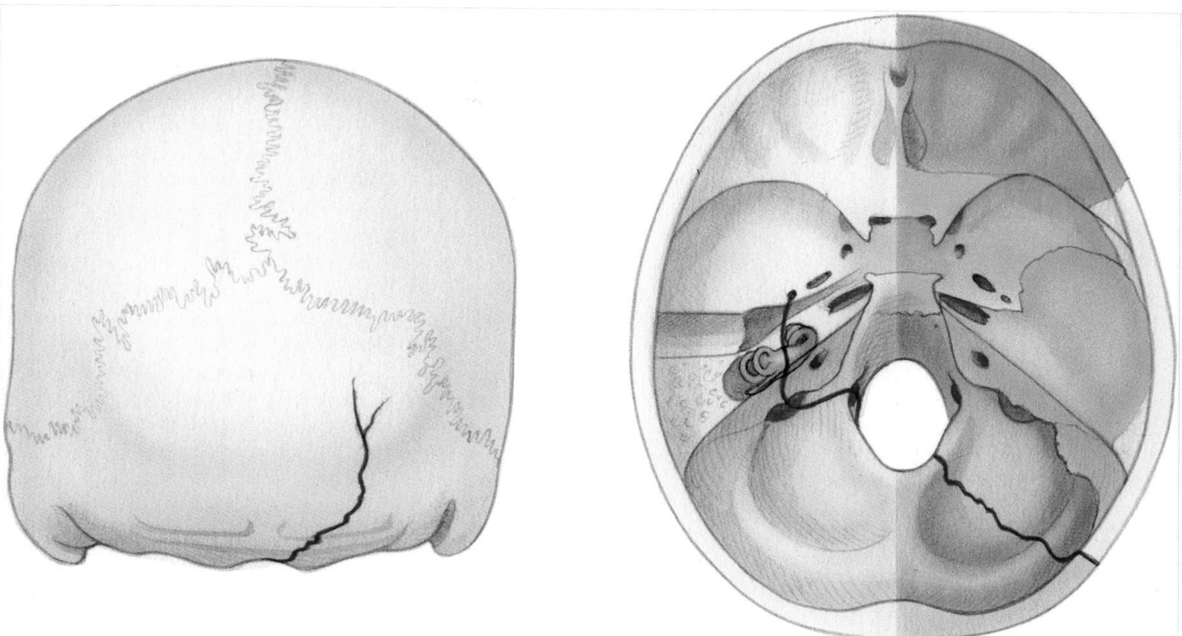

Fig. 9.3 The more common pathways of transverse fractures. (Image provided courtesy of Chris Gralapp and Robert Jackler, Department of Otolaryngology–Head and Neck Surgery, Stanford School of Medicine, California, USA)

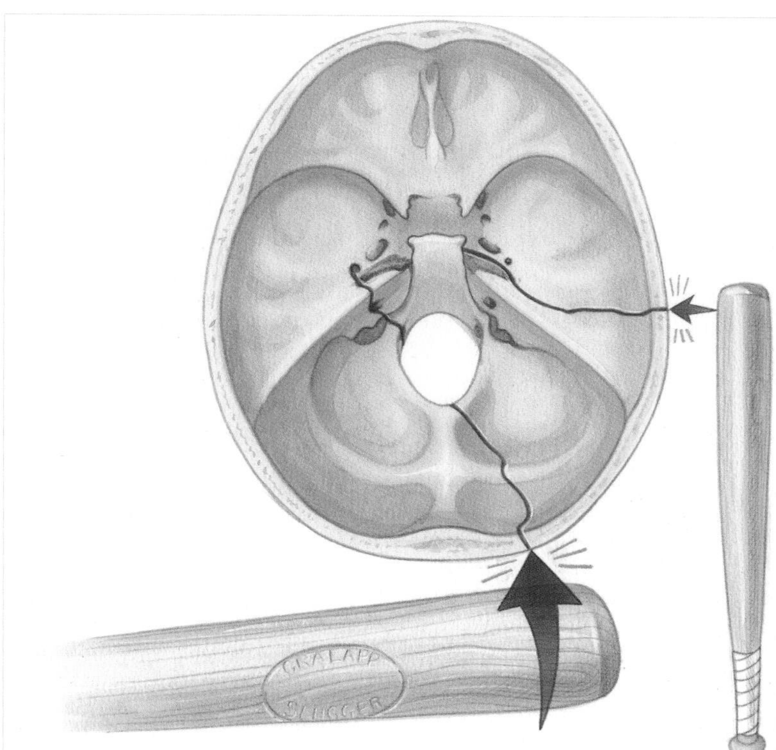

Fig. 9.4 Trauma from a lateral direction predisposes to longitudinal fracture as the fracture line hits the hard bone of the otic capsule and then is directed anteriorly. Trauma in the anterioposterior direction predisposes to transverse fracture and otic capsule violation. (Image provided courtesy of Chris Gralapp and Robert Jackler, Department of Otolaryngology–Head and Neck Surgery, Stanford School of Medicine, California, USA)

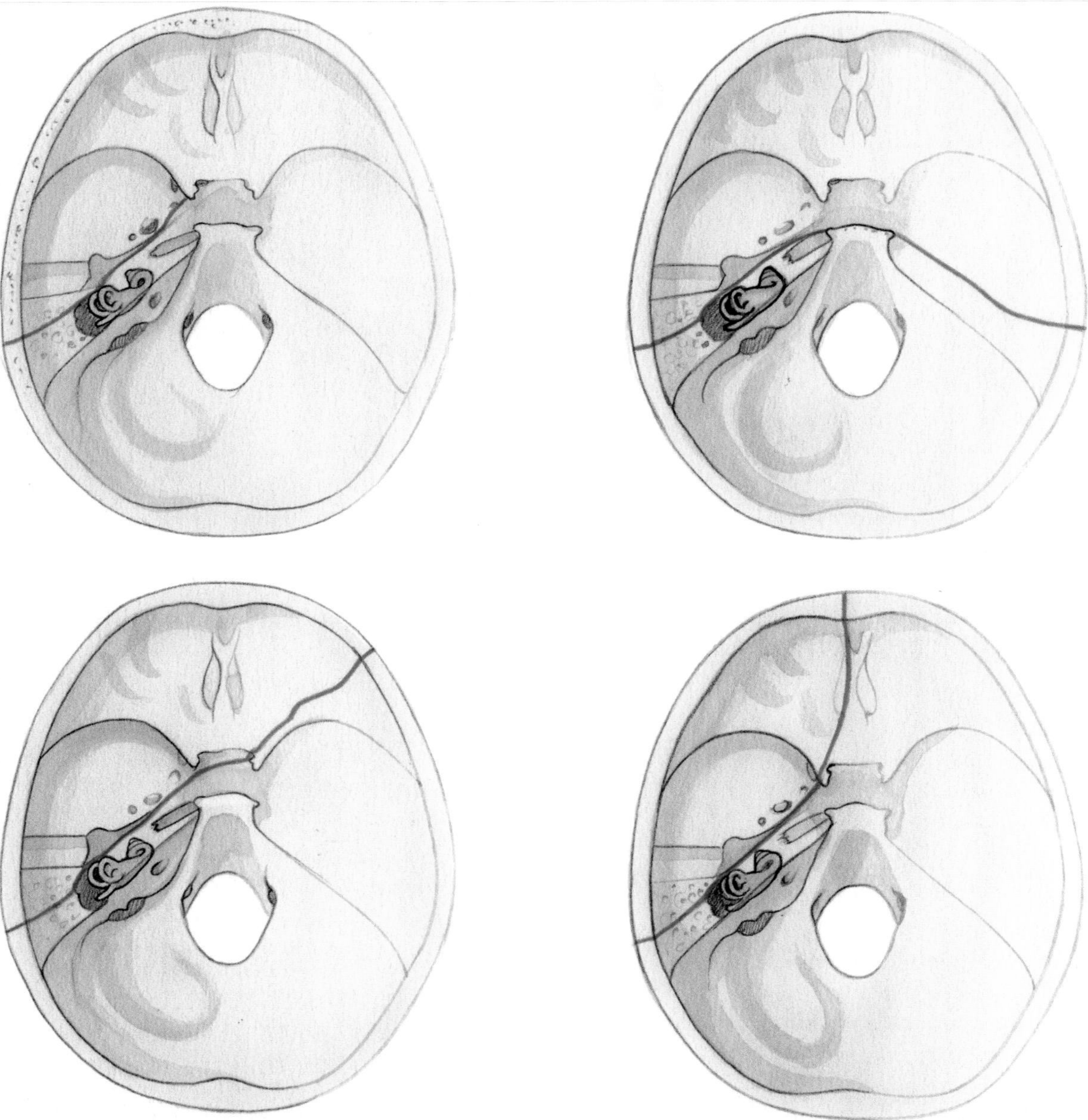

Fig. 9.5 The common pathways of longitudinal fractures. The pathway is predictable until the fracture line meets the hard clivus with force and then it is dispersed in a variety of directions. (Image provided courtesy of Chris Gralapp and Robert Jackler, Department of Otolaryngology–Head and Neck Surgery, Stanford School of Medicine, California, USA)

fractures. The etiology is most often motor vehicle accidents, assaults, falls, or gunshot injury.[14] They are more common in males, reflecting a higher incidence of trauma in males. Facial nerve injury from temporal bone trauma is less in children, hypothetically due to their more flexible skulls.[15] The perigeniculate area is the most common site (46%) of facial nerve injury in temporal bone fracture, followed by the tympanic segment, and at the second genu (12%).[16] At surgery, edema or hematoma of the facial nerve is the most common finding, but dehiscence and bone chips/spicules can also be found.[13,17,18]

> **!**
>
> The perigeniculate area is the most common site for facial nerve injury in temporal bone trauma.

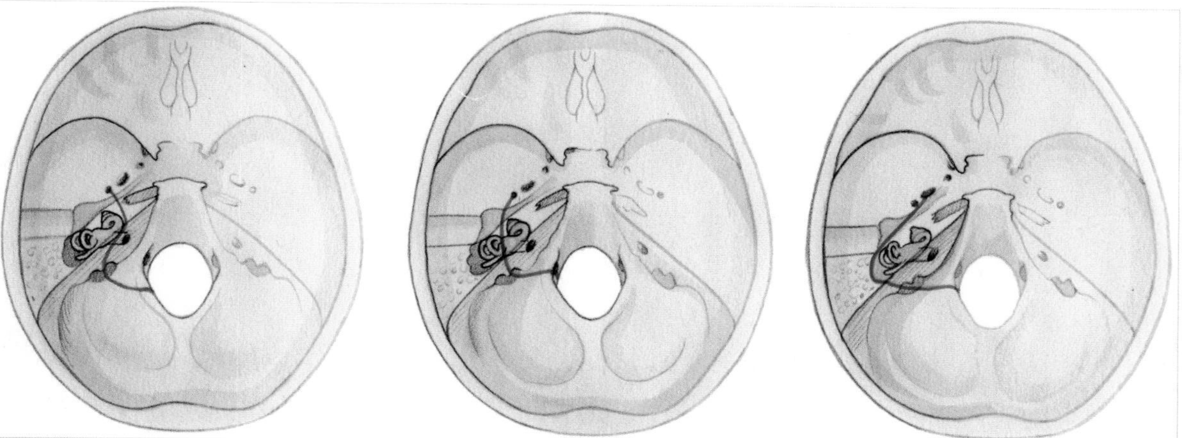

Fig. 9.6 The common pathway of transverse fractures. The hard otic capsule usually directs the fracture line around it, but with sufficient force the otic capsule is violated. (Image provided courtesy of Chris Gralapp and Robert Jackler, Department of Otolaryngology–Head and Neck Surgery, Stanford School of Medicine, California, USA)

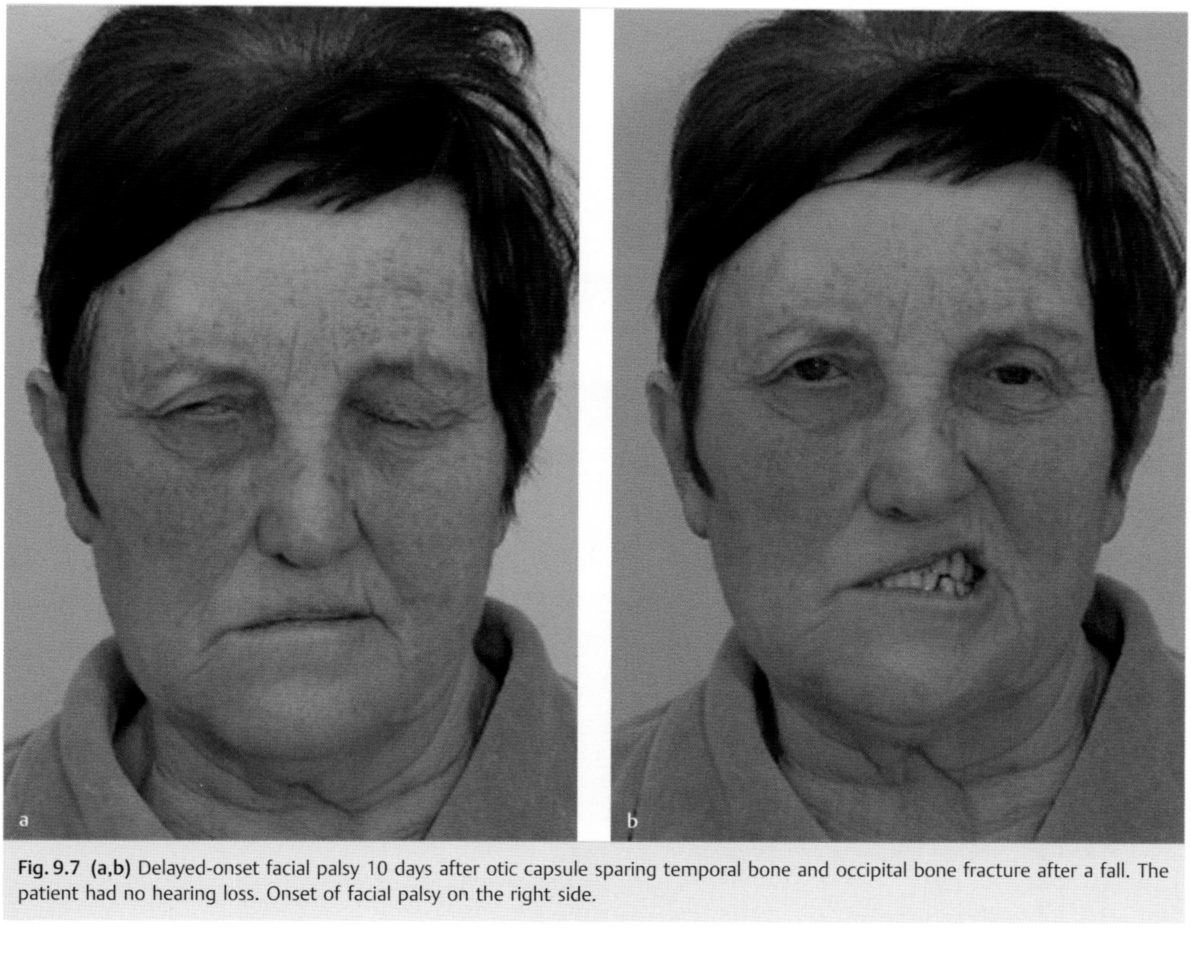

Fig. 9.7 (a,b) Delayed-onset facial palsy 10 days after otic capsule sparing temporal bone and occipital bone fracture after a fall. The patient had no hearing loss. Onset of facial palsy on the right side.

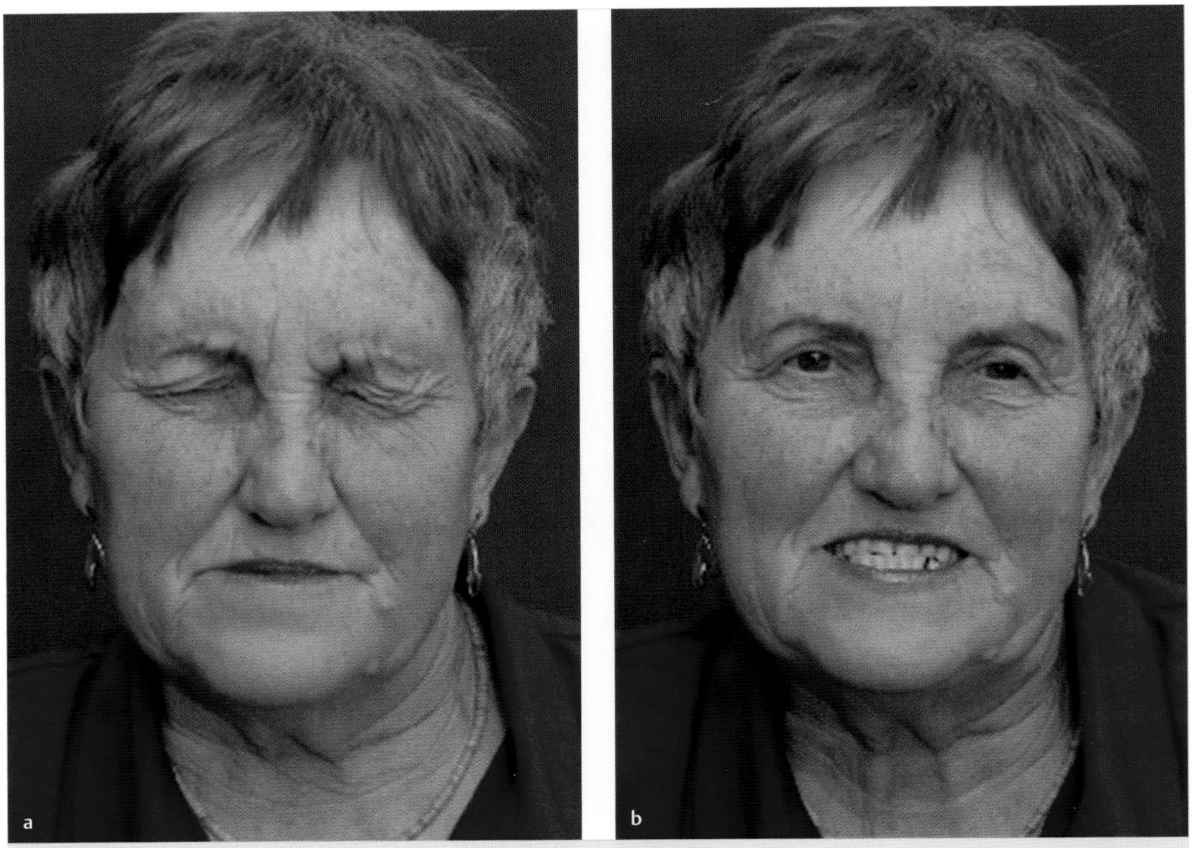

a

b

Fig. 9.8 (a,b) The patient shown in ▶ Fig. 9.7, 3 months later without surgical treatment.

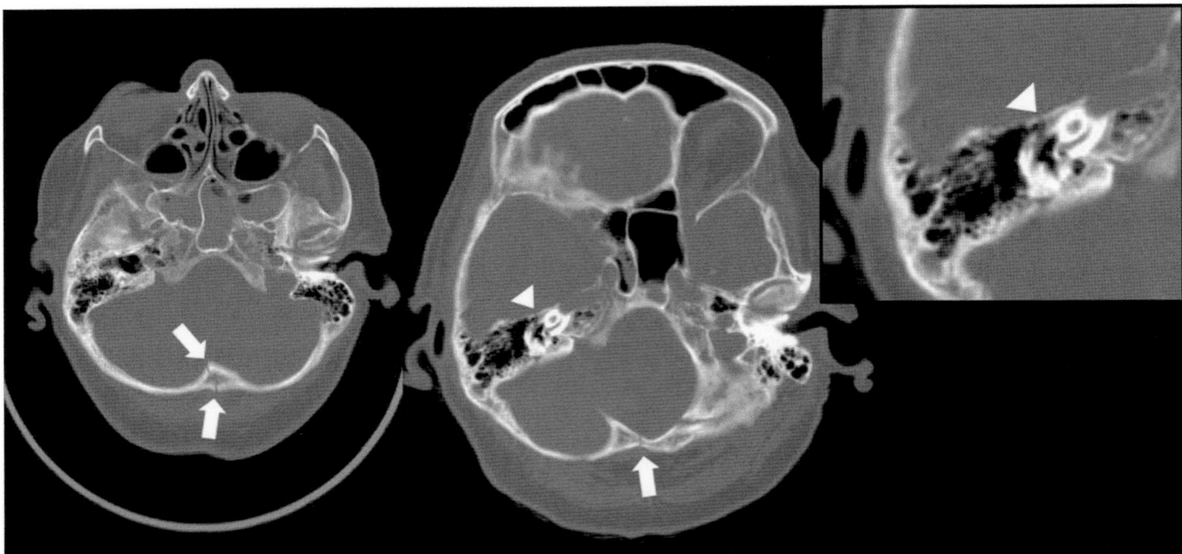

Fig. 9.9 The patient shown in ▶ Fig. 9.7 and ▶ Fig. 9.8: axial CT scan showing the occipital fracture (*arrows*) and the temporal bone fracture (*arrowheads*).

Facial nerve palsy of delayed onset occurs only if the nerve is intact and is compressed, due to edema or hematoma, within an unaccommodating bony fallopian canal. Immediate paralysis suggests discontinuity of the facial nerve until proven otherwise.[17] Findings at surgery for facial nerve injury include nerve sheath edema or hematoma, nerve transection (partial or complete), fibrosis, or bony spicules.[17]

In children, the frequency of facial nerve injuries in temporal bone trauma is lower. This is thought to be due partly to the smaller diameter of the nerve relative to that of the bony fallopian canal, which allows for greater swelling without self-compression of the facial nerve. Birth injuries are another important source of facial nerve injury in children. The overall incidence of facial nerve birth injury is 0.8 to 7.5 per 100 births, with about one-third occurring during spontaneous vaginal deliveries without instrumentation.[19]

!

Facial nerve trauma during birth can occur during spontaneous vaginal deliveries without instrumentation. The fact that no instrumentation was used does not automatically imply that the newborn has a congenital facial palsy.

Historically, the most common iatrogenic injury in otologic surgery was transection of the vertical segment using the cutting burr.[20] More recently, injury is most common in the tympanic segment[21] Most injuries (55%) occur in mastoid surgery, with it being more commonly seen in canal wall down procedures and endaural approaches.[21] The next most frequent operations causing injury include tympanoplasty (14%) and exostectomy (14%).[21]

→•

The facial nerve can pass within 1 mm of the posterior inferior tympanic annulus and caution must be used when drilling in this area.

Anatomical variations in the pathway of the facial nerve should be considered in any case of coexisting congenital ear malformation including aural atresia, auricular deformity, and inner ear dysplasia. There is an increased likelihood of an anomalous course of the facial nerve in this setting as the fallopian canal is a derivative of the second branchial arch and otic capsule, rendering the usual facial nerve landmarks useless.[22] In cholesteatoma surgery the surgeon should have heightened suspicion for facial nerve dehiscence especially when there is coexisting lateral canal fistula. The incidence of facial nerve dehiscence in this setting is 50%.[23]

!

The facial nerve is at increased risk in congenital malformations and in acquired disease with granulation tissue or cholesteatoma.

An immediate onset of facial palsy is explained by a direct lesion of the facial nerve in the moment of the trauma. In the case of delayed palsy, traumatic facial palsy may arise from secondary ischemia and/or edema surrounding the nerve. Delayed facial palsy might also result from reactivation of herpes simplex type 1 virus within the geniculate ganglion and occurs 3 to 14 days after a traumatic injury.[24]

!

Consider treatment for a possible viral reactivation, especially when there is delayed onset of the facial palsy more than 5 days after trauma.

9.4 Clinical Features

Time of onset of facial palsy is an important factor for planning treatment. If symptoms begin within the first few hours after injury, the onset is immediate. In such a case, the immediate examination discovers a facial palsy directly. In cases of delayed palsy, it implies that there was an examination before detection of the palsy that definitively demonstrated definite facial function. However, early onset can easily go unnoticed by patients and clinicians due to other effects of the trauma such as facial swelling, lacerations, and abrasions, or because more serious injuries take precedence over detailed facial examination. Determining whether facial paralysis after trauma is immediate or delayed is frequently complicated by mental status changes immediately precluding examination.

9.4.1 Intracranial Trauma

In patients with an intracranial cerebral trauma, the main symptoms are related to brain damage and the patient is seen primarily in the emergency department by neurosurgeons and neurologists. In such a situation, the otorhinolaryngologist should take care that a facial palsy is not overlooked. Most often, the otorhinolaryngologist is consulted after the initial evaluation, stabilization, and treatment has occurred. This can create issues regarding certainty regarding the time course of the facial paralysis, since the most important question is to clarify whether the palsy occurred immediately or was delayed. Intracranial trauma can lead to a central facial palsy and/or peripheral facial palsy. Damage central to the facial nucleus, when mainly the cerebrum is affected, leads to a central palsy. Damage to the brainstem can cause a central and/or a peripheral lesion.

9.4.2 Intratemporal Trauma

Intratemporal facial nerve trauma usually occurs in the setting of temporal bone fracture (blunt or penetrating) or secondary to iatrogenic injury. The management depends on the timing of presentation and whether the palsy is complete (paralysis) or incomplete (paresis). In the setting of trauma, the patient's other injuries often take precedence. When surgery is considered, the approach is dependent on the patient's hearing. In cases of temporal bone fractures, a facial palsy may be one of several clinical features. Patients with head trauma may have soft tissue injuries of the scalp, pinna, external auditory canal, and tympanic membrane. Bleeding can arise from lacerations. Clear liquid from the affected ear can be a sign of a cerebrospinal fluid leak. A torn jugular bulb or trauma to the carotid artery is a primary reason for profuse bleeding.

Facial nerve injury, sensorineural hearing loss, and cerebrospinal fluid leak are more likely to occur in otic capsule violating fractures.[25,26] A number of other injuries must also be considered. Conductive hearing loss may result from a hemotympanum, a tympanic membrane injury, or from ossicular disruption or fracture.[12] Interestingly, sensorineural hearing loss in the contralateral ear can occur months to years later. This has been attributed to "sympathetic" hearing loss, possibly due to an autoimmune reaction to outer hair cells, although the true cause is not known.[27,28] Vertigo is a common complaint thought to be due to "inner ear concussion" in otic capsule sparing fractures, or direct otic disruption and perilymph leak in otic capsule violating fractures. Most (90%) otic capsule violating fractures present with concurrent intracranial injury (including epidural hematoma and subarachnoid hemorrhage) and 9% present with sustained spinal injury.[25,29] Major vessel injury, such as from the jugular bulb or carotid artery, should be considered when there is ongoing bleeding from the ear. The higher occurrence of other severe injuries with otic capsule violating fractures is expected since higher forces are needed to disrupt the hard compact otic capsule.

The onset of facial nerve palsy in temporal bone fracture may be immediate, delayed, or unknown. Unknown onset is common when the patient is intubated and unconscious, and undergoing treatment for other injuries, and it may not be until the patient is extubated and awake that the facial injury is detected.

9.4.3 Extratemporal Trauma

The patient's clinical features depend on the localization and extent of the facial trauma. The patient may present with skin laceration and hematoma in the region of the trauma. If the parotid gland is involved in penetrating trauma, saliva leakage out of the wound can occur. If the patient does not present immediately, secondary posttraumatic development of a salivary gland swelling due to sialocele formation is common. Saliva leakage out of scar formation in patients with delayed presentation is also possible. Facial nerve injury can also occur at the same time as this penetrating trauma and the saliva can impact facial nerve repair. These injuries can be overlooked or underestimated in the midst of life-threatening situations.

The more severe the facial trauma, especially in the face of life-threatening injuries, the higher is the risk of missing or delaying the diagnosis of traumatic facial palsy.

Injuries severe enough to disrupt the salivary gland and the facial nerve have a high probability of associated vascular or skeletal damage. Gunshot injuries have a high likelihood of severe tissue damage, infection, and tissue necrosis. If the bullet goes through the face, a small external wound is commonly associated with a larger intraoral wound.

9.5 Diagnostic Work-Up

Of course, the initial ABCs of severe trauma management should always be performed first. The need for tetanus prophylaxis needs to be stressed and antibiotics should be administered. When the patient has been stabilized, the evaluation of the facial nerve can start.

If the patient is alert, a medical history will help to assess the severity of the facial nerve damage and the time course. Wounds should be irrigated and cleaned if necessary. Furthermore, it should be ruled out that the patient had a facial palsy prior to the trauma, especially defective healing or residual deficits after a former facial palsy. Most important in the diagnostic work-up are the clinical examination, electrophysiologic testing, and imaging studies. Algorithms for the management of surgical trauma and accidental trauma are presented in ▶ Fig. 9.10 and ▶ Fig. 9.11, respectively.

Note

The treatment of facial paralysis is dependent on the clinical history, electrophysiologic testing, and imaging.

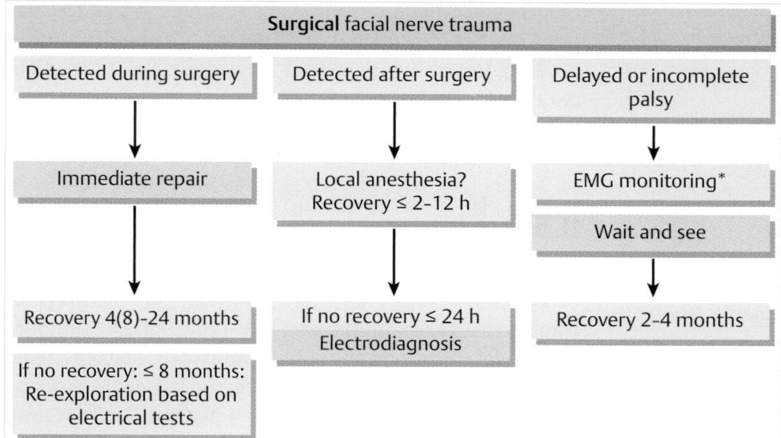

Fig. 9.10 Algorithm for the treatment of surgical facial nerve trauma. *Immediate electromyography looking for voluntary motor unit action potentials. Presence confirms nerve continuity but does not guarantee normal recovery, just that exploration will not improve outcome.

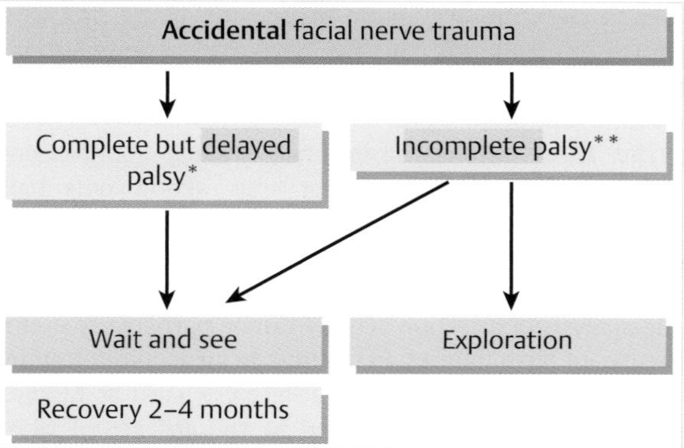

Fig. 9.11 Algorithm for the treatment of facial nerve paralysis caused by accidental trauma. *EMG and imaging are recommended if doubts exist about the delayed nature of the palsy or deterioration occurs during follow up. **Imaging should include the entire course of the facial nerve.

9.5.1 Examination

As part of the complete head and neck examination, it is important to clarify the exact localization of any external injuries. Any drainage out of the lesion site, as well as swelling of the surrounding tissue, has to be documented. Open lacerations, with concomitant facial nerve lesions, should be explored directly through the wound. Otoscopic examination or ear microscopy and hearing tests are important in cases of temporal bone trauma. Inspection of the oral cavity is mandatory to rule out combined external–internal lesions in case of gun or knife injuries. Inspection of the salivary ducts and massage of the glands are imperative in cases of salivary gland lesions to look for bloody saliva or salivary blockage. Inspection and palpation of the facial skeleton, including mandible, zygomatic arch, and maxilla, are important to look for further facial fractures.

A detailed evaluation of facial nerve motor function is the most important clinical examination; for details see Chapter 4. During the first 24 hours, and even longer in children, facial tone at rest can be normal and symmetrical. Weakening of the facial tone takes time and occurs faster in patients with complete palsy. Examination of at least the six basic mimic muscle functions (frowning, closing the eyes, wrinkling the nose, showing one's teeth, pursing the lips, and dragging down the angle of the mouth), and of the orbicularis oculi, zygomatic major, and orbicularis oris, gives an overview of complete mimic function.

In patients with an intracranial lesion, it helps to differentiate a central palsy (frowning preserved) from a complete peripheral palsy (frowning not possible); however, the physician has to be aware that an incomplete peripheral facial palsy sparing the frontal facial nerve branch can mimic a central palsy.

> ⚠
>
> In trauma cases, an incomplete peripheral facial palsy with preservation of the frontal facial nerve branch can be mistaken for a central facial palsy and vice versa.

If the patient cannot cooperate, fingernail pinches will produce grimaces in the face if the nerve is intact. In young children, facial nerve function can often be evaluated only when the child is smiling spontaneously or crying.

> ⚠
>
> Be cautious when interpreting normal or nearly normal eye closure as sign of normal or mild facial palsy only. Especially 1 to 2 days after a surgical palsy, tone and eye closure may be preserved despite a severe facial nerve lesion. Examination must include the other areas of the face so as not to be fooled into thinking that the lesion is incomplete.

Table 9.3 Important electrophysiologic test methods for evaluation of patients with facial nerve trauma

Method	Comment
Electromyography (EMG)	Method of primary choice. Most important for decision making for or against surgical exploration because investigation for pathological spontaneous activity differentiates between degenerative and nondegenerative lesion. Disadvantage: most reliable results for pathological spontaneous activity are not available until 14 days after lesion. Before that, EMG is limited to evaluation of voluntary activity
Electroneuronography (ENoG)	ENoG is helpful within the first weeks after trauma before pathological spontaneous activity might be occurring on EMG. A 90% denervation of the paralyzed mimetic musculature may be an additional parameter to indicate a surgical exploration
Transcranial magnetic stimulation (TMS)	TMS is helpful particularly in unconscious patients after head trauma. It allows identification of a conduction failure at the level of the intratemporal portion

Paralysis of unknown onset, for example when the patient has been intubated for a period of time preventing accurate assessment, is best considered as immediate paralysis.[30] The patient should then proceed to have electrophysiology and imaging to determine prognosis and whether surgical intervention would be of benefit.

9.5.2 Electrophysiology

The principles of electrical testing are covered in Chapter 6. The most important electrophysiologic methods in trauma cases are summarized in ▶ Table 9.3. Most important is electromyography (EMG), more precisely, the EMG examination of the mimic muscles with needle electrodes. With exception of cases with a distinct lesion of only one peripheral facial nerve branch, the investigation should include at least the following muscles: frontalis, orbicularis oculi, zygomatic major, orbicularis oris, and depressor anguli oris. This approach assures an investigation of all five major peripheral facial nerve branches and their target musculature.

The EMG includes insertional activity, spontaneous activity, and voluntary motor unit action potentials (VMUAPs). Insertion activity is normal in the acute phase after the trauma. A reduction of the insertion activity cannot be expected earlier than 2 to 4 months after injury. The analysis of insertion activity can be particularly useful in cases of birth injuries. In contrast to an acquired trauma during delivery, a congenital facial palsy, such as Möbius syndrome, can be characterized by the absence of facial muscles, i.e., insertion activity cannot occur in such cases (▶ Fig. 9.12, ▶ Fig. 9.13, and ▶ Fig. 9.14).

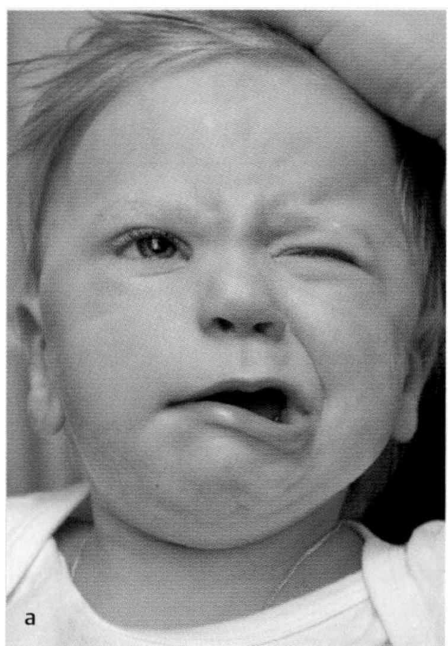
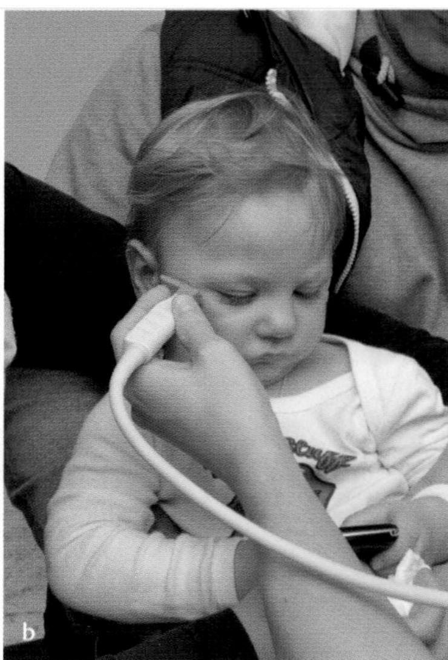
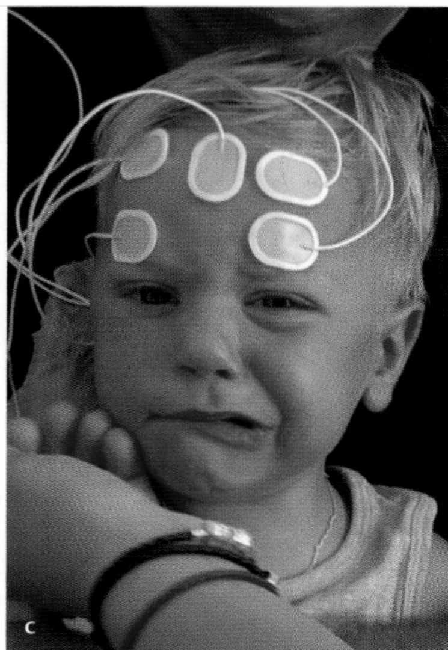

Fig. 9.12 Congenital facial palsy on the right side, without signs of synkinesis. **(a)** At the age of 1.5 years. **(b)** Ultrasound of facial muscles showing facial muscles on both sides. **(c)** Surface EMG showing activity on both sides. Based on ultrasonography and electromyography, facial muscles were verified leading to a wait-and-see approach.

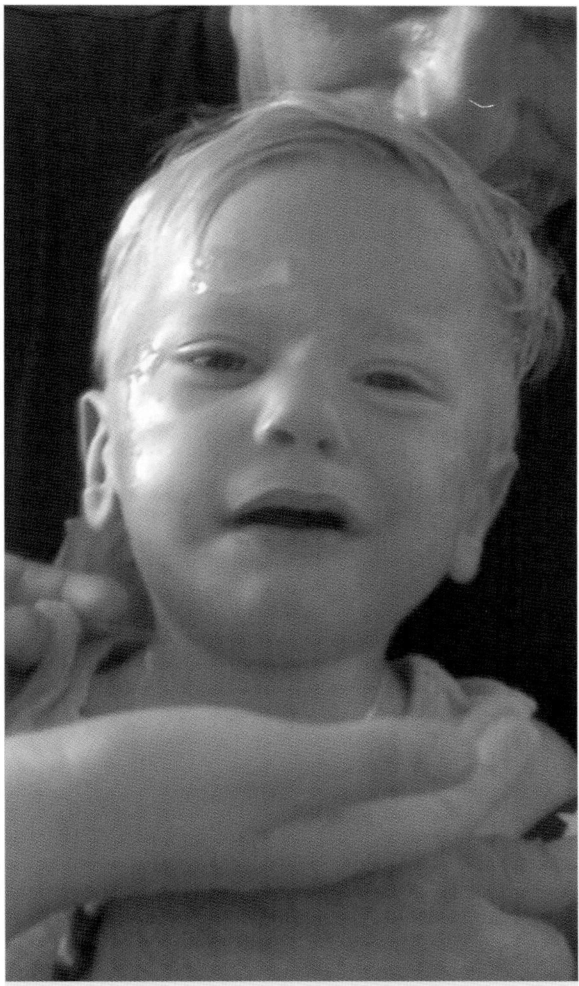

Fig. 9.13 The patient shown in ▶ Fig. 9.12, here showing obvious spontaneous improvement of facial function at the age of 2.5 years.

Pathological spontaneous activity as a sign of a degenerative lesion in cases with damage of facial nerve axons (Sunderland grade II–V) occurs greater than 14 days after the lesion. Therefore, the absence of pathological spontaneous activity within the first 14 days after onset of the trauma does not rule out a severe (degenerative) lesion.

The most reliable investigation during the acute phase (less than 14 days after onset) is the investigation of VMUAPs (▶ Fig. 9.15). The presence of VMUAPs during this early time, even on the day of the facial nerve injury, confirms that the facial nerve is intact. However, if only a zero line or single fiber activity can be detected at best, in several muscles investigated, this speaks in favor of a severe degenerative lesion. The indication for an exploration has to be considered, but should never be based solely on the electrophysiologic results. Reduction of the full interference pattern of the VMUAPs in voluntary EMG of the facial muscles indicates a nondegenerative lesion and justifies a wait-and-see strategy. It is mandatory to repeat the investigation, especially when the first investigation is performed within the first 14 days after facial nerve trauma. Stable reduced to full interference patterns during the EMG monitoring validate a conservative nonsurgical approach. It is well known that in such situations the final outcome is not worse than after facial nerve exploration and possible repair.

If available, electroneurography (ENoG) can be a helpful additional investigation within the first weeks after trauma, before spontaneous pathological activity might occur in EMG. A 90% or greater reduction of amplitude on the ENoG from the paralyzed mimic musculature can be an additional parameter to indicate the need for surgical exploration of the nerve.[9,31]

In some trauma cases, particularly in unconscious patients after head trauma, transcranial magnetic stimulation (TMS) can be helpful.[32] TMS allows identification of a conduction failure at the level of the intratemporal portion of the facial nerve, which is not accessible by electrical stimulation or other electrophysiologic tests. Hyperexcitability of the facial nerve to TMS occurs within a few hours of symptom onset, leading to a significant decrease of the compound muscle action potential in the facial muscles of the affected side. This means that if the facial nerve is lesioned in the temporal bone, TMS is directly affected, whereas preauricular stimulation via TMS or electric stimulation via ENoG can be normal or only slightly affected within the first days after trauma.

It is regarded a special situation when the trauma dates back more than 2 months or even 1 to 2 years. In such a situation EMG and investigation of the insertion activity are important. Decreased or complete loss of insertion activity suggests severe muscle atrophy and therefore indicates against the use of secondary nerve reconstruction with reanimation of the facial nerve.

9.5.3 Imaging

Imaging of the facial nerve is presented in detail in Chapter 5. Imaging of the facial nerve should be tailored to the suspected clinical localization of the lesion along the nerve's course.[33] Typically, if facial trauma is suspected to the cisternal or intracanalicular segments of the facial nerve or the pontine nuclei, contrast-enhanced magnetic resonance imaging (MRI) is indicated. If the lesion can be localized to the mastoid, tympanic, or labyrinthine segments of the facial nerve, high-resolution temporal bone computed tomography (CT) is recommended to evaluate the fallopian canal. Contrast-enhanced MRI should be performed first in cases when the palsy cannot be definitively localized.

When facial nerve palsy coexists with a temporal bone fracture, a high-resolution CT scan of the entire bony course of the facial nerve should be undertaken. When

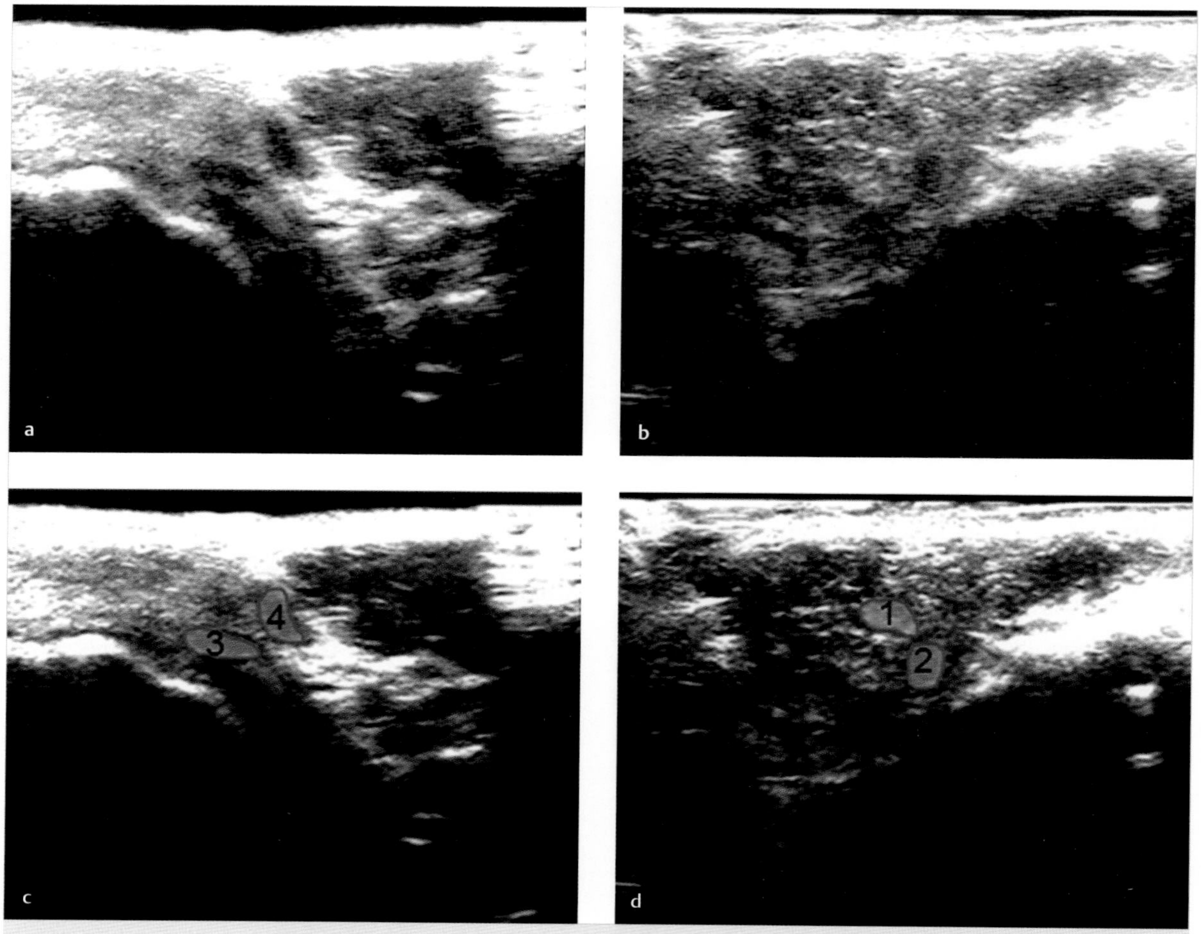

Fig. 9.14 Transverse ultrasound of (a,c) the right (paralyzed) side and (b, d) the left (healthy) side of the patient shown in ▶ Fig. 9.12. Facial muscles are identified on both sides of the face (1, 4: depressor anguli oris muscle; 2, 3: depressor labii inferioris muscle).

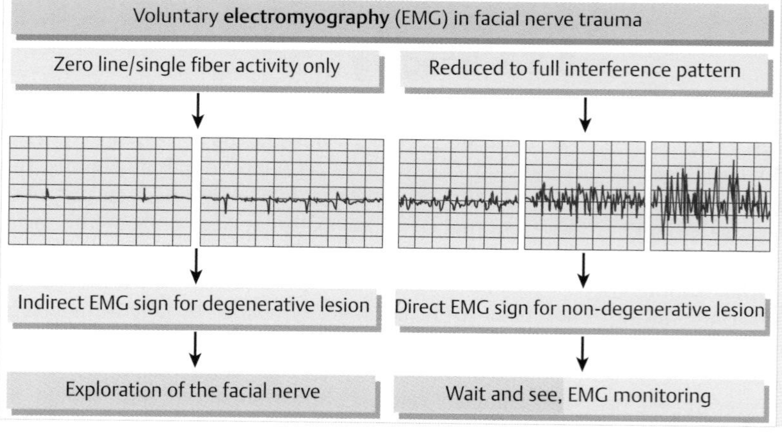

Fig. 9.15 Algorithm for the interpretation of voluntary motor unit action potentials on EMG and decision-making for or against exploration of the facial nerve and surgical nerve repair.

looking for facial injury in temporal bone fractures, a systematic approach must be taken using axial, coronal, and sagittal reformatted images. A head CT, as part of the trauma series, is usually the only imaging available. If an injury is suspected that may require intervention, the patient must be reimaged with a dedicated temporal bone CT. A fracture line extending through a portion of the fallopian canal with coexisting facial nerve palsy highlights an area of injury. A second point of injury should always be checked for, as coexisting sites of injury, such as in the perigeniculate area and the mastoid segment, occur occasionally. Significant injury to the facial nerve can occur due to shearing and stretching without any obvious fallopian canal disruption on CT.[12]

The inability to see a fracture line through the fallopian canal does not exclude it, because high-resolution computed tomography has a sensitivity of 78%.[16]

If there is a readily identifiable injury site (such as a bony spicule into the facial nerve) and paralysis of the facial nerve, no further electrophysiologic tests are needed, and the patient should proceed to surgery. If middle cranial fossa surgery is considered, MRI is recommended to assess the temporal lobe for contusion, which is often not clinically apparent.[34] MRI is also useful in detecting an encephalocele when there is a fracture involving a thin middle fossa floor. Recently, ultrasonography was established as a reliable method to depict some of the facial muscles.[35]

First clinical trials have shown that ultrasonography is a fast and reliable imaging tool to differentiate birth trauma from congenital facial palsy. In cases of birth trauma, one will find mimic muscles. Larger multicenter studies are recommended to confirm these preliminary data.

9.5.4 Facial Nerve and Facial Muscle Biopsies

Histopathology of facial nerve biopsies of the disrupted nerve stumps might be helpful during surgery for secondary facial nerve injury. A skilled pathologist is needed to examine frozen sections to determine the viability, especially of the proximal nerve stump, to avoid suturing a neuroma formation at the proximal suture site. In cases of repair more than 1 to 2 years after onset of the trauma, evaluation of the distal stump should rule out complete replacement by fibrous tissue. The degree of nerve fibrosis is more important for the functional outcome than the degree of muscle atrophy. Even a severely atrophied muscle can recover when the peripheral nerve successfully regrows into the muscle and forms new neuromuscular terminals. Nevertheless, in particular cases with long-term denervation, biopsies from selected mimic muscles might additionally help to decide for or against a secondary facial nerve repair.[36]

9.6 Treatment

Prevention is the best treatment for iatrogenic injury, with appropriate anatomical knowledge and supervised training; for instance, temporal bone laboratory dissection and experience are critical to minimizing mistakes regarding iatrogenic lesions during ear surgery. The surgeon should be aware of common injury situations and obtain patient consent informing the patient of the risk to the facial nerve during surgery.

In cases of complete nerve transection or in cases with complete facial palsy with signs of severe nerve damage, especially when the electrophysiologic tests suggest severe damage, surgical exploration is indicated. Otherwise, in cases of incomplete facial palsy or delayed onset of facial palsy, a wait-and-see approach is recommended. An overview of the treatment options is given ▶ Table 9.4.

Table 9.4 Overview of treatment options for traumatic facial nerve lesions

Method	Comment
Surgical treatment	
Primary wound treatment	Wound management is necessary as in other parts of the body. The wound treatment of contaminated wounds should be used to localize and mark the disrupted nerve stumps for later reconstruction
Primary nerve repair	Method with best functional results. Most frequent techniques: nerve grafts, nerve substitution (e.g., hypoglossal–facial jump nerve suture), combined approach. Best results are obtained after end-to-end nerve suture, but this is only possible for defects < 1 cm
Secondary nerve repair	If primary repair is not possible
Reanimation without facial nerve repair	Indicated if facial nerve repair is not possible; can be performed as primary and secondary surgery. Most frequent techniques: nerve grafts, nerve substitution (e.g., hypoglossal–facial jump nerve suture), combined approach
Nonsurgical treatment	Conservative treatment is indicated in most cases of incomplete and delayed-onset traumatic facial palsy
Adjuvant treatment	The rules for adjuvant treatment for traumatic facial palsy are the same as for all other indications of surgical facial reanimation

A special mention must be made of paralysis in the setting of gunshot injury. Surgery is often required to remove bullet fragments and manage other injuries, but the higher impact of the bullet, the higher the potential shearing forces. Watching and waiting in this group of patients increases the chance of traumatic neuroma and fibrosis.[37]

9.6.1 Nonsurgical Treatment

In cases of incomplete facial palsy or delayed onset of facial palsy there is normally no need for surgical intervention. A wait-and-see policy along with repeated electrophysiologic testing, if needed, is indicated. Administration of antibiotics is necessary in external trauma cases. For iatrogenic postoperative incomplete or delayed palsies, administration of corticosteroids has been often reported.[38] The rationale is that edema, such as in Bell's palsy, is affecting the nerve; therefore, it might be helpful to treat these patients with corticosteroids, as is standard for Bell's palsy; see Chapter 8. It must be emphasized that there is no scientific evidence that corticosteroids are more effective than a wait-and-see policy in such cases.

9.6.2 Surgical Treatment

Surgical repair of the facial nerve comprises two or three steps. Detailed surgical techniques for facial nerve reanimation are presented in Part VI. First, the extent and the localization of the nerve lesion have to be defined precisely. In cases of uncontaminated facial wounds, this step is normally combined with primary wound treatment. Second, there needs to be a decision whether a primary repair is indicated and feasible, or whether a secondary repair is indicated. The method of choice is primary repair because the final outcome is better than after secondary repair. Especially when treating small defects, it is best to combine primary wound treatment and primary nerve repair. When iatrogenic lesions are noticed by the surgeon intraoperatively, the nerve should be repaired immediately (▶ Fig. 9.16).

The nerve stimulator can still stimulate the nerve distal to the site of injury up to 72 hours after the injury, and may provide guidance to the site of injury.

If the facial palsy is not noted until the patients is postoperative, decision-making mainly depends on the surgeon's evaluation of the situation and the results of the electrophysiologic testing (see ▶ Fig. 9.10, ▶ Fig. 9.11, and ▶ Fig. 9.15). If no recovery occurs during the 4 to 8 months after primary repair, re-exploration and an attempt to treat with a secondary repair should be considered. Finally, after successful nerve repair, adjuvant surgical and nonsurgical treatment might be necessary and needs to be planned.

A special flow chart of management in cases of in temporal bone trauma is shown in ▶ Fig. 9.17. The treatment of facial nerve injury depends on the degree of injury and timing.

Primary Wound Treatment

When there are open lacerations and open wounds in the face, a facial nerve lesion can be seen sometimes directly in the depth of the wound. Otherwise, a direct exploration is necessary to locate and determine the extent of the nerve lesion.

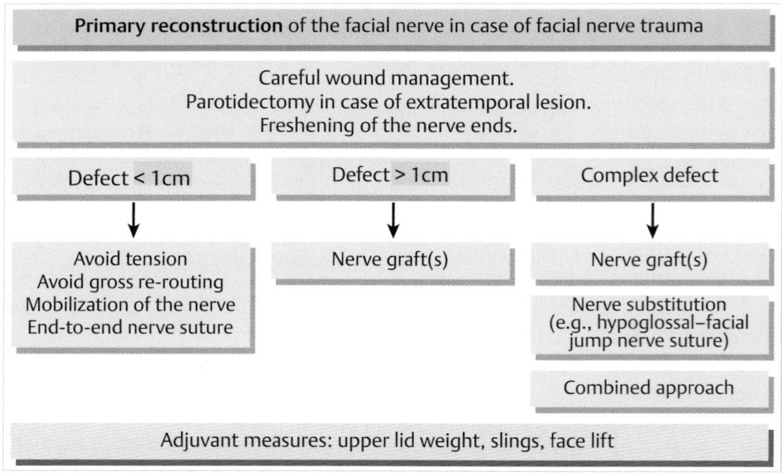

Fig. 9.16 Algorithm for choosing the optimal surgical technique for primary facial nerve repair.

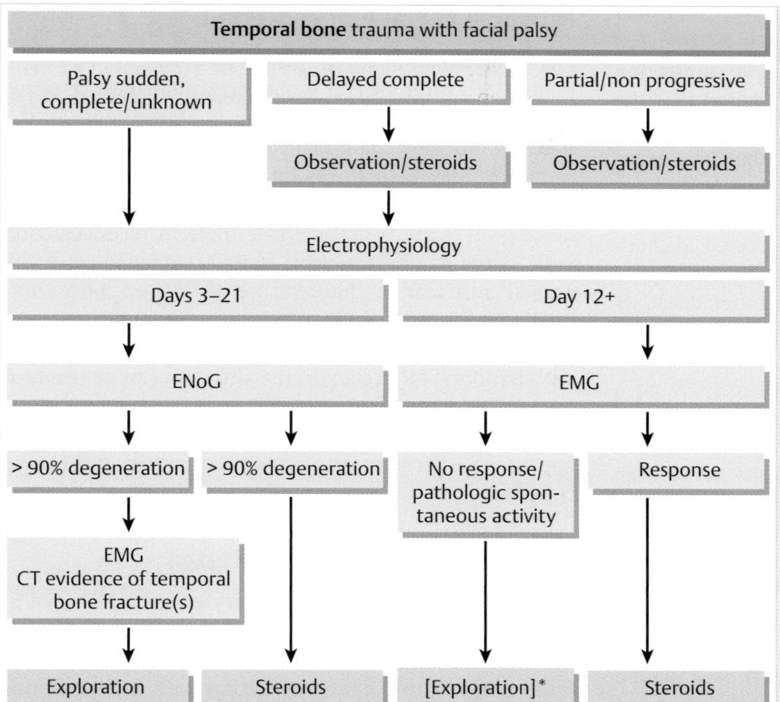

Fig. 9.17 Pathway for facial nerve injury management in temporal bone trauma. *Individual decision for or against exploration depending on electrical testing, imaging results, and time of trauma.

> In contaminated wounds the proximal and distal disrupted nerve stumps should be marked with a nonabsorbable suture or a microvascular clip. Primary repair in these circumstances can be undone by wound infection, and the reanimation surgeon does not discover this until there is no recovery observed and precious months have passed.

This allows easy re-identification of the lesion for about 4 weeks when the wound is clean and a nerve repair is planned. When the extratemporal portion of the facial nerve is affected, a parotidectomy might be necessary. In doing this procedure, one gains an optimal overview of the complete extracranial facial nerve fan and the distal nerve branches. This helps the surgeons to avoid overlooking the presence of multiple lesions.

Management in Relation to the Type of Nerve Lesion

Compression injuries are typical for injuries of the facial nerve within the temporal bone. Intraneural edema secondary to blunt trauma, traumatic hemorrhage between the bony facial nerve canal and the sheath, bone compression during manipulation of the adjacent bone, or tight packing at the end of surgery in iatrogenic cases can all result in compression damage. Clinically, compression damage leads typically to incomplete or delayed palsy. The indication for or against surgical exploration is primarily dependent on the severity of the lesion as revealed by the diagnostic work-up. Nevertheless, when compression from surgical packing might be the reason for the palsy, removing or loosening the packing should be performed immediately. Stretch injuries are typically seen during vestibular schwannoma surgery or parotid surgery. A complete disruption from stretch injuries is very rare. Nerve monitoring for cerebellopontine angle lesions is helpful for assessing the nerve at the end of surgery, as described in Chapter 15 and Chapter 18, and the parotid surgeon should stimulate the proximal facial nerve before closing. However, as in other types of injury, a complete diagnostic work-up is mandatory for unexplained or severe injury from these causes. Crush injuries are mainly seen on the extratemporal facial nerve branches when using clamps to control bleeding. Even after immediate removal of the clamps, the damage can be severe. When in doubt, the crush injury should be managed like a transection injury. Transection injuries (iatrogenic and external) and cauterizing injuries are most severe. The diagnostic tests reveal a degenerative lesion of the affected nerve branches and surgical repair is indicated with or without interposition nerve grafting.

Incomplete palsy can be managed without treatment as the prognosis is excellent. Unexpected immediate facial nerve paralysis is assumed to be a facial nerve transection until proven otherwise, and it is recommended that the patient is taken back to surgery if the situation permits. This is true even if direct visualization of the facial nerve was not achieved during surgery. In 79% of procedures leading to facial nerve injury, the facial nerve was not visualized at all.[21] CT scans should be performed to check the integrity of the inner ear and look for the site of injury. There is an old adage that the "sun should not set on a facial nerve injury"; however, we do not advocate this approach. Returning to surgery the next day, following further radiological and clinical assessment, with a rested surgical team will give the best outcome.

When returning to surgery for exploration, the degree of injury is usually underestimated.[21] If the nerve is in anatomical continuity, decompression of the fallopian canal should be performed proximal and distal to the injury site. Transection in its intratemporal course may not require approximation suture if the ends are already in approximation within the fallopian canal. When the nerve is lesioned intracranially or extratemporally, the suture technique described in the section Primary Wound Treatment is recommended to prevent tension at the repair site. If the nerve is not in anatomical continuity, reanastomosis via either direct repair or cable graft should be undertaken. If a transection is less than 50% of the diameter, only decompression should be performed.[21] As described previously, the degree of injury in this setting is usually underestimated. Cable graft techniques are available, as described previously, except when there is malignancy in the region, in which case a sural nerve graft is preferred to a greater auricular nerve graft that may have perineural invasion.

Compression iatrogenic injuries to the facial nerve can result from blunt trauma, hemorrhage within the fallopian canal, or indirect compression from packing and/or external dressing. Stretch injuries are more common in acoustic neuroma surgery when tumor bulk in the cerebellopontine angle can weigh down the facial nerve at the porus, or when dissecting the tumor within the internal auditory canal, as the facial nerve may be stretched at the meatal foramen. In both compression and stretch injuries, as long as there is anatomical continuity, the nerve should not be resected or repaired. Decompression is an option if the injury is intratemporal.

If injury is noticed during surgery or before the decision is made to return to the operating room, a colleague with suitable experience, if available, should be consulted to provide an independent viewpoint that is not colored by the stress of the situation.

Primary Facial Nerve Repair

The different options for primary repair are shown in ▶ Fig. 9.16. After careful wound cleaning the cut nerve ends are freshened and resutured end-to-end if the defect is smaller than 1 cm. Mobilization and minimal rerouting may help to obtain a tensionless situation. If extensive rerouting is necessary, this is an indication for a nerve graft (▶ Fig. 9.18). In greater defects, reconstruction with nerve graft or several grafts is needed, and the greater auricular or the sural nerve is used most commonly (▶ Fig. 9.19, ▶ Fig. 9.20, and ▶ Fig. 9.21). In complex defects, such as a complex lesion of the extratemporal facial plexus, the situation can be resolved by primary nerve graft, hypoglossal–facial jump grafting, or a combination of both techniques (combined approach). Alternatively, a cross-facial nerve graft can be considered.

Secondary Facial Nerve Repair

The different options for secondary repair are shown in ▶ Fig. 9.22. The scar tissue needs to be resected completely, resulting in fresh nerve endings. To obtain a tensionless suture, a reconstruction with interpositional graft or grafts is normally mandatory. If the nerve repair is performed 6 months or even longer after the trauma, or if it is doubtful/not possible to obtain a freshened proximal facial nerve stump, a hypoglossal–facial jump nerve anastomosis is an excellent alternative. Alternatively, a cross-nerve suture can be considered.[39]

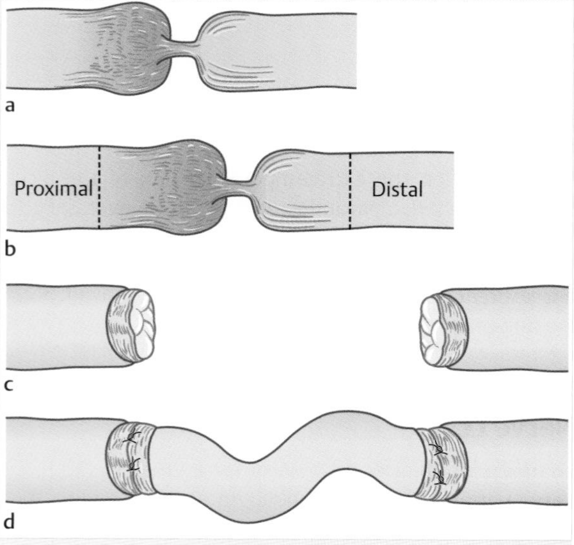

Fig. 9.18 (a–d) Trimming of lesioned facial nerve stumps and closure without tension using a small graft.

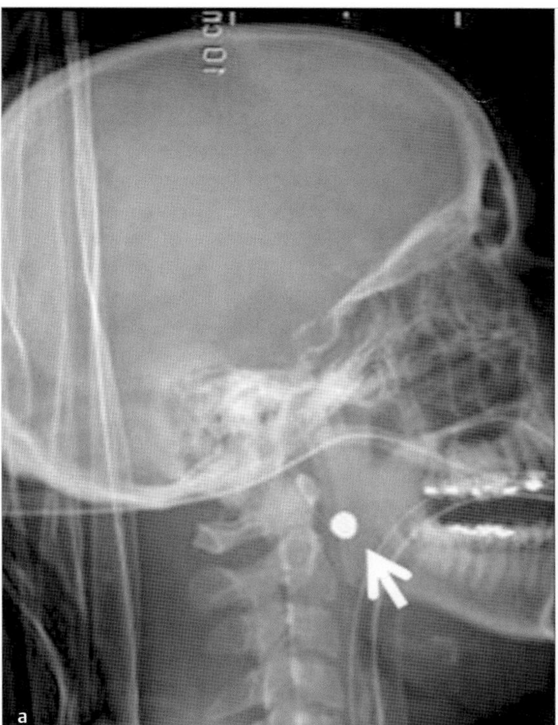
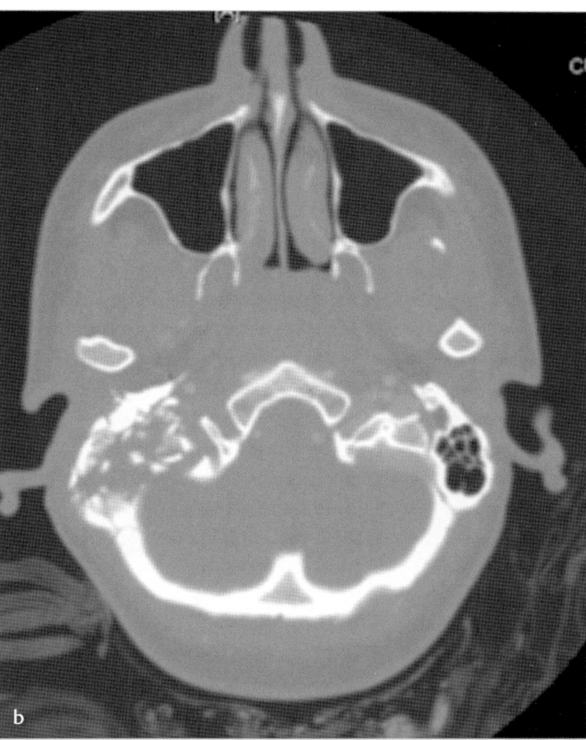

Fig. 9.19 Gunshot injury with destruction of the right mastoid and immediate complete facial palsy. (a) X-ray of the head showing the projectile (*arrow*). (b) Axial CT with complex right temporal bone fractures.

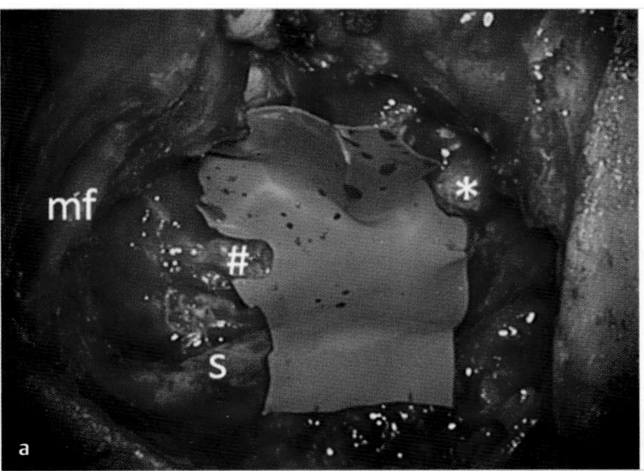

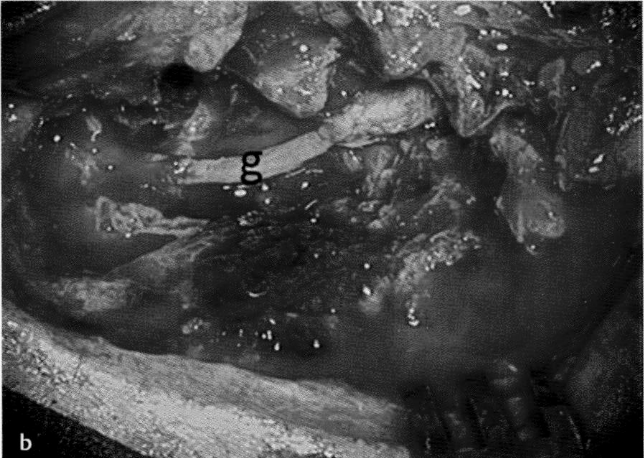

Fig. 9.20 The same patient as shown in ▶ Fig. 9.19. (a) Intraoperative site 1 day after injury. Mastoidectomy cavity, mastoid segment of the facial nerve is unidentifiable; #proximal stump; *distal stump of the facial nerve; mf, middle fossa; s, sigmoid sinus. (b) Reconstruction with graft (g) of the greater auricular nerve.

Facial Nerve Reanimation without Facial Nerve Repair

When there is disastrous destruction of the facial nerve, mainly in severe facial trauma, facial nerve repair might not be possible. Furthermore, if the trauma occurred too long ago and the diagnostic work-up argues against a secondary repair, reconstruction by regional muscle flaps, static procedures using sling techniques, or in special cases a free flap, are the method of choice; see Chapter 20 and Chapter 21.

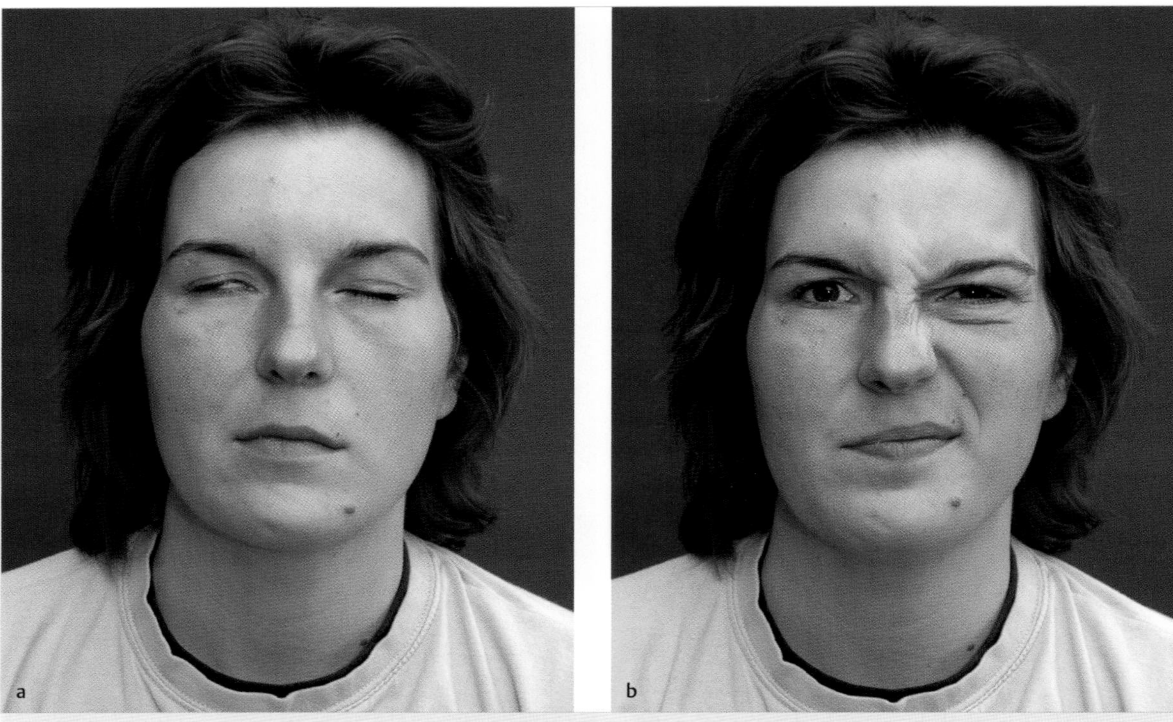

Fig. 9.21 The patient shown ► Fig. 9.19 and ► Fig. 9.20, showing recovery of the right facial nerve 10 months later.

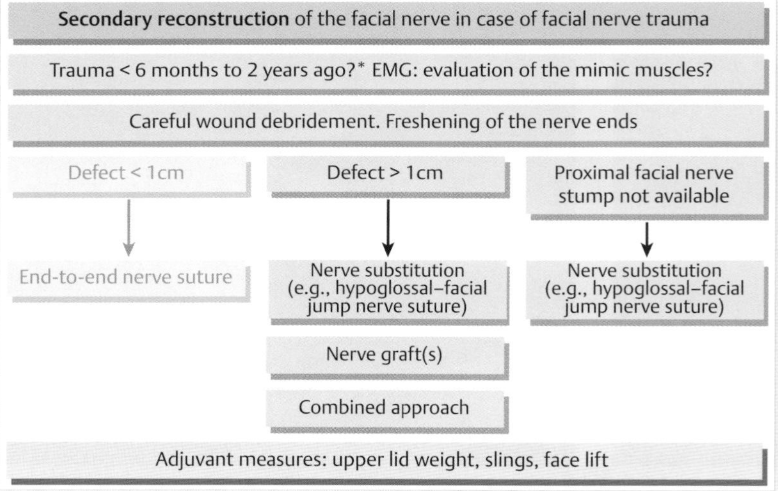

Fig. 9.22 Algorithm for choosing the optimal surgical technique for secondary facial nerve repair. Most head and neck surgeons do not recommend primary repair after more than 2 years of denervation. Only preliminary data are available to indicate the reliability of ultrasonography for assessing facial muscles. *Some centers offer reconstruction up to 6 months, and others up to 24 months, after facial nerve trauma.

Adjuvant Treatment

Adjuvant treatment in trauma cases is not different from other types of facial nerve reconstruction; see Chapter 23, Chapter 24, and Chapter 25. Reanimation of the paralytic lids should be tailored to the individual patient's deficit. Reanimation of eye closure can be combined with primary repair, secondary repair, or other types of surgical facial reanimation. Adjuvant treatment for defective healing with botulinum toxin and physical training programs are also indicated; see Chapter 25 and Chapter 26.

Special Considerations Depending on the Lesion Site

In cases of temporal bone trauma and a nonhearing ear, the translabyrinthine or transcochlear approach gives the best access to the whole length of the facial nerve and

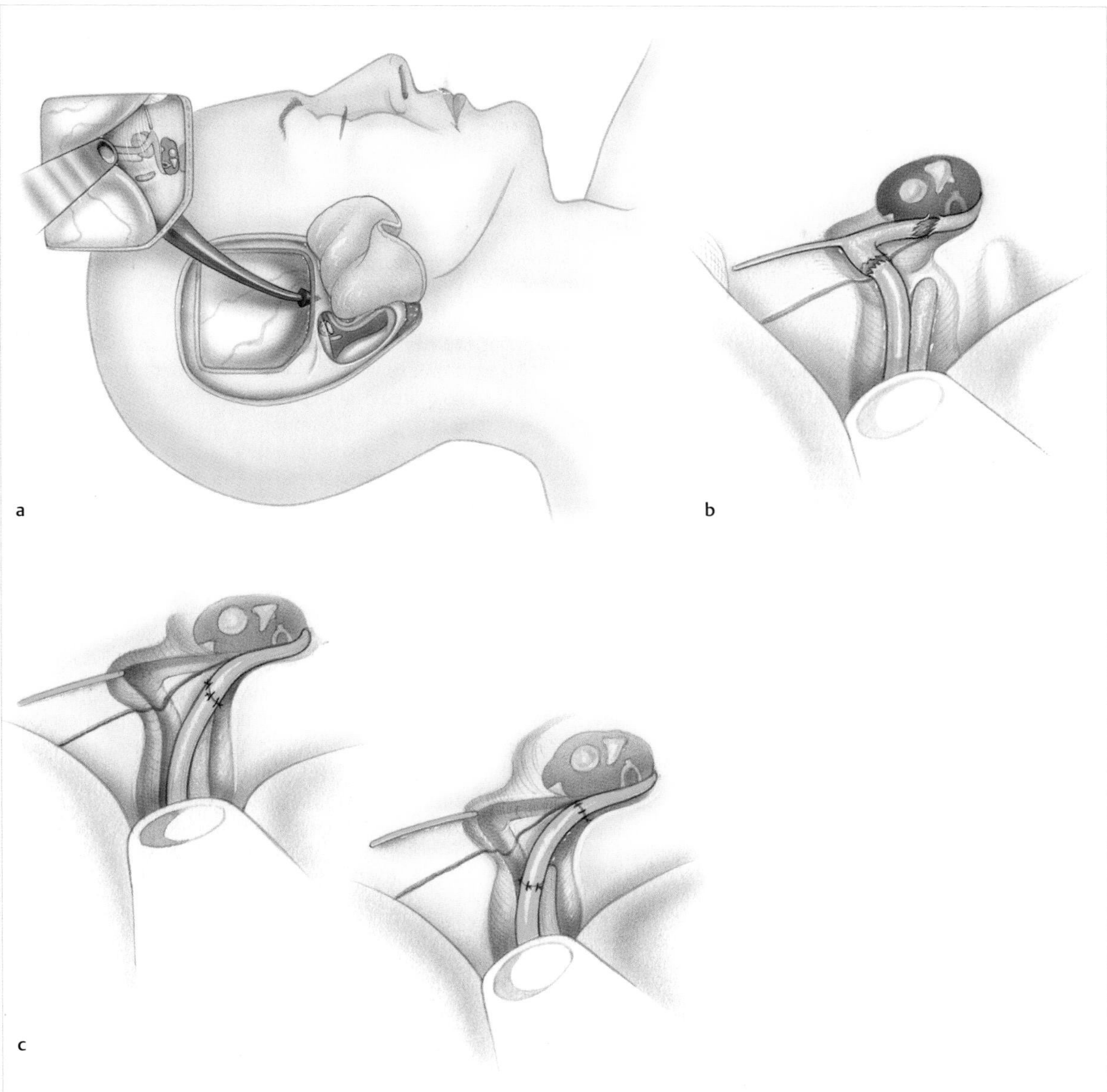

Fig. 9.23 (a) The middle fossa approach provides direct access to the perigeniculate area (b), which is the most common site of injury in temporal bone trauma. (c) The access allows either rerouting of the nerve for direct anastomoses or cable graft repair. (Image provided courtesy of Chris Gralapp and Robert Jackler, Department of Otolaryngology–Head and Neck Surgery, Stanford School of Medicine, California, USA)

avoids temporal lobe retraction. In a hearing ear, the approach depends on the site of injury but may involve a combination of a transtemporal/middle fossa approach (▶ Fig. 9.23) and a transmastoid approach. The perigeniculate area is the most common site of injury and most surgeons prefer to approach this via the middle fossa.[40,41] It may be possible to approach this area via the mastoid, but this provides inferior exposure. This must be balanced against the potential further injury that can occur from retracting an edematous temporal lobe.[41] Performing middle fossa surgery, with edematous tissues in the early posttraumatic setting, is not recommended and it is beneficial to allow time for the edema to subside.

In a nonhearing ear, the translabyrinthine or transcochlear approach provides the most direct route for repair. In a hearing ear, a combination of transmastoid and middle fossa approaches may be needed.

These patients often have other injuries preventing early surgical exploration, but, if it is undertaken within 72 hours, the facial nerve distal to the site of injury may be stimulated and assist in identification of the site of injury. After this time the motor end plate neurotransmitter stores are irreversibly deplete.[42]

During exploration, some authors have advocated dividing the greater superficial petrosal nerve to reduce the incidence of postinjury gustatory tearing (crocodile tears).[42,43]

Where possible, primary neurorrhaphy is also the gold standard for intratemporal lesion.[42] The goal is a tension-free repair, with alignment of the nerve ends. Both primary repair and cable interposition grafts tend to have better results than static or dynamic rehabilitation strategies.[44] If the decision has been made to perform a repair, any transected or crushed nerve should be resected back to the normal healthy nerve. Opening the fallopian canal and rerouting the facial nerve is an option to allow a tension-free direct anastomosis,[45] but this must be done with care as rerouting can potentially compromise the blood supply of the rerouted segment. The advantages of performing a direct anastomosis must be balanced against this potential harm to further areas of nerve.

Up to about 2 cm can be mobilized before compromising the facial nerve's blood supply within the temporal bone.[46]

When performing neurorrhaphy, the nerve ends should first be prepared so that they have a fresh clean edge, with no crushed ends. The epineural layer carries the most strength and can allow continuity of the nerve stumps and correct anatomical alignment. A small diameter, nonabsorbable suture (such as 8–0, 9–0, or 10–0 nylon) is appropriate for repair. The length can be trimmed to enable the knot to be tied more easily. Suturing the distal end first ensures that there is no accidental tension or pulling on the proximal end while suturing. Leaving the first suture cut longer allows the tie to be used to roll the nerve graft to apply further sutures. It should be noted that the facial nerve acquires it's epineurium as it becomes extradural in the labyrinthine segment, and epineural sutures proximal to this are not possible. Usually one suture here will suffice. Anastomoses proximal to this point have worse House–Brackmann outcomes.[47] The challenge of suturing within pulsating cerebrospinal fluid can be helped by stabilizing the nerve with a fenestrated suction and suturing through the fenestration.[48] After completion of the anastomoses a layer of fascia is placed over the graft area for extra support.

Epineural sutures are not possible in the intradural facial nerve.

Placing an epineural suture may be technically difficult in some situations and use of fibrin glue adhesive as an alternative is acceptable. The nerve ends should be placed in gentle apposition with the fibrin glue placed over and around the two ends. Long-term outcomes of this technique are good,[49] and many authors report that the results are as good as an epineural suture. Epineural sutures have the potential to cause a long-term foreign body reaction and induce more direct trauma through a penetrating suture. Fibrin glue may enhance conditions for regeneration. Conversely, an epineural suture provides increased repair tension and may be useful in a challenging area where movement of fluid or tissues may affect the graft area.[50]

Facial nerve repair of the intracranial segment, for instance after head trauma or vestibular schwannoma surgery, is difficult but provides the best possible outcome. If it is not performed directly intraoperatively during vestibular schwannoma surgery, an additional or secondary middle fossa or translabyrinthine approach is needed to reach the intracranial segment (as described earlier in this section). Grafting is preferred to end-to-end nerve suture. Grafting can be facilitated by use of collagen splints or other tissue adhesives to stabilize the reconstruction in the cerebellopontine angle. Connecting the nerve stumps with fibrin glue is an alternative to conventional sutures. Sutures are unnecessary to nerve grafts placed for intratemporal lesions, as the bone bed of the facial canal or a drilled new canal after rerouting stabilizes the suture sites.

Nerve reconstruction at the intracranial segment or at the intratemporal segment of the facial nerve is more easily performed with fibrin glue than with a conventional suture; see Chapter 19.

9.7 Outcome and Prognosis

Incomplete or delayed onset facial palsy treated nonoperatively has a good prognosis. Greater than 80% of the patients with delayed-onset palsy seem to recover completely within 6 to 12 weeks after onset.[14] Not much is known about the prognosis of patients with complete palsy who have the indication for surgery but who choose not to have surgery. The best results are seen after primary facial nerve repair within 30 days and end-to-end nerve suture, with only minor defective healing (House–Brackmann grade III). If the lesion site is very peripheral and only one or two branches are involved, repair can result in a complete recovery. In all other cases, moderate-to-severe defective healing will result from facial nerve repair 12 to 18 months after surgery.

!

Outcomes for incomplete and delayed palsy are excellent without surgical intervention.

If paralysis persists beyond 3 months, late decompression may have a role, with most patients returning to House–Brackmann grade I or II with decompression. One series reported 78% ($n = 9$) of patients returning to House–Brackmann grade I or II by 1 year.[51] Observation for 1 year is recommended before progressing to other interventions for facial nerve reanimation.[43] Paralysis persisting beyond 1 year should be managed with other facial reanimation techniques.

9.8 Key Points

- The differentiation between incomplete, acute, and delayed facial paralysis is key in directing the optimal treatment in patients who present with facial nerve trauma.
- Patients with traumatic but incomplete or delayed-onset facial palsy can normally be managed with conservative treatment. Primary surgery has no advantage.
- Electrophysiologic tests, especially electromyography, are important for decision making.
- In patients with temporal bone trauma and facial nerve lesion: in a nonhearing ear, the best surgical approach for repair is a translabyrinthine or transcochlear approach; in a hearing ear, the facial nerve may need to be approached by a combination of transmastoid and middle fossa approaches.
- Severe lesions need surgical exploration and surgical reanimation of the facial nerve using the general rules of facial nerve repair.
- When the nerve is in continuity, the prognosis is excellent. The best result that can be achieved by a cable graft repair is House–Brackmann grade III.

References

[1] Greywoode JD, Ho HH, Artz GJ, Heffelfinger RN. Management of traumatic facial nerve injuries. Facial Plast Surg 2010; 26: 511–518

[2] Menorca RM, Fussell TS, Elfar JC. Nerve physiology: mechanisms of injury and recovery. Hand Clin 2013; 29: 317–330

[3] Seddon H. Three types of nerve injury. Brain 1943; 66: 238–288

[4] Sunderland S. A classification of peripheral nerve injuries producing loss of function. Brain 1951; 74: 491–516

[5] Dellon AL, Mackinnon SE. Basic scientific and clinical applications of peripheral nerve regeneration. Surg Annu 1988; 20: 59–100

[6] Hohman MH, Bhama PK, Hadlock TA. Epidemiology of iatrogenic facial nerve injury: A decade of experience. Laryngoscope 2014; 124: 260–265

[7] Odebode TO, Ologe FE. Facial nerve palsy after head injury: Case incidence, causes, clinical profile and outcome. J Trauma 2006; 61: 388–391

[8] Yetiser S, Hidir Y, Gonul E. Facial nerve problems and hearing loss in patients with temporal bone fractures: demographic data. J Trauma 2008; 65: 1314–1320

[9] Kim J, Moon IS, Shim DB, Lee WS. The effect of surgical timing on functional outcomes of traumatic facial nerve paralysis. J Trauma 2010; 68: 924–929

[10] Patel A, Groppo E. Management of temporal bone trauma. Craniomaxillofac Trauma Reconstr 2010; 3: 105–113

[11] Ghorayeb BY, Yeakley JW. Temporal bone fractures: longitudinal or oblique? The case for oblique temporal bone fractures. Laryngoscope 1992; 102: 129–134

[12] Yeakley JW. Temporal bone fractures. Curr Probl Diagn Radiol 1999; 28: 65–98

[13] Hato N, Nota J, Hakuba N, Gyo K, Yanagihara N. Facial nerve decompression surgery in patients with temporal bone trauma: analysis of 66 cases. J Trauma 2011; 71: 1789–1792, discussion 1792–1793

[14] Nash JJ, Friedland DR, Boorsma KJ, Rhee JS. Management and outcomes of facial paralysis from intratemporal blunt trauma: a systematic review. Laryngoscope 2010; 120 Suppl 4: S214

[15] Lee D, Honrado C, Har-El G, Goldsmith A. Pediatric temporal bone fractures. Laryngoscope 1998; 108: 816–821

[16] Rajati M, Pezeshki Rad M, Irani S, Khorsandi MT, Motasaddi Zarandy M. Accuracy of high-resolution computed tomography in locating facial nerve injury sites in temporal bone trauma. Eur Arch Otorhinolaryngol 2013; 271: 2185: 2189

[17] Darrouzet V, Duclos JY, Liguoro D, Truilhe Y, De Bonfils C, Bebear JP. Management of facial paralysis resulting from temporal bone fractures: Our experience in 115 cases. Otolaryngol Head Neck Surg 2001; 125: 77–84

[18] Yetiser S. Total facial nerve decompression for severe traumatic facial nerve paralysis: a review of 10 cases. Int J Otolaryngol 2012; 2012: 607359

[19] Evans AK, Licameli G, Brietzke S, Whittemore K, Kenna M. Pediatric facial nerve paralysis: patients, management and outcomes. Int J Pediatr Otorhinolaryngol 2005; 69: 1521–1528

[20] Wiet RJ. Iatrogenic facial paralysis. Otolaryngol Clin North Am 1982; 15: 773–780

[21] Green JD, Jr, Shelton C, Brackmann DE. Surgical management of iatrogenic facial nerve injuries. Otolaryngol Head Neck Surg 1994; 111: 606–610

[22] Dew LA, Shelton C. Iatrogenic facial nerve injury: prevalence and predisposing factors. Ear Nose Throat J 1996; 75: 724–729

[23] Sheehy JL, Brackmann DE. Cholesteatoma surgery: management of the labyrinthine fistula—a report of 97 cases. Laryngoscope 1979; 89: 78–87

[24] Bonkowsky V, Kochanowski B, Strutz J, Pere P, Hosemann W, Arnold W. Delayed facial palsy following uneventful middle ear surgery: a herpes simplex virus type 1 reactivation? Ann Otol Rhinol Laryngol 1998; 107: 901–905

[25] Dahiya R, Keller JD, Litofsky NS, Bankey PE, Bonassar LJ, Megerian CA. Temporal bone fractures: otic capsule sparing versus otic capsule violating clinical and radiographic considerations. J Trauma 1999; 47: 1079–1083

[26] Rafferty MA, Mc Conn Walsh R, Walsh MA. A comparison of temporal bone fracture classification systems. Clin Otolaryngol 2006; 31: 287–291

[27] ten Cate WJ, Bachor E. Autoimmune-mediated sympathetic hearing loss: a case report. Otol Neurotol 2005; 26: 161–165

[28] Schindler JS, Niparko JK. Imaging quiz case 1. Transverse temporal bone fractures (left) with subsequent progressive SNHL, consistent

with sympathetic cochleolabyrinthitis. Arch Otolaryngol Head Neck Surg 1998; 124: 814–, 816–818

[29] Sun GH, Shoman NM, Samy RN, Cornelius RS, Koch BL, Pensak ML. Do contemporary temporal bone fracture classification systems reflect concurrent intracranial and cervical spine injuries? Laryngoscope 2011; 121: 929–932

[30] Brodie HA, Thompson TC. Management of complications from 820 temporal bone fractures. Am J Otol 1997; 18: 188–197

[31] Gantz BJ, Gmuer AA, Holliday M, Fisch U. Electroneurographic evaluation of the facial nerve. Method and technical problems. Ann Otol Rhinol Laryngol 1984; 93: 394–398

[32] Happe S, Bunten S. Electrical and transcranial magnetic stimulation of the facial nerve: diagnostic relevance in acute isolated facial nerve palsy. Eur Neurol 2012; 68: 304–309

[33] Gupta S, Mends F, Hagiwara M, Fatterpekar G, Roehm PC. Imaging the facial nerve: a contemporary review. Radiol Res Pract 2013; 2013: 248039

[34] Jones RM, Rothman MI, Gray WC, Zoarski GH, Mattox DE. Temporal lobe injury in temporal bone fractures. Arch Otolaryngol Head Neck Surg 2000; 126: 131–135

[35] Volk GF, Wystub N, Pohlmann M, Finkensieper M, Chalmers HJ, Guntinas-Lichius O. Quantitative ultrasonography of facial muscles. Muscle Nerve 2013; 47: 878–883

[36] Hadlock TA, Kim SW, Weinberg JS, Knox CJ, Hohman MH, Heaton JT. Quantitative analysis of muscle histologic method in rodent facial nerve injury. JAMA Facial Plast Surg 2013; 15: 141–146

[37] Bento RF, de Brito RV. Gunshot wounds to the facial nerve. Otol Neurotol 2004; 25: 1009–1013

[38] Roh JL, Park CI. A prospective, randomized trial for use of prednisolone in patients with facial nerve paralysis after parotidectomy. Am J Surg 2008; 196: 746–750

[39] Frey M, Giovanoli P. The three-stage concept to optimize the results of microsurgical reanimation of the paralyzed face. Clin Plast Surg 2002; 29: 461–482

[40] Fisch U. Facial paralysis in fractures of the petrous bone. Laryngoscope 1974; 84: 2141–2154

[41] May M. Total facial nerve exploration: transmastoid, extralabyrinthine, and subtemporal indications and results. Laryngoscope 1979; 89: 906–917

[42] Rovak JM, Tung TH, Mackinnon SE. The surgical management of facial nerve injury. Semin Plast Surg 2004; 18: 23–30

[43] Johnson F, Semaan MT, Megerian CA. Temporal bone fracture: evaluation and management in the modern era. Otolaryngol Clin North Am 2008; 41: 597–618

[44] Humphrey CD, Kriet JD. Nerve repair and cable grafting for facial paralysis. Facial Plast Surg 2008; 24: 170–176

[45] Yarbrough WG, Brownlee RE, Pillsbury HC. Primary anastomosis of extensive facial nerve defects: an anatomic study. Am J Otol 1993; 14: 238–246

[46] Gantz BJ, Rubinstein JT, Gidley P, Woodworth GG. Surgical management of Bell's palsy. Laryngoscope 1999; 109: 1177–1188

[47] Gidley PW, Gantz BJ, Rubinstein JT. Facial nerve grafts: from cerebellopontine angle and beyond. Am J Otol 1999; 20: 781–788

[48] Arriaga MA, Brackmann DE. Facial nerve repair techniques in cerebellopontine angle tumor surgery. Am J Otol 1992; 13: 356–359

[49] Bozorg Grayeli A, Mosnier I, Julien N, El Garem H, Bouccara D, Sterkers O. Long-term functional outcome in facial nerve graft by fibrin glue in the temporal bone and cerebellopontine angle. Eur Arch Otorhinolaryngol 2005; 262: 404–407

[50] Knox CJ, Hohman MH, Kleiss IJ, Weinberg JS, Heaton JT, Hadlock TA. Facial nerve repair: fibrin adhesive coaptation versus epineurial suture repair in a rodent model. Laryngoscope 2013; 123: 1618–1621

[51] Quaranta A, Campobasso G, Piazza F, Quaranta N, Salonna I. Facial nerve paralysis in temporal bone fractures: outcomes after late decompression surgery. Acta Otolaryngol 2001; 121: 652–655

10 Ramsay Hunt Syndrome

Claus Wittekindt

10.1 Introduction

Ramsay Hunt syndrome (RHS; also called Ramsay Hunt syndrome type 2, Hunt's syndrome, or herpes zoster oticus) was first described by an American neurologist James Ramsay Hunt in 1907 in a patient with otalgia associated with cutaneous and mucosal rashes. RHS is a much more serious illness than Bell's palsy, and immediate medical attention is required. Many researchers believe that Bell's palsy is caused by the herpes simplex virus type 1, which is not a causative factor of RHS. It is classified as a rare disease and is extremely rare in children. Any factor that impairs the immune system may leave a person who harbors varicella zoster virus (VZV) vulnerable to the development of RHS.[1]

10.2 Definition

RHS is a VZV infection of the geniculate ganglion of the facial nerve. It is caused by reactivation of VZV that has caused chickenpox in the same patient earlier during his/her lifetime. RHS results in paralysis of the facial nerve. It is typically associated with a red rash and blisters in or around the ear canal (▶ Fig. 10.1), but can be on the ipsilateral neck, face, roof of the mouth, lips, or dorsal tongue. The syndrome is also known as geniculate neuralgia or nervus intermedius neuralgia. It may also occur in the absence of a skin rash, a condition known as zoster sine herpete.

10.3 Epidemiology and Etiology

RHS is reported to be a rare complication of latent VZV infection. It may occur in the absence of cutaneous rash (zoster sine herpete). Remarkably, VZV has been detected by polymerase chain reaction (PCR) in the tear fluid of patients diagnosed with Bell's palsy.[2] The frequency of RHS can be estimated to account for somewhat less than 20% of facial palsies in adults. RHS is extremely rare in children younger than 6 years. The incidence of RHS among patients with HIV is unknown; however, it may occur at a higher rate than in the general population because individuals with HIV infection harbor a higher risk of VZV infection.[3] The incidence and severity increase with age. About 50% of patients are aged 60 years or older. This may be due to a decline in cellular immunity. The annual incidence rate of all types of herpes zoster is estimated to be 360 cases per 100,000 person-years. Shingles become clinically apparent in about 20% of all people at some stage in their lives. In conclusion the annual incidence rate of RHS can grossly be estimated as 1/100,000.

!

About 8% of all patients presenting with facial palsy have Ramsay Hunt syndrome and 6% of them are ≤ 18 years of age.

The syndrome is not contagious in the sense that the syndrome itself can be transmitted from one person to another; however, VZV can be found in the blisters and tears of patients with RHS and it can be transmitted to other people and cause chickenpox in those that are unvaccinated against chickenpox. Individuals with RHS should avoid contact with newborns, pregnant women, immunodepressed individuals, and people with no history of chickenpox, at least until all the blisters change to scabs.

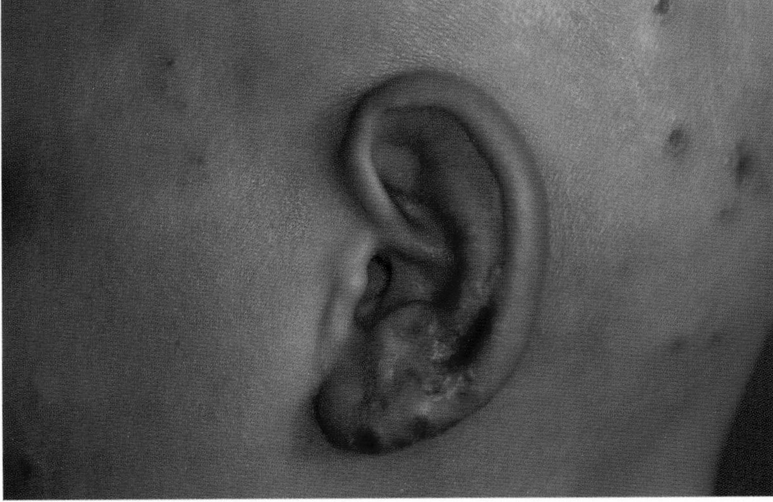

Fig. 10.1 Zoster oticus during immunosuppression caused by chemotherapy.

> ⚠
>
> Instruct the patients with Ramsay Hunt syndrome to avoid contact with newborns, pregnant women, immunodepressed individuals, and people with no history of chickenpox.

VZV infection causes two distinct clinical syndromes. Primary infection, also known as varicella or chickenpox, is a common pediatric erythematous disease characterized by a highly contagious generalized vesicular rash. The annual incidence of varicella infection has significantly declined after the introduction of mass vaccination programs in most countries of the world. After healing of chickenpox, VZV lies dormant in the nerve cell bodies and, less frequently, the non-neuronal satellite cells of the dorsal root, cranial nerve, or autonomic ganglia, and recurrence of the virus may lead to shingles. VZV reactivation involving the geniculate ganglion is the main pathophysiologic mechanism of RHS (▶ Fig. 10.2). Immunocompromised and elderly patients are more likely to develop RHS and it affects both sexes equally. However, any factor that impairs the cellular immune system can leave a person who harbours VZV vulnerable to RHS.

10.4 Clinical Features

The signs and symptoms include acute onset facial nerve paralysis, pain in the ear, loss of taste perception in the anterior two-thirds of the tongue, dry mouth and eyes, and a herpetiform erythematous vesicular rash (▶ Fig. 10.3 and ▶ Fig. 10.4). Since the cranial nerve VIII is in close proximity to the geniculate ganglion, it may also

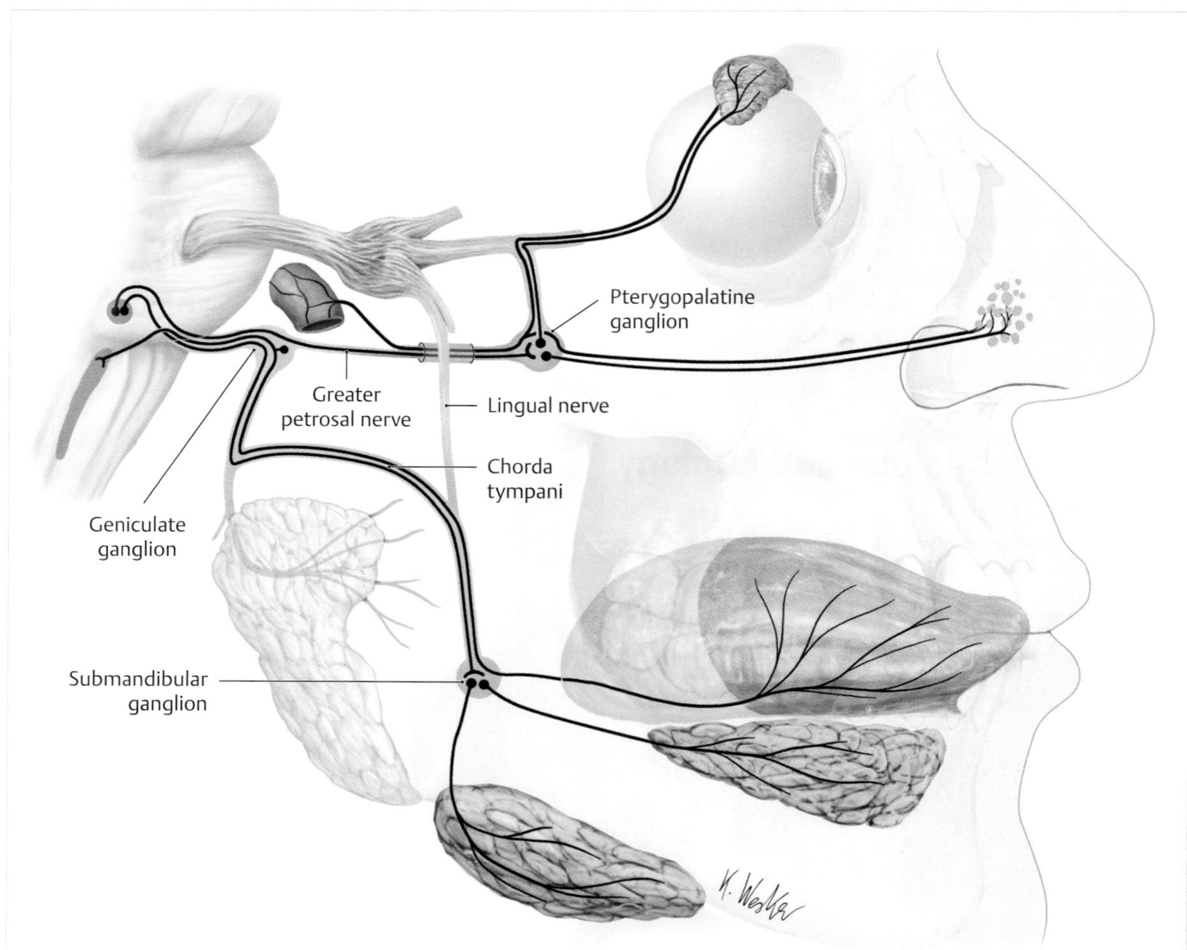

Fig. 10.2 The geniculate ganglion contains sensory neurons that innervate a skin area in the external ear and taste buds on the anterior two-thirds of the tongue. The greater petrosal nerve arises from the geniculate ganglion and contains parasympathetic fibers for the pterygopalatine ganglion. (From Atlas of Anatomy, 2nd ed., © Thieme 2012, Illustration by Karl Wesker.)

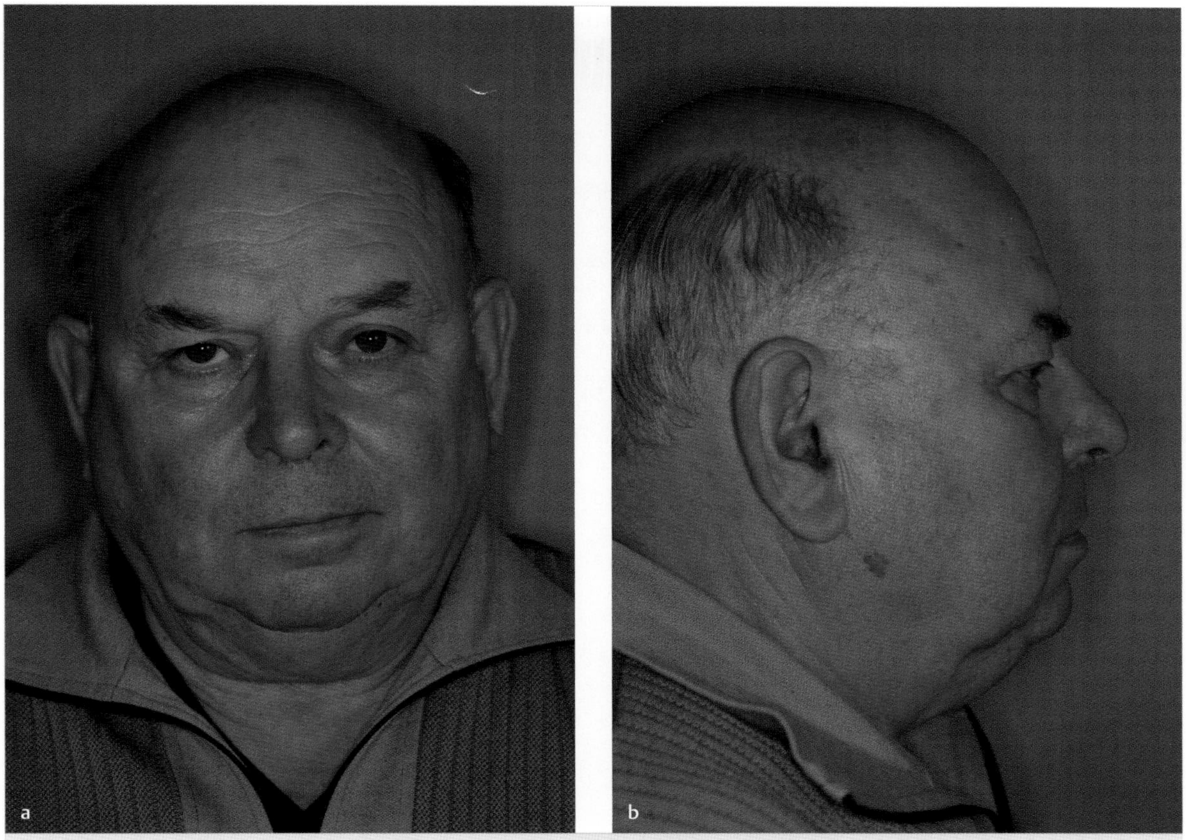

Fig. 10.3 **(a)** Incomplete paresis of the right facial nerve. **(b)** Distinct vesicular rash at the skin of the cavum of the right ear. Some cases of Bell's palsy are believed to be caused by varicella zoster virus reactivation where the vesicular rash is scant or overlooked.

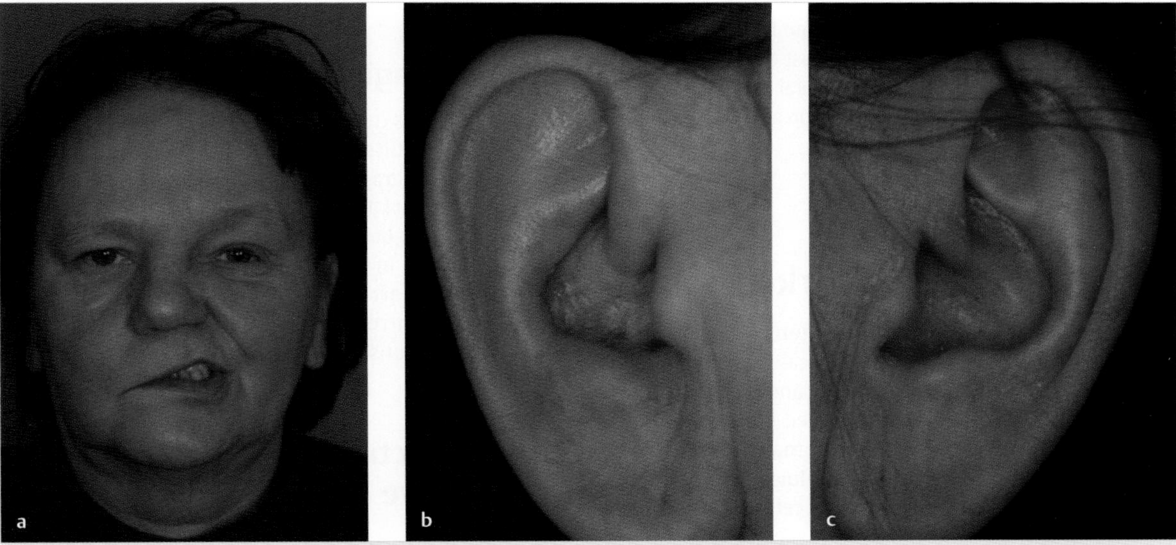

Fig. 10.4 **(a)** Complete facial nerve paresis on the right side, and **(b)** obvious exanthema of the auricle on the right side, in contrast to **(c)** normal outer ear on the left side.

Table 10.1 Clinical signs, characteristics, and clinical pecularities according to symptoms in patients with Ramsay Hunt syndrome

Symptom	Characteristics	Clinical pecularities
Pain	Paroxysmal pain within the ear, radiates outwards, often dull background pain	Usually precedes the rash by several hours or days, risk of postherpetic neuralgia is higher in old patients and females
Vesicular rash	Might be present at the ear skin or mouth (80% of patients)	Usually precedes facial paralysis, blisters of the skin may become infected
Facial paralysis	Facial palsy is more severe and often causes axon degeneration	Reaches maximum 1 week after onset, poor outcome compared with Bell's palsy
Vertigo	Spontaneous nystagmus and loss of lateral semicircular function	May continue for several months
Cochlear neuritis	Tinnitus and hearing loss are observed in 50% of patients	Expect persistent hearing loss in 25% of cases, tinnitus normally resolves without treatment

be affected, and patients may also suffer from hearing loss, tinnitus, and vertigo (▶ Table 10.1). Rare symptoms of the disease include dysarthria, gait ataxia, fever, and cervical adenopathy. Differential diagnoses include Bell's palsy, idiopathic facial pain, Lyme disease, postherpetic neuralgia, temporomandibular disorders, trigeminal neuralgia, and malignant parotid tumors. The diagnosis is challenging only when the rash does not occur or the patient is seen too late for it to be observed. The cranial nerve VIII symptoms are highly suggestive of RHS as they are almost unheard of in Bell's palsy.

!

Patients often present with face, ear, or head pain before physical findings of rash or paralysis and the diagnosis of Ramsay Hunt syndrome (RHS) should be entertained. RHS is never bilateral (Lyme disease and Bell's palsy can be). Audiovestibular symptoms suggest diagnosis of RHS is most likely. Always check the oral cavity for lesions that the patient may not mention and may not understand are related.

10.5 Diagnostic Work-Up

Diagnosis of the syndrome is most often made by observing the symptoms described in Clinical Features (painful rash in the ear and/or mouth blisters and one-sided facial paralysis). A PCR test can be performed on the fluid from the blisters to demonstrate genetic material of VZV, or VZV may be isolated from vesicle fluid and inoculated into susceptible human or monkey cells. When central nervous system complications are suspected (meningitis, meningoencephalitis, myelitis, and arteritis), lumbar puncture, after central nervous system imaging, is recommended. Audiometry usually reveals sensorineural or mixed hearing loss. Unilateral caloric weakness may be present on nystagmography.

10.5.1 Virology Testing

Viral studies include VZV isolation in conventional cell culture, which is considered the definitive diagnostic test. However, growing VZV in cell culture is difficult and is usually too slow to be clinically helpful. The sensitivity of conventional cell culture is reported to be 30 to 40%. Other tests, including electron microscopy and PCR, are generally more rapid and sensitive. The sensitivity of the conventional PCR technique is estimated to be 60%. VZV antigen detection by direct immunofluorescence assay is also possible. Antibody determinations on paired sera may be helpful in establishing the diagnosis by comparing titers at time of presentation and a few weeks later.

10.5.2 Imaging Studies

Structural lesions can be ruled out by computed tomography (CT), magnetic resonance imaging (MRI), or magnetic resonance angiography. Gadolinium enhancement of the vestibular and facial nerves on MRI has been described in RHS (▶ Fig. 10.5) but is rather nonspecific; see Chapter 5. Recent advances in clinical MRI (e.g., 3-Tesla MRI, multichannel phased array coil, three-dimensional fluid-attenuated inversion recovery [FLAIR]) allow the evaluation of subtle alterations at the level of the blood–labyrinthine barrier.[4]

10.5.3 Electrodiagnostic Tests of Facial Nerve

Electrodiagnostic methods, such as electromyography (EMG) and electroneuronography (ENoG) of facial muscles can add information regarding the extent of cranial nerve VII involvement, as well as prognostic factors

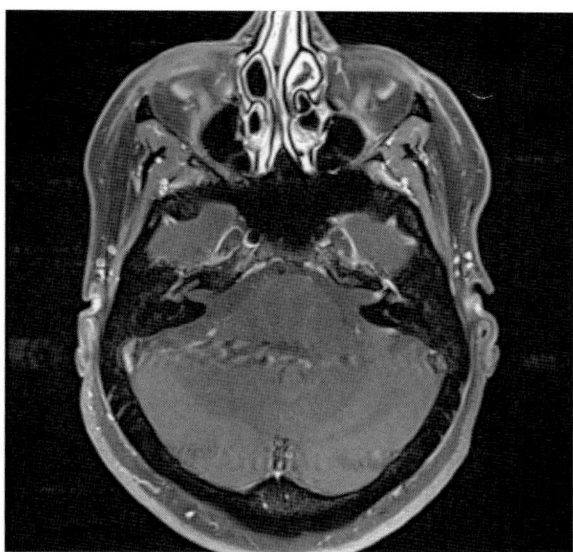

Fig. 10.5 Contrast-enhanced MRI showing enhanced signalling of the geniculate ganglion and the facial nerve in RHS.

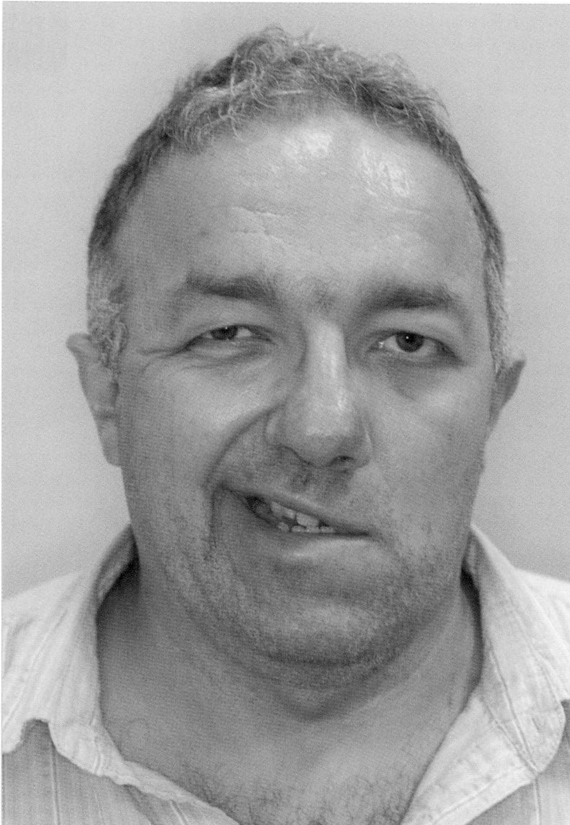

Fig. 10.6 Complete facial paralysis due to varicella zoster virus reactivation.

(► Fig. 10.6, ► Fig. 10.7, and ► Fig. 10.8); further details are given in Chapter 6. Mild injury to the facial nerve causes neuropraxia. There is decreased impulse conduction, and the outcome is favorable. Moderate injury may cause interruption of axoplasmic flow and axonotmesis. Wallerian degeneration occurs over 2 to 3 weeks. It can be detected by signs of nerve degeneration (spontaneous pathological activity in the form of positive sharp waves or fibrillation potentials) during EMG. Defective healing can thus be predicted, and misdirected axon regeneration occurs and the patient experiences prolonged recovery and synkinesis.

10.5.4 Lumbar Puncture

In the setting of a peripheral facial palsy, cerebrospinal fluid (CSF) rarely is analyzed. Although lumbar puncture is not recommended in the diagnosis of this disease, CSF findings can be helpful in confirming the diagnosis. CSF findings are reported to be abnormal in 10% patients with idiopathic peripheral facial palsy, and in > 50% of patients with RHS (pleocytosis). To summarize, CSF analysis might be helpful, although it is not recommended as a routine test. If the CSF is abnormal, a specific cause should be sought. Lumbar puncture is recommended in all patients at risk for complications (immunocompromised, pregnant women, children) or when signs suggest myelitis or encephalitis.

10.6 Treatment

Unlike Bell's palsy patients, RHS patients almost universally present for treatment because of the severe pain (it should be noted however, that 60% of Bell's patients also have pain). The treatment of the disease is not controversial but is very poorly studied. As difficult as it has been to study Bell's palsy, the study of RHS is further hampered by the fact that it is seen much less frequently. Treatment consists of antiviral agents (for example, acyclovir, valacyclovir, or famciclovir) for 7 to 10 days, steroids, and pain medication. However, only one controlled trial has been conducted in 1992. By following 15 participants, a significant reduction in sequelae was identified in RHS patients after adding acyclovir to steroids.[5] The effect of acyclovir-prednisone has also been studied in 80 RHS patients. Of 28 patients for whom treatment was begun within 3 days of onset of facial paralysis, the recovery from paralysis was complete in 21 (75%). In comparison, of 23 patients for whom treatment was begun more than 7 days after onset, recovery from facial paralysis was complete in only 7 (30%). Recovery of hearing also tended to be better after early treatment.[6] To summarize, the key to recovery from RHS is the prompt and effective treatment of VZV. The best results are reported when treatment protocols are started within about 3 days after symptoms appear.

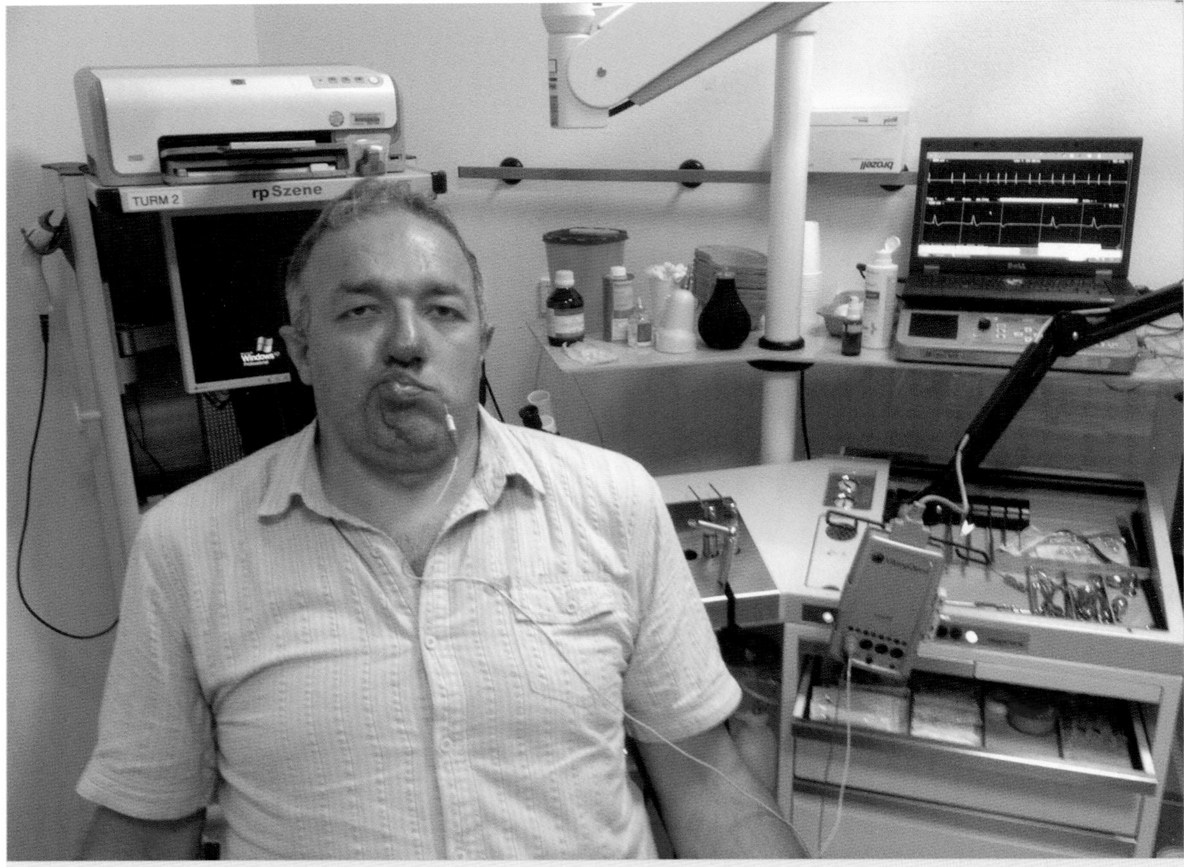

Fig. 10.7 The patient shown in ▶ Fig. 10.6, 14 days after onset of paralysis. For voluntary movements, sustained recording of action potentials indicates a favorable outcome.

> **!**
>
> Compared with Bell's palsy, patients with Ramsay Hunt syndrome are less likely to recover completely. Studies suggest that immediate treatment with steroids and antiviral agents improves the outcome.

10.6.1 Medical Treatment

- Corticosteroids and oral acyclovir are commonly used in the treatment of RHS (▶ Table 10.2).
- Combined therapy using corticosteroids plus intravenous acyclovir did not show benefit over corticosteroids alone in promoting facial nerve recovery after 6 months; however, randomized clinical trials evaluating both therapies are required.[7]
- Pain killers (opioids) and local anesthetics are well tolerated in patients experiencing acute pain.
- Vestibular suppressants may be helpful if vestibular symptoms are severe.
- As with Bell's palsy, care must be taken to prevent corneal irritation and injury.
- Antidepressants and anticonvulsants might be helpful in cases of postherpetic neuralgia or idiopathic geniculate neuralgia.

Antivirals

Antiviral medication directed against herpes viruses inhibits the replication of viral DNA. Infected cells absorb more of the antiviral medication than do normal cells and convert more of it to an active form, which prolongs its antiviral activity where it is most needed. Examples of antivirals commonly used are acyclovir (Zovirax), famciclovir (Famvir), and valacyclovir (Valtrex). Antiviral medications are recommended to be used for 7 to 10 days.

Antiviral agents may, or may not, be effective in patients with RHS.[7] On the basis of fundamental pathophysiologic principles it would seem reasonable to use them; however, these agents are associated with a number of side effects and adverse events that must be considered before they are prescribed.

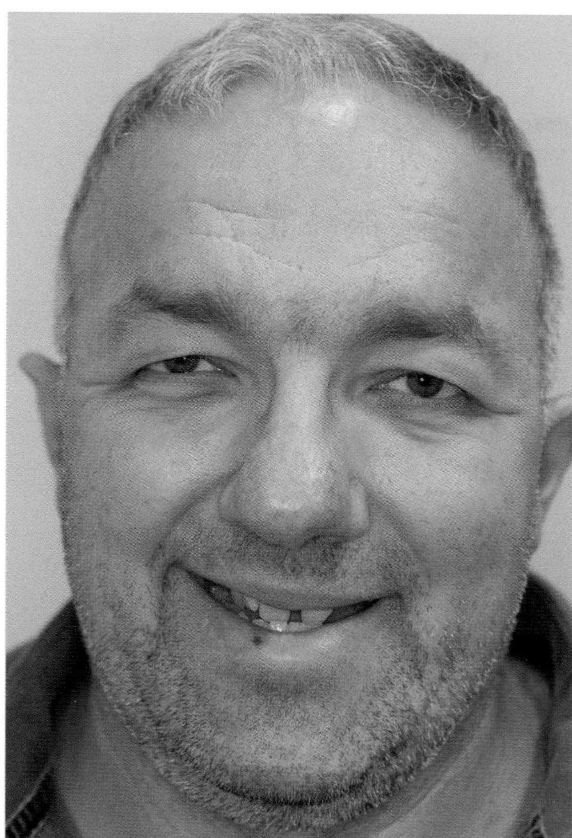

Fig. 10.8 The patient shown in ▶ Fig. 10.6 and ▶ Fig. 10.7, 2 months later, showing almost complete recovery of facial movements.

Examples of common antivirals used to treat Ramsay Hunt syndrome

- Acyclovir (Zovirax), a synthetic nucleoside analog.
- Famciclovir (Famvir), a prodrug of the antiviral agent penciclovir and a synthetic acyclic guanine derivative.
- Valacyclovir (Valtrex), the hydrochloride salt of the L-valyl ester of the antiviral drug acyclovir

Corticosteroids

Corticosteroids are used to reduce inflammation of the facial nerve (▶ Table 10.2). Their effectiveness is a matter of discussion due to the difficulty of judging how well a patient would have recovered without treatment, and the wide variety of outcome parameters when evaluating final facial nerve function.[8] Steroids (such as prednisolone/prednisone) are used at 1 mg/kg for 7 days and then tapered off. In patients at high risk, blood pressure, blood glucose, and electrolytes should be monitored throughout the treatment.

10.6.2 Treatment for Disequilibrium

Antihistamines and benzodiazepines may help reduce the effects of disequilibrium. Vestibular physical therapy might be helpful in treating loss of vestibular function.

10.6.3 Treatment for Facial Paralysis

Electrical stimulation of the facial nerves is sometimes used to aid the healing process or prevent muscle atrophy. However, it is unlikely that electrical stimulation can prevent synkinesis. Acupuncture has not been proven to be of benefit, but it might be helpful to relieve shingles pain or postherpetic neuralgia. Speech therapy by a trained therapist may be recommended to optimize speech clarity. Authors of a Cochrane database review concluded that there were limited effects of physical therapy on the outcome of facial palsy patients.[9]

10.6.4 Treatment for Pain

Painkillers might be needed, including conventional pain medication, topical lidocaine, antidepressants, and anticonvulsants. Anticonvulsants can be effective in relieving neuralgic conditions in RHS.

10.6.5 Treatment for Postherpetic Neuralgia

Treatment for postherpetic neuralgia begins with administration of antivirals during the acute phase. The antivirals acyclovir, valacyclovir, or famciclovir reduce the duration of the zoster-associated pain, which led to the assumption that antivirals also are effective preventing postherpetic neuralgia.

In a Cochrane review corticosteroids given acutely during zoster infection were described as not being effective in preventing postherpetic neuralgia.[10] A similar Cochrane review on steroids and RHS was inconclusive.[8] If postherpetic neuralgia develops, treatment focuses on relieving pain, and most patients require a combination of medication for adequate pain relief.

10.6.6 Topical Antiviral Cream

Topical antiviral cream is intended for minor mucocutaneous herpes simplex virus reactivations and plays no role in treatment of VZV reactivation or RHS.

10.6.7 Treatment for the Eye

Great care must be taken to avoid damage to the eye. Dryness may promote abrasions and ulceration of the cornea.

Table 10.2 Possible protocol for corticosteroids and antivirals when treating Ramsay Hunt syndrome

Day	Corticosteroid		Antiviral		
	Methylprednisolone, mg (IV)[a]	Methylprednisolone, mg (PO)	Acyclovir	Famciclovir	Valacyclovir
1	500	2 × 30	5 × 400 mg (PO) or 3 × 10 mg/kg (IV)	3 × 500 mg (PO)	3 × 500 mg (PO)
2	250	2 × 30	5 × 400 mg (PO) or 3 × 10 mg/kg (IV)	3 × 500 mg (PO)	3 × 500 mg (PO)
3	250	2 × 30	5 × 400 mg (PO) or 3 × 10 mg/kg (IV)	3 × 500 mg (PO)	3 × 500 mg (PO)
4	100	2 × 30	5 × 400 mg (PO) or 3 × 10 mg/kg (IV)	3 × 500 mg (PO)	3 × 500 mg (PO)
5	100	2 × 30	5 × 400 mg (PO) or 3 × 10 mg/kg (IV)	3 × 500 mg (PO)	3 × 500 mg (PO)
6	100	2 × 30	5 × 400 mg (PO) or 3 × 10 mg/kg (IV)	3 × 500 mg (PO)	3 × 500 mg (PO)
7	50[b]	2 × 30[b]	5 × 400 mg (PO) or 3 × 10 mg/kg (IV)	3 × 500 mg (PO)	3 × 500 mg (PO)

Abbreviations: IV, intravenous; PO, per oral.
Source: Adapted from Sittel et al.[17]
Notes: [a]Carrier solution (500 mL saline) may be used for IV treatment; [b]consider tapering, for example 1 week; [c]drugs with poor evidence might also be considered (pentoxifylline, vitamins).

The use of eyedrops, eye moisturizing ointment, and/or a moisture chamber, and taping the eye shut at night helps protect the eye, in particular during sleep; see Chapter 24.

10.6.8 Surgical Treatment

Surgical decompression of the facial nerve plays no role in this condition. However, long-term cases with poor defective healing may consider surgery for the paralyzed face; see Chapter 20.

10.7 Outcome and Prognosis

There is limited clinical evidence to suggest that treatment with steroids, pain medications, and antiviral agents (such as acyclovir, valacyclovir, or famciclovir) improves recovery of the facial nerve. Overall, chances of recovery are better if treatment is started within 3 days of onset of symptoms.[6] Poor prognostic factors for recovery include the following: age older than 50 years, and complete facial paralysis with signs of neural degeneration. Recovery may be complicated by misdirected reinnervation (synkinesis) primarily oral to ocular and ocular to oral but affecting the entire face. There is frequently hyperkinesis with increased resting tone in the face presenting as a deeper nasolabial fold and a sammler orbital aperture. Additionally, there may be inappropriate responses, such as tears when laughing or chewing (crocodile tears). There may also be long-term damage in hearing as full recovery only occurs in 50% of patients and residual tinnitus is commonplace. Vertigo can continue for several months after onset of RHS but often disappears after only a few weeks. RHS is not thought to recur, although some rare cases of recurrence have been reported.[11,12]

> !
> The prognosis for Ramsay Hunt syndrome is reported to be clearly worse than that for Bell's palsy.

10.7.1 Complications

Incomplete regeneration of the facial nerve is the most common complication of RHS. Involvement of cranial nerve VIII may lead rarely to persistent loss of hearing, disequilibrium, tinnitus, and/or hyperacusis. Other nerves possibly affected include the vagus, trigeminal, glossopharyngeal, oculomotor, trochlear, and abducens nerves. RHS is not associated with mortality. It is a self-limiting disease.

Neurologic Complications

Rare neurologic complications of VZV reactivation within the geniculate ganglion include granulomatous cerebral angiitis, meningoencephalitis, myelitis, Gullain–Barré syndrome, depression, postviral fatigue, and postherpetic neuralgia. Although occurrence of these complications is rare, it can result in severe consequences. In immunosuppressed patients, disseminated herpes zoster can occur due to viremia of VZV, and when seeding occurs in the internal organs, such as the lungs, liver, intestines, or brain, the fatality rate is reported to be 5 to 15%, despite antiviral therapy.[13]

Ophthalmic Zoster

When VZV is reactivated in the ophthalmic division of the trigeminal nerve, the infection is called ophthalmic zoster or herpes zoster ophthalmicus. Most frequently, vesicles appear around the orbit of the eye. Complications of ophthalmic zoster may include chronic ocular inflammation, loss of vision, and debilitating pain.

Disseminated Cutaneous Zoster

Disseminated cutaneous zoster has been defined as more than 20 vesicles outside the area of the primary and adjacent dermatomes. This complication of zoster has been described in immunocompromised persons (HIV, cancer, and patients on immunosuppressive therapy).[14] However, disseminated cutaneous zoster is rare in otherwise healthy persons who are not on immunosuppressive therapy and have no underlying cancer.

Secondary Bacterial Infection of the Vesicles

Secondary infections, including cellulitis, can be caused by the introduction of any one of many bacteria to open lesions at the site of the zoster outbreak. Such bacteria can include group A streptococci, which can cause severe infection. Good hygiene can help prevent this complication. Should such secondary bacterial infection occur, early recognition and treatment of the infection is necessary. This is most often seen in immunocompromised patients. However, open, weeping sores in any RHS patient are vulnerable to additional infection.

10.8 Prevention

The shingles vaccine effectively prevents chickenpox. Most people who get this vaccine will not get chickenpox, and thus will not harbor the virus that can later cause RHS. Clinical trials have proved that a vaccine to prevent shingles (Zostavax, Sanofi Pasteur MSD) reduces the risk of shingles, and reduces severity if one does get shingles.[15] The US Centers for Disease Control and Prevention suggests that the vaccine should be routinely given to individuals aged 60 years or older, as about 90% of the population has been exposed to chickenpox and about 20% of people that had chickenpox are likely to get shingles without the vaccine. The vaccine contains a weakened chickenpox virus.[16]

10.9 Key Points

- Ramsay Hunt syndrome (RHS) is diagnosed with clinical signs; however it may initially be indistinguishable from Bell's palsy.
- Patients often present with face, ear, or head pain before physical findings of rash or paralysis, and the diagnosis of herpes zoster oticus should be entertained.
- RHS is never bilateral (Lyme disease and Bell's palsy can be).
- Audiovestibular symptoms suggest diagnosis of RHS is most likely.
- Always check the oral cavity for lesions that the patient may not mention and may not understand are related.
- A proportion of patients with "Bell's palsy" have RHS "sine herpete."
- The outcome depends on individual risk factors, severity of the disease, and early treatment with antiviral agents and steroids.
- RHS has severe complications in some patients; risk factors are: > 50 years of age, comorbidity, and immunosuppression.
- Prevention may be possible with the shingles vaccine.

References

[1] Scott O. Herpes zoster oticus (Ramsay Hunt syndrome) [Patient.co.uk Web site]. June 22, 2011. Available at: www.patient.co.uk/doctor/herpes-zoster-oticus-ramsay-hunt-syndrome. Accessed April 6, 2014

[2] Pitkäranta A, Piiparinen H, Mannonen L, Vesaluoma M, Vaheri A. Detection of human herpesvirus 6 and varicella-zoster virus in tear fluid of patients with Bell's palsy by PCR. J Clin Microbiol 2000; 38: 2753–2755

[3] Gershon AA. Prevention and treatment of VZV infections in patients with HIV. Herpes 2001; 8: 32–36

[4] Nakata S, Mizuno T, Naganawa S et al. 3D-FLAIR MRI in facial nerve paralysis with and without audio-vestibular disorder. Acta Otolaryngol 2010; 130: 632–636

[5] Ramos Macías A, de Miguel Martínez I, Martín Sánchez AM, Gómez González JL, Martín Galán A. The incorporation of acyclovir into the treatment of peripheral paralysis. A study of 45 cases [in Spanish] Acta Otorrinolaringol Esp 1992; 43: 117–120

[6] Murakami S, Hato N, Horiuchi J, Honda N, Gyo K, Yanagihara N. Treatment of Ramsay Hunt syndrome with acyclovir-prednisone: significance of early diagnosis and treatment. Ann Neurol 1997; 41: 353–357

[7] Uscategui T, Dorée C, Chamberlain IJ, Burton MJ. Antiviral therapy for Ramsay Hunt syndrome (herpes zoster oticus with facial palsy) in adults. Cochrane Database Syst Rev 2008: CD006851

[8] Uscategui T, Doree C, Chamberlain IJ, Burton MJ. Corticosteroids as adjuvant to antiviral treatment in Ramsay Hunt syndrome (herpes zoster oticus with facial palsy) in adults. Cochrane Database Syst Rev 2008: CD006852

[9] Teixeira LJ, Valbuza JS, Prado GF. Physical therapy for Bell's palsy (idiopathic facial paralysis). Cochrane Database Syst Rev 2011: CD006283

[10] Chen N, Yang M, He L, Zhang D, Zhou M, Zhu C. Corticosteroids for preventing postherpetic neuralgia. Cochrane Database Syst Rev 2010: CD005582

[11] Coulson S, Croxson GR, Adams R, Oey V. Prognostic factors in herpes zoster oticus (ramsay hunt syndrome). Otol Neurotol 2011; 32: 1025–1030

[12] Ryu EW, Lee HY, Lee SY, Park MS, Yeo SG. Clinical manifestations and prognosis of patients with Ramsay Hunt syndrome. Am J Otolaryngol 2012; 33: 313–318

[13] Boivin G, Jovey R, Elliott CT, Patrick DM. Management and prevention of herpes zoster: A Canadian perspective. Can J Infect Dis Med Microbiol 2010; 21: 45–52

[14] Gilden DH, Kleinschmidt-DeMasters BK, LaGuardia JJ, Mahalingam R, Cohrs RJ. Neurologic complications of the reactivation of varicella-zoster virus. N Engl J Med 2000; 342: 635–645

[15] Oxman MN, Levin MJ, Johnson GR et al. Shingles Prevention Study Group. A vaccine to prevent herpes zoster and postherpetic neuralgia in older adults. N Engl J Med 2005; 352: 2271–2284

[16] Schmader KE, Levin MJ, Gnann JW, Jr et al. Efficacy, safety, and tolerability of herpes zoster vaccine in persons aged 50–59 years. Clin Infect Dis 2012; 54: 922–928

[17] Sittel C, Sittel A, Guntinas-Lichius O, Eckel HE, Stennert E. Bell's palsy: a 10-year experience with antiphlogistic-rheologic infusion therapy. Am J Otol 2000; 21: 425–432

11 Lyme Disease

Howard S. Moskowitz and Barry M. Schaitkin

11.1 Introduction

Lyme disease, also known as Lyme borreliosis, is a complex medical condition that can involve multiple body systems. Lyme disease is the most common tick-borne infectious disease in North America and in countries with moderate climates in Eurasia. The most common clinical manifestation of initial infection is erythema migrans. However, the causative pathogen can spread to other tissues and organs, which can involve a patient's skin, nervous system, joints, or heart. Facial nerve paralysis is one of the most common neurologic manifestations found in Lyme disease.

11.2 Definition

Lyme disease is an infection caused by a group of related spirochetes, *Borrelia* spp. or Lyme borrelia. These spirochetes are transmitted by specific *Ixodes* spp. ticks. Lyme disease is manifested by a multisystem inflammatory condition that is further characterized by various stages of infection with unique clinical manifestations in each stage of disease. Lyme neuroborreliosis refers to the nervous system disorders caused by *Borrelia* spp. Involvement of the nervous system, including facial palsy, occurs mainly in early localized disease as well as in chronic cases of Lyme disease.

11.3 Epidemiology and Etiology

Several endemic areas of Lyme disease have been identified in the world, and the number of patients confirmed with the disease has steadily increased in North America and Europe. In general the occurrence of Lyme disease varies largely based on environmental conditions that favor vector propagation and interactions with susceptible hosts. In the United States, Lyme disease occurs principally in the northeastern states and around the Great Lakes. In 2012, 95% of Lyme disease cases were reported from 13 states further underscoring the geographical variation in prevalence.[1] In the United States, slightly more men (53%) than women are infected. Although patients of all ages are at risk, there is a bimodal age distribution with the highest incidences found in children 5 to 9 years old and in adults 55 to 59 years old.[2] The number of confirmed cases of Lyme disease has remained high in the United States, but peaked with nearly 30,000 cases in 2009. In Europe, Lyme disease is highly endemic in southern Scandinavia and central Europe, but low in the United Kingdom. The incidence rates appear to increase from northern Europe to central Europe with the highest average annual incidence per 100,000 population found in Austria and Slovenia.[3]

Molecular characterization of the spirochetes isolated from patients in North America and Eurasia has revealed different genospecies. In North America, *Borrelia burgdorferi* is the only species of Lyme borrelia known to cause human disease. By contrast, there are at least five species of Lyme borrelia (*B. afzelii*, *B. garinii*, *B. burgdorferi*, *B. spielmanii*, and *B. bavariensis*) that have been shown to cause disease in Eurasia, all of which possess unique characteristics. This variety of causative organisms underlies a wider spectrum of possible clinical manifestations. Furthermore, this may explain some of the differences in clinical presentation.

Borrelia spp. have been shown to have a nearly complete absence of biosynthetic pathways, making them dependent on their environment for nutritional requirements.[4] The main vectors for transmission of these spirochetes are specific *Ixodes* spp. ticks: in the northeastern United States *I. scapularis* represents the predominant vector, whereas *I. pacificus* assumes this role in the western United States. By contrast, *I. ricinus* and *I. persulcatus* are the principal vectors in Europe and Asia respectively. These ticks have a four-stage life cycle (egg, larva, nymph, and adult) and feed only once during every active stage. Ticks attach to the skin of a host animal and feed for a few days. However, the risk of acquiring a *Borrelia* infection after a tick bite is low even if the tick is infected. The low transmission is partly due to the fact that a feeding period of more than 24 hours is usually needed for effective transmission of *B. burgdorferi*.[5] The need for a prolonged feeding period in order to transmit the pathogen is attributed to several linked events. Once an infected tick takes a blood meal the spirochetes increase in number and undergo phenotypic changes, which enable them to invade the host tick's salivary glands.[6] During feeding the infected tick deposits the *Borrelia* spp. into the skin of the host and the spirochetes are then able to spread from the site of inoculation.

After the feeding period has completed, the ticks drop off their host and locate near the soil surface and take several months to develop into their next developmental stage. The typical habitat for Lyme transmission usually consists of deciduous or mixed woodland. These areas usually have a substantial layer of decaying vegetation on the ground, which supports the development and survival of ticks as well as a variety of potential vertebrate reservoirs.

Lyme disease is endemic throughout the temperate zones of the northern hemisphere and is one of the most frequent vector-borne human diseases in these areas. The main vertebrate reservoirs for Lyme disease are small mammals, such as mice and some species of birds. In most tick habitats deer are important for survival since they are one of the few wild hosts that can feed sufficient numbers of adult ticks. Even though humans are incidental hosts they are the main species that develops clinical disease. The majority of cases of transmission to humans occur from late May to late September. This coincides with the increasing recreational use of areas habituated by ticks as well as the season-dependent activity of the *Ixodes* ticks.

> !
>
> Lyme disease transmission occurs mainly from May to September. The tick must generally be attached greater than 24 hours to transmit the disease.

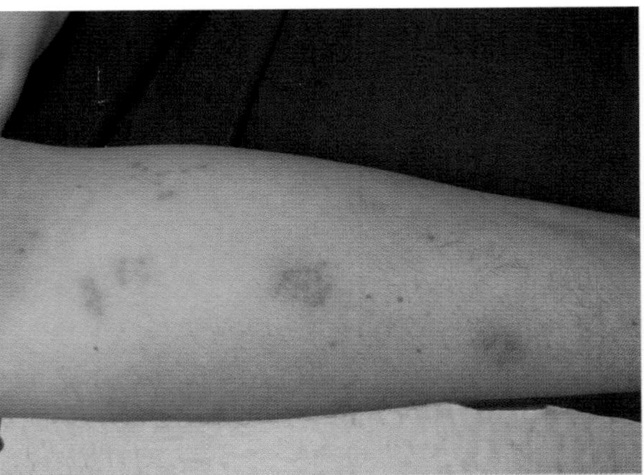

Fig. 11.1 Example of early erythema migrans lesion.

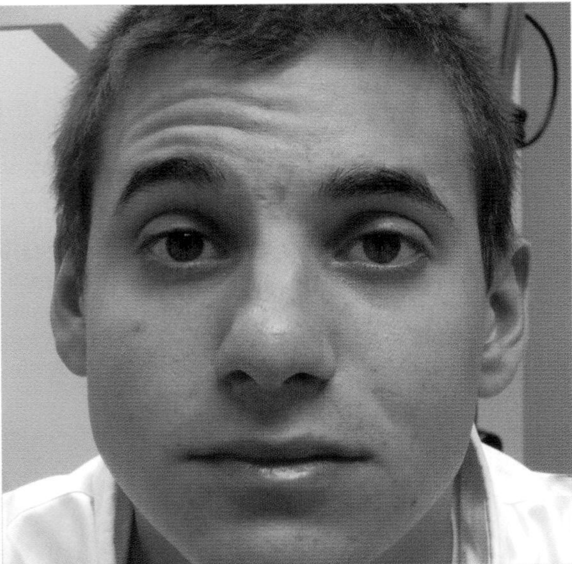

Fig. 11.2 The patient shown in ► Fig. 11.1, with typical erythema migrans facial lesions.

Once host organisms are infected the spirochetes elicit a variety of immune responses including macrophage-mediated and antibody-mediated responses. Despite these immune responses, *Borrelia* infection can still persist via a variety of phenotypic changes including downregulation of immunogenic surface-exposed proteins and rapid alteration of surface lipoproteins.[7] Interestingly, neither direct invasion of spirochetes nor production of destructive toxins is implicated in the disease manifestations. Instead it is the inflammatory reaction from the host's own immune system that is cited as the principal cause of the majority of tissue damage associated with infection.

There are several animal models of Lyme disease, but only the rhesus monkey has been shown to exhibit all of the clinical manifestations found in the human disease including early localized, early disseminated, and chronic stages. Of additional note, rhesus monkeys also develop Lyme neuroborreliosis as evidenced by cerebrospinal fluid (CSF) pleocytosis and meningeal inflammation.[8] Studies have indicated multifocal axonal degeneration without evidence of free spirochetal structures, further supporting the belief that an immune-mediated process underlies the changes associated with Lyme disease.

11.4 Clinical Features

The inflammatory process underlying Lyme disease involves multiple body systems. Cases can be further characterized by various stages of infection. Early localized infection typically manifests with an erythematous expanding skin lesion known as erythema migrans (► Fig. 11.1 and ► Fig. 11.2). Erythema migrans is the most common objective presentation of Lyme disease and is found in approximately 70 to 80% of cases.[9] However, few patients with Lyme neuroborreliosis recall a distinctive erythema migrans lesion. Early disseminated disease can be characterized by at least two erythema migrans lesions or via manifestation of associated neurologic or cardiac changes. Late-stage disease is typified by recurrent bouts of arthritis or other specific chronic neurologic manifestations such as slowly progressive encephalomyelitis.

> !
>
> Erythema migrans is the most common objective presentation of early Lyme disease.

11.5 Diagnostic Work-Up

Studies show that white blood cell counts, hemoglobin concentrations, and platelet counts of patients with Lyme disease are usually normal. Erythrocyte sedimentation rates can be slightly raised in all stages of Lyme disease, but significantly elevated values are uncommon. CSF fluid examination in Lyme neuroborreliosis often reveals a pleocytosis with more than 90% lymphocytes, raised protein concentration, and normal glucose concentration.

Clinical diagnosis can be made with good certainty in cases with prototypical erythema migrans without the need for supporting laboratory investigations. At this initial stage of infection serological antibodies for Lyme disease are infrequently positive. However, confirmatory serological testing can be performed 2 to 6 weeks later if needed.

The main challenges to the laboratory diagnosis of Lyme disease relate to the difficulty to confirm the presence of *Borrelia* spp. using conventional microbiological methods. Microscopy has very little practical utility, although spirochetes can be detected from skin lesions. However, in patients without skin lesions, there is a sparsity of organisms found in extracutaneous tissues, limiting the efficacy of direct detection methods. In these cases, serology is generally preferred to verify infection.

Serological testing has been a controversial topic for definitive diagnosis. In an attempt to improve the consistency and validity of positive serological tests, the US Centers for Disease Control and Prevention (CDC) in association with other agencies recommended a two-tiered approach for diagnosis, particularly in cases without the distinctive erythema migrans initial lesion. These guidelines recommended a first stage of testing with a sensitive enzyme-linked immunosorbent assay (ELISA). In cases with positive ELISA testing, IgM and IgG immunoblots can then be performed on the same serum sample for conclusive diagnosis. However, there are also reports of false-positive responses with high background rates of seropositivity in highly endemic areas.[10]

!

In patients without erythema migrans a two-tiered approach is recommended:

1. Enzyme-linked immunosorbent assay (ELISA) testing.
2. IgM and IgG immunoblots on the same sample if ELISA is positive.

A positive Lyme antibody test in blood is indicative only of exposure, which may be current or previous. Thus, Lyme antibodies can be found by coincidence in asymptomatic individuals. The mere presence of antibodies to the spirochete does not establish the presence of an ongoing infection. Furthermore, the presence of antibodies does not prove that coexisting symptoms and signs are due to Lyme disease. Unfortunately, there is no current assay that is able to definitively discriminate between an active infection and past exposure. Considering these limitations the overuse of Lyme serology almost certainly leads to a considerable overdiagnosis.

Additional studies have looked into the expanded utility of polymerase chain reaction (PCR) from a variety of samples for detection of spirochetal DNA and positive results can support the diagnosis. However, PCR has been found to be most sensitive from skin samples of patients who have erythema migrans and microbiological confirmation is generally not needed at this stage.

A positive *Borrelia* antibody test in blood is indicative only of exposure, which may be current or previous. The presence of antibodies to the spirochete does not establish the presence of an ongoing infection. There is no current assay that is able to definitively discriminate between an active infection and past exposure.

11.6 Treatment

Borrelia spp. have been generally found to be susceptible to tetracyclines, most penicillins, many second-generation and third-generation cephalosporins, and macrolides via in vitro studies. Accordingly, doxycycline, amoxicillin, and cefuroxime are highly effective and are preferred agents for early localized Lyme disease and are administered in order to prevent dissemination and the development of later sequelae (▶ Table 11.1 and ▶ Table 11.2). The preferred parenteral drug for Lyme disease is ceftriaxone, not only because of its high activity against *Borrelia* in vitro, but also because it can cross the blood–brain barrier well and has a long serum half-life. Alternative choices for parenteral antibiotics are cefotaxime and penicillin.

11.7 Outcomes and Prognosis

When Lyme disease involves the nervous system it is often referred to as Lyme neuroborreliosis and most commonly manifests as various cranial or peripheral neuropathies or meningitis. The diagnosis of Lyme neuroborreliosis generally requires laboratory confirmation with pleocytosis in the CSF and intrathecally produced *Borrelia*-specific antibodies, since neurologic signs and symptoms may not be specific. Cerebrospinal inflammation due to other causes of subacute and chronic meningitis must be ruled out, particularly neurosarcoidosis, and meningeal lymphomatosis and carcinomatosis. Chronic Lyme neuroborreliosis may be confused with primary progressive spinal multiple sclerosis and stroke-like syndromes. Intrathecal antibody production can be used for a definite diagnosis, but it has a low sensitivity in the earliest phase of the disease. A positive CSF antibody test

Table 11.1 Recommended treatment routes for Lyme disease according to clinical features

Clinical symptom	Preferred route	Duration (days)
Erythema migrans	Oral	10–21
Cranial nerve involvement	Oral	10–21
Arthritis	Oral	14–28
Cardiac disease	Intravenous	14–21
Late neurologic	Intravenous	14–28

Table 11.2 Common treatment regimens for Lyme disease according to route of administration

Route	Treatment regimen
Oral	Doxycycline[a] 100 mg two times daily
	Amoxicillin 500 mg three times daily
	Cefuroxime 500 mg two times daily
Intravenous	Ceftriaxone 2 g daily
	Cefotaxime 2 g every 8 hours

Dosages should be weight-based for children.
[a]Doxycycline is contraindicated in children under 8 years of age, as well as in pregnant and breastfeeding women.

with concomitant CSF inflammation is currently the best laboratory evidence of active Lyme neuroborreliosis. The frequency of Lyme neuroborreliosis is not surprising given that the frequency of spirochetemia in early disease exceeds 40%.[11]

> The diagnosis of Lyme neuroborreliosis generally requires laboratory confirmation with pleocytosis in the cerebrospinal fluid and intrathecally produced *Borrelia*-specific antibodies, since neurologic signs and symptoms may not be specific.

Of all potential involved cranial nerves, Lyme disease most commonly affects the facial nerve, accounting for upward of 80% of all Lyme-related cranial nerve neuropathies.[12] Facial palsy associated with Lyme disease can be found in early disseminated or late-stage disease. In some patients acute facial nerve palsy has been reported to be the only manifestation of the disease. Historically, there have been numerous cited causes of acquired peripheral facial palsy, including a variety of infections (otitis media, mastoiditis), temporal bone trauma, malignancy, and idiopathic causes (Bell's palsy). Of these, Bell's palsy is believed to constitute the largest group, causing 60 to 75% of cases of peripheral facial palsy. However, over the past several decades the prevalence of Lyme disease has increased likely in part due to improved knowledge of and testing for this disease entity. In endemic areas, Lyme disease has become one of the most commonly identified causes of acquired facial palsy especially among children.

The molecular basis of the neurotropism of *Borrelia* has yet to be elucidated. It usually takes 2 to 4 weeks after the primary infection to develop Lyme neuroborreliosis. The spread of the spirochete to the nervous system has been speculated to be hematogenous, but a transneural spread from the site of entry along peripheral nerves to the nerve roots, meninges, and subarachnoid space is also possible. There have been reports of topographical association of the location of a preceding tick bite and the site of first neurologic signs. Furthermore, a rat model revealed ipsilateral neuritis of peripheral nerves following local inoculation of *Borrelia* spirochetes; however, none of the rats developed a facial palsy or other symptoms of Lyme disease during the course of experiments.[13]

There is an exceptional amount of heterogeneity regarding the incidence of Lyme disease, specifically causing facial nerve palsy. This variation is due to many factors, most notably geography as many studies are focused on areas where *Borrelia* is an endemic infection. The prevalence of Lyme disease among patients with facial palsy varies widely between published series. In several published studies on adults, the prevalence of Lyme disease facial palsy has ranged from very low prevalence to up to one-quarter of cases. An initial large study in an endemic area reported that 101 of 951 patients with Lyme disease developed facial paralysis at some point during their illness.[14] The prevalence of Lyme disease facial palsy in children with facial palsy seems to be considerably higher with upward of two-thirds of such patients having Lyme disease. However, the reason for this apparent increased frequency is currently unknown.

There is considerable debate about the most appropriate diagnostic and therapeutic management strategy for Lyme facial palsy. Some authorities recommend that all such patients should undergo lumbar puncture to guide treatment. Although most patients have evidence of central nervous system involvement on examination of CSF, no markers have been specifically identified that are indicative of poor prognosis. Additionally, much of the published experience of patients with Lyme neuroborreliosis is from Europe where different species of *Borrelia* are known to cause Lyme disease.

11.7.1 Lyme Facial Palsy versus Bell's Palsy

Bell's palsy refers to a peripheral facial palsy of unknown origin and is generally conceived as a diagnosis of exclusion. The clinical differentiation between Bell's palsy and a facial palsy due to Lyme neuroborreliosis is generally made through clinical evaluation as both disease entities have a differing clinical picture. The evaluation should take note of preceding and concomitant general symptoms, most notably for radicular pains, headache, and presence of other motor deficits, as cases of Lyme typically have a higher occurrence of neurologic symptoms outside the facial palsy. Although some studies have suggested the use of a history of tick bite as a differentiating feature, a reported history of tick bite is typically uncommon even in cases of definite Lyme neuroborreliosis.[15] Accordingly, the absence of a tick bite does not exclude Lyme disease.

CSF analysis of leukocytes, albumin, and glucose can be obtained within hours. Although antibodies to *Borrelia* in serum and CSF are often helpful in the diagnosis, it generally takes several days to obtain these results. There are studies where Lyme neuroborreliosis is the most common cause of bilateral facial nerve palsy, and it has been cited to occur bilaterally in up to one-quarter of cases.[14] In studies of bilateral facial paralysis either Lyme disease or Bell's palsy is generally most common depending on many factors including age of the patient, geographic location, and even the frequency of testing. Finally, although electrophysiologic studies have been applied in order to differentiate between the different causes of Bell's palsy, the results to date have not shown to be conclusive.

> !
>
> Lyme disease and Bell's palsy are among the most frequent causes of bilateral facial paralysis.

The optimal treatment for a patient with facial palsy depends on the etiology, which is often unknown at the time of initial patient presentation. For facial palsy due to Lyme disease most infectious disease experts recommend antibiotic therapy, although it is unclear whether there is a difference in outcomes for oral versus intravenous therapy. For Bell's palsy, corticosteroids are widely accepted as proper management, but varying data exist for the role of concomitant antiviral medication.

11.7.2 Studies on Lyme Facial Palsy

Given the difficulties with definitive diagnosis of Lyme disease, studies have attempted to further refine the ability to accurately assess which patients have a facial palsy that is due to Lyme disease. Peltomaa et al (2002) looked for the presence of Lyme disease and associated risk factors in a large series of consecutive patients with facial nerve paralysis.[16] In their analysis of 503 consecutive patients with acute facial palsy, 11 patients were found to have Lyme disease. Patients with evidence of Lyme disease were more commonly found to have fever, headache, enlarged cervical lymph nodes, bilateral paralysis, and arthralgia as compared with patients without evidence of Lyme. They utilized logistic regression modeling and found that the combination of variables that best predicted the occurrence of Lyme disease in patients with facial palsy were summer season at the onset of facial paralysis, presence of enlarged cervical lymph nodes, and arthralgia. Furthermore, total paralysis of facial nerves, recurrent facial paralysis, and hyperacusis were the best combination of variables that predicted a poor outcome.

> !
>
> Factors that suggest Lyme disease as the diagnosis of acute facial paralysis are onset in the summer season, presence of enlarged cervical lymph nodes, headaches, and arthralgias.

Many other studies have focused on outcomes following a facial palsy due to Lyme disease. In 2011, Kowalski et al reported on a retrospective double-cohort study to analyze outcomes in patients with Lyme facial palsy treated with oral antibiotics that were matched to controls with early localized Lyme disease without facial palsy.[17] Of the 15 patients with Lyme facial palsy, 14 regained nerve function. Long-term outcomes between the two groups were similar, although patients with facial palsy reported significantly more fatigue.

Kalish and colleagues (2001) chose 84 randomly selected patients from the Lyme, Connecticut region with a prior history of erythema migrans, facial palsy, or Lyme arthritis 10 to 20 years prior, and 30 uninfected control subjects, in order to assess the long-term sequelae from acute disease.[18] The patients in the three study groups and the control group did not differ significantly in current symptoms or neuropsychologic test results. However, patients selected for a prior history of facial palsy frequently had more widespread nervous system involvement and more often had residual facial nerve or peripheral nerve deficits. Moreover, they found that patients with facial palsy who did not receive antibiotics for acute disease had more joint pain and sleep difficulty, and lower scores on the body pain index and standardized physical component scores, than did patients with facial palsy who received antibiotics. Accordingly, although the overall current health status of each patient group was satisfactory, long-term sequelae were more clearly apparent among patients with facial palsy who did not receive antibiotics for acute disease. Furthermore, 7 of the 31 patients who originally presented with Lyme facial palsy had residual facial weakness on long-term follow-up; of the 7 patients with residual weakness, only 6 exhibited mild weakness.

In a study of a different design, Ljostad et al (2005) studied 69 patients with peripheral facial nerve palsy.[19] Patients were followed prospectively for 5 years. Only seven patients were found to have Lyme disease as the underlying etiology. All of these patients though had additional neurologic symptoms. These neurologic symptoms were diverse and included tinnitus, slight ataxia, slight hemiparesis, hyperesthesia, and diplopia, as well as residual facial palsy. In addition, 87% had associated constitutional complaints. Thus, Lyme disease was found to be an infrequent cause of facial palsy unless the patient also exhibited additional neurologic or constitutional symptoms.

Although frequently cited as an important component of the diagnosis of facial palsy due to Lyme disease, studies focusing on data from lumbar punctures are lacking. In a recent study, Bremell and Hagberg analyzed records of patients with peripheral facial palsy who had undergone lumbar puncture.[15] Patients were classified as Bell's palsy, definite Lyme neuroborreliosis, or possible Lyme neuroborreliosis, on the basis of the presence of *Borrelia* antibodies in serum and CSF and preceding erythema migrans. Patients with definite Lyme neuroborreliosis most commonly developed symptoms during the second half of the year, with a peak in August. In contrast, patients with Bell's palsy fell ill with a much more even distribution over the course of the year. Patients with definite Lyme neuroborreliosis were also found to have significantly more neurologic symptoms outside of the facial palsy, including radicular pain as well as sense disturbances, and significantly higher levels of mononuclear cells and albumin in their CSF. Furthermore, the absence of any cases outside the peak season also served as evidence that the incubation period for Lyme disease is rarely more than a couple of weeks.

In an effort to look for Lyme disease as a potential coinfective process in patients found to have either varicella zoster virus (VZV) reactivation or Bell's palsy, Furuta et al (2001) analyzed 113 patients with acute peripheral facial paralysis.[20] They found that 5 of 81 patients with Bell's palsy, 1 of 32 patients with VZV reactivation, and 1 of 58 control subjects exhibited both IgM and IgG antibodies to *Borrelia*, a difference that was not statistically significant. However, three of the five patients in the Bell's palsy group exhibited headache or general fatigue, suggesting an association between facial palsy and Lyme borreliosis in these patients. The low prevalence of positive *Borrelia* titers was also an interesting finding, because the study was performed in one of the areas that is endemic for Lyme disease in Japan. In addition, they found evidence for cross-reactivity to *B. afzelii* in IgM blots in patients with herpes simplex virus 1 reactivation, suggesting that these data must be interpreted with caution for accurate diagnosis.

11.7.3 Studies on Lyme Facial Palsy Focusing on Children

Data on etiology, outcome as well as treatment for acute facial palsy specifically as it pertains to children, have been more limited until recently. Much of the original data addressing this question in the pediatric population is more than 20 years old and was generated in an era before Lyme disease was more fully recognized and evaluated. A review in 1981 of 170 patients with facial nerve paralysis ranging in age from birth to 18 years found that idiopathic palsy was the most common etiology (42%), followed by trauma, infection, congenital causes, and neoplasm.[21] However, new data on incidence, etiology, and natural course of this disease are crucial to provide pertinent advice for parents.

Nigrovic et al (2008) sought to describe diagnostic predictors in children by looking at children with facial palsy who were evaluated in the emergency department of a tertiary care pediatric center. Of 420 patients with facial palsy, 313 patients with peripheral facial palsy were evaluated for Lyme disease and 106 were found to have Lyme disease. In the 46 children with an erythema migrans rash, the rash preceded the onset of the facial palsy in all cases, in accordance with general understanding of the disease progression. The prevalence of Lyme disease among patients with facial palsy in this cohort was somewhat lower than other pediatric series, which might be due to the fact that there is a different subset of patients that is evaluated in the emergency department for facial palsy.

Nigrovic et al (2008) found Lyme disease facial palsy to be independently associated with onset of symptoms during peak Lyme disease season, presence of fever, and history of headache. [22]Furthermore, both the onset of symptoms during the Lyme disease season and presence of headache remained significant independent predictors for children who did not have meningitis. Bilateral facial palsy was also found to be an independent predictor of Lyme disease in children, but was not validated by the authors' final multivariate analysis.

In a similar study, Fine and colleagues looked at children who presented with facial nerve palsy and tried to create a model for predicting Lyme disease as the causative factor.[23] In their study, they analyzed data from 264 children. The children had peripheral facial palsy and were evaluated for Lyme disease. Of particular note, a diagnosis of Lyme was found in 65% of children from high-risk counties in Massachusetts during peak Lyme disease season as compared with 5% for those children who did not have both geographic and seasonal risk factors. Of the patients with both seasonal and geographic risk factors, 100% of the patients with two clinical factors were found to have Lyme disease. Furthermore, factors that were independently associated with Lyme disease facial palsy were timing from June to November, residence in a high-risk area, fever, and headache. The authors created a prediction tool that incorporated the geographic and seasonal risk that was able to identify all cases. In contrast, clinical experts correctly treated only 68 of 94 patients with Lyme disease facial palsy.

Up to 90% of children with Lyme disease facial palsy have been found to demonstrate abnormal CSF findings indicative of a central nervous system infection.[24] Accordingly, many authors view lumbar puncture and associated studies of CSF as serving an important role in the definitive diagnosis of Lyme disease despite the invasive nature of this test. Tveitnes et al (2007) studied children admitted for acute facial palsy who were investigated with lumbar puncture.[25] In that study, 115 children were included and 65% were found to have Lyme neuroborreliosis. In accordance with other studies, all patients were diagnosed between May and November. Furthermore, lymphocytic meningitis was found in all but one patient.

!

Many authorities, especially pediatricians, view lumbar puncture and associated studies of cerebrospinal fluid as an important diagnostic tool for the definitive diagnosis of Lyme disease.

Historically, most facial palsies in children have been suggested to resolve completely without any residual symptoms. To further clarify this issue, several recent studies have looked into long-term recovery after acute facial palsy in children. Jenke et al (2011) investigated 106 children with facial palsy.[26] All of the patients with Lyme disease were treated with 14 days of intravenous antibiotics. Long-term follow data were available for only 23 of the 25 patients with Lyme disease, and 95.7% had full resolution of facial palsy by the end of 12 weeks. Overall, faster recovery was noted in younger children independent of disease etiology. The rate of recovery did not differ significantly depending on age or etiology, with complete recovery in more than 97% of the cases. However, although not statistically significant, many children with Lyme neuroborreliosis achieved initial faster recovery as compared with those with idiopathic facial palsy.

!

Children with acute facial paralysis have a very good prognosis, but not all have a complete recovery.

Similar results were found by Drack and Weissert in their retrospective study of 84 children with peripheral facial palsy.[27] In that cohort, Lyme neuroborreliosis was found in 26 cases. Between the months of June and November, the number of cases with Lyme neuroborreliosis rose to 53.3%, while there were no cases of Lyme disease between the months of January and April. The patients with Lyme disease were treated with intravenous antibiotics for 14 to 21 days. Of the 26 patients, 25 showed complete recovery from their facial palsy, with only one patient showing mild (House–Brackmann grade II) residual weakness. Patients with Lyme disease showed a higher recovery rate than those with other infections or idiopathic causes (96% as compared with 88%).

However, Bagger-Sjoback et al (2005) revealed that in contrast to some previously cited dogma, not all children with facial palsy attributed to Lyme disease will recover completely.[28] Of 255 patients they studied who were originally diagnosed with Lyme disease, 132 had signs of facial palsy. Of those who originally had facial palsy, 118 responded to a questionnaire 3 to 5 years later, and 15 of these patients reported a residual facial palsy. Furthermore, 13 of the 15 consented to examination. On physical examination four patients of these patients were found to have normal facial nerve function, while the other nine patients exhibited mild weakness of the facial nerve (House–Brackmann grade II).

Similarly, Skogman et al (2012) found higher rates of persistent facial nerve dysfunction after they analyzed the data from 84 children with confirmed Lyme neuroborreliosis who underwent a neurologic reexamination after a median of 5 years.[29] Objective neurologic findings were found in 16 children. The majority of these children had persistent facial nerve palsy ($n = 11$), but other motor or sensory deficits were also found ($n = 5$). Facial nerve dysfunction was moderate in the 11 cases of residual facial nerve palsy (House–Brackmann grades III to IV), but no child had a severe or total loss of facial nerve function. Some children also showed signs of vestibular nerve dysfunction, either via caloric testing, head shaking nystagmus, or end-gaze nystagmus.

Prognostic factors for total recovery of facial nerve palsy have not been fully identified in children. Skogman and colleagues attempted to clarify this issue by analyzing the results from medium-term follow-up after children developed acute facial palsy.[30] In that study, although the majority of the patients were diagnosed with Lyme neuroborreliosis, some of the children included in the study did not have Lyme disease, which somewhat complicates the data. Out of 27 children, 21 had a full recovery of facial nerve function. However, six children exhibited mild-to-moderate residual impairment of facial nerve function. The authors did not find a correlation between residual facial palsy and gender, age, treatment, or other symptoms.

A study in 2010 found that children could have Lyme neuroborreliosis even if they had an initial normal neurologic examination.[31] In that study, the Dutch Paediatric Surveillance System was used to find registered cases of childhood neuroborreliosis. Reporting pediatricians were contacted and received a detailed questionnaire. In total, 78 of the 89 patients reported had complete documentation, of which 66 met the strict case definition for Lyme neuroborreliosis. At presentation, 52 children had at least one objective neurologic sign, but 14 patients had no neurologic signs at physical examination. Facial palsy was one of the presenting symptoms in 47 patients and the only symptom in 9 children. Of the 14 patients without objective neurologic signs at initial physical examination, 3 had transient and fully reversible neurologic symptoms of facial asymmetry and two reported changes in personality and paresthesia. The number of subjective complaints was higher in patients without objective neurologic signs at diagnosis. Thus, there is a need to suspect Lyme disease in children with typical antecedents and multiple symptoms even if there are no corresponding neurologic signs on initial physical examination.

11.7.4 Overview of Lyme Facial Palsy Studies

There are many methodological issues that must be taken into account when the aggregate pool of data from studies on facial palsy in Lyme disease is analyzed. With regard to geography, the significantly higher prevalence of Lyme disease in endemic areas is well documented. Accordingly, many studies with large numbers of patients with Lyme disease are accrued from these areas. It is therefore important to integrate this into decision algorithms as attempts to generalize these quoted prevalence numbers to areas with significantly lower prevalence of Lyme disease may skew diagnostic and treatment decisions.

The prevalence of Lyme disease is also significantly higher in months where vector–host interactions are optimized. Accordingly, this should assume an important role in patient work-up as the likelihood of Lyme disease at other times of the year seems significantly less likely. However, this potential diagnosis must still be closely considered as there is evidence that Lyme neuroborreliosis occurs after a period of latency between the time of infection to the onset of symptoms. Accordingly, in patients with a history or physical examination suggestive of Lyme disease, there should be strong consideration of testing for Lyme disease even during the colder seasons.

> **!**
>
> The prevalence of Lyme disease is significantly higher in months where vector–host interactions are optimized. Accordingly, this should assume an important role in patient work-up.

An additional important issue is that studies vary in terms of how Lyme disease is diagnosed and whether to attribute the acute facial palsy to Lyme disease even with serological or CSF evidence of *Borrelia*. Importantly, although many studies use strict criteria set by the CDC or other similar authorities, other studies rely on less-specific criteria. Differences in diagnostic parameters will have a direct effect on the overall frequency of facial palsies that are attributed to Lyme disease, which in turn will have an impact on models or decision algorithms. Although ELISAs are a fundamental part of the CDC's two-tiered diagnostic system, some ELISAs have been shown to produce high false-positive rates. Also, the presence of seropositive control subjects in the endemic area suggests that some incidental seropositivity may exist in the patient groups. In addition, since herpes simplex virus 1 or VZV reactivation are major causes of acute facial palsy in all geographic areas, IgM immunoblots for *Borrelia* antibodies should be carefully evaluated since cross-reactivity in IgM immunoblots can be seen in patients without subsequent IgG seroconversion.[20]

Accordingly, in cases where the facial palsy is the only clinical manifestation of disease, the relationship between facial palsy and Lyme disease remains speculative by serological testing alone. Even setting aside diagnostic issues, it is presently not possible to definitively state that even though a patient tests positive for Lyme disease that their associated facial palsy is directly or even indirectly caused by that infection.

> **⚠**
>
> In cases of facial palsy where this is the only clinical manifestation of disease, the relationship between facial palsy and Lyme disease remains speculative by serological testing alone.

At the present time there are no rapid tests available for Lyme disease for immediate diagnosis to assess for the treatment options. Even if tests are ordered, the results are not generally known for several days, and this requires physicians to choose among treatment options without definitive test results. Although studies have not definitively shown that such a delay results in poorer outcomes, accurate tools that can predict or strongly favor a diagnosis could be of great importance as underdiagnosis of Lyme disease could be associated with disease progression and further complications, whereas overdiagnosis could lead to excessive antibiotic use.

Given the prevalence and potentially serious nature of the clinical manifestations of Lyme disease, there has also been considerable interest in the prevention of disease. Vaccination has been shown to be a highly effective way to control the spread of disease. Several antigenic subunits of *B. burgdorferi* have been evaluated for their vaccine potential. To date, most clinical effort has focused on the OspA lipoprotein, which is abundantly expressed by the spirochete. A recombinant OspA vaccine was developed that was found to prevent most definitive cases of Lyme disease.[32] In 1998, LYMErix became available to the public but it was withdrawn from the market in 2002 because of poor sales and concern for an association with autoimmune arthritis.[33] Yet given the potential impact on healthcare there has been a renewed interest in vaccination against Lyme disease. A novel vaccine may have more widespread utility as it targets additional OspA serotypes and epitopes to *Borrelia* spp. in addition to *B. burgdorferi* that are known to cause Lyme disease in other areas of the world. A recent phase I/II study indicated that a multivalent OspA vaccine may be an effective intervention for prevention of Lyme disease.[34] Continued clinical efficacy in larger studies will be needed to assess long-term viability as a clinical solution to this problem.

The cumulative data support several important criteria that should favor a diagnosis of Lyme disease. A diagnosis of Lyme disease should be strongly considered in endemic areas, during peak Lyme disease season, in children, and in those with associated signs and symptoms (particularly headache, as erythema migrans may not be found). Strong consideration for empiric antibiotics in such cases should be made even before serological testing results are available. Furthermore, long-term follow-up is strongly encouraged as patients may show residual facial weakness.

!

Strong consideration for testing for Lyme disease in patients with facial palsy should be given for the following situations:

- Presence of erythema migrans.
- Lives in or recently traveled to an endemic region.
- Onset during months of May to September.
- Presence of fever, headaches, arthralgia, cervical adenopathy, radicular pain, or other neurologic symptoms.
- Bilateral facial paralysis.

11.8 Key Points

- Lyme disease is caused by a group of related spirochetes.
- Erythema migrans is strongly associated with the condition but is not always detected.
- The US Centers for Disease Control and Prevention recommends a two-tiered testing strategy for diagnosis.
- Testing is complicated by seropositive controls in endemic areas, and by its very nature showing exposure rather than a definitive causative factor.
- Headache, fever arthralgias, cervical adenopathy, endemic locations, and summer season should raise suspicion for testing.
- Antibiotics are generally accepted as the preferred treatment of choice.

References

[1] Centers for Disease Control and Prevention. Lyme disease. 2014. Available at: www.cdc.gov/lyme/stats/index.html. Accessed: April 8, 2014

[2] Bacon RM, Kugeler KJ, Mead PS Centers for Disease Control and Prevention (CDC). Surveillance for Lyme disease—United States, 1992–2006. MMWR Surveill Summ 2008; 57: 1–9

[3] EUCALB. European Union concerted action on Lyme borreliosis. 2014. Available at www.eucalb.com. Accessed: April 8, 2014

[4] Margolis N, Hogan D, Tilly K, Rosa PA. Plasmid location of Borrelia purine biosynthesis gene homologs. J Bacteriol 1994; 176: 6427–6432

[5] Meiners T, Hammer B, Göbel UB, Kahl O. Determining the tick scutal index allows assessment of tick feeding duration and estimation of infection risk with Borrelia burgdorferi sensu lato in a person bitten by an Ixodes ricinus nymph. Int J Med Microbiol 2006; 296 Suppl 40: 103–107

[6] Schwan TG, Piesman J. Vector interactions and molecular adaptations of Lyme disease and relapsing fever spirochetes associated with transmission by ticks. Emerg Infect Dis 2002; 8: 115–121

[7] Liang FT, Yan J, Mbow ML et al. Borrelia burgdorferi changes its surface antigenic expression in response to host immune responses. Infect Immun 2004; 72: 5759–5767

[8] England JD, Bohm RP, Jr, Roberts ED, Philipp MT. Lyme neuroborreliosis in the rhesus monkey. Semin Neurol 1997; 17: 53–56

[9] Wright WF, Riedel DJ, Talwani R, Gilliam BL. Diagnosis and management of Lyme disease. Am Fam Physician 2012; 85: 1086–1093

[10] Hilton E, DeVoti J, Benach JL et al. Seroprevalence and seroconversion for tick-borne diseases in a high-risk population in the northeast United States. Am J Med 1999; 106: 404–409

[11] Wormser GP, McKenna D, Carlin J et al. Brief communication: hematogenous dissemination in early Lyme disease. Ann Intern Med 2005; 142: 751–755

[12] Reik L. Lyme Disease and the Nervous System. New York, NY: Thieme Medical; 1991

[13] Eiffert H, Karsten A, Schlott T et al. Acute peripheral facial palsy in Lyme disease—a distal neuritis at the infection site. Neuropediatrics 2004; 35: 267–273

[14] Clark JR, Carlson RD, Sasaki CT, Pachner AR, Steere AC. Facial paralysis in Lyme disease. Laryngoscope 1985; 95: 1341–1345

[15] Bremell D, Hagberg L. Clinical characteristics and cerebrospinal fluid parameters in patients with peripheral facial palsy caused by Lyme neuroborreliosis compared with facial palsy of unknown origin (Bell's palsy). BMC Infect Dis 2011; 11: 215

[16] Peltomaa M, Pyykkö I, Seppälä I, Viljanen M. Lyme borreliosis and facial paralysis—a prospective analysis of risk factors and outcome. Am J Otolaryngol 2002; 23: 125–132

[17] Kowalski TJ, Berth WL, Mathiason MA, Agger WA. Oral antibiotic treatment and long-term outcomes of Lyme facial nerve palsy. Infection 2011; 39: 239–245

[18] Kalish RA, Kaplan RF, Taylor E, Jones-Woodward L, Workman K, Steere AC. Evaluation of study patients with Lyme disease, 10–20-year follow-up. J Infect Dis 2001; 183: 453–460

[19] Ljøstad U, Økstad S, Topstad T, Mygland A, Monstad P. Acute peripheral facial palsy in adults. J Neurol 2005; 252: 672–676

[20] Furuta Y, Kawabata H, Ohtani F, Watanabe H. Western blot analysis for diagnosis of Lyme disease in acute facial palsy. Laryngoscope 2001; 111: 719–723

[21] May M, Fria TJ, Blumenthal F, Curtin H. Facial paralysis in children: differential diagnosis. Otolaryngol Head Neck Surg 1981; 89: 841–848

[22] Nigrovic LE, Thompson AD, Fine AM, Kimia A. Clinical predictors of Lyme disease among children with a peripheral facial palsy at an emergency department in a Lyme disease-endemic area. Pediatrics 2008; 122: e1080–e1085

[23] Fine AM, Brownstein JS, Nigrovic LE et al. Integrating spatial epidemiology into a decision model for evaluation of facial palsy in children. Arch Pediatr Adolesc Med 2011; 165: 61–67

[24] Belman AL, Reynolds L, Preston T, Postels D, Grimson R, Coyle PK. Cerebrospinal fluid findings in children with Lyme disease-associated facial nerve palsy. Arch Pediatr Adolesc Med 1997; 151: 1224–1228

[25] Tveitnes D, Øymar K, Natås O. Acute facial nerve palsy in children: how often is it lyme borreliosis? Scand J Infect Dis 2007; 39: 425–431

[26] Jenke AC, Stoek LM, Zilbauer M, Wirth S, Borusiak P. Facial palsy: etiology, outcome and management in children. Eur J Paediatr Neurol 2011; 15: 209–213

[27] Drack FD, Weissert M. Outcome of peripheral facial palsy in children —a catamnestic study. Eur J Paediatr Neurol 2013; 17: 185–191

[28] Bagger-Sjöbäck D, Remahl S, Ericsson M. Long-term outcome of facial palsy in neuroborreliosis. Otol Neurotol 2005; 26: 790–795

[29] Skogman BH, Glimåker K, Nordwall M, Vrethem M, Ödkvist L, Forsberg P. Long-term clinical outcome after Lyme neuroborreliosis in childhood. Pediatrics 2012; 130: 262–269

[30] Skogman BH, Croner S, Ödkvist L. Acute facial palsy in children—a 2-year follow-up study with focus on Lyme neuroborreliosis. Int J Pediatr Otorhinolaryngol 2003; 67: 597–602

[31] Broekhuijsen-van Henten DM, Braun KP, Wolfs TF. Clinical presentation of childhood neuroborreliosis; neurological examination may be normal. Arch Dis Child 2010; 95: 910–914

[32] Steere AC, Sikand VK, Meurice F et al. Lyme Disease Vaccine Study Group. Vaccination against Lyme disease with recombinant Borrelia burgdorferi outer-surface lipoprotein A with adjuvant. N Engl J Med 1998; 339: 209–215

[33] Barrett PN, Portsmouth D. The need for a new vaccine against Lyme borreliosis. Expert Rev Vaccines 2013; 12: 101–103

[34] Wressnigg N, Pöllabauer EM, Aichinger G et al. Safety and immunogenicity of a novel multivalent OspA vaccine against Lyme borreliosis in healthy adults: a double-blind, randomised, dose-escalation phase 1/2 trial. Lancet Infect Dis 2013; 13: 680–689

12 Pediatric Facial Nerve Palsies

Kristen M. Davidge, J. Michael Hendry, Ronald Zuker, and Gregory H. Borschel

12.1 Introduction

This chapter focuses on congenital facial paralysis. Here, the authors review the definition and etiologies of congenital facial paralysis, both syndromic and nonsyndromic. Notable syndromes, such as Möbius syndrome, are highlighted. The assessment of a child presenting with facial paralysis is discussed, including important features on history and physical examination and relevant investigations. The chapter concludes with a discussion of treatment options, with a particular focus on operative management as this is the mainstay in congenital facial paralysis.

Facial nerve paralysis (FNP) in children represents a unique spectrum of pathology that requires special consideration. In addition to controlling critical functions such as blinking and oral competence, the facial nerve plays an integral role in nonverbal communication and emotional expression. When facial nerve palsy occurs in children, physical, social, and psychological development may be affected over the long term. Secure attachment between children and caregivers can be negatively impacted during infancy, and social stigmatization can occur later in life.[1] This is particularly true of congenital facial nerve paralysis, where early recognition, correct diagnosis, and appropriate intervention are important to prevent these negative outcomes.[2,3] The challenge of the pediatric facial reconstructive surgeon is therefore to restore spontaneous and symmetric expression that fosters interpersonal relationships and normal psychosocial development.

In this chapter, the authors focus on the management of congenital facial nerve paralysis. Acquired etiologies of facial nerve paralysis in children will be discussed briefly, but evaluation and treatment of these conditions are similar to those for adults and they are covered in detail elsewhere in this book.

12.2 Definition

It is important to address the controversy in the literature that centers on the distinction between developmental and congenital FNP. Some authors reserve the term congenital FNP to describe only those resulting from birth trauma, at or near the time of delivery.[3] The distinction is important because of its prognostic significance, but is misleading because it implies that there is something that distinguishes perinatal birth trauma from other traumatic facial nerve injuries. Conversely, to restrict the definition to include only developmental abnormalities underemphasizes the important role that heritability has in pathogenesis.

Here, congenital FNP is defined as unilateral or bilateral FNP present at birth due to hereditary or in utero developmental factors.

> **!**
>
> Here, congenital facial nerve palsy is defined as unilateral or bilateral facial nerve paralysis present at birth due to hereditary or in utero developmental factors.

12.3 Epidemiology

The estimated incidence of pediatric FNP varies broadly from 1.5 to 64 cases per 1,000 live births depending on the definitions used.[3,4] Acquired etiologies are most prevalent, and are classified and managed as in adults. Common acquired etiologies in children include Bell's palsy, as described in Chapter 8, Lyme disease, as described in Chapter 11, other infections such as acute otitis media, intracranial tumors such as ependymoma or medulloblastoma, and blunt trauma.[5]

Perinatal injury to the facial nerve also occurs at an incidence of 1.8 in 1,000 live births, owing to the superficial position of the stylomastoid foramen and the soft, compressible mastoid bone overlying the vulnerable neonatal facial nerve.[3–6] Fortunately, FNP resulting from birth trauma has a favorable prognosis with full recovery expected in 89 to 100% of individuals.[2,4,5] This is in part due to the fact that the temporal bone is relatively soft in the newborn and so fracture and transection of the nerve is very rare. Management often begins with simple observation for a minimum of 1 year, after which rehabilitation algorithms are no different from those for adult injury; see Chapter 9.[4]

> **!**
>
> The risk of perinatal trauma of the facial nerve is mainly related to the superficial position of the stylomastoid foramen and the soft, compressible mastoid bone overlying the vulnerable neonatal facial nerve.

Congenital facial palsies comprise 8 to 11% of all cases of pediatric FNP, with an estimated population incidence of 1 in 8,860.[4,5,7–9] They are of particular interest because they carry a very poor prognosis in the absence of surgical intervention and can have a lasting impact on the child's development.[10] Children with congenital FNP will often experience language, social, and functional impairment to varying degrees depending on the underlying pathology. Issues such as nasal dysarthria and delayed language development can occur in as many as 50% of those with bilateral facial nerve paralysis.[11] Hearing loss is not uncommon and may hinder normal intellectual and language development.[11]

> !
>
> Congenital facial palsies have a bad prognosis without surgical intervention, whereas perinatal injuries to the facial nerve have a favorable prognosis.

12.4 Etiology

Congenital FNPs are thought to arise from the maldevelopment of any component of the central or peripheral structures that relate to the facial nerve and its function. Specifically, they can result from facial nuclear agenesis, facial nuclear hypoplasia or dysplasia, impaired facial nerve development, or primary.[3,12,13] Among those with congenital FNP, facial nuclear abnormalities are present in approximately 50% of patients, and 10% demonstrate complete nuclear agenesis.[6] Pathology of the facial nerve and canal can be seen in as many as 30% of patients undergoing computed tomography (CT), including early termination of the facial nerve at the internal auditory meatus, horizontal or pyramidal.[14,15]

Clinically, congenital FNP can be classified as syndromic or nonsyndromic. The most common syndromes associated with congenital FNP include Möbius syndrome, hemifacial microsomia, and Goldenhar's syndrome, although several other associations exist (i.e., CHARGE syndrome). Nonsyndromic congenital FNP includes neonatal asymmetric crying facies and isolated (hereditary) facial nerve palsy.

12.4.1 Möbius Syndrome

The earliest descriptions of Möbius syndrome date back to the work of von Graefe in the 1880s, and were subsequently elaborated by Paul Julius Möbius in 1888. Namely, he described a syndrome characterized by bilateral facial nerve palsy and concurrent impaired ocular abduction.[11,16–20] Other terms applied to this condition include Möbius sequence, facial diplegia, and oromandibular limb hypogenesis.[19]

Epidemiology and Etiology

Möbius syndrome is rare, with an estimated annual incidence of 4 per 189,000 live births.[11,16,20] Framing the disease as a developmental sequence more accurately describes the early embryonic insults that lead to the characteristic features of Möbius syndrome.[19] However, much controversy surrounds the exact developmental defect that gives rise to the Möbius phenotype. Undoubtedly, the etiology is multifactorial and involves some combination of embryonic brainstem ischemia, fetal teratogen exposure, and hereditary disease transmission.[13,21,22] These developmental insults manifest as brainstem nuclear hypoplasia, secondary nuclear degeneration, or brainstem atrophy.[22,23]

The vascular hypotheses emphasize the likely occurrence of ischemic injury to the fetal brainstem resulting from subclavian artery maldevelopment.[11,22,23] The most compelling evidence for this theory are the focal brainstem calcifications observed on CT in the region of cranial nerve motor nuclei in up to 71% of patients with Möbius syndrome.[17] Such calcifications are highly suggestive of prior ischemic injury and necrosis.[17,22–25] The degree of brainstem necrosis can range in severity and location from the mid-pons to the rostral medulla, where the most extreme cases are not compatible with life.[18] Opponents of the vascular etiology argue that global ischemic injury to the brainstem and sporadic location of calcifications cannot explain the focal pathogenesis of Möbius syndrome and the associated limb.[11,13]

Möbius syndrome has also been associated with varied teratogenic exposures, including gestational hyperthermia, electric shock, chorionic villus sampling, illicit drugs, thalidomide, and ergotamine.[16] A strong correlation has also been observed between Möbius syndrome and the abortifacient medication misoprostol, with an odds ratio of 30.[26]

Finally, a genetic component to Möbius syndrome is suggested by several multigeneration familial cases of the disease that occur in an autosomal-dominant, autosomal-recessive, and X-linked inheritance pattern.[19,21] Genetic loci linked with the Möbius phenotype include 3q21–22, 10q21–22, and 13q12. These loci are believed to encompass a series of homeobox genes (genes regulating early morphogenesis) that may control the patterning of the facial nucleus, among other structures.[16,21,27]

Clinical Features

The hallmark features of Möbius syndrome are paralysis of the facial and abducens nerves, resulting in loss of facial expression and impaired lateral gaze respectively (▶ Fig. 12.1).[13,28] Large case series estimate that facial nerve paralysis is bilateral in 92% and unilateral in 8%.[11] Facial nerve paralysis is complete in approximately one-third of patients, but most patients demonstrate relative sparing of the lower face.[11] Other cranial nerves can be involved, most commonly the hypoglossal and oculomotor nerves, and in severe cases global brainstem atrophy and corticospinal tract maldevelopment may be present.

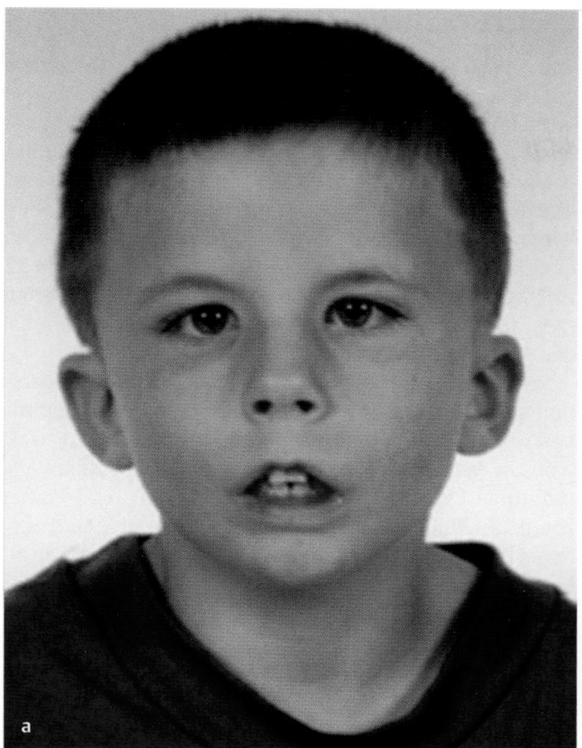
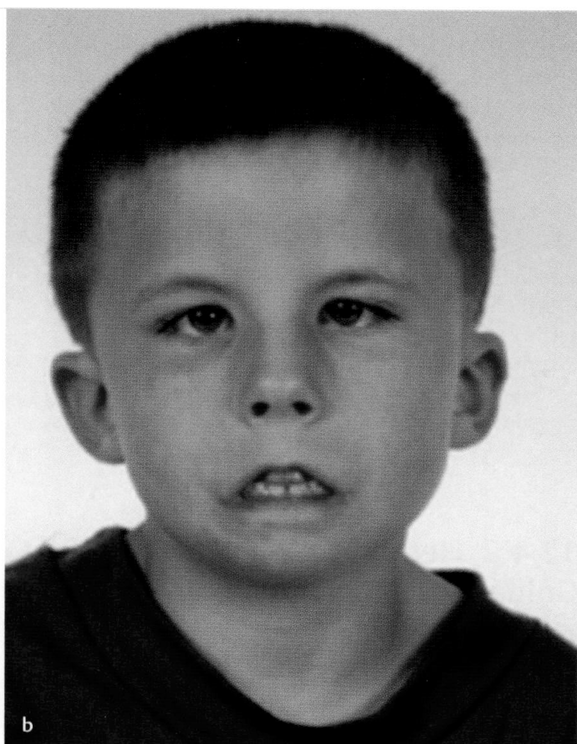

Fig. 12.1 A patient with Möbius syndrome with bilateral facial nerve paralysis: **(a)** at rest, and **(b)** during smiling.

> **!**
>
> If a congenital facial nerve palsy is combined with a palsy of the abducens nerve, rule out Möbius syndrome.

Typical facial dysmorphology associated with Möbius syndrome includes: prominent epicanthal folds (89%), flattened nasal bridge (81%), micrognathia (64%), high-arched palate (61%), cleft lip or palate, external ear defects, bifid uvula, microglossia, and microstomia. Limb malformations are also common and include the Poland deformity (40–86%), talipes equinovarus (club foot) (28%), syndactyly, brachydactyly, ectrodactyly, and other phalangeal deformations.[11–13,17,18,21,22,28] Specific ocular features in addition to the abducens nerve palsy include Duane's retraction syndrome and congenital fibrosis of the extraocular muscles.[11]

The combined malformations experienced by patients with Möbius syndrome can lead to substantial morbidity. Palatal and pharyngeal dysfunction can often contribute to feeding difficulties early in life.[11,12] Later on, this may translate into speech difficulties arising from flaccid dysarthria or velopharyngeal insufficiency.[16] Functional problems such as disabled suckling and swallowing, palatal weakness, and regurgitation can also occur, and may necessitate placement of a gastrostomy tube to maintain proper nutrition.[11] Cerebellar and corticospinal tract involvement can lead to poor motor development, poor skill acquisition, and coordination problems.[11,12,16] It is estimated that 82 to 100% of patients with Möbius syndrome demonstrate impairment in either fine or gross motor coordination.[11]

Intellectual disability as a primary symptom of Möbius syndrome is a subject of controversy. Historically, rates of primary intellectual disability within this population ranged from 0 to 75%,[11,18,21] yet given the heterogeneity in methodologies, study population, and intellectual evaluation these estimates should be regarded critically. The only prospective evaluation examining intellectual capacity in patients with Möbius syndrome revealed average verbal subtest scores, but lower than average IQ scores that were underestimated due to poor physical performance scores.[29] The incidence of true mental retardation (IQ < 70) from the study was 9%. Several studies report that these patients will go on to scholastic achievements and gainful employment, despite ocular and/or physical disability.[16] Emotional communication is also hindered by the lack of expressive facial gestures.[16] As a result, these patients are at higher risk of experiencing rejection, low self-esteem, and behavioral problems.[16]

Lastly, strong associations between Möbius syndrome and autism have been suggested, with a prevalence of approximately 30 to 40%.[19,30] The correlation is even stronger in cases of Möbius syndrome with true concurrent intellectual disability.[30] Caution is required when interpreting these conclusions however, because the evaluation of autism in patients with Möbius syndrome is confounded by the lack of facial expression, impaired eye contact, and developmental delay.[16]

Möbius syndrome, especially when occurring bilaterally, demonstrates impressively how important facial expression is for emotional expression and nonverbal communication. Therefore, diagnostics and therapy of communicative and emotional disabilities are highly recommended; see Chapter 14 for further information.

12.4.2 Hemifacial Microsomia and Goldenhar's Syndrome

Gorlin provided the initial description of hemifacial microsomia as a heterogeneous disorder involving unilateral or bilateral bony and soft tissue facial hypoplasia, auricular defects, and skin tags/pits.[31] Essentially, hemifacial microsomia and Goldenhar's syndrome lie on a spectrum of first and second branchial arch malformations, and both may have facial nerve involvement.[3,32] Hemifacial microsomia is typically unilateral (bilateral in up to 30%), whereas Goldenhar's syndrome is bilateral and is additionally characterized by epibulbar dermoids, as well as vertebral, cardiac, and renal anomalies. Owing to these features, Goldenhar's syndrome has also been termed oculo-auriculo-vertebral dysplasia.[3,31]

!

Hemifacial microsomia is typically unilateral, whereas Goldenhar's syndrome is bilateral.

Epidemiology and Etiology

Hemifacial microsomia is one of the most common craniofacial dysostoses, with an estimated population incidence of 1 in 5,600 live births and a male-to-female ratio of 1:1.[33] Goldenhar's syndrome has an overall reported incidence in the literature of 1 in 3,500 to 25,000 live births and a male-to-female ratio of 3:2, but strong epidemiologic data are lacking.[32,34]

Dysplasia of the first and second branchial arches is thought to occur sporadically, although hereditary cases have been reported.[32] Several etiologic factors, such as vascular disruption, maternal diabetes, teratogens, and free radical generation, have been proposed and supported in the literature.[3]

Clinical Features

The clinical features of hemifacial microsomia are varied, but include preauricular skin tags and fistulae, conductive hearing loss, microtia/anotia, mandibulomaxillary hypoplasia, ocular hypoplasia, micropthalmia/anopthalmia, ocular dysmotility, cleft palate or high-arched palate, macrostomia, hypoplasia of masticatory muscles, and hypoplastic facial muscles.[3,31,33] The reported incidence of unilateral facial palsy in this population ranges from 22 to 50%,[31,33,35] with bilateral facial nerve paralysis being rare. Involvement of other cranial nerves and global developmental delay has also been reported.

Systemic features include cardiac anomalies (i.e., coarctation of the aorta), renal anomalies (i.e., agenesis, hydronephrosis), and vertebral anomalies (i.e., fused ribs, scoliosis, vertebral dysplasia).[34] Patients with Goldenhar's syndrome specifically present with bilateral facial anomalies, bulbar epidermoids or lipodermoids, and vertebral anomalies, in addition to the other features of hemifacial microsomia.

12.4.3 Neonatal Asymmetric Crying Faces

Congenital paralysis of the lower lip depressor muscles was first described by Parmelee in 1932, but Pape and Pickering coined the term *neonatal asymmetric crying facies* (NACF) in 1972.[36] Indeed, paralysis of the marginal mandibular branch of the facial nerve supplying the mentalis, depressor labii inferioris, and depressor anguli oris leads to inability to depress the lower lip, and marked asymmetry when crying.[36] Several other descriptors have also been applied to this condition, including congenital unilateral lower lip palsy, and congenital hypoplasia of the depressor anguli oris muscle.[3,37,38]

Epidemiology and Etiology

Estimations of population incidence range from 0.31 to 0.8% in case series from Israel and Greece.[37–39] The paralysis can be neural (20%) or muscular (80%) in origin.[3,40]

Clinical Features

The classic presentation of NACF is a child who has a symmetrical facial appearance at rest but demonstrates asymmetric depression of the lower lip during animation of the face (▶ Fig. 12.2).[3] The underlying paralysis of the marginal mandibular branch of the facial nerve supplying the mentalis, depressor labii inferioris, and depressor anguli oris can be confirmed by electromyography (EMG); details are given in Chapter 6. Imaging studies, easy and fast by sonography, can also confirm the lack of the typical and circumscribed lack of facial muscle function; see Chapter 5.The remainder of facial nerve function, including forehead wrinkling, nasolabial fold depth,

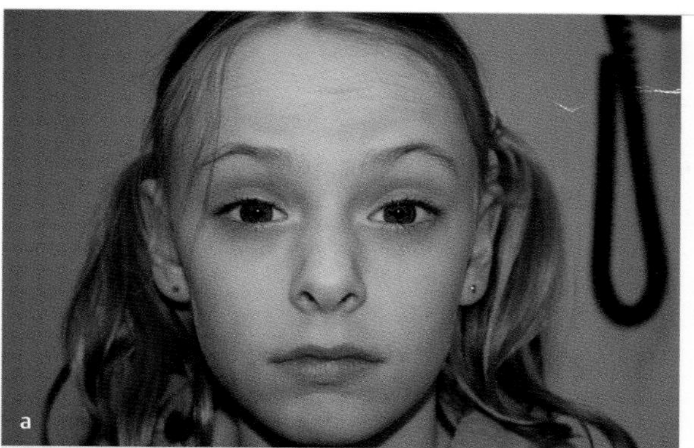

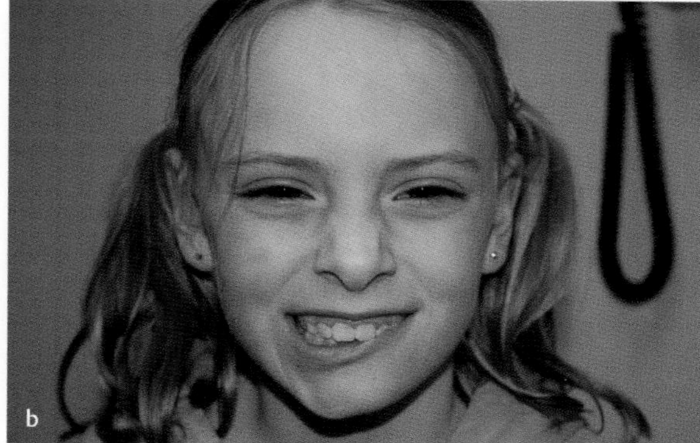

Fig. 12.2 A patient with neonatal asymmetric crying facies, with left-sided paralysis of the marginal mandibular branch of the facial nerve: (a) at rest, and (b) during smiling.

and eyelid closure, all remain intact.[38,41] As such, the implications of NACF are predominantly aesthetic in nature with limited to no impact on speech development or feeding in infancy.

Associated congenital anomalies have been variably reported in NACF, with recent estimates suggesting coexisting anomalies in 9.4% of cases.[38,41] Reported associations include cardiac anomalies, neuroblastoma, mediastinal teratoma, trisomy 18, and neurofibromatosis type 1. Lower lip paralysis has also been reported in approximately 14% of patients with 22q11 deletion syndrome,[41] and the coincidence of cardiac malformations and congenital lower lip palsy has been termed Caylor cardiofacial syndrome.[3,37,41] However, the true incidence of major malformations in patients with NACF and the role of routine screening remains controversial.[36,39]

12.4.4 Hereditary Congenital Facial Nerve Paralysis

Isolated congenital paralysis of the facial nerve has been termed hereditary congenital facial nerve paralysis (HFCP), and has been recently distinguished from Möbius syndrome by the absence of other cranial nerve involvement, and orofacial or limb malformations.[12] Facial paralysis is typically bilateral but asymmetric in severity and distribution.[12]

Case studies have demonstrated familial, autosomal dominant inheritance patterns with magnetic resonance image (MRI) evidence of hypoplasia of cranial nerve VII or partial agenesis of the facial nucleus as a potential cause.[12] Linkage analyses from several large families have established a causative locus for HCFP on the long arm of 3q21-q22.[27] Pathologic evaluation has revealed a marked, but isolated, decrease in the number of neurons in the facial motor nucleus with a corresponding underdeveloped facial nerve.[12,25] In HFCP, pathology is restricted to the facial nuclei, as opposed to Möbius syndrome where the lesion results from maldevelopment of the entire lower brainstem, posterior fossa, or corticospinal.[13] Indeed, Jemec et al found that 27% of patients in their case series had central, facial nuclear pathology on MRI when isolated unilateral facial palsy was their only symptom.[6]

12.5 Diagnostic Work-Up

12.5.1 History

When a child presents with facial paralysis, the most important aspect of the history is to determine the onset and progression of paralysis so as to differentiate congenital from acquired causes for prognostic and treatment purposes.[15,42] Indeed, congenital (i.e., "developmental") facial paralysis is present at birth, does not improve over time, and there is no potential to reinnervate the native facial musculature as it is absent or severely atrophic. The nature and distribution of facial asymmetries should be established from the parents and/or child, with particular attention to functional problems such as eyelid closure, gaze abnormalities, feeding, weight gain, and drooling. Any prior or ongoing treatments for facial paralysis should be noted. A birth and developmental history, along with a review of systems, will help identify associated anomalies that may require further investigation. A family history of congenital facial paralysis may point to hereditary or syndromic causes.

12.5.2 Physical Examination

The approach to the physical examination for facial nerve paralysis in children is similar to that in adults, but in the neonate and young child this examination will be limited to careful observation. Serial examinations may be helpful in these situations, and may show changes in facial nerve function over time if a noncongenital etiology is suspected.

A detailed assessment of facial nerve function should be performed, including the presence or absence of adequate corneal protection and oral competence, and the distribution and severity of paralysis. Facial nerve grading scales are less useful in congenital facial nerve palsy, but have applicability in pediatric patients with acquired paralysis.[42] Cranial nerve examination, inspection for dysmorphic features, and upper limb examination are important to identify coexisting anomalies and syndromic associations. Evaluation of potential donor nerves (i.e., nerve to the masseter muscle), donor muscles (i.e., gracilis), and recipient vessels (i.e., facial artery) is important for surgical planning when considering facial reanimation. Importantly, facial vascular anatomy may be aberrant in Möbius syndrome and hemifacial.[3,28] Children may “underperform” in the office, and photos and videos of facial expression acquired by the parents are often helpful.

!

During basic examination, do not forget to evaluate the potential donor nerves (i.e., nerve to the masseter muscle), donor muscles (i.e., gracilis), and recipient vessels (i.e., facial artery) as this is important for surgical planning when considering facial reanimation.

12.5.3 Investigations

The role of diagnostic testing in congenital facial nerve paralysis is limited. Electrodiagnostic testing can be a challenge in the pediatric population, but may be useful in differentiating birth trauma from congenital causes in the newborn. Indeed, since facial muscles are absent in congenital cases, insertional activity on EMG will be absent; see Chapter 6.[43] Imaging studies, such as CT or MRI, may be useful for diagnosis in pediatric patients when a noncongenital cause is suspected, or to confirm absence of the facial nerve or musculature in congenital cases.[25] Preoperative imaging prior to facial reanimation may also be warranted in complex congenital cases, such as hemifacial microsomia, to better delineate soft tissue and vascular anatomy.

12.6 Treatment

Management of congenital facial nerve palsy differs from that for acquired facial paralysis. In congenital cases, facial nerve function has no capacity to recover spontaneously and thus the mainstay of treatment is operative. Primary facial nerve reconstruction (i.e., nerve transfers, nerve grafting, direct muscle neurotization) is not possible since the muscles of facial expression are absent or severely atrophic, and thus delayed reconstruction is the sole option for reanimation. Furthermore, surgical procedures for upper face animation such as eye closure and brow elevation are rarely required in congenital facial paralysis owing to adaptation of the ocular and periocular structures from birth.[42] Indeed, lubrication of the cornea with an ointment or drops, if required, is usually sufficient. The primary focus of surgical reconstruction in congenital cases is therefore to restore a spontaneous and dynamic smile.

!

In congenital cases, facial nerve function has no capacity to recover spontaneously and thus the mainstay of treatment is operative.Primary facial nerve reconstruction is not possible since the muscles of facial expression are absent or severely atrophic. The best option for restoration is free functional muscle transfer.

12.6.1 Addressing the Lower Face

Dynamic reconstruction is the gold standard for restoration of smile in congenital complete facial nerve paralysis. Although static procedures of the lower face can provide symmetry at rest, they do not animate the face and are of little value in this population where the overarching goal is to restore spontaneous facial expression. Both regional muscle transfers, as described in Chapter 21, and free muscle transfer as described in Chapter 22, have been described for facial reanimation, but the former are not preferred for smile restoration owing to their suboptimal line of pull, inadequate excursion, and resultant contour deformity.[44]

The best option for restoration of smile in congenital facial paralysis is free functional muscle transfer. Multiple muscle donors have been utilized, including the gracilis, latissimus dorsi, pectoralis minor, rectus abdominis, and extensor carpi radialis brevis.[44] The authors' preference is the gracilis muscle because of its expendability, minimal donor morbidity with a well-hidden scar, ease of harvest, consistent neurovascular anatomy allowing reliable debulking of the flap, and ability to be harvested simultaneous with facial exposure. Potential donor nerves for innervation of the free muscle transfer include a cross-face nerve graft (CFNG) and the masseteric nerve, a branch of the mandibular nerve (V3) (► Fig. 12.3). There is ongoing debate as to which of these donor nerves produces superior outcomes for smile reanimation, and they each have their advantages and disadvantages (► Table 12.1).[45,46] In unilateral facial paralysis, the authors' preference is to use a two-stage CFNG to optimize spontaneity of expression and simplify postoperative motor reeducation for the child. In bilateral cases, such as Möbius syndrome, CFNG is not an option and the nerve to the masseter muscle becomes the donor of choice.

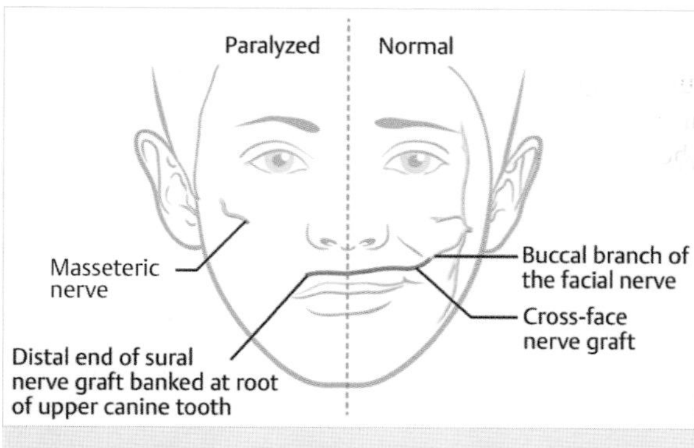

Fig. 12.3 Donor nerve options for powering a free gracilis muscle transfer include a cross-face nerve graft and the masseteric nerve.

> **!**
>
> For unilateral cases, potential donor nerves for innervation of the free muscle transfer include a cross-face nerve graft and the masseteric nerve. In bilateral cases the masseteric nerve is the donor of choice.

Table 12.1 Advantages and disadvantages of innervation sources for vascularized muscle transfers

Innervation source	Advantages	Disadvantages
Cross-face nerve graft	Spontaneous smile	• Two operative procedures • Nerve graft required • Less power • Less predictable outcome • Synkinesis • Potential to downgrade normal facial nerve
Masseteric nerve	• One-stage procedure • Direct nerve coaptation • Powerful	• Spontaneity more difficult to achieve but possible • Involuntary smile with chewing • Theoretical potential to weaken bite (but rarely seen)

The authors' preferred timing for facial reanimation in congenital cases is around 5 to 6 years of age, in order to restore facial expression for the school years. At younger ages, the child will have difficulty participating in postoperative rehabilitation and the technical complexity of free tissue transfer increases. When a CFNG is planned, this may be performed at 4 years of age so that the reconstruction can be completed at 5 years. In bilateral facial nerve palsy, there is a wait at least 3 to 4 months between reanimation procedures. However, particularly in congenital cases, the timing of facial reanimation may be influenced by the presence of other congenital anomalies. For example, in hemifacial microsomia, facial skeletal reconstruction may take priority and will influence the positioning and tension of a free muscle transfer for facial reanimation.

> **!**
>
> The interval in a two-stage cross-face nerve graft (CFNG) between the CFNG and the free muscle transfer is at least 3 to 4 months.

Partial congenital facial paralysis with present but inadequate excursion of the oral commissure on one side can be a challenge to manage. Options include biofeedback exercises to strengthen to affected side, as described in Chapter 26, botulinum toxin injection, as described in Chapter 25, to reduce the strength of the unaffected side (or lesser affected side in bilateral cases), and dynamic free vascularized muscle transfer to augment the existing function on the affected side. In the latter situation, problems with excessive bulk in the cheek and excessive tone at rest postoperatively can occur.

> **!**
>
> The preferred timing for facial reanimation in congenital cases is around 5 to 6 years of age, to restore facial expression for the school years. At younger ages, the child will have difficulty participating in postoperative rehabilitation and the technical complexity of free tissue transfer increases.

Authors' Preferred Technique for Cross-Face Nerve Graft

The authors' preferred technique for CFNG is shown in ▸ Fig. 12.4, and described as follows:

1. A preauricular incision is made on the side of the normally functioning facial nerve.
2. A cheek flap is raised in the subcutaneous plane and is carried anterior to the parotid gland.
3. As branches of the facial nerve are identified, they are stimulated with a nerve stimulator to determine their primary function. The facial nerve branches of interest are those that predominantly supply the upper lip and commissure elevators. Nerve branches that depress or retract the commissure should be avoided, but it is almost impossible to avoid some eye motion with upper

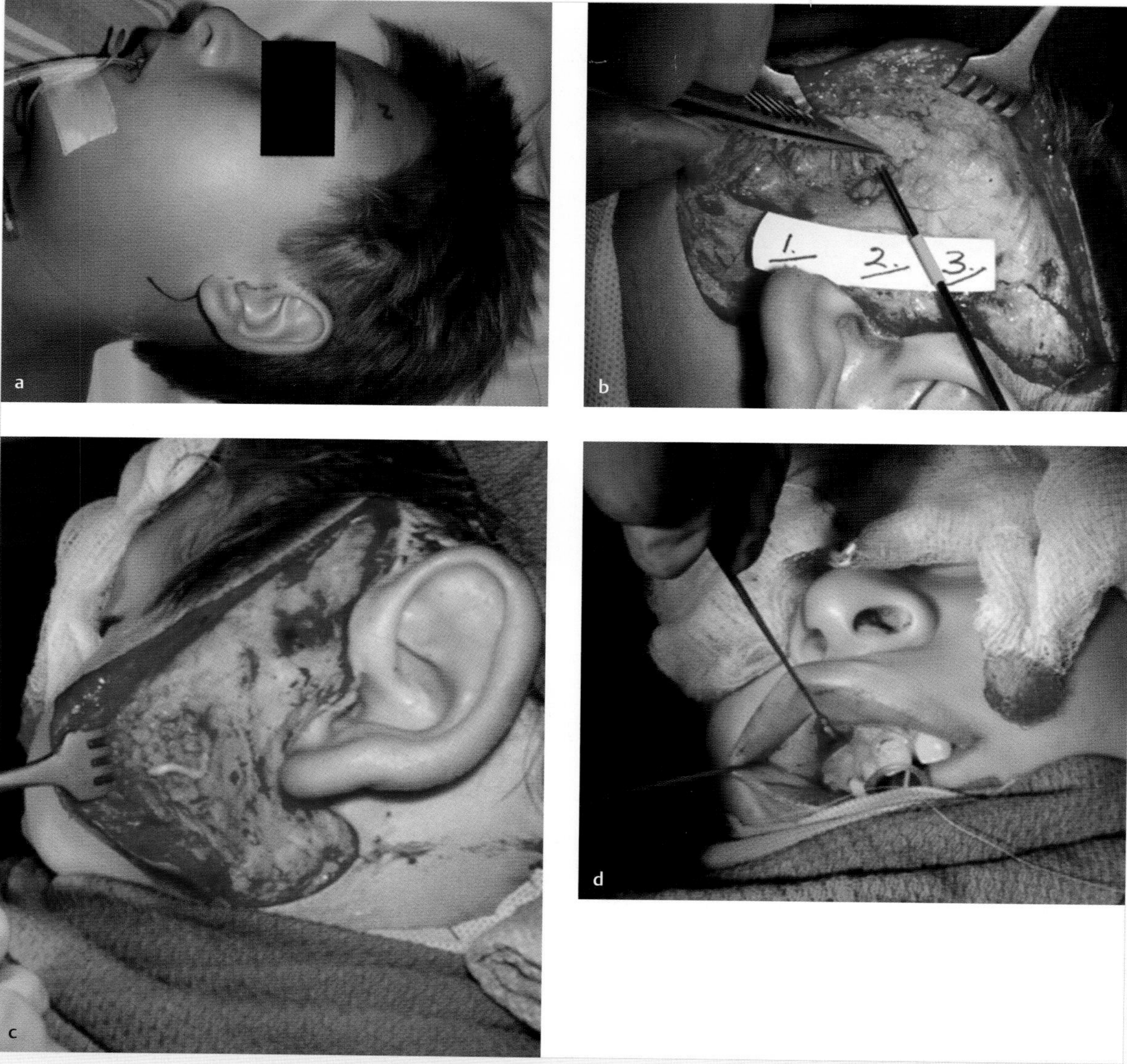

Fig. 12.4 Surgical approach to cross-face nerve graft. **(a)** Design of the preauricular incision for access to the unaffected facial nerve for cross-face nerve grafting (note the 'N' drawn preoperatively on the left forehead to indicate the normal, nonparalyzed side). **(b)** Identification of three branches of the facial nerve, which are being stimulated to determine which facial muscles they innervate. **(c)** Coaptation of the sural nerve graft to the donor facial nerve branches. **(d)** Banking of the distal end of the cross-face nerve graft in the upper buccal sulcus at the level of the canine tooth.

lip elevation. Indeed, specificity of motion only occurs more distally, when the nerve branches have become very small. It is better to select a larger nerve branch within or just anterior to the parotid so that a greater number of axons will be delivered to the recipient muscle, and adequate commissure excursion can be achieved.

4. Once a nerve branch of interest has been identified, it is critical to ensure that one or more of the remaining branches also stimulates the upper lip and commissure elevators so as not to downgrade function on the normal side.
5. A sural nerve graft is harvested through three transverse incisions in the posterior leg. The graft is reversed, and the distal end is coapted to the donor facial nerve branch. A subcutaneous tunnel is then made across the upper lip to the contralateral upper gingival buccal sulcus, where a small intraoral incision is made.
6. The proximal end of the sural nerve graft is delivered into this incision and marked with a 5–0

polypropylene stitch and a hemoclip to facilitate identification at the time of free muscle transfer.
7. The intraoral and skin incisions are then reapproximated.

Authors' Preferred Technique for Free Functional Gracilis Transfer

The authors' preferred technique for free functional gracilis transfer is described as follows:

1. Preoperatively, the nasolabial creases are marked and in unilateral cases the vector and excursion of smile on the unaffected side are measured and marked.[47] The facial dissection and gracilis muscle harvest proceed simultaneously using a two-team approach.
2. Gracilis muscle harvest: the leg is positioned with the hip abducted and externally rotated, and the knee flexed. A line from the pubic symphysis to the medial femoral condyle is marked with a dotted line, and a longitudinal incision is placed 1 to 2 cm posterior to this line. The incision is approximately 10 cm in length, and overlies the proximal gracilis muscle. In children, the gracilis muscle can also usually be palpated, which facilitates placement of the incision.
3. Dissection is carried down to muscle fascia. Occasionally, the surgeon will see a musculocutaneous perforator exiting the gracilis muscle, which aids in the identification of the vascular pedicle. The plane between the adductor longus and gracilis muscles is opened from distal to proximal, and the ascending branches of the medial femoral circumflex vessels are identified entering the deep surface of gracilis.
4. The vascular pedicle courses at right angles to the gracilis muscle, whereas the anterior branch of the obturator nerve courses at 45 degrees to muscle superior to the vessels (▸ Fig. 12.5). The vascular pedicle is dissected to its origin from the profunda femoris, and the nerve is similarly traced proximally. Once the neurovascular pedicle is identified, the muscle is carefully dissected circumferentially.
5. Only one-third to one-half of the circumference of the gracilis muscle is required, which varies based on patient age and muscle size. A critical step in harvesting the gracilis for facial reanimation is trimming of the muscle to avoid excessive bulk (▸ Fig. 12.6). Generally, the pedicle enters the gracilis muscle anteriorly on its deep surface, but occasionally it will enter more centrally. In either case, the posterior aspect of the muscle can often be safely trimmed.
6. The functioning length of required muscle is determined by measuring the distance from the oral commissure to the helical root when the commissure is positioned at the same level as the contralateral unaffected side. We then add 2 cm to this functioning length to accommodate for suturing at either end of the muscle. The required length of the gracilis muscle is usually centered on its vascular pedicle, but can be altered to facilitate the vascular anastomosis or minimize time to reinnervation.
7. While the muscle is still in situ, mattress sutures are placed along the entire edge of the gracilis that will be inserted into the oral commissure and upper lip; these will prevent the anchoring sutures to the oral commissure from sliding through the gracilis muscle over time. Other centers place alternate forms of bolster into the muscle for the same purpose, such as running sutures or gastrointestinal staples. The critical component is the security of the fixation of the anchoring sutures, because should the muscle migrate laterally the problem becomes very difficult to correct secondarily.

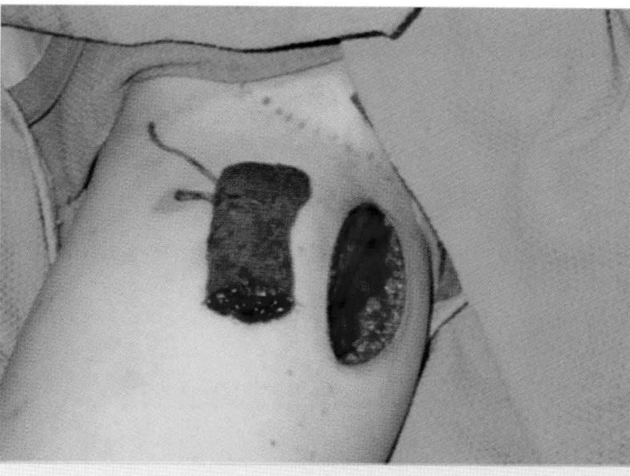

Fig. 12.5 Harvested free gracilis muscle from the right medial thigh. Note how the nerve runs in a superolateral direction approximately 1 cm above the vascular pedicle.

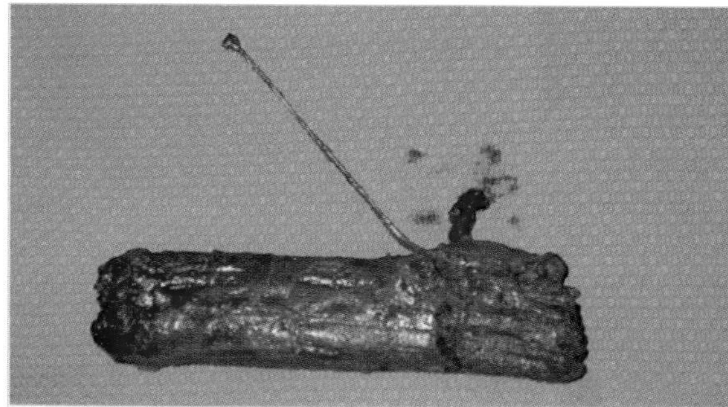

Fig. 12.6 Trimming of the gracilis muscle is a critical step to avoiding excess bulk in the cheek.

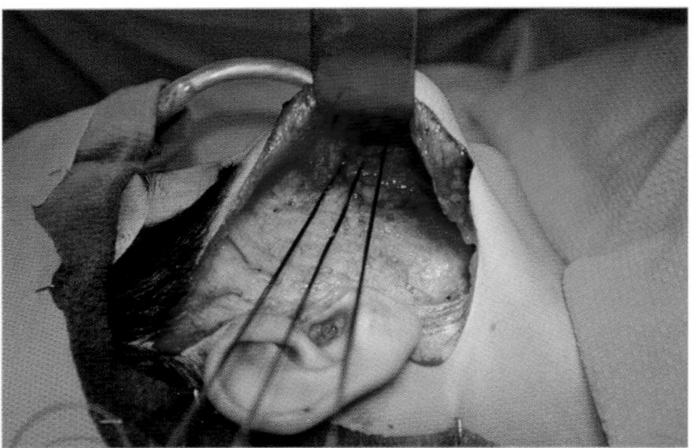

Fig. 12.7 Placement of the anchoring sutures at the oral commissure for securing the gracilis muscle.

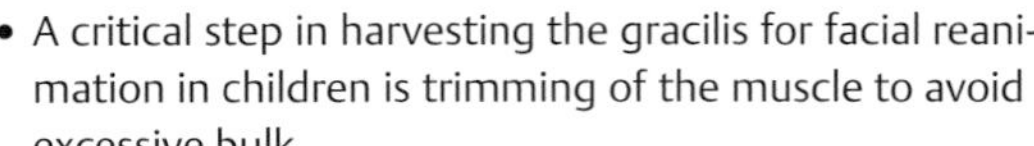

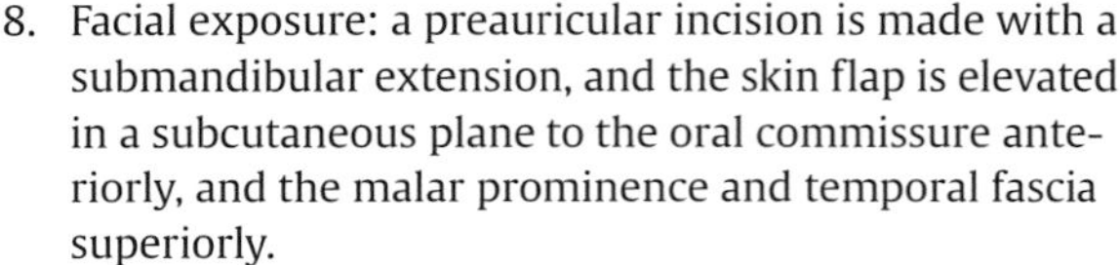

- A critical step in harvesting the gracilis for facial reanimation in children is trimming of the muscle to avoid excessive bulk.
- It is critical to attach the gracilis in a way that assures secure fixation. Different centers employ different techniques.

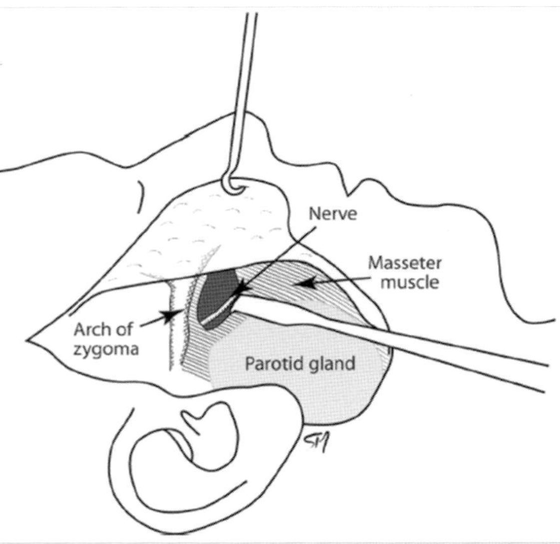

Fig. 12.8 Surgical approach to the masseteric nerve. A transverse incision is made inferior and parallel to the zygomatic arch. The nerve lies on the deep surface of the masseter muscle, coursing anteriorly and inferiorly. Use of the nerve stimulator helps to identify the nerve. (Reproduced with permission from Fattah A, Borschel GH, Manktelow RT, Bezuhly M, Zuker RM. Facial palsy and reconstruction. Plast Reconstr Surg 2012;129(2):340e–352e.)

8. Facial exposure: a preauricular incision is made with a submandibular extension, and the skin flap is elevated in a subcutaneous plane to the oral commissure anteriorly, and the malar prominence and temporal fascia superiorly.
9. In congenital cases, finding the right dissection plane can be difficult owing to the absence of facial musculature; in these situations, the facial artery can serve as a useful guide. Maneuvers to assist with reducing bulk in the cheek include carefully trimming excess subcutaneous fat from the cheek flap and resection of the buccal fat pad.
10. The anchoring sutures for the gracilis are then placed. Often, one anchoring suture is placed at the oral commissure, and two in the upper lip using a no. 1 or no. 2 absorbable suture (▶ Fig. 12.7). Additionally, a suture can be placed in the lateral lower lip when there is a droop of the oral commissure at rest. Accurate placement of these anchoring sutures is a critical step. When traction is applied to the sutures, the resulting nasolabial crease should be well defined and located at the same distance from the oral commissure as the contralateral side. Unnatural lip eversion or lip inversion will result if the anchoring sutures are placed too superficial or too deep, respectively.
11. The facial vessels are then identified and prepared for anastomosis. The facial vein is located just anterior to masseter muscle, whereas the facial artery lies anterior to facial vein and courses toward the oral commissure. The facial vein is transected superiorly and the facial artery is transected distally (anteriorly); this allows the vessels to be reflected posteriorly to facilitate the microvascular anastomoses. The facial vasculature can be anomalous in congenital cases, and alternative vessels such as the transverse facial vein and superficial temporal vessels can be utilized if necessary.
12. When a CFNG has been performed, the banked sural nerve is exposed through the pre-existing upper buccal sulcus incision and the nerve coaptation will be performed intraorally.
13. When the masseteric nerve is utilized, an incision is made parallel and approximately one fingerbreadth inferior to the zygomatic arch (▶ Fig. 12.8 and ▶ Fig. 12.9). Dissection is carried down to the deep surface of the masseter. The motor nerve lies on the deep surface of the muscle, courses anterior and inferior, and is located about 3 cm anterior to the helical root.[48] A nerve stimulator can help identify the nerve. Once the nerve is identified, it is traced through muscle, divided, and transposed superiorly so that the nerve coaptation can be performed more superficially. The motor nerve to the masseter muscle has one large fascicle and is generally a good size match to the obturator nerve.
14. Gracilis inset (▶ Fig. 12.10): the gracilis muscle is then transplanted into the face and secured to the

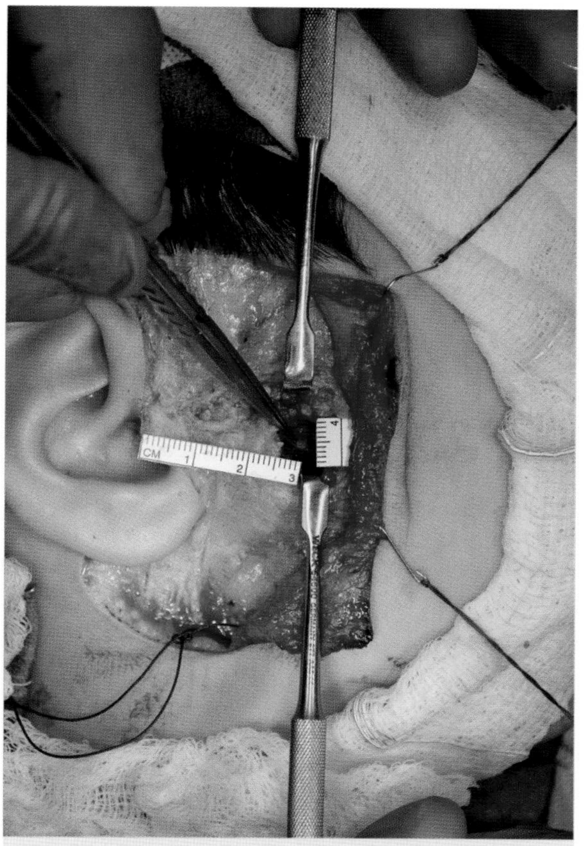

Fig. 12.9 The masseteric nerve can be found approximately 3 cm anterior to the helical root and 1 cm inferior to the zygomatic arch.

anchoring sutures in the lip first. The vessel repair is performed next under the operating microscope. In most cases, the venous anastomosis is completed before the arterial anastomosis. Great care is taken to ensure that there is no twisting or kinking of donor or recipient vessels.

15. A tension-free epineurial repair of the obturator nerve to the donor nerve is then completed. When possible, the obturator nerve should be shortened to reduce time to gracilis reinnervation.
16. Lastly, the origin of the gracilis muscle is secured to the temporal fascia with 1–0 absorbable suture. Spreading out the muscle over the width of the temporal fascia to the helical root posteriorly is helpful in reducing bulk (▶ Fig. 12.11). The muscle should lie along the same vector as the contralateral smile, and should course below the malar prominence (which also assists in reducing bulk). The tension of the gracilis is set so that the oral commissure barely moves and matches the contralateral side at rest.
17. Once the gracilis inset is completed, a Penrose drain is placed through a retroauricular stab incision and the skin edges are reapproximated in a tension-free manner. An oral commissure hook-shaped splint is placed and secured to the scalp to protect the gracilis inset (▶ Fig. 12.12). This is fashioned from thermoplastic material by the therapist.

Postoperative Care

As with any free tissue transfer, good pain control, adequate hydration, and avoidance of vasoconstricting

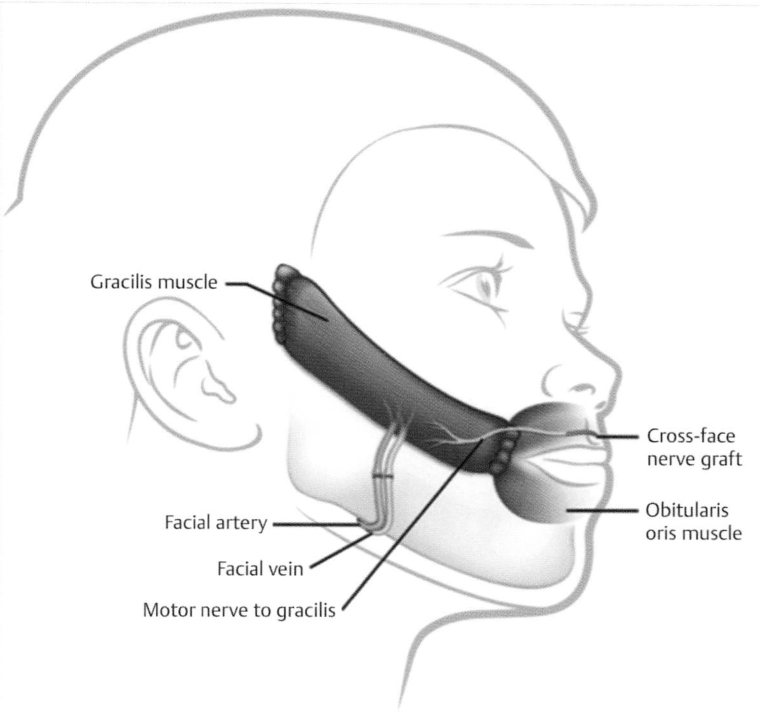

Fig. 12.10 Diagram showing the orientation of the gracilis muscle as part of a two-stage procedure. Note the obturator nerve running towards the cross-face nerve graft that was previously banked in the upper buccal sulcus.

substances (i.e., caffeine) is important in the postoperative period. Flap monitoring is not routinely performed in our center, but others use Doppler ultrasound imaging. Perioperative antibiotics are given, but no anticoagulation. The child is maintained on bed rest for 1 day and is then gradually mobilized. Any pressure or contact over the face is avoided for 6 weeks.

Reinnervation of the gracilis muscle is first seen at approximately 8 to 10 weeks when the nerve to masseter is the donor, and at 5 to 6 months when a CFNG is utilized. Once the muscle begins moving (and reinnervation occurs), rehabilitation exercises are initiated to assist in achieving smile symmetry and spontaneity. This involves practicing the smile motion in front of a mirror two to three times a day for 4 to 5 minutes apiece for a total duration of approximately 6 months. A spontaneous smile is expected following a CFNG, but is more challenging to attain with a masseter nerve donor.

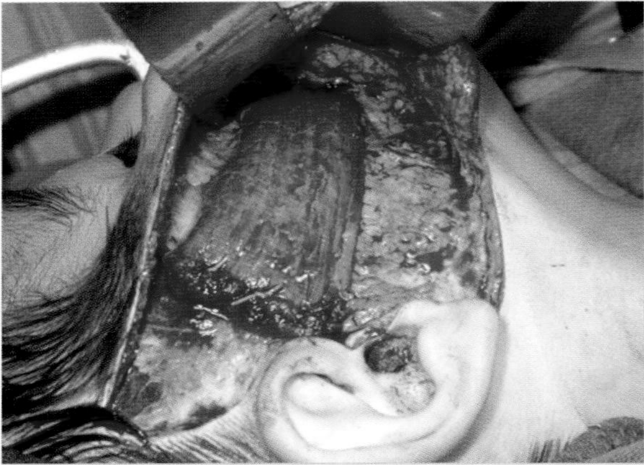

Fig. 12.11 The final inset of the gracilis muscle following suturing of the origin of the gracilis to the temporal fascia.

> **!**
>
> Reinnervation of the gracilis muscle is first seen at about 8 to 10 weeks when the nerve to the masseter muscle is the donor, and at 5 to 6 months when a cross-face nerve graft is utilized.

Complications

Early complications include bleeding, infection, and vessel thrombosis; fortunately these are all rare occurrences. Infection usually manifests as an abscess deep the gracilis muscle and in close proximity to the vascular repair, necessitating return to the operating room for irrigation and debridement. Perioperative antibiotics and frequent intraoperative irrigation have assisted in preventing this eventuality.

Late complications are often more difficult to correct.[42, 49] Excess bulk in the cheek is one of the more common patient complaints. Generally, there is a wait several months for the edema to resolve prior to committing to a secondary debulking procedure, such as thinning the cheek flap, buccal fat excision, and/or tangential resection of the gracilis muscle (taking care not to disrupt the vascular supply to the flap). Other complications include disruption of the gracilis muscle from the oral commissure, which is rare but challenging to correct, and excess tension on the oral commissure. The latter can be corrected by releasing the gracilis origin at the temporal region to allow the gracilis to shift anteriorly and reduce the pull on the commissure. Inadequate excursion of the gracilis can be a result of reduced muscle viability and fibrosis, poor neural regeneration, or insufficient postoperative rehabilitation. Treatment consists of biofeedback and/or electrical stimulation. In severe cases of insufficient motion, the muscle can be removed and replaced with a

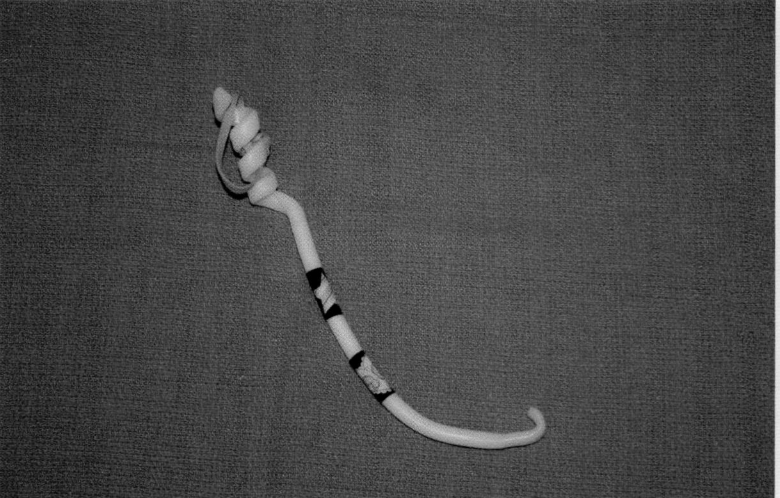

Fig. 12.12 Oral commissure hook to protect the gracilis muscle inset.

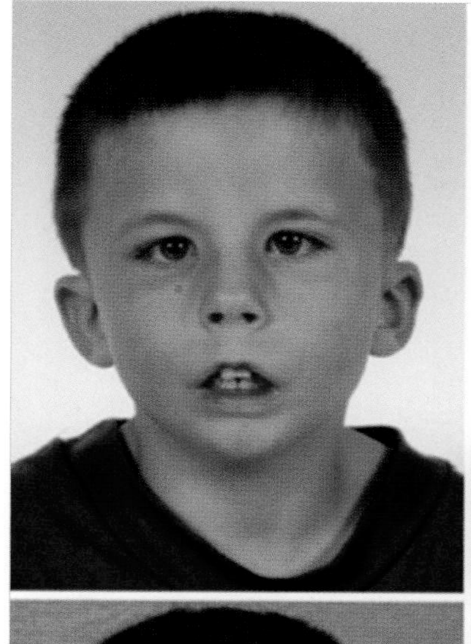
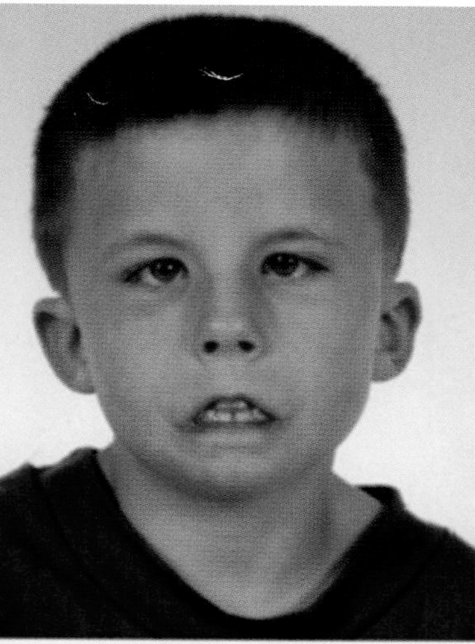
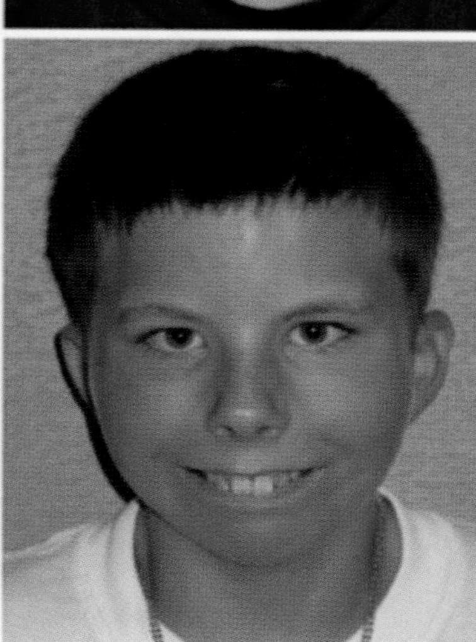

Fig. 12.13 A patient with Möbius syndrome with bilateral facial paralysis. Preoperative views at rest (top, left) and with smiling (top, right) show that activity of the lower divisions of the facial nerve resulted in a grimace rather than smile. Bilateral, staged free gracilis transfers were performed for restoration of the smile using the masseteric nerves as donor nerves. Postoperative views at rest (bottom, left) and while smiling (bottom, right) show that symmetry of the smile and nasolabial crease was achieved by careful suture placement in the commissure. (Reproduced with permission from Fattah A, Borschel GH, Manktelow RT, Bezuhly M, Zuker RM. Facial palsy and reconstruction. Plast Reconstr Surg 2012;129(2):340e–352e.)

new muscle with a different innervation source. Others have recommended augmentation of the transplanted muscle with temporalis muscle.[49]

!

Bulk in the cheek is one of the more common patient complaints; but wait several months for the edema to resolve prior to committing to a secondary debulking procedure.

Outcomes

Dynamic reconstruction of the smile with free tissue transfer can dramatically improve the child's appearance and ability to express him/herself. With our current surgical techniques, one can reliably create a natural-looking smile that mirrors the contralateral side (▶ Fig. 12.13 and ▶ Fig. 12.14). However, the child's appearance and function are rarely perfect. Despite our best efforts, the nasolabial crease often remains deficient in its upper third, the excursion of the commissure is not perfectly symmetric (especially with a CFNG), and spontaneity may not be achieved (especially with the nerve to the masseter muscle). Even when the excursion is excellent, there may be a delay in initiation of the smile on the reconstructed side that leads to slight asymmetry with animation.

12.6.2 Neonatal Asymmetric Crying Facies

The simplest approach to restore symmetry during animation in children with NACF is to paralyze the functioning lower lip depressors on the unaffected side using botulinum toxin (▶ Fig. 12.15).[44] While the effect is temporary, it can be repeated and will allow the patient and/or family to visualize the effect of the paralysis. Often, symmetry is markedly improved with this approach.[50] If

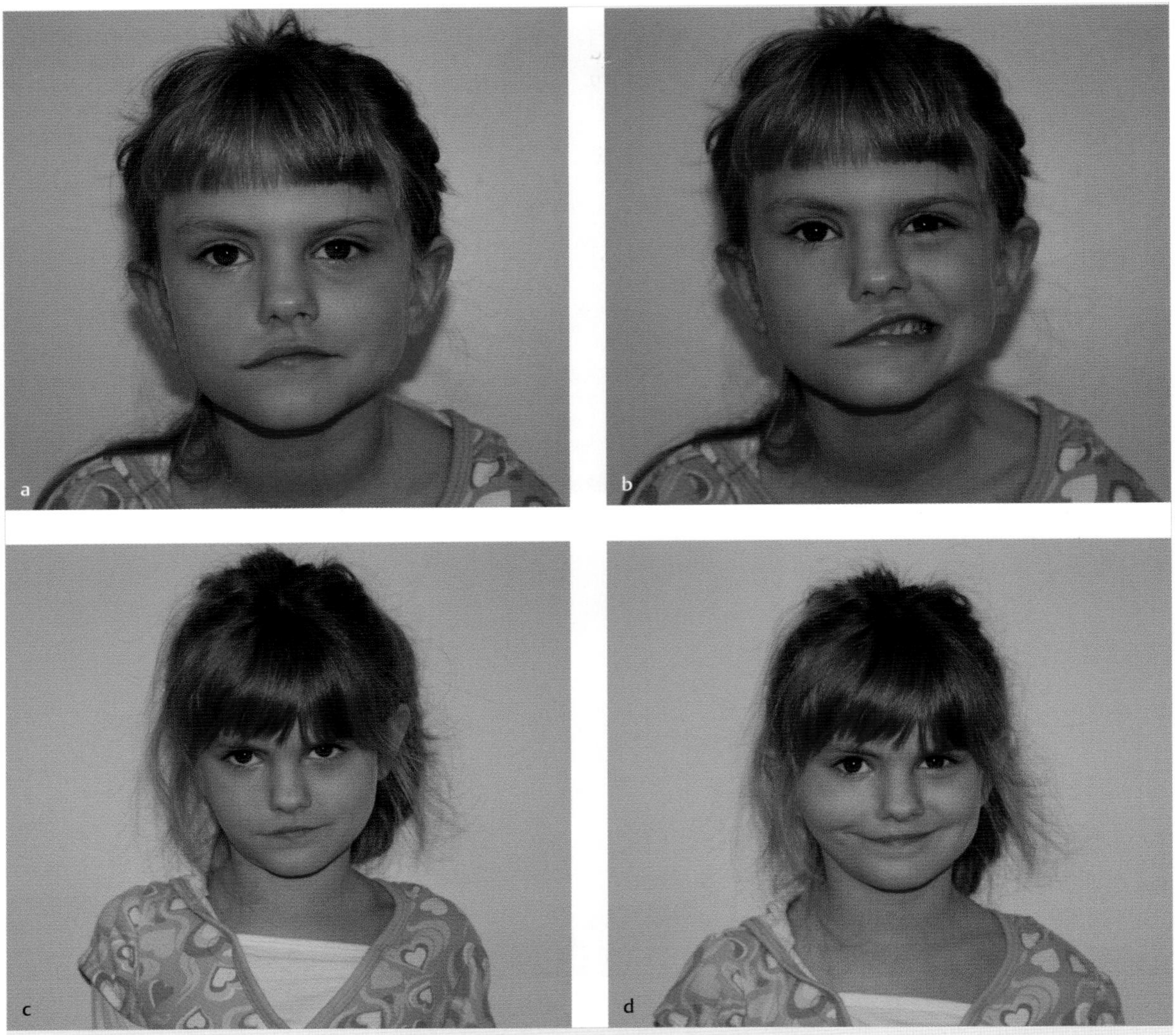

Fig. 12.14 A patient with right incomplete congenital unilateral facial paralysis. Preoperatively, asymmetry is noted: **(a)** at rest, and **(b)** while smiling. Reconstruction was performed using a free gracilis transfer powered by the ipsilateral masseter nerve. Postoperative results show improved symmetry at rest and restoration of smile on the right side: **(c)** at rest, and **(d)** while smiling. At 9 weeks postoperatively, note the slight excess bulk in the right cheek, which was later revised.

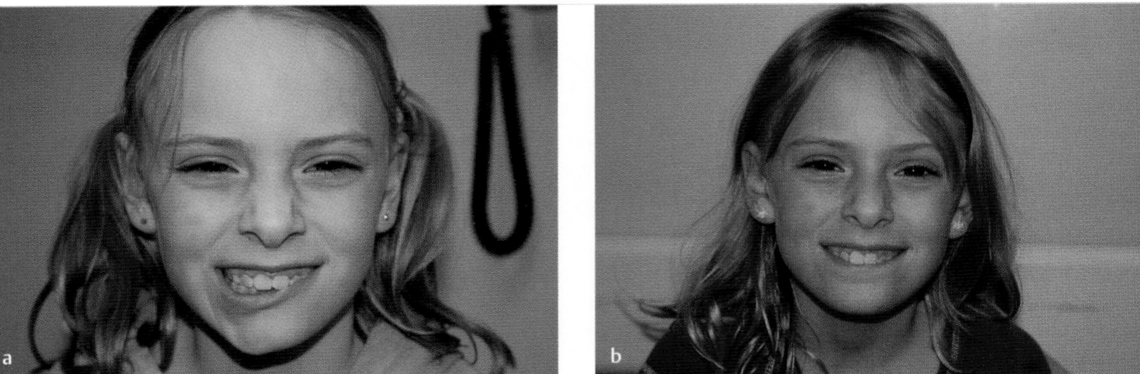

Fig. 12.15 A patient with left-sided paralysis of the marginal mandibular branch of the facial nerve: **(a)** preinjection of Botox, and **(b)** postinjection of Botox into the unaffected (right) lower lip depressors.

a more permanent solution is desired, myectomy of the functioning depressor anguli oris can be performed through an intraoral approach. Some authors have also proposed dynamic restoration of lower lip function using local muscle flaps, such as anterior digastric and platysma flaps; see Chapter 27 for details[51]; however these procedures are technically challenging, create visible scars, and the results are variable.

12.6.3 Acquired Facial Paralysis in the Pediatric Population

The management of acquired facial paralysis in children is dependent on etiology and timing of presentation, and follows the same algorithm for upper and lower face reconstruction as in the adult population (which is discussed in detail in Part VI of this book).[52] What differs is the prognosis for nerve recovery. Indeed, axonal regeneration occurs more rapidly in children and the distance to target muscles is shorter. Every effort should therefore be expended to restore innervation to the native facial musculature in situations where spontaneous recovery does not occur, or is not expected to occur as in traumatic lacerations. The window for reinnervation of native musculature can be up to 12 to 18 months in children. When no distal facial nerve is available, direct neurotization of the facial musculature using the ipsilateral proximal facial nerve stump or a cross-face nerve graft can generate sufficient tone in the pediatric population to maintain symmetry at rest.[3,52]

12.7 Key Points

- Congenital facial paralysis is caused by maldevelopment of central and/or peripheral structures relating to the facial nerve or facial musculature. It can occur sporadically, or can be found in association with syndromes such as Möbius syndrome.
- Evaluation of the patient is critical in differentiating congenital from acquired causes of pediatric facial paralysis, and for perioperative planning.
- The mainstay of treatment of congenital facial paralysis is operative, since there is no capacity for spontaneous recovery.
- Dynamic reconstruction of the smile is the gold standard for congenital facial paralysis, with our preferred approach being a free segmental gracilis transfer powered by a cross-face nerve graft (unilateral cases) or the masseteric nerve (bilateral cases).

References

[1] Terzis JK, Anesti K. Experience with developmental facial paralysis: part II. Outcomes of reconstruction. Plast Reconstr Surg 2012; 129: 66e–80e

[2] Jackson CG. Facial Nerve Paralysis: Diagnosis and Treatment of Lower Motor Neuron Facial Nerve Lesions and Facial Paralysis. Rochester, MN: American Academy of Otolaryngology—Head and Neck Surgery Foundation Inc. 1986:38–40

[3] Terzis JK, Anesti K. Developmental facial paralysis: a review. J Plast Reconstr Aesthet Surg 2011; 64: 1318–1333

[4] Falco NA, Eriksson E. Facial nerve palsy in the newborn: incidence and outcome. Plast Reconstr Surg 1990; 85: 1–4

[5] Yılmaz U, Cubukçu D, Yılmaz TS, Akıncı G, Ozcan M, Güzel O. Peripheral facial palsy in children. J Child Neurol 2014; 29: 1473–1478

[6] Jemec B, Grobbelaar AO, Harrison DH. The abnormal nucleus as a cause of congenital facial palsy. Arch Dis Child 2000; 83: 256–258

[7] Evans AK, Licameli G, Brietzke S, Whittemore K, Kenna M. Pediatric facial nerve paralysis: patients, management and outcomes. Int J Pediatr Otorhinolaryngol 2005; 69: 1521–1528

[8] Grundfast KM, Guarisco JL, Thomsen JR, Koch B. Diverse etiologies of facial paralysis in children. Int J Pediatr Otorhinolaryngol 1990; 19: 223–239

[9] Pavlou E, Gkampeta A, Arampatzi M. Facial nerve palsy in childhood. Brain Dev 2011; 33: 644–650

[10] Toelle SP, Boltshauser E. Long-term outcome in children with congenital unilateral facial nerve palsy. Neuropediatrics 2001; 32: 130–135

[11] Verzijl HT F M, van der Zwaag B, Cruysberg JRM, Padberg GW. Möbius syndrome redefined: a syndrome of rhombencephalic maldevelopment. Neurology 2003; 61: 327–333

[12] Alrashdi IS, Rich P, Patton MA. A family with hereditary congenital facial paresis and a brief review of the literature. Clin Dysmorphol 2010; 19: 198–201

[13] Verzijl HTFM, van der Zwaag B, Lammens M, ten Donkelaar HJ, Padberg GW. The neuropathology of hereditary congenital facial palsy vs Möbius syndrome. Neurology 2005; 64: 649–653

[14] Saito H, Takeda T, Kishimoto S. Neonatal facial nerve defect. Acta Otolaryngol Suppl 1994; 510: 77–81

[15] Terzis JK, Anesti K. Experience with developmental facial paralysis: Part I. Diagnosis and associated stigmata. Plast Reconstr Surg 2011; 128: 488e–497e

[16] Briegel W. Neuropsychiatric findings of Möbius sequence—a review. Clin Genet 2006; 70: 91–97

[17] Dooley JM, Stewart WA, Hayden JD, Therrien A. Brainstem calcification in Möbius syndrome. Pediatr Neurol 2004; 30: 39–41

[18] Ghabrial R, Versace P, Kourt G, Lipson A, Martin F. Möbius' syndrome: features and etiology. J Pediatr Ophthalmol Strabismus 1998; 35: 304–311, quiz 327–328

[19] Miller MT, Strömland K. The Möbius sequence: a relook. J AAPOS 1999; 3: 199–208

[20] Woollard ACS, Harrison DH, Grobbelaar AO. An approach to bilateral facial paralysis. J Plast Reconstr Aesthet Surg 2010; 63: 1557–1560

[21] Kremer H, Kuyt LP, van den Helm B et al. Localization of a gene for Möbius syndrome to chromosome 3q by linkage analysis in a Dutch family. Hum Mol Genet 1996; 5: 1367–1371

[22] St Charles S, DiMario FJ, Jr, Grunnet ML. Möbius sequence: further in vivo support for the subclavian artery supply disruption sequence. Am J Med Genet 1993; 47: 289–293

[23] Govaert P, Vanhaesebrouck P, De Praeter C, Fränkel U, Leroy J. Moebius sequence and prenatal brainstem ischemia. Pediatrics 1989; 84: 570–573

[24] Lammens M, Moerman Ph, Fryns JP et al. Neuropathological findings in Moebius syndrome. Clin Genet 1998; 54: 136–141

[25] Verzijl HTFM, Valk J, de Vries R, Padberg GW. Radiologic evidence for absence of the facial nerve in Möbius syndrome. Neurology 2005; 64: 849–855

[26] Pastuszak AL, Schüler L, Speck-Martins CE et al. Use of misoprostol during pregnancy and Möbius' syndrome in infants. N Engl J Med 1998; 338: 1881–1885

[27] Verzijl HT, van den Helm B, Veldman B et al. A second gene for autosomal dominant Möbius syndrome is localized to chromosome 10q, in a Dutch family. Am J Hum Genet 1999; 65: 752–756

[28] Singham J, Manktelow R, Zuker RM. Möbius syndrome. Semin Plast Surg 2004; 18: 39–46

[29] Briegel W, Schimek M, Knapp D, Holderbach R, Wenzel P, Knapp E-M. Cognitive evaluation in children and adolescents with Möbius sequence. Child Care Health Dev 2009; 35: 650–655

[30] Johansson M, Wentz E, Fernell E, Strömland K, Miller MT, Gillberg C. Autistic spectrum disorders in Möbius sequence: a comprehensive study of 25 individuals. Dev Med Child Neurol 2001; 43: 338–345

[31] Bassila MK, Goldberg R. The association of facial palsy and/or sensorineural hearing loss in patients with hemifacial microsomia. Cleft Palate J 1989; 26: 287–291

[32] Kokavec R. Goldenhar syndrome with various clinical manifestations. Cleft Palate Craniofac J 2006; 43: 628–634

[33] Carvalho GJ, Song CS, Vargervik K, Lalwani AK. Auditory and facial nerve dysfunction in patients with hemifacial microsomia. Arch Otolaryngol Head Neck Surg 1999; 125: 209–212

[34] Berker N, Acaroğlu G, Soykan E. Goldenhar's Syndrome (oculo-auriculo-vertebral dysplasia) with congenital facial nerve palsy. Yonsei Med J 2004; 45: 157–160

[35] Wang R, Martínez-Frías ML, Graham JM, Jr. Infants of diabetic mothers are at increased risk for the oculo-auriculo-vertebral sequence: A case-based and case-control approach. J Pediatr 2002; 141: 611–617

[36] Pape KE, Pickering D. Asymmetric crying facies: an index of other congenital anomalies. J Pediatr 1972; 81: 21–30

[37] Kobayashi T. Congenital unilateral lower lip palsy. Acta Otolaryngol 1979; 88: 303–309

[38] Lahat E, Heyman E, Barkay A, Goldberg M. Asymmetric crying facies and associated congenital anomalies: prospective study and review of the literature. J Child Neurol 2000; 15: 808–810

[39] Perlman M, Reisner SH. Asymmetric crying facies and congenital anomalies. Arch Dis Child 1973; 48: 627–629

[40] Renault F. Facial electromyography in newborn and young infants with congenital facial weakness. Dev Med Child Neurol 2001; 43: 421–427

[41] Pasick C, McDonald-McGinn DM, Simbolon C, Low D, Zackai E, Jackson O. Asymmetric crying facies in the 22q11.2 deletion syndrome: implications for future screening. Clin Pediatr (Phila) 2013; 52: 1144–1148

[42] Marcus JR, Borschel GH, Zuker RM. Facial paralysis and facial reanimation. In: Bentz ML, Bauer BS, Zuker RM, eds. Principles and Practice of Pediatric Plastic Surgery. Vol. 2. Boca Raton, FL: CRC Press; 2007

[43] May M. Facial paralysis at birth: medicolegal and clinical implications. Am J Otol 1995; 16: 711–712

[44] Fattah A, Borschel GH, Manktelow RT, Bezuhly M, Zuker RM. Facial palsy and reconstruction. Plast Reconstr Surg 2012; 129: 340e–352e

[45] Bae Y-C, Zuker RM, Manktelow RT, Wade S. A comparison of commissure excursion following gracilis muscle transplantation for facial paralysis using a cross-face nerve graft versus the motor nerve to the masseter nerve. Plast Reconstr Surg 2006; 117: 2407–2413

[46] Lifchez SD, Matloub HS, Gosain AK. Cortical adaptation to restoration of smiling after free muscle transfer innervated by the nerve to the masseter. Plast Reconstr Surg 2005; 115: 1472–1479, discussion 1480–1482

[47] Manktelow RT, Zuker RM, Tomat LR. Facial paralysis measurement with a handheld ruler. Plast Reconstr Surg 2008; 121: 435–442

[48] Borschel GH, Kawamura DH, Kasukurthi R, Hunter DA, Zuker RM, Woo AS. The motor nerve to the masseter muscle: an anatomic and histomorphometric study to facilitate its use in facial reanimation. J Plast Reconstr Aesthet Surg 2012; 65: 363–366

[49] Terzis JK, Olivares FS. Secondary surgery in paediatric facial paralysis reanimation. J Plast Reconstr Aesthet Surg 2010; 63: 1794–1806

[50] Manktelow RT. Microsurgical strategies in 74 patients for restoration of dynamic depressor muscle mechanism: a neglected target in facial reanimation. Plast Reconstr Surg 2000; 105: 1932–1934

[51] Terzis JK, Kalantarian B. Microsurgical strategies in 74 patients for restoration of dynamic depressor muscle mechanism: a neglected target in facial reanimation. Plast Reconstr Surg 2000; 105: 1917–1931, discussion 1932–1934

[52] Fattah A, Borschel GH, Zuker RM. Reconstruction of facial nerve injuries in children. J Craniofac Surg 2011; 22: 782–788

Part IV

Importance of the Facial Nerve for Communication and Emotion

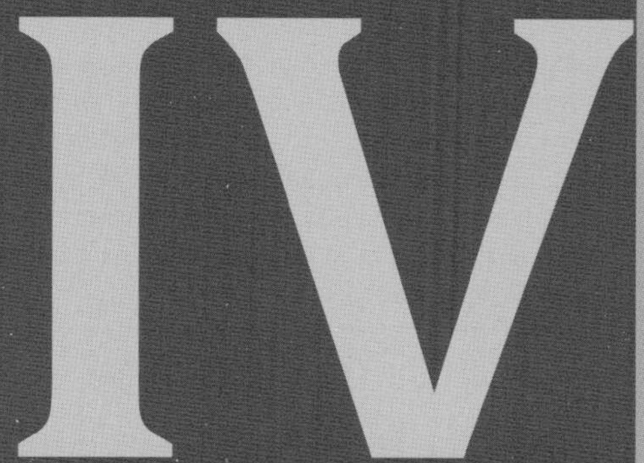

13 Psychological Exploration of Emotional, Communicative, and Social Impairments in Patients with Facial Impairments

Christian Dobel and Orlando Guntinas-Lichius

13.1 Introduction

Facial paresis is in many cases not a life-threatening disease, but it is certainly life altering. It cannot be hidden and is very often stigmatizing, which leads to social withdrawal, isolation, and a severe reduction in quality of life. The medical community is only beginning to understand all the psychological ramifications of facial paresis, but for the patient it can equal or exceed the physical aspects. Nevertheless, the universal interest of observers of patients with facial paresis is obvious when one considers the many ritual masks identified from different cultures that clearly display symptoms of this disorder. Similarly, it is present in our western cultures in characters such as "Two-Face", who is well known from graphic novels and movies.

> !
>
> In contrast to the motor deficits of a facial palsy, there is a lack of knowledge of the psychological and communication dysfunction related to the palsy. The reason might be that patients with facial palsy are normally seen by only medical physicians and not by psychologists.

With regard to a patient's medical case history, physicians typically ask for symptoms such as impaired food intake, diminished ability to articulate, impairments of the eyes, hyperacusis etc. The diagnostic procedures and methods are targeted towards these symptoms and, as a consequence, to therapeutic approaches as well. Psychological aspects and their consequences, which are extremely important to the patient, may become overlooked. Recent overviews of the topic still tend to focus primarily on the various pharmaceuticals and reconstructive and physical therapy approaches without including psychological assessment.[1–3]

> !
>
> Psychological aspects and consequences of the palsy are normally not addressed by the physician. Although relevant for the patient, these aspects are often overlooked and underestimated.

In this chapter, the authors provide the current knowledge of emotional, communication, and social aspects of facial paresis and how to explore these in patients with this disorder. Only by employing such an approach can the disorder be fully understood.

13.2 Emotions as a Core of Human Interactions

While emotions are used in common language synonymously with feelings or affect, there is general agreement in the scientific community that emotions consist of different components, i.e., how the person feels, and also their physiological and neurophysiologic correlates, and how they are expressed in gesture and language and what actions they entail; for more extensive reading on the topic, see Oatley 2006[4]. At least since Charles Darwin,[5] faces have held a specific role in communication both in animals and in humans. Faces convey information about identity, gender, and age, and also about the emotional state of a person. This information is retrieved almost effortlessly and automatically by a dedicated neurocognitive network for facial processing. This happens within the first 200 milliseconds after a face is perceived.[6,7] One of the most famous books on emotions is *The Expression of the Emotions in Man and Animal* by Darwin.[5] For Darwin, emotional expressions showed a continuity from lower animals to adult humans. While certain facial expressions might not be functional now, they were, in his view, for our ancestors. As an example, sneering in humans, in whom the teeth are partially uncovered on one side, finds its root in snarling and the preparation to bite. As such, Darwin saw emotional expression as a crucial and core feature of human interaction:

> "The movements of expression in the face and body, whatever their origin may have been, are in themselves of much importance for our welfare. They serve as the first means of communication between the mother and her infant; she smiles approval, and thus encourages her child on the right path, or frowns disapproval. We readily perceive sympathy in others by their expression." (Darwin 1872, p. 359[5].)

From a developmental perspective this citation from 1872 is already emphasizing the importance of emotional expression to develop long-standing and intense relationships between children and mothers, i.e., the so-called attachment.[8] By drawing on their biological origins, Darwin is already emphasizing the universality of emotional expressions, i.e., that it is not necessary to learn them and that they are culturally independent. These characteristics were taken up later by Paul Ekman who proposed the universal presence of six basic emotions (happiness, anger, disgust, fear, sadness, and surprise) in all humans. These and other important concepts for understanding the role of emotional expression for human interaction are summarized in ▶ Table 13.1. The pattern of facial muscle activity of a specific emotional expression is so similar in all cultures that it can be readily recognized by persons from other cultures.[9] Nevertheless, there are some very recent findings demonstrating that the quality to recognize emotions is situation dependent and context dependent.[10,11]

!

One can imagine that congenital facial palsy might influence the development of relationships between a child and his/her parents although this has not been investigated so far.

Taken together, this brief introduction emphasizes the importance of emotional facial expression for social interactions. As a main channel to communicate emotional states, faces are of the utmost importance to be comprehended by others and to be integrated in satisfying and rich emotional relationships. While the altered ability to produce emotional expressions has without doubt a strong impact on the perception of other persons of oneself, there are strong reasons to assume that they also have a causal impact on one's own emotions.

!

It is not just that impaired emotional expression of a patient with facial palsy has an influence on the perception of others. It is also very important for the patient to understand that the deficit might have an impact on his/her own emotional state.

13.3 Understanding Own and Others' Emotions

One fundamental issue in the investigation of social interactions concerns the question of how human and nonhuman primates know about mental (thoughts, intentions,

Table 13.1 Important concepts on emotions and their relation to human interaction with impact on patients with facial palsy

Concept	Comment
Ekman's six basic emotions	Based on the ideas by Charles Darwin, Paul Ekman provided empirical evidence that six facial expressions are recognized universally in diverse cultures across all ages: anger, disgust, fear, happiness, sadness, and surprise. This led to the development of stimulus material that is used worldwide
Mirror neurons	Mirror neurons were first described in the premotor cortex of monkeys. They fire when an individual performs an action, but also if it perceives the same action performed by another individual. In humans it was shown, for example, that the insula is active both when a person sees a face displaying disgust and also when he/she experiences disgust. The mirror neuron system is conceived as the necessary basis to develop empathy
Shared manifold hypothesis	Interacting persons share several mental states such as somatic sensations or emotions. The responsible neural correlate is the mirror neuron system that invokes a sort of simulation process on a functional level. This in turn results in the sense of similarity of oneself with others
Facial feedback hypothesis	Charles Darwin was among the first to propose that physiological changes (e.g., specific movements of the facial muscles) have a direct impact on emotion. The theory was tested and supported in several studies in which the facial muscles were experimentally manipulated by, for example, inducing a facial muscular pattern similar to smiling. This pattern induced higher ratings of funniness for cartoons. Other evidence was provided by injection of botulinum toxin into facial muscles responsible for expression of emotion
Emotional contagion	Emotional contagion described the phenomenon that two interacting individuals tend to express the same emotions. This can be observed in mothers and their children. The induction of emotions seems to happen in a conscious or unconscious manner. The synchronization of emotions is important for personal relationships. It is assumed that mirror neurons play a crucial part in this mechanism

etc.) and emotional states in other members of their species (or even in members of other species). After all, there is a great variability in the openly perceivable signals and even more variability in their interpretation; for an introduction to this see Baron-Cohen 1997[12]. Nevertheless, there is by and large agreement how certain signals should be interpreted. We all know, for example, that looking at something or somebody is an expression of interest. But we also know that looking at something when we daydream is not a cue for attention.

A milestone in the search to solve this question was the discovery of mirror neurons located in parietofrontal and limbic regions. These neurons fire not only if a subject, being human or a nonhuman primate, *performs* a specific behavior, but also when he *observes* the very same behavior.[13,14]

!

Mirror neurons in the parietofrontal and limbic regions are activated when we perform an emotional expression, and also when we see the equivalent expression in the face of our counterpart. It is not known whether the mirror neuron system is altered in patients with facial palsy.

This principle was not only found for actions, but all sorts of social and emotional processes such as the recognition of emotional faces. Because the very same neural networks are involved in the perception of one's own mental states as in the mental states of others, this mechanism allows one to interpret actions, intentions, and emotions in our social partners. As such the involved cortical structures were later termed the "social brain." Thus, understanding other peoples' minds involves a sort of simulation process and is thought of as a prerequisite to develop empathy. Such processes are described by the "shared manifold hypothesis."[15]

Nevertheless, even though this explains how others perceive emotional facial expressions, this still leaves open the question how emotions arise from the perception of oneself. This issue was already brought forth by one of the founders of modern psychology, William James in the 18th century (and similarly by the neuroanatomist Karl Lange). James and Lange wondered, for example, if we cry because we are sad or if we are sad because we cry. Common sense lets us favor the second hypothesis, but there is some evidence for the first which became famous as the James–Lange theory; for a review, see Lang 1994[16]. The theory proposes that specific physiological changes (e.g., a muscular process) precede and in fact directly cause the experience of emotions.

"My thesis on the contrary is that the bodily changes follow directly the perception of the exciting fact, and that our feeling of the same changes as they occur is the emotion." (James 1884, page 13[17])

Even though this theory did not remain without objection (e.g., by Walter Cannon,[18] one of the students of William James), it had a very strong influence on emotion research and was also applied to the processing of emotional expressions in faces. Building on the James–Lange theory, the "facial feedback hypothesis" claims that movement of one's own face directly influences emotional experience. This hypothesis is supported by a series of findings. In the "directed facial action task" participants are told to follow muscle-by-muscle instructions in order to reach one of the six basic emotions proposed by Ekman. As an example they were told to:

1. Wrinkle their nose.
2. Raise their upper lip.
3. Open their mouth and stick out their tongue.

Importantly, participants were not told that this represents the muscular facial pattern for "disgust." While they held this facial gesture autonomic measures were taken. The results demonstrated that the portrayed negative emotions (anger, disgust, fear) evoked stronger sympathetic activity compared with positive emotions,[19] which is in line with the predictions made by the James-Lange theory. Other experimental approaches provided evidence that specific voluntary movements and positions of the facial muscles lead to altered emotional perceptions. Another example is that German readers judged stories that they read aloud as less positive if they contained many /ü/. This is an umlaut articulated similar to the English /oo/ and which involves protruding the lips, i. e., the opposite of a smiling movement.[20] Further evidence was brought forth by a famous study in which participants would either hold a pen between the teeth without touching it with the lips, or hold it with the lips only. The first condition leads to the contraction of the zygomatic major muscle and the risorius muscle, which are both muscles that are strongly involved in smiling. In contrast, the second condition activates the orbicularis oris muscle, which is incompatible with smiling. In line with the facial feedback hypothesis, the participants holding the pen between their teeth judged cartoons as funnier than persons holding it in their lips.[21] Further support for the facial feedback hypothesis was given by a study that used injections of botulinum toxin into the facial muscles,[22] which demonstrated that changing the expression also altered the patient's emotional state.

!

The facial feedback hypothesis addresses the unanswered question of whether facial palsy limits the spectrum of emotional perception of the patient.

Taken together, these studies provide evidence that changes in the facial muscle activity evoke voluntary (by holding a pen between the lips, etc.) or involuntary (by injection of botulinum toxin) movement that has a strong influence on how people feel. These results suggest that the emotional perception is likewise altered in patients suffering from facial palsy. At the same time, the shared manifold hypothesis predicts that people who interact with patients with facial palsy are more strongly influenced by the displayed facial expression, assuming they understand the emotion behind it even when it differs from how the patient actually verbalizes their feelings. Modern theories integrating language production and comprehension[23] stress that speakers monitor the mental states of listeners in an online fashion, and adjust their utterances accordingly. This mechanism ensures that speakers are well understood and that knowledge and mental states of listeners are taken into account when speakers plan what to say. Thus, even on this macroscopic level of language processing, emotions play a major role. This is one reason why facial palsy leads to social and communication problems. As another factor, mimic and verbal expressions of emotions often lead to "emotional contagion," i.e., that other persons become "infected" by our emotional states and often involuntarily imitate them.[24,25]

As examples of neutral and emotional faces, ► Fig. 13.1 displays several patients that were asked to display a neutral face and to smile.

Obviously, facial paresis has a very strong influence on social interactions about which patients often complain. Unfortunately, there are currently only very few studies that address this problem. It is to date not clear if the mimic interaction is just physically very exhausting, and what the role of stigmatization is and to what degree emotional perception and expression are altered; as an exception see, for example, Keillor 2002[26]. How these concepts can be used for therapeutic approaches is the topic of Chapter 14.

In the following sections, the authors address psychological changes in patients with facial palsy in order to make the practitioner sensitive to these issues. It is recommended that the reader considers them when generating medical case reports.

13.4 Psychological Changes After Facial Palsy

Even though there has not been much research on changes in interpersonal communication and emotional perception, there are some reports that suggest potential problematic issues (Box 13.1). Psychological parameters should be screened during interviews with patients and counseling may be suggested as needed. Many patients with facial palsy have the impression that they cannot express emotions satisfactorily.[27] This influences the ability to automatically evoke emotions in other persons, which was referred to as "emotional contagion" in Understanding Own and Others' Emotions As this plays a more dominant role in women than in men,[28] gender-specific differences in the patient population can be expected also. The necessary screening and emotional support can be provided by personnel with substantial medical training and experience with facial paralysis.

Box 13.1 Most important emotional changes in patients with facial palsy

- Patients have the impression that they cannot express emotions satisfactorily.
- Expressions of patients are often perceived as negative even when the patients smile.
- Patients with facial palsy avoid making eye contact more frequently than healthy subjects.
- Patients with facial palsy are at risk of developing depressive symptoms resulting frequently in social avoidance and isolation.
- Patients suffer more frequently from distress anxiety than the normal population.
- Quality of life is significantly reduced in patients with acute and chronic facial palsy.

There are hints that women and men with facial palsy are differently affected by the handicap to express emotions, but this has not been explored scientifically in detail.

Importantly, the impression of patients that they cannot express emotions appropriately is supported by the judgment of observers.[29] While faces of normal persons were rated neutral when they displayed a neutral expression and positive when they smiled, this was not so for faces with facial palsy. Their expression was most often classified as negative even when they smiled (► Fig. 13.2).

Accordingly, the majority of patients in a British study[30] reported that they are negatively and often even aggressively evaluated by strangers. Patients for whom such hurtful comments persisted even after surgery and therapy were more likely to develop depressive symptoms resulting frequently in social avoidance and isolation.

!

Reactive depression is an important consequence of facial palsy that is normally not addressed by the physician who is focused on the motor deficits resulting from the palsy.

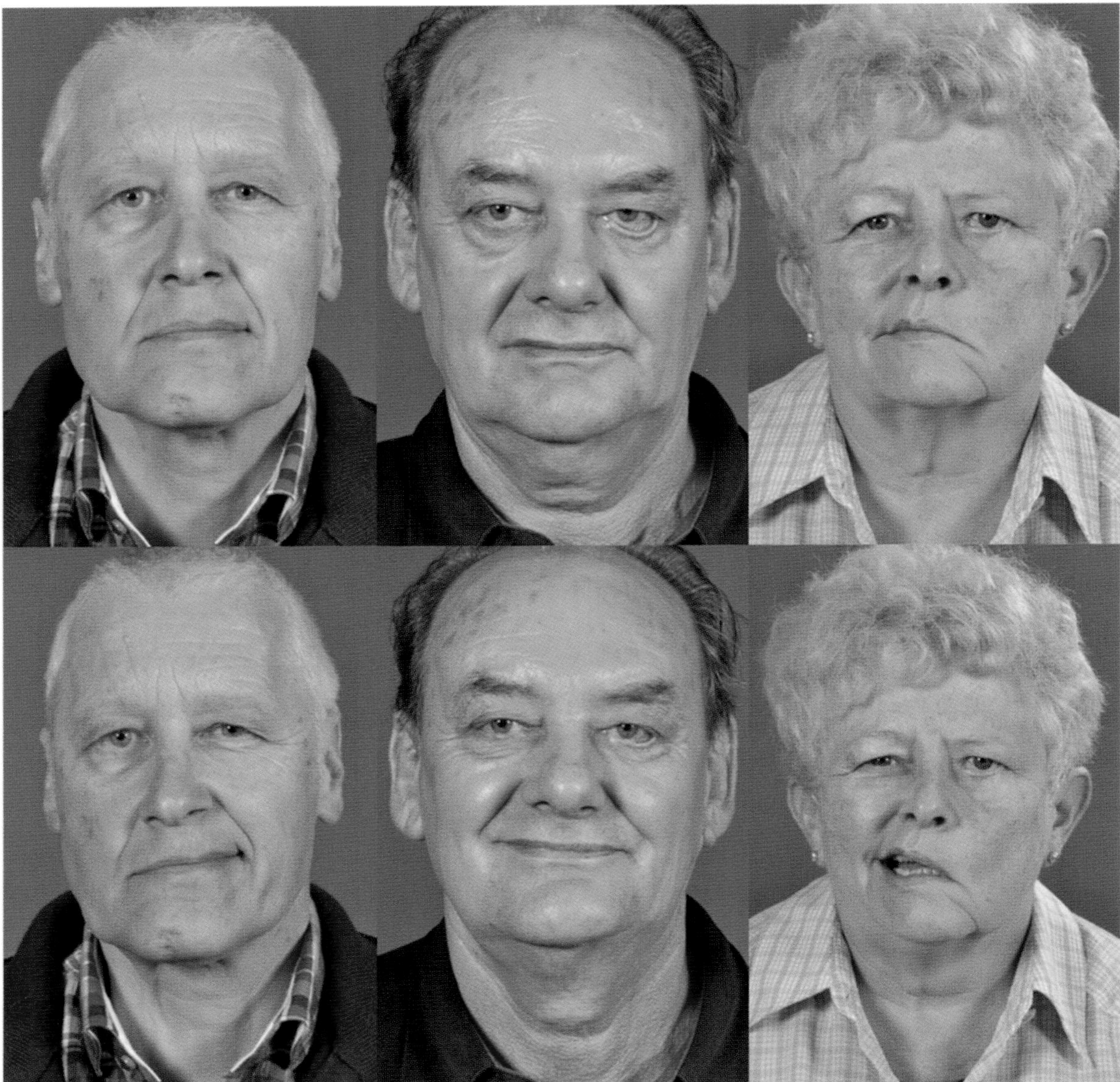

Fig. 13.1 Examples of patients with different severity of unilateral facial palsy at rest (top row) and when smiling spontaneously (bottom row). Depending on the severity of the palsy, smiling appears more or less normal, or significantly altered. (Reproduced with permission from Dobel C, Miltner WH, Witte OW, Volk GF, Guntinas-Lichius O. Emotional impact of facial palsy [in German]. Laryngorhinootologie 2013;92(1):9–23.)

Individuals with facial paralysis are also judged as less attractive than controls, and smiling does not result in a more positive evaluation, which is normally the case.[31] However, it is encouraging that facial reanimation leads to a more normalized classification of faces in repose and to more positive evaluations when patients smile.[32] Similarly, attractiveness increases and faces become evaluated more positively.[33] Those studies from 2012 and 2014 further stress the effectiveness of facial reanimation surgery and also point out that surgeons should not only aim for functional restoration, but also for the improvement to express emotions.

!

Facial reanimation surgery does not only improve motor function but can also enrich the capabilities to express emotions and impact how the patient is perceived.

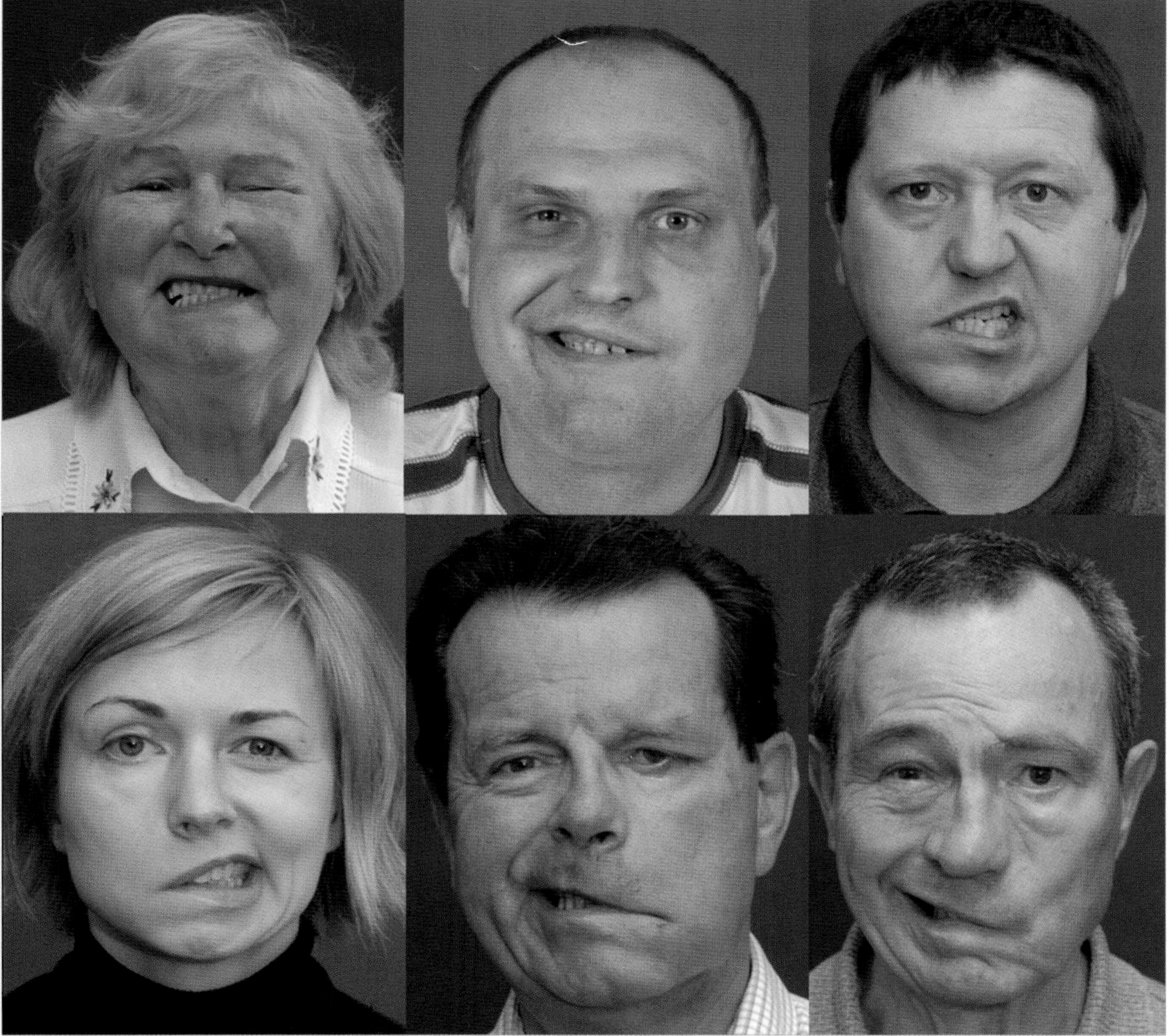

Fig. 13.2 Examples of patients with acute peripheral facial palsy (top row) and chronic facial palsy (bottom row) when asked to produce a smile (voluntary smiling). (Reproduced with permission from Dobel C, Miltner WH, Witte OW, Volk GF, Guntinas-Lichius O. Emotional impact of facial palsy [in German]. Laryngorhinootologie 2013;92(1):9–23.)

Similar reports for the penalty of facial malformation exist[34] for other disorders (e.g., after facial lesions or facial surgery for removal of tumors). Those studies show that disfigured faces are an immense burden to the patient and lead to a large amount of stigmatization. In most cases it cannot be hidden and we are made constantly aware of our looks when we are confronted with our mirror images during daily routines. Similarly, as mentioned previously, faces with lesions displaying a neutral expression are most often classified as sad or angry. In contrast, faces without lesions are more often judged as positive even if in repose.[34] These patients try to compensate for their facial disfigurement by overly friendly and overly helpful behavior. Strangers avoid direct eye contact and, as in patients with facial paresis, social avoidance and isolation are a frequent outcome in patients with facial disfigurement.[35] To what degree patients with facial disfigurement and patients with facial palsy differ in their social and emotional behavior has not been studied so far.

Given the severe stigmatization and the often involved social isolation, it is not surprising that many patients suffer from distress, anxiety, and depression.[36,37] Patients with chronic palsy are especially prone to develop depression.[37,38] This severe disorder (International Statistical Classification of Diseases and Related Health Problems 10th Revision [ICD-10] F32) is characterized by continuous low mood, reduction of energy, and loss of interest in enjoyable activities. Self-esteem and self-confidence are often severely affected. In a current British study about one-third of the patients investigated

($N = 103$, both chronic and acute) displayed significant signs of anxiety and depression.[39] Interestingly, there were correlations between the patients' perception of the severity of facial palsy and the level of measured distress. This correlation did not exist for the actual clinical severity and thus stresses the importance of asking patients for their perception of the illness.

Although there might be a correlation between severity of the palsy and the patient's distress, the patient's perception of the severity is a more important determinant of the development of severe depressive symptoms.

Not surprisingly, patients with facial paresis report a general reduction in quality of life,[27] which appears for them often even more weary than their physical limitations. A recent review[40] surveyed 598 articles and found 28 questionnaires assessing facial paralysis with regard to patient-reported outcome measures. Only three of the questionnaires fulfill the necessary psychometric qualities: the Facial Clinimetric Evaluation Scale,[41] the Facial Disability Index,[42] and a questionnaire developed to study aberrant facial nerve regeneration; for more details on the questionnaires see Chapter 7 and Chapter 14. The authors strongly stress the need for the development of further instruments to learn more about how patients feel their quality of life has changed.

!

Measure quality of life in patients with facial palsy using validated questionnaires.

This seems even more relevant given that quality of life measures improve after a whole range of treatment approaches, i.e., reconstructive facial surgery,[43] treatment of symptoms with botulinum toxin,[44] and the implantation of weights in the upper eyelid[45] (as well as physical therapy).[46,47] While these are certainly encouraging results, it should be kept in mind that the changes of quality of life after interventions might also be due to improvement in coping with the original disorder responsible for the paresis.

In conclusion, facial paresis has not only physical, but also very strong psychological consequences on emotion, communication, and social life. Even though this is covered only marginally in the literature, it is of high importance for the patient and should be considered in outcome measures. There is already some evidence that therapeutic approaches alleviate the psychological consequences and improve the quality of life. It is recommended that patients are screened and receive counseling for these symptoms if it is deemed necessary, based on the behavior problems described in Box 13.2.

Box 13.2 Recommendations for screening and counseling of psychological symptoms and problematic behaviors in patients with facial palsy

- Ask for the loss of ability to produce emotional contagion in other persons
- Ask for the impression that feelings and emotions cannot be expressed satisfactorily
- Report of incidences where the patient was confronted in a hurtful and aggressive way because of his or her looks
- Ask for avoidance of social contacts and social isolation
- Ask for the impression of negative evaluation by others
- Ask and quantify higher levels of distress, anxiety, and signs of depression
- Quantify changes in quality of life

13.5 Key Points

- Facial palsy has not only a severe impact on facial motor functions, but also on social and emotional interactions. These psychological aspects of the disorder are often underestimated and should be addressed in research and clinical practice.
- Emotions have a biological origin and possess universal properties across all cultures and ages. They have important functions for survival, and they are crucial for social interactions and to establish relationships. Emotions are closely tied to physiological processes and many investigators believe that physiological changes have a direct impact on emotions.
- The mirror neuron system is active when the same action is performed or perceived by a human or nonhuman primate. Based on a simulation process, it is presumably the necessary neural correlate to develop empathy, to distinguish between self and others, and to get a sense for similarity between oneself and others.
- Patients with facial palsy often suffer from depression and increased anxiety. Their quality of life is reduced and they report social isolation and withdrawal. Several treatments have led to an increase in quality of life. Thus, measures of quality of life and of depression and anxiety constitute important outcome measures.

References

[1] Melvin TA, Limb CJ. Overview of facial paralysis: current concepts. Facial Plast Surg 2008; 24: 155–163

[2] Sardesai MG, Moe K. Recent progress in facial paralysis: advances and obstacles. Curr Opin Otolaryngol Head Neck Surg 2010; 18: 266–271

[3] Lindsay RW, Robinson M, Hadlock TA. Comprehensive facial rehabilitation improves function in people with facial paralysis: a 5-year experience at the Massachusetts Eye and Ear Infirmary. Phys Ther 2010; 90: 391–397

[4] Oatley K, Keltner D, Jenkins MJ. Understanding Emotion. Oxford: Blackwell Publishing; 2006

[5] Darwin C. The Expression of the Emotions in Man and Animals. London: John Murray; 1872

[6] Bruce V, Young A. Understanding face recognition. Br J Psychol 1986; 77: 305–327

[7] Haxby JV, Hoffman EA, Gobbini MI. The distributed human neural system for face perception. Trends Cogn Sci 2000; 4: 223–233

[8] Bowlby J. Attachment. Attachment and Loss Vol. 1. 2nd edn. New York, NY: Basic Books; [1969] (1999)

[9] Ekman P. Facial expression and emotion. Am Psychol 1993; 48: 384–392

[10] Aviezer H, Hassin RR, Ryan J et al. Angry, disgusted, or afraid? Studies on the malleability of emotion perception. Psychol Sci 2008; 19: 724–732

[11] Aviezer H, Bentin S, Dudarev V, Hassin RR. The automaticity of emotional face-context integration. Emotion 2011; 11: 1406–1414

[12] Baron-Cohen S. Mindblindness: An Essay on Autism and Theory of Mind. Cambridge, MA: MIT Press; 1997

[13] Schulte-Rüther M, Markowitsch HJ, Fink GR, Piefke M. Mirror neuron and theory of mind mechanisms involved in face-to-face interactions: a functional magnetic resonance imaging approach to empathy. J Cogn Neurosci 2007; 19: 1354–1372

[14] Cattaneo L, Rizzolatti G. The mirror neuron system. Arch Neurol 2009; 66: 557–560

[15] Gallese V. The roots of empathy: the shared manifold hypothesis and the neural basis of intersubjectivity. Psychopathology 2003; 36: 171–180

[16] Lang PJ. The varieties of emotional experience: a meditation on James-Lange theory. Psychol Rev 1994; 101: 211–221

[17] James W. What is an emotion? Mind 1884; 9: 188–205

[18] Cannon WB. The James-Lange theory of emotions: a critical examination and an alternative theory. By Walter B. Cannon, 1927. Am J Psychol 1987; 100: 567–586

[19] Levenson RW, Ekman P, Friesen WV. Voluntary facial action generates emotion-specific autonomic nervous system activity. Psychophysiology 1990; 27: 363–384

[20] Zajonc RB, Murphy ST, Inglehart M. Feeling and facial efference: implications of the vascular theory of emotion. Psychol Rev 1989; 96: 395–416

[21] Strack F, Martin LL, Stepper S. Inhibiting and facilitating conditions of the human smile: a nonobtrusive test of the facial feedback hypothesis. J Pers Soc Psychol 1988; 54: 768–777

[22] Davis JI, Senghas A, Brandt F, Ochsner KN. The effects of BOTOX injections on emotional experience. Emotion 2010; 10: 433–440

[23] Levelt WJM. Speaking: From Intention to Articulation. Cambridge, MA: MIT Press; 1989

[24] Wild B, Erb M, Bartels M. Are emotions contagious? Evoked emotions while viewing emotionally expressive faces: quality, quantity, time course and gender differences. Psychiatry Res 2001; 102: 109–124

[25] Falkenberg I, Bartels M, Wild B. Keep smiling! Facial reactions to emotional stimuli and their relationship to emotional contagion in patients with schizophrenia. Eur Arch Psychiatry Clin Neurosci 2008; 258: 245–253

[26] Keillor JM, Barrett AM, Crucian GP, Kortenkamp S, Heilman KM. Emotional experience and perception in the absence of facial feedback. J Int Neuropsychol Soc 2002; 8: 130–135

[27] Coulson SE, O'Dwyer NJ, Adams RD, Croxson GR. Expression of emotion and quality of life after facial nerve paralysis. Otol Neurotol 2004; 25: 1014–1019

[28] Sonnby-Borgström M, Jönsson P, Svensson O. Gender differences in facial imitation and verbally reported emotional contagion from spontaneous to emotionally regulated processing levels. Scand J Psychol 2008; 49: 111–122

[29] Ishii LE, Godoy A, Encarnacion CO, Byrne PJ, Boahene KD, Ishii M. What faces reveal: impaired affect display in facial paralysis. Laryngoscope 2011; 121: 1138–1143

[30] Bradbury ET, Simons W, Sanders R. Psychological and social factors in reconstructive surgery for hemi-facial palsy. J Plast Reconstr Aesthet Surg 2006; 59: 272–278

[31] Ishii L, Godoy A, Encarnacion CO, Byrne PJ, Boahene KD, Ishii M. Not just another face in the crowd: society's perceptions of facial paralysis. Laryngoscope 2012; 122: 533–538

[32] Dey JK, Ishii M, Boahene KDO, Byrne PJ, Ishii LE. Facial reanimation surgery restores affect display. Otol Neurotol 2014; 35: 182–187

[33] Dey JK, Ishii M, Boahene KDO, Byrne PJ, Ishii LE. Changing perception: facial reanimation surgery improves attractiveness and decreases negative facial perception. Laryngoscope 2014; 124: 84–90

[34] Godoy A, Ishii M, Byrne PJ, Boahene KD, Encarnacion CO, Ishii LE. How facial lesions impact attractiveness and perception: differential effects of size and location. Laryngoscope 2011; 121: 2542–2547

[35] Macgregor FC. Facial disfigurement: problems and management of social interaction and implications for mental health. Aesthetic Plast Surg 1990; 14: 249–257

[36] Brach JS, VanSwearingen J, Delitto A, Johnson PC. Impairment and disability in patients with facial neuromuscular dysfunction. Otolaryngol Head Neck Surg 1997; 117: 315–321

[37] VanSwearingen JM, Cohn JF, Turnbull J, Mrzai T, Johnson P. Psychological distress: linking impairment with disability in facial neuromotor disorders. Otolaryngol Head Neck Surg 1998; 118: 790–796

[38] Vanswearingen J. Facial rehabilitation: a neuromuscular reeducation, patient-centered approach. Facial Plast Surg 2008; 24: 250–259

[39] Fu L, Bundy C, Sadiq SA. Psychological distress in people with disfigurement from facial palsy. Eye (Lond) 2011; 25: 1322–1326

[40] Ho AL, Scott AM, Klassen AF, Cano SJ, Pusic AL, Van Laeken N. Measuring quality of life and patient satisfaction in facial paralysis patients: a systematic review of patient-reported outcome measures. Plast Reconstr Surg 2012; 130: 91–99

[41] Kahn JB, Gliklich RE, Boyev KP, Stewart MG, Metson RB, McKenna MJ. Validation of a patient-graded instrument for facial nerve paralysis: the FaCE scale. Laryngoscope 2001; 111: 387–398

[42] VanSwearingen JM, Brach JS. The Facial Disability Index: reliability and validity of a disability assessment instrument for disorders of the facial neuromuscular system. Phys Ther 1996; 76: 1288–1298, discussion 1298–1300

[43] Guntinas-Lichius O, Straesser A, Streppel M. Quality of life after facial nerve repair. Laryngoscope 2007; 117: 421–426

[44] Henstrom DK, Lindsay RW, Cheney ML, Hadlock TA. Surgical treatment of the periocular complex and improvement of quality of life in patients with facial paralysis. Arch Facial Plast Surg 2011; 13: 125–128

[45] Salles AG, Toledo PN, Ferreira MC. Botulinum toxin injection in long-standing facial paralysis patients: improvement of facial symmetry observed up to 6 months. Aesthetic Plast Surg 2009; 33: 582–590

[46] Beurskens CH, Heymans PG. Physiotherapy in patients with facial nerve paresis: description of outcomes. Am J Otolaryngol 2004; 25: 394–400

[47] Pereira LM, Obara K, Dias JM, Menacho MO, Lavado EL, Cardoso JR. Facial exercise therapy for facial palsy: systematic review and meta-analysis. Clin Rehabil 2011; 25: 649–658

14 Diagnostic and Therapeutic Approaches to Emotional and Social Impairments in Patients with Facial Paresis

Christian Dobel and Orlando Guntinas-Lichius

14.1 Introduction

Chapter 13 explored the psychological aspects that often come along with facial paresis. These issues are often overlooked and underestimated by the physician even though they are of great importance for patients. The psychological consequences range from changed abilities to express emotions, to encounters of aggressive and hurtful incidences, to severe depression and anxiety, and as such are often accompanied by avoidance of social contacts and isolation. Thus, not surprisingly, the perceived quality of life is reduced. Similar effects have been observed for other disorders resulting in facial disfigurement, but there is a general lack of awareness for these psychological processes.

In this chapter, the authors summarize the diagnostic methods and procedures that exist to assess the psychological consequences of facial palsy and the therapeutic approaches that can be taken. While some of these methods and approaches are empirically well established and are used frequently in several medical fields, others call for systematic investigations and research.

> **!**
>
> Many patients with facial palsy suffer not only from a lack of motor function but equally, or even more so, from the psychological implications. This is best detected using a psychological assessment tool.

14.2 Diagnosis of Emotional and Social Symptoms

14.2.1 Assessment of General Anxiety, Social Anxiety, and Distress

Measuring individual levels of anxiety and distress has a long history in psychological research. In addition to physiological measures (skin conductance, pulse, blood pressure, etc.), behavioral measures (self-reports of alcohol and drug consumption, sleeping patterns, etc.) and especially questionnaires are the most prominent tools to assess anxiety and distress. While questionnaires lack the comprehensiveness and specificity of individual psychological testing or a detailed medical examination, they may serve as standardized tools that are easily applicable and feasible in most clinical settings; see ▶ Table 14.1 for an overview of questionnaires.

Symptom Checklist 90

One of the most widely used instruments to measure psychological distress for clinical and research purposes is the Symptom Checklist 90 (SCL-90-R).[1] The SCL-90-R is a self-report instrument to evaluate a broad range of psychological concerns. It consists of 90 items (each on a five-point Likert scale) and can be completed within 15 minutes. Nine primary symptom dimensions are assessed (somatization, obsessive-compulsive, interpersonal sensitivity, depression, anxiety, hostility, phobic anxiety, paranoid ideation, and psychoticism). These dimensions yield three global distress indices: the global severity index, the positive symptom total, and the positive symptom distress index. The existing norms are gender-keyed and exist for community nonpatients, psychiatric outpatients, psychiatric inpatients, and adolescent nonpatients. The SCL-90-R exists in over 24 languages and is used worldwide. Due to its high psychometric quality regarding reliability and validity, the SCL-90-R is used not only for individual assessment, but also to measure treatment outcome and therapeutic progress. This instrument can be administered and analyzed electronically. For patients with facial palsy it is a very useful instrument to get an impression of the amount of general distress due to the illness.

> The Symptom Checklist 90 is a reliable 15-minute self-administered instrument providing an overview of the level of distress of the patient related to their facial palsy

State-Trait Anxiety Inventory

In contrast to the SCL-90-R, the State-Trait Anxiety Inventory (STAI)[2] puts a focus on anxiety. While stress is often accompanied by feelings of tension and anxiety, they do not refer to the same construct. The STAI is also a self-administered questionnaire, which can be completed within 10 minutes. It consists of 40 questions on a four-point Likert scale. The psychometric quality is high and

Table 14.1 List and characteristics of important questionnaires and scales for the diagnosis of stress, social anxiety, depression, and quality of life

Name (abbreviation)	What does it measure?	Available languages
General aspects of health and perceived impairment of a disease		
Symptom Checklist 90 (SCL-90) and revised version (SCL-90-R)	Subjectively perceived psychological and/or physical impairment and burden of a disorder	English, Spanish, French, German
Short Form Health Survey (SF-36)	Broad measure of health status	More than 50
Anxiety in general and social anxiety		
State-Trait Anxiety Inventory (STAI)	State anxiety about events and anxiety as a stable personality characteristic	English, Spanish, French, German, Chinese, Danish, Dutch, Finnish, Italian, Norwegian, Portuguese, Swedish, Thai
Liebowitz Social Anxiety Scale (LSAS)	Fear and avoidance of a variety of social situations	English, Spanish, French, Hebrew, Turkish, German
Social Interaction Anxiety Scale (SIAS) and Social Phobia Scale (SPS)	Fear of being scrutinized by others (SPS) and fear of social interactions (SIAS)	English, Spanish, German
Depression		
Beck Depression Inventory (BDI)	General symptoms of depression	Multiple including Arabic, Chinese, Japanese
Hospital Anxiety and Depression Scale (HADS)	Anxiety and depression in persons with physical illness	Multiple including Arabic and Chinese
Specific measures for neuromuscular disorders		
Facial Disability Index (FDI)	Perceived impairment due to a neuromuscular disorder	English, Spanish, Swedish, Italian
Facial Clinimetric Evaluation (FaCE)	Facial impairment and disability	English
All measures are self-report measures that are easy applicable, validated, and can be complemented in a few minutes.		

retesting is possible. One of the advantages of this instrument is the assessment of transient feelings of anxiety (i. e., state dependent on situations) as well as a general proneness to anxiety (i.e., trait anxiety as a personal characteristic stable over time and situations). Thus, the measurement of state anxiety gives the clinician an impression of how well the patient deals with his/her current situation and the illness. In contrast, trait anxiety tells the clinician about illness-independent characteristics of a patient and the general level of his/her anxiety. Thus, the STAI is a very useful tool for clinicians to distinguish state and trait anxiety. Similar to the SCL-90-R, there are versions in several languages and norms exist for various populations.

> **!**
>
> The State-Trait Anxiety Inventory can be used to obtain a measure of the general level of anxiety of the patient.

It was outlined in the Introduction to this chapter that avoidance of social situations and social isolation may accompany the physical aspects of facial palsy. As such the authors recommend some questionnaires and scales that have been specifically developed for the diagnosis of social anxiety.

Liebowitz Social Anxiety Scale

The Liebowitz Social Anxiety Scale (LSAS)[3] is a brief questionnaire that measures the degree to which persons fear and avoid social situations. While the original version was administered by clinicians, there is also a self-administered version (LSAS-SR) that is probably more suitable for the physician caring for patients with facial paralysis.[4] It consists of 24 questions with two subscales (fear and avoidance) in which the patients has to answer on a four-point Likert scale to what level he/she fears and avoids specific social situations such as eating and drinking in public. He/she is asked to answer the questions with regard to the past week. The scoring scale categorizes the responses in five steps from no/mild to very severe social anxiety. Several online versions exist on the internet (for instance: http://www.socialanxietysupport.com/disorder/liebowitz/) and thus it is an easily applicable instrument that has found wide use in clinical and research settings.

Social Interaction Anxiety Scale and Social Phobia Scale

The Social Interaction Anxiety Scale (SIAS) and Social Phobia Scale (SPS) are two companion scales to measure different aspects of social phobia.[5] While the SPS measures the patients' fear of being evaluated during routine activities like eating and drinking, the SIAS focuses on more general social interactions. Usually, the two scales are administered together. Both scales have 20 items with a five-point Likert scale that can be completed and scored within several minutes. There are cut-off scores to indicate social phobia or more generalized social anxiety. The scales have very good psychometric qualities, and provide good internal consistency and test–retest reliability. They do not correlate with symptoms of depression, state and trait anxiety, locus of control, and social desirability. The scales were proven to respond to treatment success and thus they are recommended to be used for clinical and research applications.

14.2.2 Assessment of Depressive Symptoms

Beck Depression Inventory

The Beck Depression Inventory (BDI)[6] is a multiple-choice self-report inventory that is widely used in clinical practice as well as in research to measure the severity of depressive symptoms. The BDI is often used to monitor changes over time and the response of patients to treatment and therapy. It consists of 21 questions and can be administered within 10 minutes. The answers vary in intensity and are scored accordingly (e.g., 0, I do not feel sad; 1, I feel sad; 2, I am sad all the time and I can't snap out of it; 3, I am so sad or unhappy that I can't stand it). The BDI measures somatic aspects of depression (fatigue, loss of energy, lack of interest in sex, etc.) as well as affective aspects (feelings of being punished, guilt, etc.). There are currently three versions. In contrast to the original BDI, BDI-IA improved the ease of use, but the questionnaire did not address several symptoms for depression specified in the *Diagnostic and Statistical Manual of Mental Disorders*, 3rd edition (DSM-III). This and other criticisms were addressed in the revised version BDI-II.[7] BDI-II correlates highly with the Hamilton Rating Scale for Depression (HRSD),[8] which is used by trained clinicians to evaluate depressive symptoms of patients. There is also a short version of the BDI: BDI-FS (fast screen)[9] in which the somatic criteria have been removed. This was done in order to improve the diagnostic validity of this instrument for patients with illnesses in which the inclusion of the somatic criteria would have led to an overestimation of depression (e.g., multiple sclerosis, chronic pain, drug abuse) As for the instruments described above, versions of the BDI exist for multiple languages.

Note that if patients score high on the item on suicidal ideation, caution is warranted and it is recommended that a trained psychotherapist becomes involved. This is especially the case if a patient also reaches high levels on the Beck Hopelessness Scale (BHS).[10] This brief self-report instrument consists of 20 items that measure negative feelings and attitudes towards the future.

> The Beck Depression Inventory in its different versions is an international standardized tool to assess depressive symptoms of patients with facial palsy. If a patient exhibits suicidal thoughts and feelings of hopelessness, a psychiatrist or psychotherapist should always be involved.

Hospital Anxiety and Depression Scale

The Hospital Anxiety and Depression Scale (HADS) was developed to measure depression and anxiety in patients experiencing health problems.[11] It is quite brief and consists of 14 items: half devoted to the measurement of anxiety and half to depression. The items put a special focus on somatic aspects of depression and anxiety (fatigue, insomnia, or hypersomnia) that are also common in other health problems. In contrast to the methods described previously, it is not as thoroughly investigated and validated, but it is nevertheless used in a large number of clinical studies.[12]

> !
>
> The Hospital Anxiety and Depression Scale is an instrument to quickly assess anxiety and depressive symptoms at the same time. Although widely used, it does not have the validity of the more comprehensive questionnaires described above.

14.2.3 Assessment of Quality of Life and Social Functioning

Short Form Health Survey

For the assessment of quality of life, the Short Form Health Survey (SF-36) is an instrument that is widely employed; see Chapter 7. It consists of eight sections (vitality, physical functioning, bodily pain, general health perceptions, physical role functioning, emotional role functioning, social role functioning, and mental health). The administration of the test requires 5 to 10 minutes and can be given by persons with basic training in psychometrics and statistics. The SF-36 is most often used to measure individual health status, the impact and burden of an illness on a patient's life, as well as the effectiveness of treatment. It has been repeatedly used in national health surveys and there are versions in different languages as well as normative data for several countries and different populations.[13] The psychometric qualities of the instrument are good. The questionnaire has been used in patients with facial palsy and facial nerve reconstruction.[14] Even though facial function improved after nerve repair, patients reported impaired quality of life. This serves as an example that the psychological burden of a disease does not always run in parallel with the physical impairments. In such cases we recommend consulting a psychotherapist.

!

The Short Form Health Survey is the gold standard to measure general quality of life. A considerable advantage is that data exist from a variety of diseases making it possible to compare patients with facial palsy with those with other maladies.

Facial Disability Index and Facial Clinimetric Evaluation

While the SF-36 was designed to cover a broad range of health problems including impairments in social functioning, two questionnaires exist that were specifically designed for patients with facial neuromuscular disorders: the Facial Disability Index (FDI)[15] and the Facial Clinimetric Evaluation (FaCE).[16] FDI is administered by a clinician and FaCE is self-administered; both questionnaires are described in detail in Chapter 7. They contain several questions regarding physical impairments, but also the reduction of social activities following the illness. FDI is focused more on oral functions while FaCE covers different functions relevant for specific parts of the face. Thus, FaCE is somewhat more detailed, but both can be completed within 10 minutes. For FDI, there are currently English, Spanish,[17] Swedish,[18] and Italian[19] versions, and a German version is currently validated.[20]

As described in more detail in Chapter 13, these tests have been used in patients with facial palsy and they have demonstrated that an improvement of quality of life can be registered after treatment.

The Facial Disability Index and the Facial Clinimetric Evaluation instrument measure how quality of life is affected by the facial palsy more specifically than the measures obtained by the more global Short Form Health Survey instrument.

Given the usability, the psychometric qualities of these instruments, as well as the importance for patients, it is highly recommended to use them for research, and also in daily practice, especially to monitor effectiveness of therapeutic measures.

In contrast to the instruments described above, the assessment of emotional changes in patients with facial paresis has not been specifically investigated and the instruments able to do this need to be developed and evaluated systematically.

!

A standard validated instrument to measure emotional changes in patients with facial palsy is lacking.

14.2.4 Guidance for Clinicians

Having presented these different measures and scales, the question arises of which are recommended for frequent use and daily practice. It is suggested that each patient is asked in a first interview or in follow-up sessions which physical and psychological consequences are most difficult and inhibiting. If a patient does not mention any psychological symptoms himself/herself, the clinician should ask directly if he feels depressed or overly anxious in social situations. To get more precise measures, we suggest applying BDI–II, and if someone reaches moderate-to-high levels for suicidal ideation BHS should be administered in addition. In cases where a patient scores high on suicidal ideation and/or hopelessness, a trained psychotherapist should be consulted immediately. Because social isolation and withdrawal is frequent in patients with facial palsy, it is suggested that SIAS and SPS is also measured in every patient, or, alternatively, LSAS. SIAS and SPS give a somewhat more detailed image of social behavior and they possess very good psychometric qualities. Thus, for research questions they seem favorable. SF-36 measures quality of life with a very broad view and gives the clinician a more general impression of the burden of the disease. Even though FDI and FaCE are not as widely used as the other instruments, the authors recommend their use in every patient, because they are specifically designed for patients with disorders of the facial muscles. All of the measures described above can be used to monitor and track the effectiveness of treatment and surgery and can be applied repeatedly. This has been done for various disorders. If the clinicians have the impression that the physical aspects of facial lesions improved after treatment, but the psychological ones did not, it is suggested that colleagues from psychosomatic or psychiatric departments are consulted. The other mentioned measures are highly useful for research and/or to get a more detailed and broader image if a

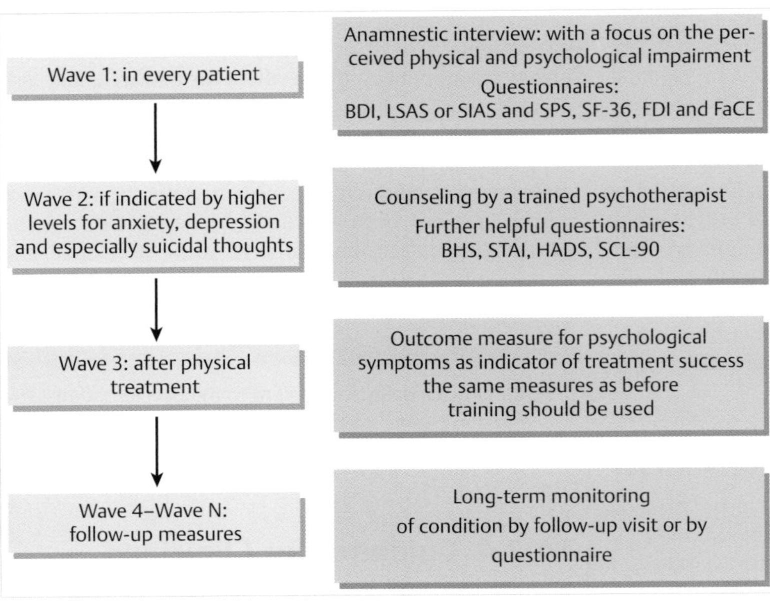

Fig. 14.1 Flowchart for the diagnosis of anxiety and depression in patients with facial palsy. BDI, Beck Depression Inventory; BHS, Beck Hopelessness Scale; FaCE, Facial Clinimetric Evaluation; FDI, Facial Disability Index; HADS, Hospital Anxiety and Depression Scale; LSAS, Liebowitz Social Anxiety Scale; SCL-90, Symptom Checklist 90; SF-36, Short Form Health Survey; SIAS, Social Interaction Anxiety Scale; SPS, Social Phobia Scale; STAI, State-Trait Anxiety Inventory.

patient scores high on measures of depression and anxiety. A flowchart is presented in ▶ Fig. 14.1.

> **!**
>
> If facial motor functions improve but psychological function of the patients does not improve, it is recommended that the patient is referred to a psychologist.

14.3 Assessment of Emotional Functions

The ability to express different emotions can be assessed by directly asking patients to express basic emotions ("Please show me how you look surprised/happy/angry," etc.). Alternatively a context can be provided for which an appropriate emotional face should be shown ("Imagine that you greet dear family members that you haven't seen for a long time. Can you show me how you would do that?"). These events can be taken by the treating physician as an indication of which emotions are particularly impaired and inhibited. There are online courses provided by Paul Ekman (http://www.paulekman.com/product-category/face-training/) in which the ability to recognize even subtle emotions can be strengthened.

Given the dissociation between voluntary and spontaneous emotional expression in facial paresis, psychologists/psychiatrists often measure emotional expressions in a more spontaneous manner, e.g., in response to film clips, videos, or similar material. This also allows videorecording the patient to document changes in response to treatment. Ratings from several raters can be used to document the perceived changes in an objective manner using Self-Assessment Manikins, which are described later in this section.

As outlined in Chapter 13, because of the importance of expressing emotions, the authors recommend performing a validated instrument evaluation in each patient and especially if surgery is used to reestablish improved functioning.

> **!**
>
> Emotional expression is different from simple facial motor function. A patient might have improved motor function after facial nerve reconstruction but emotional expression might not have been improved in the same manner.

The authors also propose that practitioners measure the perception of emotional faces, e.g., the classic examples from Ekman and Friesen[21] are the basis on which the "Ekman 60 Faces Test" was developed.[22] Alternatively, there are several other databases containing emotional faces for which norms from different populations have been recorded.[23,24] Notably, there is also a database for emotional faces that were taken in a natural, conversational context.[25] Because these pictures were taken repeatedly, with different intensities and from different angles, they give the researcher and clinician the possibility for repeated assessments without the danger of presenting the very same material twice. To rate the emotional quality of all kinds of emotional stimuli, a widely used method, in addition to a mere classification, is the measurement of arousal (how calm or arousing a stimulus is) and valence (if a stimulus is perceived as positive or negative). For this purpose, Self-Assessment Manikins are usually employed,[26] i.e., little graphic figures expressing somatic arousal or positive/negative emotions. Participants are asked to mark their emotional reaction (arousal or valence) on a continuous scale in response to each item. Using these measures clinicians and researchers can easily determine which aspects of emotional perception are altered.

Taken together, the authors encourage clinicians to determine with established instruments, and also in an explorative way, which emotional and social changes patients perceive in themselves and in others. They should also be asked if they have encountered hurtful and stigmatizing situations based on their looks. If necessary, counsel should be provided by trained therapists.

14.4 Therapeutic Approaches to Address Emotional and Social Changes

Given the importance of intact emotional expression for the social life of patients, the authors suggest exploring the patient's ability to express emotions for therapeutic purposes also. As already proposed by others,[27] treating clinicians and surgeons should not only target the re-establishment of mere physical functions, but also the ability to express emotions. If a detailed investigation is performed in which emotional expressions are particularly impaired, this can provide the basis for standard physical therapy.[28] It is recommended that the perception of both the patients and their relatives is taken into account. Studies analyzing the effect of psychological therapy in patients with facial palsy have not yet been published.

To make patients and their relatives more sensitive to these psychological issues, it is possible to establish group sessions and family training. These are easy to establish and have proven useful in other contexts such as in depression[29] and anxiety disorders.[30] They seem particularly advisable if the measures recommended above give an indication of heightened levels of depression and anxiety. Patients and their relatives can be taught how to express emotions by means other than the face. Verbal expression and body language are particularly highly recommended. Relatives can then give feedback if an intended emotion was well communicated and perceived. Such efforts can be supported by professional actors that can teach which verbal means and which gestures are particularly suited to provoke emotional contagion. Emotional contagion describes the tendency for two individuals to emotionally converge. Similar approaches for mime therapy have been well documented and evaluated.[31] Unfortunately, to date, patients with facial paralysis have not received family therapy to the extent that it is has been used in other emotional conditions. The authors recommend that this is addressed in future research.

> **!**
>
> So far there has been a failure of integrating the relatives of the patients into therapy as is standard in many other comparable diseases.

For the recovery of motor function after stroke, one of the most successful therapies is Constraint-Induced Movement Therapy.[32,33] In this therapy patients are forced to intensively use the affected body part while at the same time movements of the unaffected body parts are strongly restricted; more details are given in Chapter 26. As a consequence patients cannot but use the affected body part and the learned nonuse of body parts is avoided. Such an approach in the rehabilitation of facial palsy can be enhanced by biofeedback and the use of surface electromyography.[34] To gain the most from such approaches, it is necessary that patients train by themselves in a very intense manner and thus are only occasionally supervised by therapists. Their progress can be monitored in an automated computer-based way. Most computers have a camera and the recorded videos can be transmitted to the treating physician to evaluate progress. Based on recent findings regarding the facial feedback hypothesis; see Chapter 13, it is expected that improvements in expressing positive emotions will parallel improved wellbeing and reduced depressive symptoms.[35]

14.5 Key Points

- Several easily applicable and well-documented methods exist to measure depression, anxiety, and quality of life. These measures should be used for clinical and research purposes, especially to document improvement after treatment.
- In addition to a first explorative interview, we recommend to use the at least one of the following instruments: the Beck Depression Inventory II, the Social Interaction Anxiety Scale, and the Social Phobia Scale (alternatively the Liebowitz Social Anxiety Scale) as measures for depression and social fear in each patient. The Short Form Health Survey is a broader instrument to get an impression of the perceived quality of life.
- If patients score high on suicidal ideation and hopelessness, trained psychiatrists or psychotherapists should become involved.
- Apart from physical improvement, treatment should also focus on improvement of expression of facial emotions. Thus, the ability to express emotions and its response to treatment must be assessed. This can be done on photographs or videos of patients using Self-Assess-

ment Manikins. Nevertheless, such issues must be addressed in future research.

- Even though they have not been investigated intensively, it seems advisable to incorporate emotional factors in treatment.

References

[1] Derogatis LR, Savitz KL. The SCL-90-R, brief symptom inventory, and matching clinical rating scales. In: Maruish ME, ed. The Use of Psychological Testing for Treatment Planning and Outcomes Assessment. Mahwah, NJ: Erlbaum; 1999:679–724

[2] Spielberger CD, Gorsuch RL, Lushene R, Vagg PR, Jacobs GA. Manual for the State-Trait Anxiety Inventory. Palo Alto, CA: Consulting Psychologists Press; 1983

[3] Liebowitz MR. Social phobia. Mod Probl Pharmacopsychiatry 1987; 22: 141–173

[4] Rytwinski NK, Fresco DM, Heimberg RG et al. Screening for social anxiety disorder with the self-report version of the Liebowitz Social Anxiety Scale. Depress Anxiety 2009; 26: 34–38

[5] Mattick RP, Clarke JC. Development and validation of measures of social phobia scrutiny fear and social interaction anxiety. Behav Res Ther 1998; 36: 455–470

[6] Beck AT, Ward CH, Mendelson M, Mock J, Erbaugh J. An inventory for measuring depression. Arch Gen Psychiatry 1961; 4: 561–571

[7] Beck AT, Steer RA, Ball R, Ranieri W. Comparison of Beck depression inventories -IA and -II in psychiatric outpatients. J Pers Assess 1996; 67: 588–597

[8] Hamilton M. Rating depressive patients. J Clin Psychiatry 1980; 41: 21–24

[9] Beck AT, Steer RA, Brown GK. BDI-Fast Screen for Medical Patients, Manual. San Antonio, TX: The Psychological Corporation; 2000

[10] Beck AT. Beck Hopelessness Scale. San Antonio, TX: The Psychological Corporation; 1988

[11] Zigmond AS, Snaith RP. The hospital anxiety and depression scale. Acta Psychiatr Scand 1983; 67: 361–370

[12] Bjelland I, Dahl AA, Haug TT, Neckelmann D. The validity of the Hospital Anxiety and Depression Scale. An updated literature review. J Psychosom Res 2002; 52: 69–77

[13] Ware JE Jr, Kosinski M, Keller SD. SF 36 Physical and Mental Health Summary Scales: A User's Manual. Boston, MA: The Health Institute; 1994

[14] Guntinas-Lichius O, Straesser A, Streppel M. Quality of life after facial nerve repair. Laryngoscope 2007; 117: 421–426

[15] VanSwearingen JM, Brach JS. The Facial Disability Index: reliability and validity of a disability assessment instrument for disorders of the facial neuromuscular system. Phys Ther 1996; 76: 1288–1298, discussion 1298–1300

[16] Kahn JB, Gliklich RE, Boyev KP, Stewart MG, Metson RB, McKenna MJ. Validation of a patient-graded instrument for facial nerve paralysis: the FaCE scale. Laryngoscope 2001; 111: 387–398

[17] Gonzalez-Cardero E, Infante-Cossio P, Cayuela A, Acosta-Feria M, Gutierrez-Perez JL. Facial disability index (FDI): adaptation to Spanish, reliability and validity. Med Oral Patol Oral Cir Bucal 2012; 17: e1006–e1012

[18] Marsk E, Hammarstedt-Nordenvall L, Engström M, Jonsson L, Hultcrantz M. Validation of a Swedish version of the Facial Disability Index (FDI) and the Facial Clinimetric Evaluation (FaCE) scale. Acta Otolaryngol 2013; 133: 662–669

[19] Pavese C, Cecini M, Camerino N et al. Functional and social limitations after facial palsy: expanded and independent validation of the Italian version of the facial disability index. Phys Ther 2014; 94: 1327–1336

[20] Dobel C, Miltner WHR, Witte OW, Volk GF, Guntinas-Lichius O. Emotional impact of facial palsy [in German] Laryngorhinootologie 2013; 92: 9–23

[21] Ekman P, Friesen W. Pictures of Facial Affect. Palo Alto, CA: Consulting Psychologists Press; 1976

[22] Diehl-Schmid J, Pohl C, Ruprecht C, Wagenpfeil S, Foerstl H, Kurz A. The Ekman 60 Faces Test as a diagnostic instrument in frontotemporal dementia. Arch Clin Neuropsychol 2007; 22: 459–464

[23] Kennedy KM, Hope K, Raz N. Life span adult faces: norms for age, familiarity, memorability, mood, and picture quality. Exp Aging Res 2009; 35: 268–275

[24] Ebner NC, Riediger M, Lindenberger U. FACES—a database of facial expressions in young, middle-aged, and older women and men: development and validation. Behav Res Methods 2010; 42: 351–362

[25] Kaulard K, Cunningham DW, Bülthoff HH, Wallraven C. The MPI facial expression database—a validated database of emotional and conversational facial expressions. PLoS ONE 2012; 7: e32321

[26] Lang PJ. Behavioral treatment and biobehavioral assessment: computer applications. In: Sidowski B, Johnson JH, Williams TA, eds. Technology in Mental Health Care Delivery Systems. Norwood, NJ: Ablex; 1980

[27] Vanswearingen J. Facial rehabilitation: a neuromuscular reeducation, patient-centered approach. Facial Plast Surg 2008; 24: 250–259

[28] Pereira LM, Obara K, Dias JM, Menacho MO, Lavado EL, Cardoso JR. Facial exercise therapy for facial palsy: systematic review and meta-analysis. Clin Rehabil 2011; 25: 649–658

[29] Luciano M, Del Vecchio V, Giacco D, De Rosa C, Malangone C, Fiorillo A. A 'family affair'? The impact of family psychoeducational interventions on depression. Expert Rev Neurother 2012; 12: 83–91, quiz 92

[30] Chambless DL. Adjunctive couple and family intervention for patients with anxiety disorders. J Clin Psychol 2012; 68: 548–560

[31] Beurskens CH, Heymans PG. Mime therapy improves facial symmetry in people with long-term facial nerve paresis: a randomised controlled trial. Aust J Physiother 2006; 52: 177–183

[32] Miltner WH, Bauder H, Sommer M, Dettmers C, Taub E. Effects of constraint-induced movement therapy on patients with chronic motor deficits after stroke: a replication. Stroke 1999; 30: 586–592

[33] Morris DM, Taub E. Constraint-induced movement therapy. In: O'Sullivan SB, Schmitz TJ, eds. Improving Functional Outcome in Physical Rehabilitation. Philadelphia, PA: F.A. Davis; 2012

[34] Brown DM, Nahai F, Wolf S, Basmajian JV. Electromyographic biofeedback in the reeducation of facial palsy. Am J Phys Med 1978; 57: 183–190

[35] Lewis MB. Exploring the positive and negative implications of facial feedback. Emotion 2012; 12: 852–859

Part V

Surgery around the Facial Nerve

V

15 Intraoperative Facial Nerve Monitoring

Brent J. Benscoter and Jack M. Kartush

15.1 Introduction

The facial nerve is at risk of iatrogenic injury in many surgical procedures. Because even the most experienced surgeon may inadvertently injure the nerve, intraoperative neurophysiologic monitoring (IOM) has evolved as a helpful adjunct to reduce the incidence of neural trauma. While monitoring is clearly not a substitute for training and experience, facial nerve monitoring is now commonplace in neurotology and has become increasingly used in many otologic and head and neck procedures.

There is a growing industry of technologists specifically trained to assist surgeons in the operating room, especially for complex, multimodality monitoring such as the use of electromyography (EMG) in conjunction with somatosensory evoked potentials (SSEPs) and transcranial motor evoked potentials during scoliosis surgery.

In contrast, the surgeon typically performs single modality monitoring such as facial or recurrent laryngeal EMG. This requires that the surgeon be trained in both the technical and the interpretive aspects of monitoring because "poor monitoring is worse than no monitoring."[1–3,4–6] Poor monitoring is akin to a soldier relying on a faulty minesweeper—in both circumstances, improper methods or interpretation may actually increase the chance of an adverse outcome by leading to a false sense of security.

Training has not kept pace with the expanding clinical use of IOM. Facial nerve monitoring began to be slowly adopted about 30 years ago but has since had a logarithmic rise in use—without a concomitant rise in IOM training. Not uncommonly, staff and residents learn by word of mouth as the senior resident hurriedly describes electrode placement to the junior resident during preoperative preparation of the patient. Such cursory, on the job, training has led to regrettable deficiencies in both the technical and the interpretive knowledge base for many surgeons, which can result in suboptimal monitoring. To assure the highest level of monitoring, university teaching and private hospital programs must develop a core curriculum of surgeon-directed monitoring with standardized departmental protocols.

This chapter will focus on the neurophysiology of monitoring, technical methods, and common interpretive pitfalls that are often encountered. Understanding and applying these principles in combination with sound surgical technique can minimize the risk of facial nerve injury.

> **!**
>
> There is an urgent need to develop a core curriculum of surgeon-directed facial nerve monitoring with standardized departmental protocols to ensure optimal usage of nerve monitoring.

15.2 History

It is of value to review the history of facial nerve monitoring in order to understand how present-day features and standards have evolved. Facial nerve monitoring was first reported in 1898 by Krause (published by Krause in an English translation in 1912).[7] He used galvanic stimulation and visual facial muscle observation during a cochlear nerve section for tinnitus. In the 1940s, Olivecrona attempted to preserve the facial nerve during acoustic neuroma surgery. He also used a stimulator while a nurse watched for visible facial movement.[8] Advances were made in the 1960s with Parsons,[9] Jako,[10] and Hilger[11] who all independently reported on dedicated monitors to use during otologic and parotid surgery. Jako's method was of interest because it used a mechanical transducer placed on the patient's cheek to assess the response rather than rely on visual inspection.[9] Hilger subsequently also developed a mechanical transducer, which was later enhanced by Silverstein in 1985 (WR Electronics).

EMG monitoring was not described until 1979 by Delgado, who used it for acoustic neuroma surgery.[12] EMG recording has since become the most commonly used method of monitoring due to the increased sensitivity obtained using intramuscular needle electrodes versus a motion detector.

In 1980, Jack Kartush, MD, David Lilly, PhD, and Malcolm Graham, MD, modified an auditory brain stem neurophysiologic device (Amplaid) to allow electric facial nerve stimulation and EMG recording. The normal acoustic signal calibrated in decibels required conversion to constant-current electric stimulation. Audiologists were brought into the operating room to set up the complex equipment array and verbally report to the surgeon anytime they saw an EMG response on the oscilloscope. Of interest, this subsequently led many other audiologists to enter this new field.

Neurologists have long performed EMG by observing not just the visual representation on an oscilloscope but also the acoustic representation when displayed through a loudspeaker. In 1982 Sugita added the benefit of acoustic display of the facial EMG response to directly alert the surgeon rather than relying on another individual to constantly gaze at the oscilloscope.[13]

In 1983, Kartush and Richard Prass, MD, engaged Nicolet Biomedical Company to develop a dedicated constant-current facial nerve monitor with EMG recording displayed both visually and acoustically to allow direct realtime feedback to the surgeon. The device was intended to be simple and focused to reduce complexity and obviate the need to "boot up" a generic computer and related software applications. "Intelligent" features were designed such as electrocautery artifact suppression and alarms to warn the surgeon of disconnected electrodes or high impedances. An electronic gate was implemented to silence the stimulus artifact to prevent the surgeon from confusing the stimulus sound with the response sound. In addition, the raw EMG was also converted to an audible tone to highlight the response in the noisy operating room environment. The response tones had different pitches to let the surgeon know from which EMG channel the response originated. The response tones were also programmed to correlate their volume with the amplitude of the EMG response. To implement the design, Nicolet in turn engaged the departments of otolaryngology at the Massachusetts Eye and Ear Infirmary and Stanford University. This device became known as the nerve integrity monitor (NIM). Dedicated nerve stimulators optimized for microsurgery were also developed. The technology was transferred to Xomed, which itself was later purchased by Medtronic. In 1984, Dr Aage Moller designed a constant-voltage facial nerve stimulator with acoustic display of the response (Grass Corporation). Unfortunately, the device was quickly removed from the market due to liability concerns. In 1992, Michael Gleeson, MD, Tony Strong, MD, and Christopher Hovey developed the Neurosign monitor—a facial nerve stimulator with auditory display and light-emitting diode (LED) lights instead of an oscilloscope to provide a simplified representation of the response's amplitude (Neurosign, The Magstim Company Ltd).

Numerous other dedicated devices have subsequently been designed, but as the monitoring field has expanded to include multimodality monitoring for brain, spine, and vascular procedures, most of these latter day products have been designed with an extraordinary number of features to accommodate many different surgical procedures. However, the inherent complexity that a feature-rich set engenders typically mandates the services of a trained technologist or neurophysiologist. To meet the educational needs of a growing number of individuals with diverse backgrounds engaged in monitoring, Kartush founded the American Society of Neurophysiological Monitoring (ASNM) in 1989. The ASNM provides a forum for education and develops quality standards for practice and training.

15.3 Clinical Application

Avoidance of facial nerve injury is a primary concern across many disciplines including otology, skull base surgery, head and neck surgery, and neurologic surgery. There is no substitute for sound microsurgical skills and thorough knowledge of intracranial, temporal, and extratemporal anatomy of the facial nerve. However, the inherent complexity of the nerve, combined with pathology such as cholesteatoma or tumor, poses challenges with dissection and at times identification of the facial nerve. Great advances have been made over the last century in reducing surgical morbidity and mortality by adopting the operative microscope. Neurophysiologic monitoring may further minimize the risk of nerve injury.

> !
>
> Facial nerve monitoring is of interest for otology, skull base surgery, head and neck surgery, and neurologic surgery. It is routinely used in vestibular schwannoma surgery. Its use in other areas is increasingly common but because there is a lack of equipoise by many surgeons, it is unlikely that a randomized control study will ever be performed for monitoring during mastoid surgery.

There are three main goals of monitoring. First and foremost is nerve identification via "triggered EMG" (electric stimulation), which is of particular value when pathology or anomalies distort the usual anatomical landmarks. Second, monitoring can detect injury during surgical maneuvers. Intramuscular needle EMG recording can allow early detection of stretch or ischemic injury that may not otherwise be apparent to the surgeon. Third, postdissection stimulation can confirm the function of the nerve prior to closure.

Many studies have demonstrated improved postoperative facial nerve outcomes with use of intraoperative monitoring in skull base surgery.[14–18] This led the National Institutes of Health in 1991 to recommend facial monitoring during acoustic neuroma (vestibular schwannoma) surgery.[19]

The impact of facial nerve monitoring during routine otologic surgery is less studied and somewhat controversial. Some surgeons prefer to use monitoring selectively, i.e., higher risk cases. However, it is not always possible to predict severity of disease or the presence of anomalies beforehand. Furthermore, some studies have shown that there is a significant risk of iatrogenic facial nerve injury during presumably minor cases, e.g., canaloplasty for exostoses.[20]

For routine otologic surgery, some state that monitoring helps less-experienced surgeons and residents to avoid injury. Others argue that it gives a false sense of security encouraging a more aggressive, unwarranted surgical approach. These are similar arguments that were posited before monitoring was accepted for skull base surgery. In a survey more than a decade ago to identify the facial nerve monitoring practices in the United States, the authors found that out of 223 respondents, 75% had access to monitoring, but only 32% thought it was a requirement.[21] In a study looking at the prevalence of facial nerve dehiscence in 262 cases, 10% of primary surgeries were found to have a visual dehiscent facial nerve, while double that (20%) of revision cases had a dehiscence. Using electrical stimulation with a threshold set at 1 volt being the difference between dehiscent or bony covered, 53% of primary surgeries and 96% of revision surgeries had a dehiscence.[22] In terms of cost, it was estimated that the cost of monitoring was between US$222.73 and US$525.00 per case. The authors argued that this cost was offset by the avoidance of the high management costs of facial nerve paralysis.[23] Finally, a "best practice" review article concluded that current evidence suggests that monitoring is of value in identifying the facial nerve that is at risk during middle ear and mastoid surgery, and it is also cost effective.[24]

Forty years ago, McCabe proclaimed the use of electric stimulation during parotidectomy as an absolute essential, i.e., a sine qua non.[25] At the time, McCabe referred to facial nerve stimulation with visual observation of the muscle contractions. Today, that method may still be used by some, although, increasingly, facial nerve monitors are used to more accurately record and document small responses that may not be visible to the eye. In a 2005 survey of 1,548 otolaryngologists in the United States, 78.5% of surgeons reported using intraoperative monitoring without stimulators, while 21.5% used nerve stimulators without EMG monitoring. There was no statistically significant association between the use of monitoring in current practice and a history of inadvertent permanent facial nerve injury. The authors concluded that though there was a growing trend to use facial nerve monitoring, there was not a prospective, randomized clinical study to examine efficacy.[26] However, a survey published in 2014, focused on North American otologists in the American Neurotology Society, has demonstrated that nearly 90% of the respondents are now routinely using facial nerve monitoring during mastoid surgery.[27] Furthermore, 95% of these surgeons monitor every cochlear implant surgery.

15.4 Physiology

EMG is the recording technique most widely used today for monitoring the facial nerve. This relies on the compound muscle action potential (CMAP) generated by muscles supplied by the facial nerve; for details on neurophysiology, see Chapter 2, and for electrophysiologic diagnostics, see Chapter 6. As a nerve is stimulated, depolarization potentials propagate distally to the motor end plates. Multiple potentials emanating from the muscle fibers are observed as a CMAP on the monitor. Using the muscle action potential as opposed to the nerve action potential, an order of magnitude larger response can be observed due to the natural amplifying effect of the muscle response.

An important part of EMG testing is to assess a potential site of injury. Nerve conduction is tested by electrical stimulation applied proximal to the area in question while the response is measured distally. Even in the case of an obviously injured nerve, if stimulation is applied distal to the site of injury, the nerve may respond normally acutely. This is because distal axonal degeneration is a progressive process of Wallerian degeneration that can take 48 to 72 hours before the distal nerve becomes affected. An injured nerve stimulated proximal to the injury may exhibit reductions in amplitude and prolonged latency. Stimulating proximal to an injured nerve may require increasing current to elicit a response. This is often due to a physiological conduction block (neuropraxia) and physically injured neural elements (axonotmesis or neurotmesis) that may occur after significant surgical trauma.[28]

In performing site of injury testing, it is important that stimulation be precise to prevent technical and interpretive errors. Too high a level of monopolar stimulation could result in a false-positive error with inadvertent current spreading from the probe tip through soft tissue *around* the site of injury rather than *through* the injured nerve segment—a phenomenon referred to as "current jump." To avoid this error, either a bipolar stimulator should be used or only low-to-moderate current intensities with a fine-tipped monopolar stimulator.

!

Too high a level of monopolar stimulation can result in a false-positive error with inadvertent current spreading from the probe tip through soft tissue *around* the site of injury rather than *through* the injured nerve segment—a phenomenon referred to as "current jump."

EMG responses may be detected during continuous free-running monitoring or during active electrical stimulation. Continuous free-running EMG is a passive way to monitor throughout the surgery. It is of greatest benefit during direct facial nerve manipulations, such as during acoustic tumor resection when surgical maneuvers may deform the nerve and create EMG potentials secondary to trauma. Passive monitoring is of lesser value when the surgeon has yet to identify the nerve.

Passive monitoring = continuous free-running electromyography during surgery

Active monitoring = passive monitoring plus active electrical stimulation

Table 15.1 The two main types of compound muscle action potential signals during facial nerve monitoring

"Burst" potentials	"Train" potentials
A single polyphasic response due to activation of multiple motor units at the same time	Asynchronous firing of multiple motor units
Occur with direct mechanical stimulation	Last seconds to minutes depending on the severity of injury
Have a characteristic visual single wave and an audible "click" or "beep	Show multiple irregular waves
	Prolonged audible sound similar to an airplane propeller

There are two main types of CMAP signals that can occur during continuous recording (▶ Table 15.1).[29] The first is the "burst" potential, which represents a single polyphasic response due to activation of multiple motor units at the same time (▶ Fig. 15.1). Burst potentials can occur with direct mechanical stimulation of the nerve and are usually represented on the monitor by both a characteristic visual single wave and an audible "click" or "beep." This sound alerts the surgeon and provides instantaneous feedback of irritation. The second type of response during free-running EMG monitoring is a "train" potential. This is caused by asynchronous firing of multiple motor units and can last seconds to minutes depending on the severity of injury. The monitor displays multiple irregular waves (▶ Fig. 15.2) with an audible sound similar to an airplane propeller. Thermal or stretch injury often causes a "train" response, and increasing severity of injury will produce a longer response until the nerve electrically recovers. This should alert the surgeon to halt dissection to minimize further trauma. Occasionally one channel of recording will produce a prolonged "train" response after injury that obscures new responses from being detected in the other channel. The "noisy" channel can be temporarily silenced on the monitor so that only the quiet channel is used for monitoring—but the surgeon should be forewarned that monitoring will be less accurate under these conditions. Consequently, the muted channel should be turned back on as soon as is feasible.

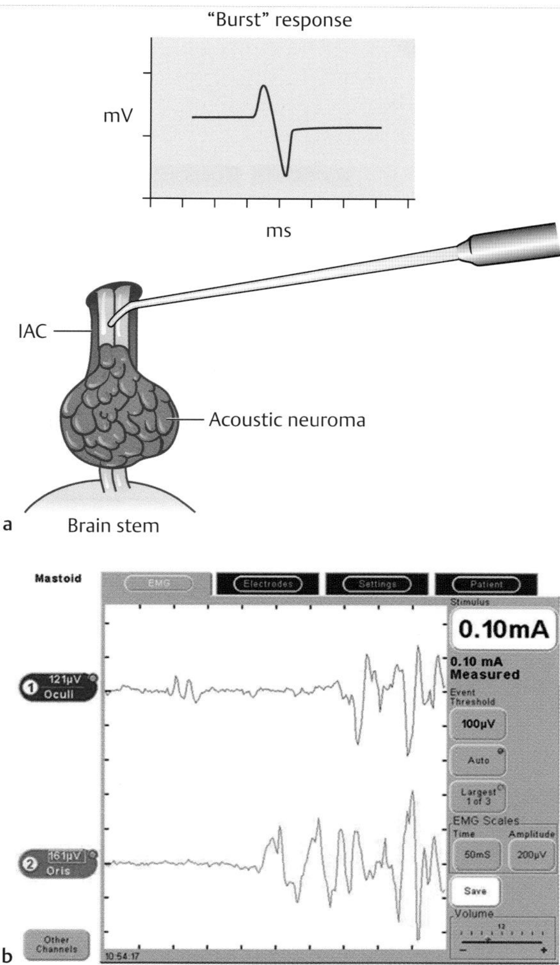

Fig. 15.1 (a,b) "Burst" potential, representing a single polyphasic electromyography response due to activation of multiple motor units simultaneously. IAC, internal auditory canal. (Adapted with permission from Kartush JM. Electroneurography and intraoperative facial monitoring in contemporary neurotology. Otolaryngol Head Neck Surg 1989;101(4):496–503.)

> **!**
>
> If "train" responses occur, the dissection should be temporarily halted to seek a cause and minimize trauma or ischemia.

Other reasons for response include stimuli from the laser, cautery, vibration, cold irrigation, or patient-initiated movement from lightened anesthesia. Gradual thermal injury from the laser or cautery may produce a slow increase in the baseline. It is important to remember that electrocautery creates high levels of electrical artifact that prevent accurate monitoring during those periods. High levels of cautery may injure the nerve without any subsequent EMG potentials. Therefore, following a potentially risky application of cautery adjacent to the facial nerve, it is prudent to stimulate the nerve proximally to assure that its response to electric stimulation remains unchanged.

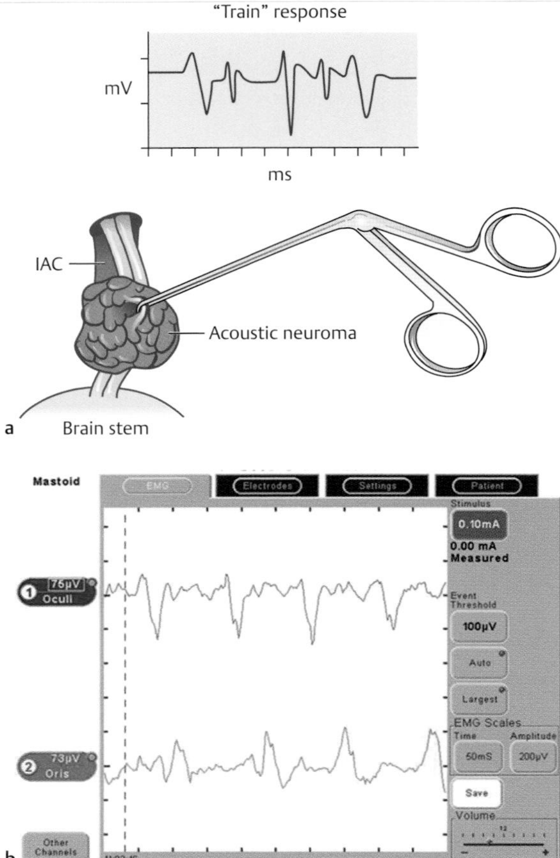

Fig. 15.2 (a,b) "Train" potential, representing asynchronous firing of multiple motor units. IAC, internal auditory canal. (Adapted with permission from Kartush JM. Electroneurography and intraoperative facial monitoring in contemporary neurotology. Otolaryngol Head Neck Surg 1989;101(4):496–503.)

!

Electrocautery creates electrical artifacts that often mask electromyography responses on the monitor. Stimulation after cautery near the nerve is prudent to assure neural integrity has not been compromised.

Vibration from drill potentials close to the nerve may cause a "train" response that ceases immediately after stopping the drill (▶ Fig. 15.3). "Train responses" caused by temperature or concentration changes from irrigations can be worrisome but cause no permanent harm. Nonetheless, even if a loud train response is believed to be due simply to cold irrigation, it may be prudent to defer surgical manipulations until the train response ceases in order to avoid missing small pertinent responses that could be buried in the noisy baseline.

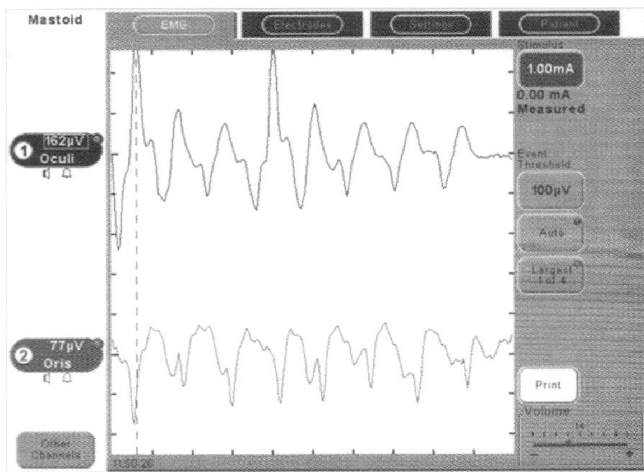

Fig. 15.3 Drill potentials causing asynchronous stimulation of the facial nerve resembling a "train potential." (Adapted with permission from Kartush JM. Electroneurography and intraoperative facial monitoring in contemporary neurotology. Otolaryngol Head Neck Surg 1989;101(4):496–503.)

While "passive" monitoring refers to listening for only trauma-induced EMG responses, "active" monitoring refers to the frequent use of titrated levels of electric stimulation to assess both the nerve's location and its ongoing integrity, especially after potentially risky maneuvers adjacent to the nerve, e.g., cautery, laser, or drilling. Such use of stimulation to actively map and reassess nerve integrity is essential to maximize the benefits of IOM.

Monitors are typically set to stimulate the nerve with a frequency around five pulses per second. Thus, electrically induced responses are acoustically recognized by the surgeon via the loudspeaker by having the same regular, rapid frequency—referred to as pulse tones, in contrast to the burst and train tones described previously.

In otologic surgery, depending upon where the nerve is stimulated, the EMG response occurs approximately 6 to 7 milliseconds after the stimulus artifact, This brief time interval is too short to be distinguished by the human ear so that the stimulus and response acoustically would be perceived to occur simultaneously. This problem is typically resolved by most surgeon-directed, facial nerve–focused devices by automatic silencing of the loudspeaker for approximately 3 milliseconds following the stimulus. This mutes the stimulus artifact but unmutes in time for just the response to be heard. With this feature, if pulsed tones are heard, the surgeon knows they represent an actual EMG muscle response. Without automatic speaker muting (typically absent on multimodality devices), the surgeon is wholly dependent upon the technologist's interpretation of the visual EMG display.

The current level is "titrated," i.e., dynamically adjusted from 0.05 to 2 mA depending on the proximity to the nerve and intervening soft tissue or bone. It is common in otologic and parotid surgery to stimulate starting at 0.8 mA, as this will usually stimulate through a thin shell of fallopian canal bone near the tympanic segment. In contrast, exposed bare nerve, such as during proximal stimulation at the brainstem, often requires 0.05 mA only. Typically, the stimulator is set to a pulse duration of 100 microseconds. Stimulus efficacy is, to some extent, dependent on both current intensity and stimulus duration. Therefore, elevations in stimulus duration, e.g., 200 microseconds, would require lesser current levels to obtain a similar tissue effect.

Typical initial stimulus parameters:

- Stimulation frequency: 5 Hz
- Stimulation current: start at approximately 0.8 mA and titrate up or down as clinically indicated
- Maximum current: 2 to 3 mA depending on proximity of the nerve and the presence of intervening tissue

Multiple stimulating instruments are available in both bipolar and monopolar types. Bipolar stimulators have the advantage of *specificity*—stimulating a discrete area between the two tips maximizes stimulus precision. For example, this would be useful in surgery at the internal auditory canal to differentiate between the facial nerve and vestibular nerve. In contrast, the increased *sensitivity* of monopolar stimulation is optimal for general mapping of the nerve's location. However, its precision can be improved by dynamically lowering the current as the dissection moves closer to the nerve.

- Monopolar stimulator—optimal for general mapping of the facial nerve's location.
- Bipolar stimulator—better for precise stimulation of a discrete area.

Conventional instruments can be used to dissect tumors or cholesteatoma off the facial nerve, but sharp dissection may not elicit an EMG response until after transection or severe injury has occurred. Kartush Stimulating Instruments (KSIs) are a particular variant of monopolar stimulators that allow *simultaneous* stimulation during surgical dissection (► Fig. 15.4).

With stimulating instruments, an electrically evoked CMAP will be produced to continuously confirm nerve integrity and location. While most standard stimulators have insulation down to an exposed tip, the stimulating instruments must have an adequate cutting edge. For this, a larger amount of the tip must remain noninsulated. The surgeon must keep this in mind, as the chance of current shunting is higher. Increasing the current can overcome the shunting, but, as noted, overly high stimulation levels

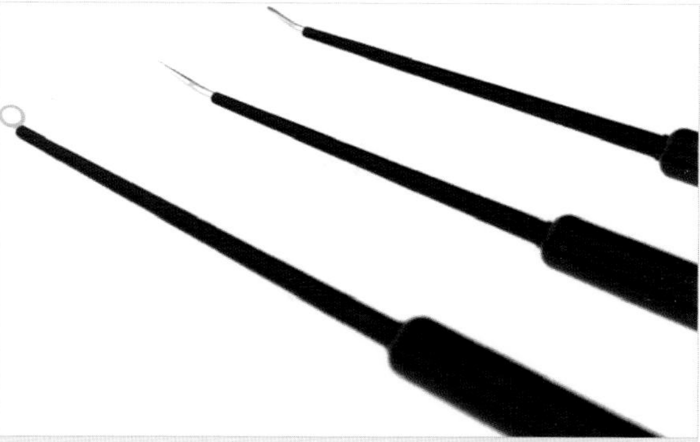

Fig. 15.4 Kartush Stimulating Instruments. These instruments connect directly to the stimulator, which allows simultaneous monopolar mapping during sharp surgical dissection (Magstim/ Neurosign). (Reproduced with permission of Jack M. Kartush, MD.)

can result in a false-positive error due to current shunting thorough adjacent tissue. Some instruments such as the stimulating round curette have had a hole created in the center to minimize the surface area and current shunting. Conversely, probes with insulation flush to the tip will have less current shunting into adjacent liquids, but must be carefully placed directly perpendicular on the nerve to avoid a false-negative error from inadequate current delivery.

15.5 Training

For monitoring to be effective, the surgeon must correctly interpret the neurophysiologic responses.[1] Furthermore, if the surgeon takes on the additional responsibility of electrode and device setup, additional training is required on the technical components of IOM. Meticulous attention must be paid to anesthesia, the device, the electrical parameters, and the electrodes. Some hospitals and surgeons perform monitoring in conjunction with a technologist. These individuals must be specially trained and ideally have passed certification in monitoring (Certification in Neurophysiological Intraoperative Monitoring). Certification for more advanced skills including interpretation can be obtained by taking an examination to become certified as a Diplomat of the American Board of Neurophysiological Monitoring.

At many institutions, however, surgeons often perform both the technical and interpretive aspects of monitoring without any formal training. For example, junior resident physicians often have had lessons filtered down from senior residents, none of whom may have had any formal IOM training. Other times, surgeons may have had only a brief explanation of setup by a medical device company representative. Finally, in some cases a hospital will have a separate department, such as neurology or anesthesiology, to provide monitoring. Even when assistants are present during monitoring, it is incumbent on the surgeon to understand the technical foundation sufficiently to be able to properly interpret responses and to troubleshoot for possible false-positive and false-negative errors.

Most monitoring devices provide both visual and auditory feedback. The visual representation of the EMG on an oscilloscope can help differentiate artifact from true neural responses. Auditory feedback is important because the surgeons receive direct realtime feedback, which they can immediately correlate with their own ongoing surgical maneuvers. They need not rely on a technologist to provide the feedback, who, even with the best of intentions, can momentarily be distracted during a long case and miss an important response. A well-trained technologist or neurophysiologist, however, can be of immeasurable benefit in assuring proper setup and assisting with troubleshooting while the surgeon focuses on the procedure.

Checklists have been documented to improve safety in complex fields including aviation and nuclear energy. Furthermore, complex tasks can benefit from written, standardized protocols. Until recently, the concept of adopting written standards has been a difficult one for physicians who have been concerned that such publications may stifle the practice of medicine and could be used as a tool against physicians during malpractice litigation. The American Society of Anesthesiologists set an important landmark by adopting "Standards For Basic Anesthesia Monitoring" in 1986.[30] One of its once controversial components was the recommendation that pulse oximetry be considered mandatory for continuous of monitoring oxygenation. It has since proven beneficial for both patients and anesthesia practitioners. It is suggested that the field of IOM would likewise benefit from accepted minimal standards and advise development of a uniform core curriculum for surgeons in training.[27,31]

Intraoperative monitoring of the recurrent laryngeal nerve is being performed with increasing frequency often using identical monitors and instrumentation as in facial nerve surgery. An international thyroid study group has had similar concerns about the nonuniformity of recurrent laryngeal nerve monitoring protocols and has recently published an international standards guideline.[32] Clearly, a similar statement of guidelines for facial monitoring is overdue.

Otolaryngology and other specialties are now beginning to develop clinical guidelines, although the choice of prioritizing topics can be somewhat perplexing. The American Academy of Otolaryngology—Head and Neck Surgery Foundation has, for example, created a 21-page evidence-based guideline on removing ear wax—yet no similar document has been created for neurophysiologic monitoring.[33] In the interim, nonsurgical societies have created their own recommended guidelines which are being used as critical references during litigation. Until surgical societies publish their own guidelines, surgeons should strongly consider reviewing these published references.[34,35]

15.5.1 Technical Setup

Video examples of the nerve monitoring protocol steps (▶Video 15.1 to ▶Video 15.15) are available at www.jkartush.com and at the Thieme MediaCenter.

Assuring proper intraoperative monitoring techniques with checklists and protocols will enhance the quality of patient care and increase the surgeon's ability to rely on the neurophysiologic data conveyed by technologists or interpreted directly by the surgeon. Over the decades, the authors' team has evolved a 13-step protocol to ensure proper EMG monitoring setup (▶ Table 15.2). These steps should be followed similar to a "time-out" in the operating room or a preflight checklist prior to airplane takeoff. Video examples demonstrating key steps in facial nerve monitoring (▶Video 15.1 to ▶15.15) can be accessed at www.jkartush.com and at the Thieme MediaCenter.

Anesthetic Considerations

Communicate with the anesthesiologist to ensure proper induction medications. Long-acting paralytics should be avoided as they make monitoring the CMAP impossible. Short-acting paralytics can be used for intubation. However, because of the rare patient with pseudocholinesterase deficiency, even short-acting paralytics can sometimes have extremely long half-lives, which can interfere with monitoring. Therefore, baseline facial nerve testing as well as train-of-four peripheral nerve EMG testing can ensure that any paralytic agent has been completely metabolized.

Proper Use of Local Anesthetic

If local anesthetics such as lidocaine inadvertently contact the facial nerve, the nerve will be unresponsive for hours. This not only can result in a frightening, temporary postoperative facial palsy, but intraoperative monitoring will be rendered useless because a chemically paralyzed nerve will be unable to respond to either electric or mechanical stimuli. Consequently, even severe injury to the nerve will go unrecognized. The only way to confirm that the nerve has not been inadvertently infiltrated with local anesthesia is to obtain an early baseline response as detailed in Obtain a Baseline Response. With parotid and otologic surgery, lidocaine should not be allowed to infiltrate around the stylomastoid foramen. This may be a particular problem in young children with a less-developed mastoid tip, causing the facial nerve to be in a more superficial position than in adults. When injecting the ear

Table 15.2 Kartush facial nerve monitoring protocol

Step		Check box ✓
1	Consult with anesthesia to avoid long-acting muscle relaxants	
2	Avoid local anesthetic near the facial nerve	
3	Demonstrate absence of neuromuscular blockade via: • Train-of-four • Transcutaneous facial nerve stimulation or • Facial nerve stimulation within the operative field	
4	Assure that the monitor's loudspeaker is set at a volume sufficient to be heard over the operating room's ambient noise	
5	Perform a tap test	
6	Check electrode impedance	
7	Check stimulus current flow through soft tissue	
8	Obtain a baseline facial nerve response to stimulus	
9	Electrically map the location of the nerve	
10	Selectively use monopolar, bipolar, or stimulating instruments	
11	Titrate stimulus current based on nerve location and surrounding tissue (bone, soft tissue, blood, spinal fluid)	
12	Obtain a final proximal facial nerve response to stimulus prior to closure	
13	Generate a brief written report (can be within operative report): • Confirm adherence to protocol • Highlight key events	

canal, local anesthetic can infiltrate into the middle ear through a tympanic membrane perforation or myringotomy tube, which can paralyze a dehiscent facial nerve. If anesthetic visibly flows into the middle ear, immediate saline irrigation followed by suctioning can be of benefit. To avoid this inadvertent lidocaine paralysis of the facial nerve when a tympanic membrane perforation is present, saline-soaked gelfoam is placed through the perforation prior to injections. Note, however, that it is possible for lidocaine injected into the ear canal skin to occasionally enter the middle ear subcutaneously, i.e., without a perforation.

!

Long-acting paralytics used by the anesthesiologist or local anesthesia injected by the surgeon may compromise or even completely preclude effective facial nerve monitoring.

Proper Electrode Placement

In otologic, neurotologic, and neurosurgery, two-channel EMG nerve monitoring is sufficient for monitoring responses generated from the facial nerve prior to its extratemporal branching. In comparison with two-channel monitoring, four-channel monitoring has the advantage to independently monitor not just eye and mouth, but also forehead and lower lip. This might be superior in surgery of the facial nerve branches, e.g., for parotid surgery. Intramuscular needle electrodes are inserted in a paired manner in the superior portion of the orbicularis oris and orbicularis oculi (▶ Fig. 15.5). Care should be taken to avoid inadvertent injury to the orbit—the eyelids should be taped shut prior to placing electrodes. Two additional electrodes are placed near the sternum: one serves as the ground, and the other as a return (anode) for the monopolar nerve stimulator. Finally, a wire is dropped from the sterile field to be attached to the stimulator output. This wire is for cathode (negative) stimulation, which is more effective than anode (positive) stimulation. Colored electrodes are used to help differentiate the cables. The authors' long-standing protocol has been adopted by many practioners: blue for orbicularis oculi, red for orbicularis oris, green for ground, white for anode, and black for cathodal stimulation. The mnemonic is "blue eyes, red lips, green ground, black stim."

Check Recording Electrode Impedance

Surgeons should know how to assess electrode impedance for their specific device. The interelectrode impedance should be less than 2 kOhm, and the individual

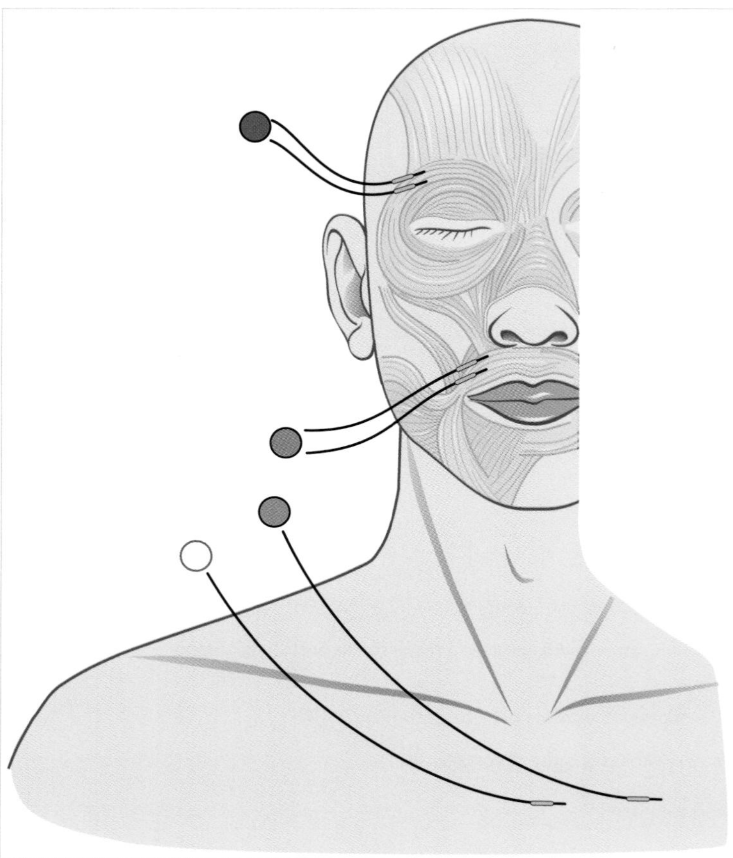

Fig. 15.5 For two-channel recording, intramuscular needle electrodes are inserted in a paired manner in the superior portion of the orbicularis oris and orbicularis oculi. Particular care should be taken to avoid inadvertent injury to the eye during placement as well as during removal of the electrodes at the end of the procedure. Additional electrodes are placed over the sternum. Consistent color coding of electrodes reduces setup errors: blue, eyes; red, lips; green, ground; white, anode. (Adapted with permission from Kartush JM. Electroneurography and intraoperative facial monitoring in contemporary neurotology. Otolaryngol Head Neck Surg 1989;101(4):496–503.)

electrodes should be less than 5 kOhm. Impedance may be elevated with poor needle position or faulty electrodes. The electrodes should be adjusted or replaced to ensure low impedance.

The "Tap Test"

Once intramuscular needle electrodes have been inserted, tapping on the overlying skin will typically create an audible and visual response on the monitoring device. This maneuver can be used to assess the integrity of the connection from the electrodes to the machine and confirm that the loudspeaker is set at an appropriate volume for the operating room. Note, however, that the tap test is only an electrical artifact—it is *not* a true CMAP. Therefore, the user should not assume that hearing a tap test response means that the entire system and nerve are fully functioning. The tap test's artifactual response will be present even if nerve or muscle is temporarily paralyzed due to lidocaine or muscle relaxant. Consequently, the user should understand that while this test is useful, it is only providing limited information and should not be presumed to be a confirmation that the entire system is functioning correctly.

Confirm Current Flow

The stimulator should be attached and used to touch soft tissue or wet bone away from the nerve, which should result in 100% of the current returned to the monitor. Most monitors will display this information visually and/or audibly with a characteristic sound that is distinct from the response tone. This is an essential test that confirms proper flow of the stimulus with return of current from the patient and then through the recording electrodes. However, this test does *not* exclude persistent muscle relaxants or a chemically paralyzed nerve.

Obtain a Baseline Response

Stimulate on or around the facial nerve with sufficient current to elicit a response. Once such a baseline response is obtained, the surgeon has obtained absolute confirmation that not only is the system functioning properly, but also that the facial nerve and muscles have not been inadvertently paralyzed with medications. This is best performed early in the surgery prior to any risky manipulations around the nerve. Microdehiscences of the fallopian canal are common along the tympanic segment so a response can be often obtained at a stimulus setting of less than 1 mA even though the nerve appears covered in bone. The surgeon should not hesitate to increase the stimulus current up to 2 to 2.5 mA to obtain a baseline response—modern monitoring devices use pulsed constant-current stimulation, which have demonstrated no evidence of injury at these levels when used for the brief durations of surgical monitoring. Dedicated facial nerve monitors typically have a safe maximum current level of 5 mA. Do use caution, however, when stimulating with a multimodality device because these products have the ability to stimulate at very high levels that are sometimes needed during spine surgery. The distance from the nerve and the amount of tissue between the nerve and stimulator will affect the current level necessary to elicit a response. Typically, the nerve in the tympanic segment covered by bone with tiny dehiscences will stimulate at 0.8 mA, though it may need to be turned up to 1 to 2 mA if soft tissue, cerebrospinal fluid (CSF), or blood is present. In comparison, the nerve will readily respond to only 0.05 mA when stimulated directly in the cerebellopontine angle. Once a baseline response is obtained, current intensity should be turned down to the minimum current necessary to achieve a consistent response. During tympanomastoid surgery, a Kartush Stimulating Curved Needle is thin enough that it can be used to reach through the antrum or around the ossicles to stimulate at the second genu or tympanic portion of the facial nerve to obtain a baseline response.

The senior author (JMK) has noted that litigation for iatrogenic facial nerve injury is increasingly focusing on failure to monitor *correctly*, rather than failure to monitor; there is more on medicolegal aspects concerning the facial nerve in Chapter 28. The most common focus of monitoring negligence points to failure to stimulate, i.e., failure to check current flow and/or baseline response. Under these circumstances, the surgeon often reports having "hooked up the monitor" but never having stimulated, erroneously assuming that only passively listening for trauma responses would be sufficient.

In addition to the aforementioned setup protocol, during the procedure, the surgeon can maximize the use of IOM by adhering to principles of "active" instead of "passive" monitoring. With passive monitoring, the surgeon listens only for potentials induced by trauma. With active monitoring, the surgeon uses electric stimulation to optimize: (1) nerve location, (2) ongoing awareness of nerve proximity, and (3) confirmation of nerve integrity after dissection and prior to wound closure. Active monitoring is aided by the use of KSIs that allow the surgeon to operate and stimulate simultaneously. Many types of dedicated monopolar and bipolar probes are also available although, unlike stimulating surgical instruments, they require the surgeon to discontinue their dissection, switch to the probe, stimulate, and then switch back to dissecting tools. The specifics of active monitoring vary based on procedure and the severity of pathology or anatomic anomalies. For example, during tympanomastoid surgery with only a small attic cholesteatoma and no anatomic anomalies, the surgeon may only require a few brief moments of stimulation: (1) current flow check on soft tissue, (2) baseline stimulation of tympanic facial nerve, and (3) end-of-dissection stimulation prior to closure. In contrast, during resection of a 4-cm acoustic tumor, using stimulating instruments throughout the tumor dissection allows ongoing updates to the surgeon on nerve location and nerve integrity.

Table 15.3 Typical errors during facial nerve monitoring

Error	Possible cause
False-positive response	Inadvertent stimulation of adjacent structures = "current jump"
False-negative response	Stimulating through blood or fluid, causing "current shunting"
	Inadequate facial nerve stimulation
	Severe injury precluding depolarization
	Complete transection of the nerve
	Technical problems

15.6 Troubleshooting/Pitfalls

Whether or not a technologist is employed to assist with the technical aspects of monitoring, an in-depth understanding of IOM is essential to troubleshoot when the results of monitoring are in conflict with anatomical findings.

Errors can be seen on both the stimulation as well as the recording sides (▶ Table 15.3). *False-positive* responses can occur by inadvertent stimulation of adjacent structures—a phenomenon described earlier as "current jump." This occurs when stimulation current spreads from an adjacent structure to the nerve (▶ Fig. 15.6). This can cause a surgeon to misidentify the nerve, or to become hesitant around the incorrect structure. Accuracy can be improved by switching to bipolar stimulation or by reducing the current intensity of a precise monopolar stimulator.

False-negative responses can occur when stimulating through blood or fluid, causing "current shunting." This draws current away from the intended target. In general, current shunting is readily minimized by simple insulation of the stimulus probes and aspiration of any significant fluid, e.g., blood, CSF, irrigation (▶ Fig. 15.7).

Lack of response to stimulation may be due to purely technical issues or may be due to injury. Examples include: (1) inadequate facial nerve stimulation, (2) severe injury precluding depolarization, (3) complete

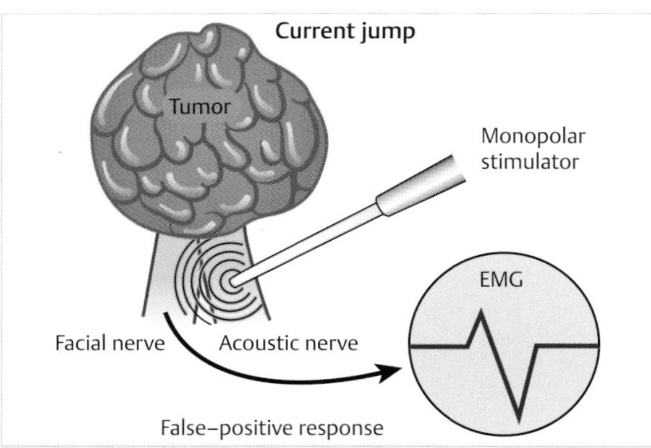

Fig. 15.6 False-positive nerve response due to stimulation of adjacent structures, known as "current jump." EMG, electromyography. (Adapted with permission of Jack M. Kartush, MD.)

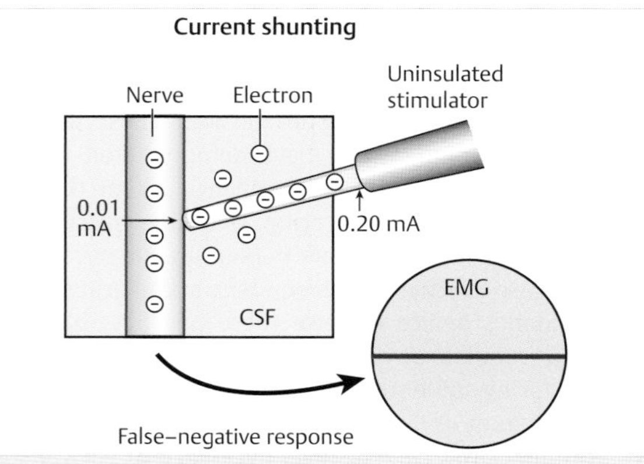

Fig. 15.7 False-negative response due to "current shunting" through cerebrospinal fluid (CSF). EMG, electromyography. (Adapted with permission of Jack M. Kartush, MD.)

transection of the nerve, or (4) technical problems. When in doubt, electrical stimulation of the facial nerve both proximal and distal to the site of dissection should be performed to assess its integrity. In addition to the aforementioned stimulus errors, failure to obtain facial responses can include anesthesia issues, errors in setup, or equipment malfunction. ▶ Table 15.4 lists common problems and possible solutions. Incorrect setup of the electrodes can occur anywhere from placement through the skin, to the receiver box located next to the operating table, or at the input into the monitor. Multimodality monitoring devices allow many types of sophisticated monitoring paradigms—but increased complexity can also lead to additional causes of user error. Failure to record responses has been encountered with software misallocation of stimuli and recording channels.

Because of these numerous causes of failure to record a response, the surgeon needs to be extremely careful in ruling out technical malfunction before concluding that a nerve has been so severely injured that surgical repair may be indicated. In particular, failure to respond to stimulation should not, by itself, be used as a determinant to resect and graft an unresponsive nerve segment. Instead, this measure is typically taken only in conjunction with significant visualized physical disruption of the nerve.[26]

As an example of a false-positive error, Sugita and Kobayashi reported on one case in which the facial nerve was inadvertently cut because stimulation of the trigeminal nerve resulted in contraction of the muscles of mastication. A motion detector was used for recording, and this was not able to differentiate between jaw movement and contraction of the facial musculature.[12]

Some patients with a normal response to electrical stimulation at the end of surgery may develop a delayed facial paralysis. This is especially true with acoustic neuroma resection. Such instances do not represent a failure of monitoring but instead reflect postoperative (and postmonitoring) changes to the nerve. At this time, there appears to be no indicator to routinely predict this phenomenon although multiple episodes of lengthy train

Table 15.4 Checklist for intraoperative facial monitoring problems

Problem	Possible solution/cause
Current jump	Lower the current intensity or use bipolar stimulation
Current shunting	Insulated stimulator, aspirate adjacent fluids
Cautery artifact noise	Muting circuit
Cautery precludes monitoring	Visualize or palpate the face
Laser heating effect	Monitor baseline amplitude
Saline cooling	Warm saline with "blood warmer"
Stimulus artifact	Increase "stimulus ignore" time; exclude an overcharged capacitor
Static discharge	Use insulated instruments
No response to stimulation	• Power off • Current intensity too low • Current measured too low • Electrode impedance too high • Electrode disconnected • Current shunting • Threshold setting too high • Volume too low • Muscle relaxant used • Local anesthetic on nerve • "Stimulus ignore" too long • Nerve not contacted • Other cranial nerve/tissue • Nerve injured

potentials during acoustic tumor surgery are likely to reflect microtrauma and ischemic episodes that increase the likelihood of postoperative edema and ischemia. Delayed facial palsy may also be due to reactivation of latent viral particles.[36] To help minimize the delayed ischemic effects of facial nerve edema, some surgeons perform decompression of the facial nerve at the meatal foramen during the translabyrinthine and middle cranial fossa approach to allow room for swelling.[37]

15.7 Further Study

Although optimal monitoring is dependent upon the surgeon having proper training in the technical and interpretive aspects of monitoring, there are unfortunately scant resources to which surgeons may turn. Ironically, one of the first books published on monitoring was focused on otology and head and neck surgery—but it is no longer in print.[1] Other ear, nose and throat-specific articles are available but are dispersed among numerous articles and book chapters.

Currently available monitoring texts are most often focused on multimodality monitoring for brain and spine with an emphasis on SSEP, motor evoked potentials, and electroencephalography modalities—rather than facial and recurrent laryngeal nerve monitoring. Therefore, surgeons may wish to consider the ASNM online webinar on New Practice Guidelines in Facial Nerve Monitoring. The original webinar presented by the senior author (JMK) in 2014 was videorecorded allowing surgeons to cost-effectively learn critical standards. Taking such a course not only earns continuing medical education credit, but allows the surgeon to have objective documentation of monitoring-specific training that can be of future value when sought by third parties.[31] Additional information on impending standards of care and the need for national monitoring guidelines due to increasing use by otologists is reviewed in the Triological Society's online publication, ENT Today.[27]

15.8 Key Points

- The benefits of facial nerve monitoring during cerebellopontine angle surgery are well established, making monitoring a virtual standard in the United States.
- Monitoring during routine otologic surgery and parotidectomy is becoming increasingly common although there is a lack of prospective trials demonstrating the benefits of routine nerve monitoring. However, such studies are unlikely to ever be performed.
- Because poor monitoring is worse than no monitoring, it is incumbent on surgeons as well as technologists to assure that they have proper training in both the technical and interpretive components of intraoperative neurophysiologic monitoring.
- Use of standard procedures, training, and checklists can help to achieve this goal.[35,36]

References

[1] Kartush JM. Intraoperative facial nerve monitoring: otology, neurotology and skull base surgery. In: Bouchard KR, ed. Neuromonitoring in Otology and Head and Neck Surgery. New York: Raven Press; 1992:99–120

[2] Kartush JM. Electroneurography and intraoperative facial monitoring in contemporary neurotology. Otolaryngol Head Neck Surg 1989; 101: 496–503

[3] Hong R, Kartush M. Acoustic neuroma neurophysiologic correlates: facial and recurrent laryngeal nerves before, during, and after surgery. Otolaryngol Clin North Am. 2012;45(2):291–306, xvii–xviii

[4] Porter R, Kartush J. Diagnosis, evaluation and treatment of facial nerve disorders. In: Kirtane MV, de Souza C, Sanna M, Devaiah A., eds. Otology and Neurotology. Delhi, Stuttgart, New York: Thieme; 2013:Chapter 30

[5] Kartush J, Lee A. Intraoperative monitoring. In: Babu S, ed. Practical Neurotology for the Otolaryngologist. San Diego, CA: Plural Publishing; 2012:165–191

[6] Kartush JM. Presidential address. American Society of Neurophysiological Monitoring meeting, Detroit, Michigan, 1989

[7] Krause F. Surgery of the Brain and Spinal Cord, Based on Personal Experiences. New York: Rebman; 1912:738–743

[8] Givre A, Olivecrona H. Surgical experiences with acoustic tumors. J Neurosurg 1949; 6: 396–407

[9] Parsons RC. Electrical stimulation of the facial nerve. Laryngoscope 1966; 76: 391–406

[10] Jako G. Facial nerve monitor. Trans Am Acad Ophthalmol Otolaryngol 1975; 69: 340–342

[11] Hilger JA. Facial nerve stimulator. Trans Am Acad Ophthalmol Otolaryngol 1964; 68: 74–76

[12] Delgado TE, Buchheit WA, Rosenholtz HR, Chrissian S. Intraoperative monitoring of facial muscle evoked responses obtained by intracranial stimulation of the facial nerve: a more accurate technique for facial nerve dissection. Neurosurgery 1979; 4: 418–420

[13] Sugita K, Kobayashi S. Technical and instrumental improvements in the surgical treatment of acoustic neurinomas. J Neurosurg 1982; 57: 747–752

[14] Dickins JR, Graham SS. A comparison of facial nerve monitoring systems in cerebellopontine angle surgery. Am J Otol 1991; 12: 1–6

[15] Harner SG, Daube JR, Ebersold MJ, Beatty CW. Improved preservation of facial nerve function with use of electrical monitoring during removal of acoustic neuromas. Mayo Clin Proc 1987; 62: 92–102

[16] Kwartler JA, Luxford WM, Atkins J, Shelton C. Facial nerve monitoring in acoustic tumor surgery. Otolaryngol Head Neck Surg 1991; 104: 814–817

[17] Magliulo G, Petti R, Vingolo GM, Cristofari P, Ronzoni R. Facial nerve monitoring in skull base surgery. J Laryngol Otol 1994; 108: 557–559

[18] Silverstein H, Rosenberg SI, Flanzer J, Seidman MD. Intraoperative facial nerve monitoring in acoustic neuroma surgery. Am J Otol 1993; 14: 524–532

[19] National Institutes of Health. Consensus Statement: Acoustic Neuroma. Presented at the NIH Consensus Development Conference, Bethesda, MD, 1991

[20] Green JD, Jr, Shelton C, Brackmann DE. Iatrogenic facial nerve injury during otologic surgery. Laryngoscope 1994; 104: 922–926

[21] Greenberg JS, Manolidis S, Stewart MG, Kahn JB. Facial nerve monitoring in chronic ear surgery: US practice patterns. Otolaryngol Head Neck Surg 2002; 126: 108–114

[22] Noss RS, Lalwani AK, Yingling CD. Facial nerve monitoring in middle ear and mastoid surgery. Laryngoscope 2001; 111: 831–836

[23] Wilson L, Lin E, Lalwani A. Cost-effectiveness of intraoperative facial nerve monitoring in middle ear or mastoid surgery. Laryngoscope 2003; 113: 1736–1745

[24] Heman-Ackah SE, Gupta S, Lalwani AK. Is facial nerve integrity monitoring of value in chronic ear surgery? Laryngoscope 2013; 123: 2–3
[25] McCabe BF. Injuries to the facial nerve. Laryngoscope 1972; 82: 1891–1896
[26] Lowry TR, Gal TJ, Brennan JA. Patterns of use of facial nerve monitoring during parotid gland surgery. Otolaryngol Head Neck Surg 2005; 133: 313–318
[27] Bronstein D. Otologists report greater widespread use of intra-operative facial nerve monitoring. ENT Today. May 1, 2014. Available at: http://www.enttoday.org/article/otologists-report-greater-widespread-use-of-intra-operative-facial-nerve-monitoring/. Accessed April 11, 2015
[28] Kircher ML, Kartush JM. Pitfalls in intraoperative nerve monitoring during vestibular schwannoma surgery. Neurosurg Focus 2012; 33: E5
[29] Prass RL, Lüders H. Acoustic (loudspeaker) facial electromyographic monitoring: Part 1. Evoked electromyographic activity during acoustic neuroma resection. Neurosurgery 1986; 19: 392–400
[30] American Society of Anesthesiologists. Standards for Basic Anesthetic Monitoring. American Society of Anesthesiologists Committee on Standards and Practice Parameters 1986
[31] Kartush JM. Webinar: New practice guidelines in facial nerve monitoring. ASNM, June 2014. Available at: www.asnm.org/event/id/440608/Webinar-New-Practice-Guidelines-in-Facial-Nerve-Monitoring.htm. Accessed April 11, 2015
[32] Randolph GW, Dralle H, Abdullah H et al. International Intraoperative Monitoring Study Group. Electrophysiologic recurrent laryngeal nerve monitoring during thyroid and parathyroid surgery: international standards guideline statement. Laryngoscope 2011; 121 Suppl 1: S1–S16
[33] Roland PS, Smith TL, Schwartz SR et al. Clinical practice guideline: cerumen impaction. Otolaryngol Head Neck Surg 2008; 139 Suppl 2: S1–S21
[34] American Society of Electroneurodiagnostic Technicians, Inc. National Competency Skill Standards For Performing Intraoperative Neurophysiologic Monitoring. 2011. Available at http://www.aset.org/files/public/IONM_National_Competency_Skill_Standards_Approved_2011.pdf
[35] Skinner SA, Cohen BA, Morledge DE et al. Practice guidelines for the supervising professional: intraoperative neurophysiological monitoring. J Clin Monit Comput 2014; 28: 103–111
[36] Gianoli GJ, Kartush JM. Delayed facial palsy after acoustic neuroma resection: the role of viral reactivation. Am J Otol 1996; 17: 625–629
[37] Kartush JM, Graham MD, LaRouere MJ. Meatal decompression following acoustic neuroma resection: minimizing delayed facial palsy. Laryngoscope 1991; 101 6pt1: 674–675

16 Tumors Affecting the Facial Nerve

John P. Leonetti, Sam J. Marzo, and Matthew L. Kircher

16.1 Introduction

The facial nerve innervates all the muscles responsible for the expression of human emotions. Proper and symmetric function of the facial nerve is both a cosmetic and a physical necessity. Inability to close one's eye can result in severe ocular complications, while the emotionless face can lead to disabling psychological and emotional dysfunction.

While Bell's palsy may account for 75 to 80% of all cases of unilateral facial paralysis, neoplastic invasion of cranial nerve VII can be the cause of this finding in 7 to 10% of these patients.[1]

The purpose of this chapter is to provide an algorithm for the diagnosis and management of patients with facial paralysis caused by a neoplasm in an effort to help the clinician avoid a delay in diagnosis associated with the inappropriate assignment of "Bell's palsy" to all patients with unilateral facial paralysis (▶ Fig. 16.1). The special features of facial nerve schwannoma will also be presented in detail in a subchapter.

> **!**
>
> Bell's palsy or idiopathic facial paralysis generally occurs rapidly and is maximal within 1 week affecting all branches of the facial nerve. Gradual-onset and/or partial facial weakness are usually due to neoplastic invasion of the facial nerve.

16.2 Surgical Anatomy

When considering the possibility of facial paralysis due to a tumor, it is helpful to divide the course of the facial nerve into three segments. The *intradural* segment is that portion of the facial nerve from the brainstem to the fundus of the internal auditory canal. The *intratemporal* segment of cranial nerve VII is the portion from the geniculate ganglion to the stylomastoid foramen. The *extratemporal* segment is defined as the main trunk of the extracranial facial nerve and the peripheral branches. The clinical presentation and radiographic assessment are more easily understood with this practical designation of these three segments of the facial nerve.

> **!**
>
> Isolated brain neoplasms causing partial facial paralysis and an upper motor neuropathy are extremely rare.

16.3 Clinical Features

16.3.1 Presenting Symptoms

All patients with neoplastic invasion of the facial nerve will eventually present with ocular or mild speech difficulties as partial facial weakness or twitching progresses to full facial paralysis over a matter of days, weeks, or months. The onset of facial paralysis is rarely acute, as in

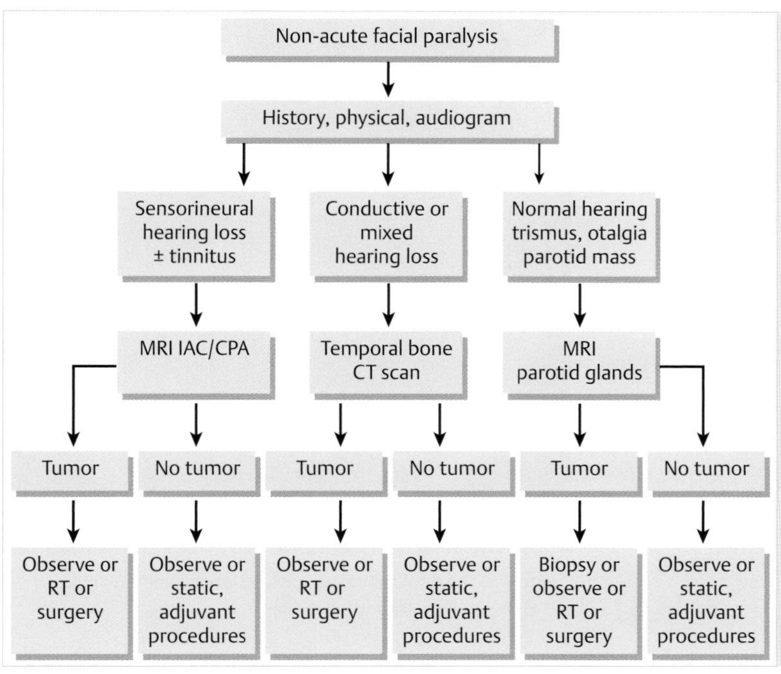

Fig. 16.1 Diagnostic and management algorithm for patients with tumors affecting the facial nerve. CPA, cerebellopontine angle; IAC, internal auditory canal; RT, radiotherapy.

Bell's palsy, and will vary in length of time according to the location and histology of the tumor.

Intradural tumors may also cause facial numbness, hearing loss, and tinnitus. Intratemporal lesions may cause hearing loss and pain, but are less likely to cause facial numbness, trismus, or tinnitus. Extratemporal neoplasms are usually malignant parotid tumors that also cause pain and trismus. ▶ Table 16.1 is a summary of the symptoms associated with neoplastic facial paralysis in a series of 221 patients.[2]

!

The hearing loss in patients with intradural tumors is sensorineural while patients with intratemporal tumors have a conductive or mixed hearing loss.

16.3.2 Presenting Signs

Facial paralysis in patients with intradural or intratemporal tumors is generally very gradual in onset, and may begin as intermittent twitching, but eventually involves the entire ipsilateral face. Extratemporal tumors of the parotid gland may cause gradual-onset facial weakness (facial neuroma) but most patients present with rapid (nonacute) facial weakness of a division or the main trunk of the nerve. Facial, temporal, or scalp skin cancers can cause paralysis of individual peripheral facial nerve branches, which can progress proximally to eventually affect the entire nerve. Intradural neoplasms may cause trigeminal nerve weakness (decreased corneal or facial sensitivity) or lower cranial (IX–XII) nerve palsies.

Intratemporal lesions may involve the ear canal or middle ear with anterior extension into the parotid gland. Extratemporal lesions are most often malignant parotid tumors with invasion of peripheral branches or the main trunk of the facial nerve. Temporomandibular involvement will lead to trismus, and palpable or subclinical cervical lymph nodes can also be present (▶ Table 16.2).

Table 16.1 Associated symptoms found in 221 patients with neoplastic-related facial paralysis

Symptom	Extratemporal	Intradural	Intratemporal
Facial weakness	All patients	All patients	All patients
Facial numbness	22	2	0
Pain	7	12	107
Trismus	0	3	41
Hearing loss	37	41	0
Tinnitus	16	4	0

!

Transcranial tumors may cause a combination of facial nerve signs and symptoms depending upon the size and location of the neoplasm.

16.4 Diagnostic Work-Up

The clinical evaluation of a patient with nonacute facial paralysis will determine the need for additional diagnostic studies. Patients with suspected tumors of the intradural or extratemporal regions should undergo magnetic resonance imaging (MRI) with contrast to determine the location, size, and vascularity of the tumor (▶ Fig. 16.2 and ▶ Fig. 16.3). Intratemporal tumors are more accurately assessed with thin-cut, high-resolution computed

Table 16.2 Associated signs found in 221 patients with neoplastic-related facial paralysis

Sign	Extratemporal	Intradural	Intratemporal
Facial weakness	All patients	All patients	All patients
Parotid mass	0	3	93
Ear mass	0	46	9
Cranial nerve V	25	6	8
Cranial nerve IX–XII	10	2	0

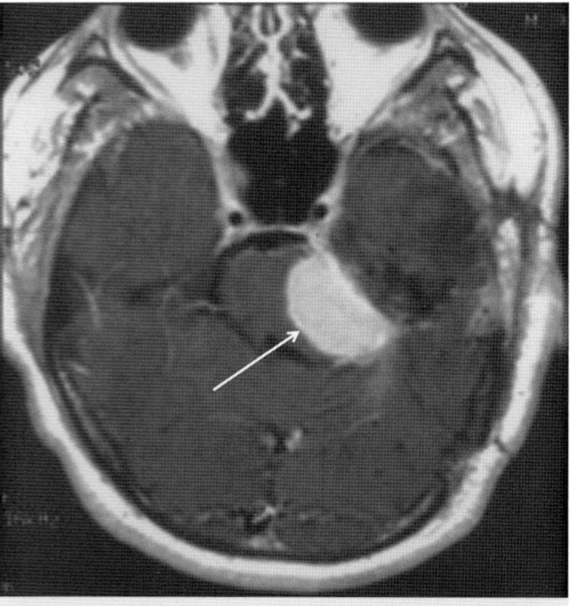

Fig. 16.2 Axial MRI showing a left cerebellopontine angle meningioma causing facial paralysis.

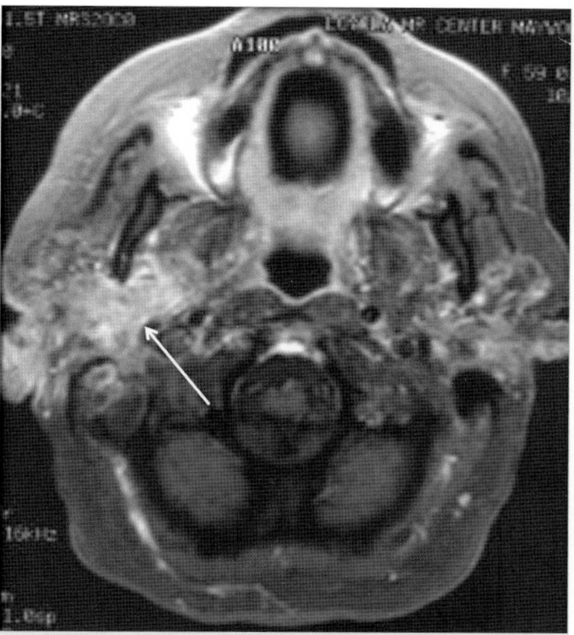

Fig. 16.3 Axial MRI showing a right parotid malignancy causing facial paralysis.

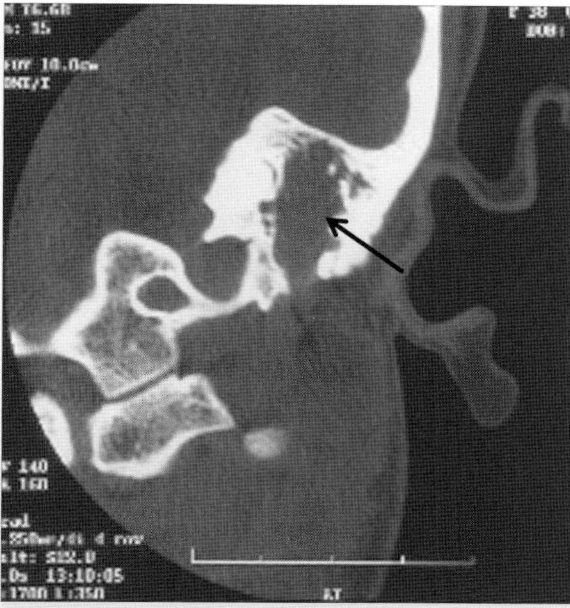

Fig. 16.4 Coronal CT image demonstrating a left facial neuroma.

tomography (CT) scanning of the temporal bone (▶ Fig. 16.4); see also Chapter 5. Cerebral angiography is utilized in patients with suspected vascular tumors that may be preoperatively embolized or in patients who might require sigmoid sinus, jugular bulb, or carotid artery sacrifice (▶ Fig. 16.5).

Preoperative tissue diagnosis of intradural or intratemporal tumors is rarely needed. Fine needle aspiration cytology (FNAC) should only be utilized in patients with extratemporal tumors if the result of the FNAC will alter the ultimate management of the patient; see Chapter 4.

Pure-tone and speech discrimination audiometry must be obtained if the tumor location involves the cochlear nerve, the labyrinth, the ossicular chain, or the external auditory canal. A preoperative auditory brainstem response should be performed if intraoperative eighth nerve monitoring will be utilized to help preserve hearing during the extirpation of an intradural tumor.

The tumor histology relative to the anatomic location of origin is shown in ▶ Table 16.3.

> !
>
> The tumors listed in ▶ Table 16.3 are based upon a series review of 221 patients. Case reports from an extensive literature review are likely to demonstrate a large number of rare primary or metastatic tumors that may also result in neoplastic-related facial paralysis.

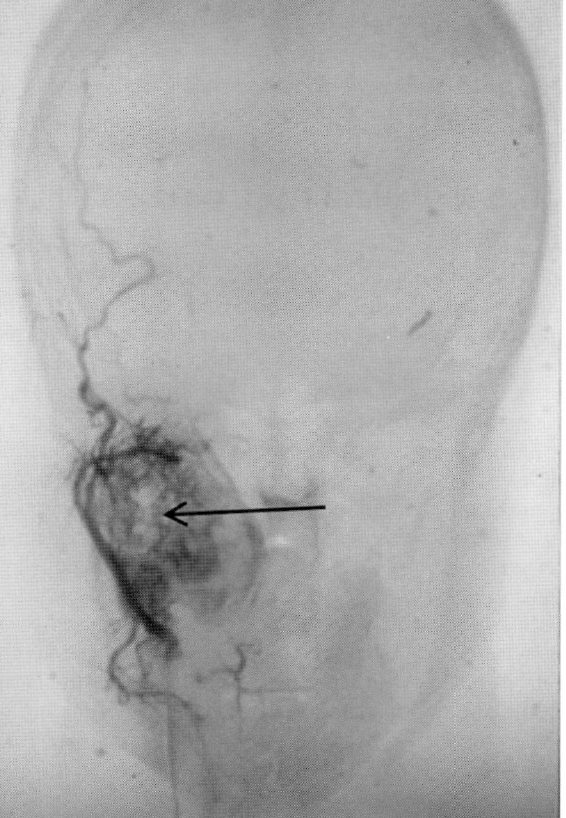

Fig. 16.5 Cerebral angiogram showing a right glomus jugulare that caused facial paralysis.

Table 16.3 Tumor histology and site of origin in 221 patients with neoplastic-related facial paralysis

Intradural		Intratemporal		Extratemporal	
Facial neuroma	17	Glomus tumor	21	Adenoid cystic carcinoma	43
Meningioma	13	Facial neuroma	15	Mucoepidermoid carcinoma	42
Hemangioma	3	Cholesteatoma	12	Squamous cell carcinoma	21
Epidermoid	3	Squamous cell carcinoma	4	Carcinoma ex-pleomorphic	16
Lipoma	1	Rhabdomyosarcoma	2	Cutaneous carcinoma	5
Meningiosarcoma	1	Adenocarcinoma	1	Facial neuroma	1
Total	38	Total	55	Total	128

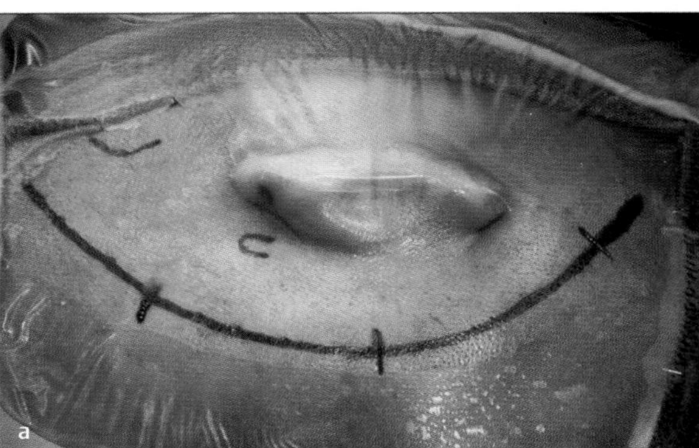

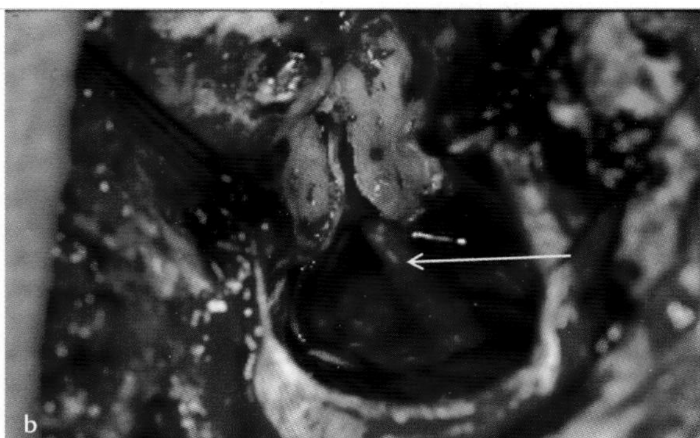

Fig. 16.6 Cerebellopontine angle meningioma: **(a)** accessed via a right translabyrinthine approach, and **(b)** with facial nerve interposition graft (*arrow*).

16.5 Surgical Approaches

A variety of transtemporal approaches can be employed alone, or in a combined fashion, in the extirpation of isolated or transcranial tumors causing facial paralysis.[3–9] Intradural tumors of the cerebellopontine angle, internal auditory canal, petrous apex, or clivus can be resected by using one or any combination of the translabyrinthine, retrosigmoid, middle cranial fossa, or petrosal approach(es).

Extratemporal tumors may be resected with a parotidectomy alone or in conjunction with a subtotal petrosectomy or infratemporal fossa approach. The infratemporal fossa approach may be performed with a preauricular or postauricular incision. With significant temporal bone extension of disease, the postauricular incision is utilized with an ear canal oversew to enable concurrent temporal bone resection. Transtemporal techniques may be necessary in order to obtain a tumor-free margin of the facial nerve, the ear canal, or the middle ear. A sampling of these surgical approaches is provided in ▶ Fig. 16.6, ▶ Fig. 16.7, ▶ Fig. 16.8, ▶ Fig. 16.9 and ▶ Fig. 16.10.

A preauricular modified Blair incision is utilized for infratemporal access in cases without significant disease involvement of the temporal bone. A parotidectomy exposure with superior transposition of the facial nerve and transcervical dissection along the styloid process often provides adequate exposure to the infratemporal skull base. In situations where an extratemporal lesion extends near the stylomastoid foramen, the skin flap is elevated posteriorly over the mastoid tip, and a mastoidectomy is performed to allow identification of the mastoid segment of the facial nerve for sampling and/or grafting.

In situations where subtemporal access is required, the incision may also be extended superiorly into a hemicoronal design. This incision extends to the level of the deep layer of the temporal fascia with preservation of the superficial temporal artery when possible. The incision continues in front of the tragus and onto the face in a plane superficial to the superficial musculoaponeurotic system and into the neck in a subplatysmal plane. Neck dissection allows identification and preservation of neurovascular structures including proximal control of the internal carotid artery.

Dissection proceeds superficial to the superficial layer of the deep temporal fascia until approximately 2 cm superior to the palpated zygoma. At this point, an incision is made through the superficial layer of the deep temporal fascia along an imaginary line from the superior orbital rim to the zygomatic root exposing the underlying

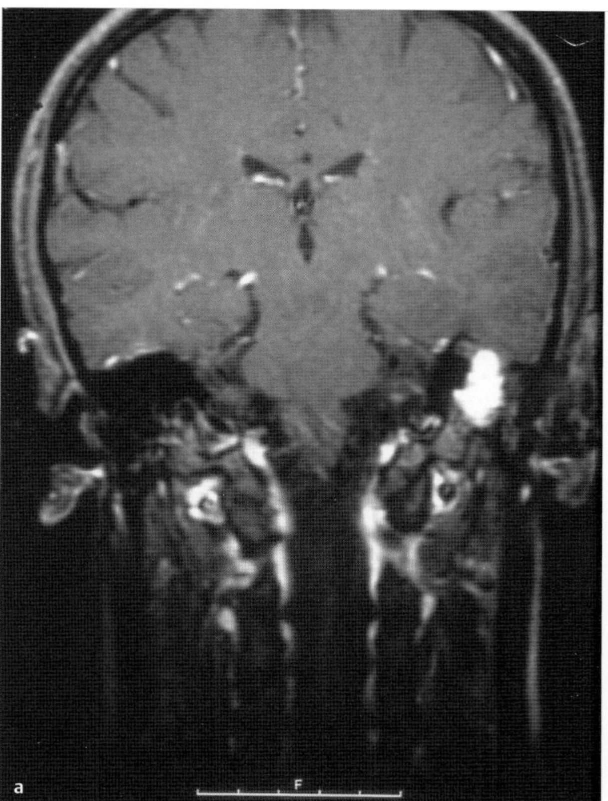

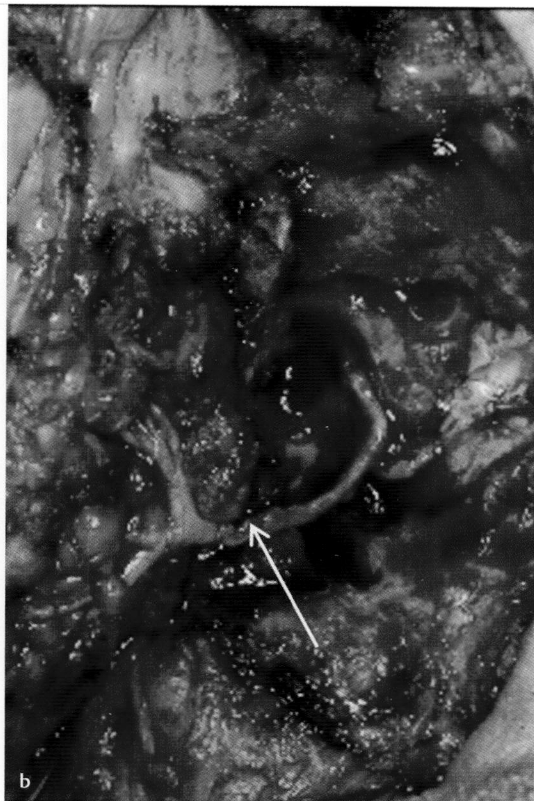

Fig. 16.7 Facial neuroma (a) resected via a left transtemporal approach, and (b) with sural nerve interposition graft (*arrow*).

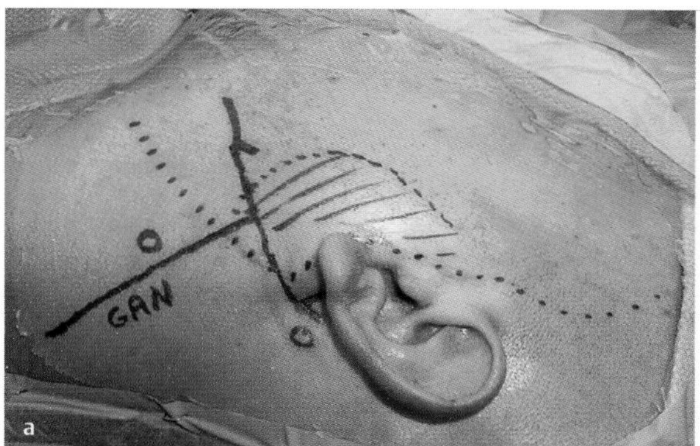

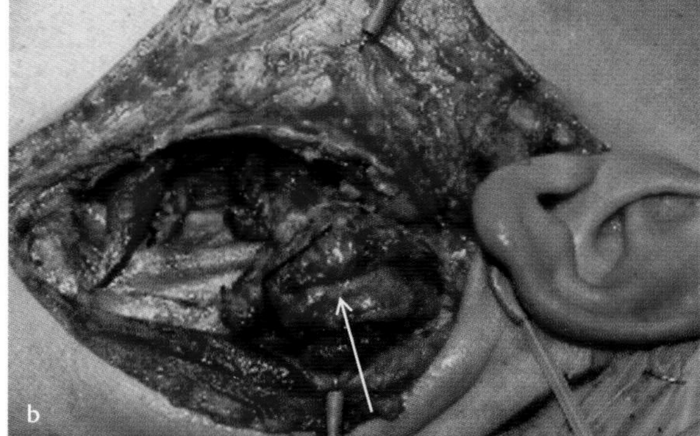

Fig. 16.8 (a) Preoperative, and (b) midoperative photographs of left parotidectomy with cervical lymphadenectomy for a mucoepidermoid carcinoma (*arrow*) causing preoperative facial paralysis. GAN, greater auricular nerve location.

temporal fat pad. Elevation proceeds in this plane down to the zygoma to protect the overlying frontal branch of the facial nerve. An incision is made in the zygomatic periosteum and further subperiosteal dissection exposes the orbitozygomatic complex.

The temporalis muscle may be incised superiorly and bluntly elevated off the temporal fossa maintaining a superior cuff of muscle for resuturing back into position. Orbitozygomatic osteotomies and/or temporal craniotomies may then be performed as needed to achieve exposure. A mandibular coronoidectomy also increases the inferior arc of temporalis muscle rotation.

Dissection along the infratemporal skull base continues bluntly identifying the lateral pterygoid plate, foramen ovale, foramen spinosum, and the spine of the sphenoid bone. Mandibular condylectomy and/or resection of the glenoid fossa using a large cutting burr with division of V3 and middle meningeal vessels allow access to the petrous carotid artery.

16.6 Facial Nerve Management

On rare occasions the facial nerve or a peripheral segment of the facial nerve can be preserved without jeopardizing the tumor-free margin. For example, saving the upper division of the facial nerve when only the lower division is invaded by a malignant parotid tumor, or saving viable vertical segment facial nerve fibers when the medial surface of the mastoid segment has been invaded by a glomus jugulare tumor. In most cases, however, a more significant portion of the facial nerve will be resected as part of complete tumor extirpation. Facial nerve repair is presented in detail in Chapter 20.

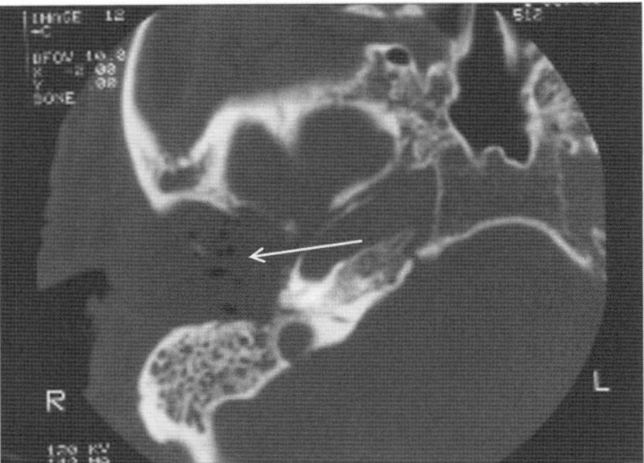

Fig. 16.9 Recurrent temporal bone cancer (*arrow*) causing facial paralysis.

16.6.1 Primary Neurorrhaphy

This allows the best clinical result, provided the neural repair is tension free and performed with meticulous technique to prevent connective tissue ingrowth through the neurorrhaphy. Unfortunately, this option is rarely possible due to the extent of the disease at presentation.

16.6.2 Interposition Graft

The greater auricular nerve can be utilized to repair defects of 6 to 8 cm in length while the sural nerve is usually employed to bridge a gap of longer lengths (► Fig. 16.11).[10]

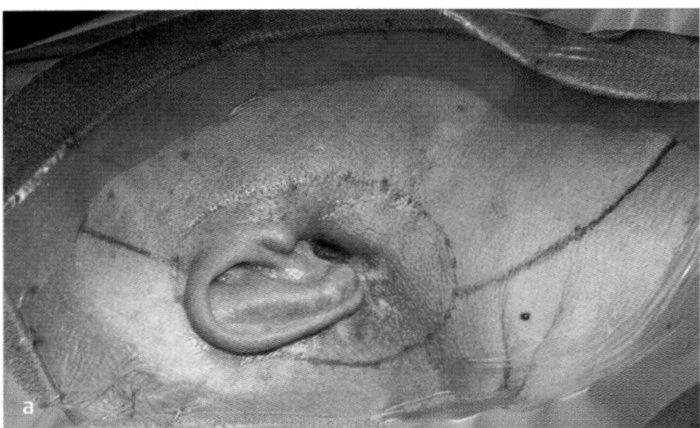

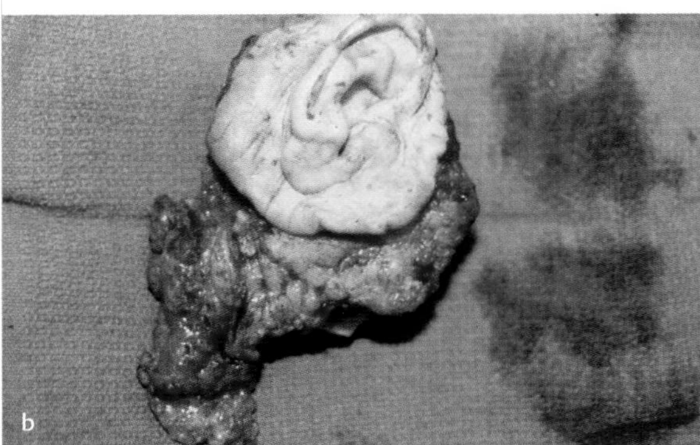

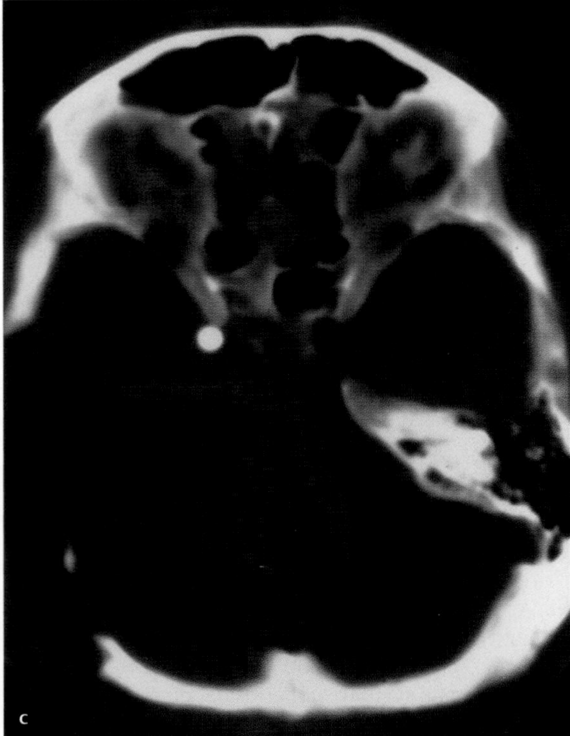

Fig. 16.10 Right combined lateral skull resection of temporal bone cancer causing facial paralysis; see ► Fig. 16.9. **(a)** Preoperative site marked. **(b)** En bloc surgical resection. **(c)** Postoperative CT scan demonstrating resected bony margins.

16.6.3 Hypoglossal–Facial Anastomosis

The split 12–7 technique allows for good facial tone, some dynamic facial function, and spared tongue movement on the operative side. This technique is used when the proximal facial nerve has been resected, but the distal nerve and facial musculature are viable.[11]

16.6.4 Microvascular Free Flap

Musculature free tissue transfer is used when the proximal facial nerve is available and tumor free, but the peripheral facial nerve and musculature have been resected. A variety of donor muscles have been utilized such as the rectus abdominis, the serratus anterior, and the gracilis muscle. This technique allows natural lower face movement as well as aesthetic recontouring of the operative defect.[12]

16.6.5 Cross-Facial Graft

The sural nerve can be interposed between a branch or division of the contralateral facial nerve and the distal trunk of the resected facial nerve to restore more natural facial movement. This technique can also be combined in a delayed fashion with a microvascular free flap if the distal facial nerve and musculature are resected.[13]

Examples of these reconstructive techniques are shown in ▶ Fig. 16.12, ▶ Fig. 16.13 and ▶ Fig. 16.14.

16.7 Facial Schwannoma

A special mention will be made here regarding facial schwannomas. These are rare neoplasms arising from the Schwann cell sheath that may occur anywhere along the course of the facial nerve.[14] This diversity of tumor location and proximity to neurovascular structures creates a variety of clinical signs and symptoms depending on the facial nerve segment and nearby anatomy involved.

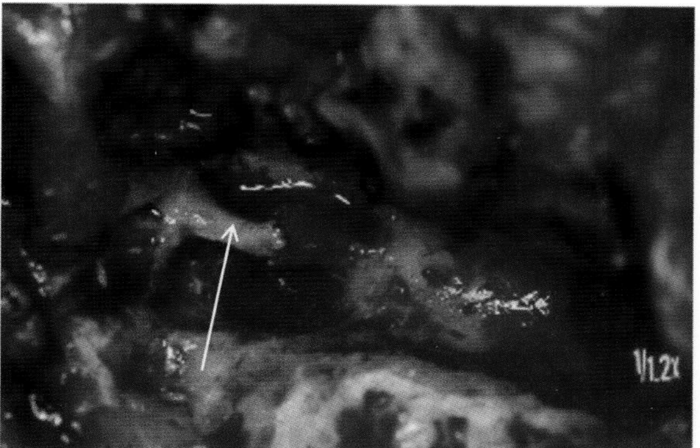

Fig. 16.11 Interposition greater auricular nerve graft (*arrow*) following facial nerve resection and parotidectomy with subtotal petrosectomy for adenoid cystic carcinoma.

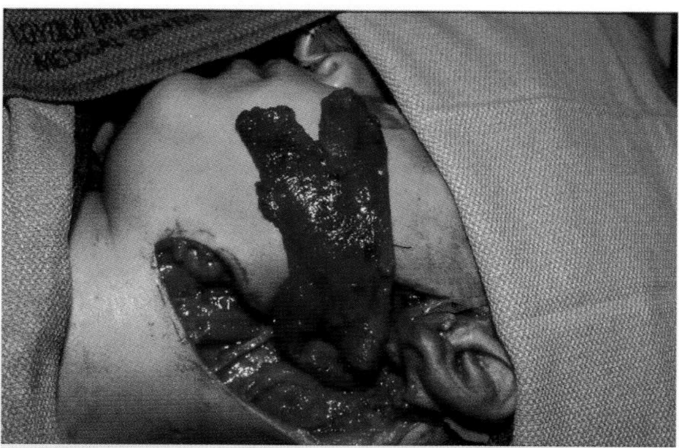

Fig. 16.13 Serratus anterior free flap for defect reconstruction and lower facial reanimation following adenoid cystic carcinoma resection.

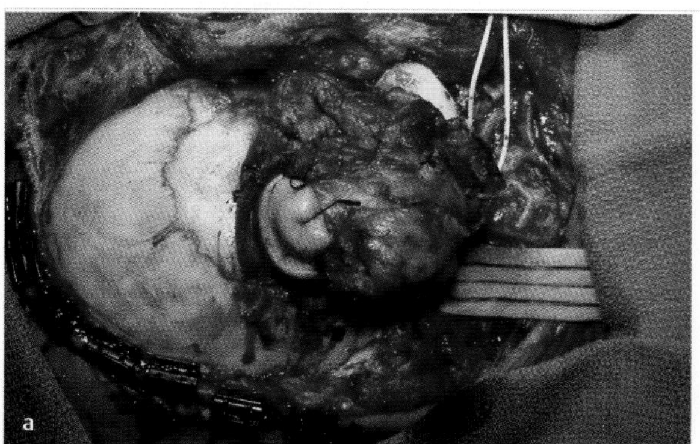

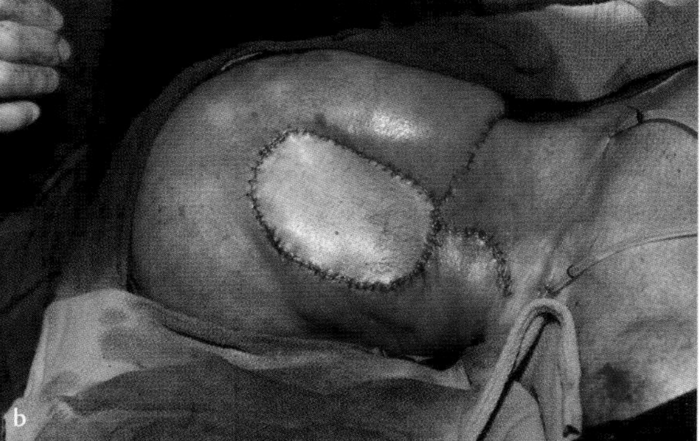

Fig. 16.12 (a,b) Rectus abdominis free flap following the resection of a temporal bone cancer.

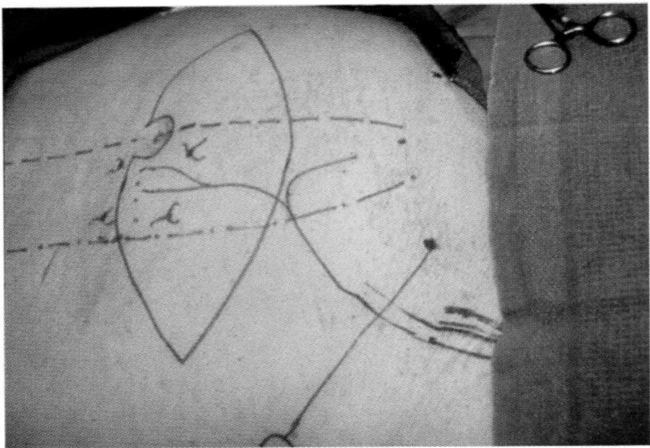

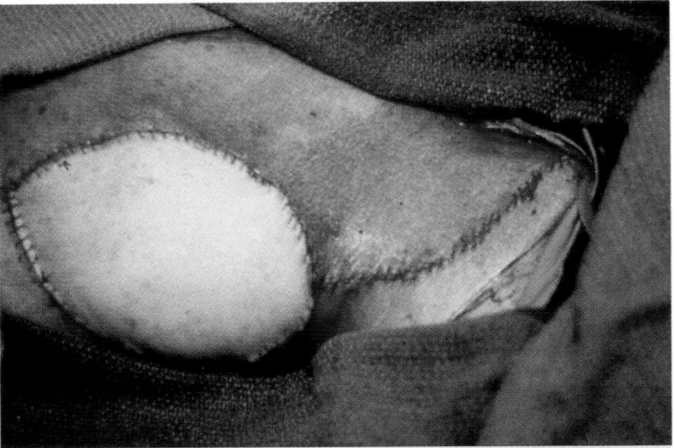

Fig. 16.14 Rectus abdominis free-flap reconstruction following a total parotidectomy with temporal bone resection.

Common presenting symptoms include facial palsy, hearing loss, and tinnitus, although clinical manifestations can be largely varied between patients.[15] Tumors in the parotid region may present as a mass with a slowly progressive facial palsy. Middle ear involvement may lead to conductive hearing loss while lesions of the cerebellopontine angle present with sensorineural hearing loss, tinnitus, and/or dysequilibrium similar to an acoustic neuroma.

> ⚠
>
> A tumor in the parotid gland with slowly progressive facial palsy or even without facial palsy can be a facial nerve schwannoma. If the intraparotid facial nerve and its branches cannot be exposed in continuity during parotid tumor surgery, think of the differential diagnosis of a facial schwannoma.

Due to identical histological makeup, facial schwannomas and vestibular schwannomas share the same imaging characteristics. Tumor extension along the fallopian canal helps to distinguish these two lesions and usually indicates a primary facial neoplasm such as schwannoma or hemangioma. Unlike hemangiomas of the facial nerve, schwannomas do not typically produce facial weakness until the tumors are very large.

Treatment options for facial schwannomas include observation, surgical decompression, tumor resection, or radiotherapy. Nerve grafting is performed at the time of resection if possible. Preoperative facial nerve function will largely determine the course of action except in rare cases where large tumors causing brainstem compression require resection. In cases without risk of brainstem compression, most practitioners will wait until facial nerve dysfunction deteriorates to a House–Brackmann grade III or worse before resecting the tumor and grafting. Decompression of the tumor can be done when function deteriorates to a House–Brackmann grade II in an attempt to preserve facial function. Likewise, radiotherapy may be advocated before or after surgery in an attempt to provide tumor growth control with preservation of residual facial function.[16]

> If a facial schwannoma tumor resection is planned, the involved facial nerve segment has to be resected. Peeling of the tumor with the purpose to preserve some facial nerve fibers is not appropriate and does not lead to better postoperative facial nerve function than accurate nerve grafting.

16.8 Adjuvant Procedures

Static slings can be used to provide lower and midface tone, while oculoplastic eyelid procedures such as upper eyelid weight implants and lower eyelid shortening procedures are used to assist in eyelid closure and reduce the risk of corneal injury; more details are given in Chapter 21 and Chapter 24).[17]

Facial retraining physical therapy, as described in Chapter 26, can assist in the optimum neural recovery while botulinum toxin injection, as described in Chapter 25, can provide short-term relief from synkinetic facial dystonia.[18]

16.9 Key Points

- Facial paresis or paralysis that develops over longer than 48 hours may be caused by a tumor.
- A careful history of the onset of the facial paralysis should be obtained from the patient and, if possible, from other family members or friends.
- A complete head and neck, cranial nerve, and microscopic otoscopy is likely to uncover the origin of the tumor.

- Magnetic resonance imaging, computed tomography, and occasionally a cerebral angiogram will define the location, size, vascularity, and sometimes the likely tumor histology.
- A variety of head and neck, otologic, lateral skull base, and reconstructive operative techniques can be used to safely resect these tumors, reconstitute the defect, and reanimate the paralyzed face.
- Beware of the incorrect diagnosis of "atypical Bell's palsy" as this may in reality be a wolf in sheep's clothing.

References

[1] Marzo SJ, Leonetti JP, Petruzelli GJ. Facial paralysis caused by malignant skull base neoplasms. Neurosurg Focus 2002; 12: e2

[2] Leonetti JP, Marzo SJ, Anderson DA, Sappington JM. Neoplastic causes for non-acute facial paralysis. Ear Nose Throat J

[3] Leonetti JP, Anderson DE, Marzo SJ, Origitano TC, Schuman R. The preauricular subtemporal approach for transcranial petrous apex tumors. Otol Neurotol 2008; 29: 380–383

[4] Abdel Aziz KM, Sanan A, van Loveren HR, Tew JM, Jr, Keller JT, Pensak ML. Petroclival meningiomas: predictive parameters for transpetrosal approaches. Neurosurgery 2000; 47: 139–150, discussion 150–152

[5] Fisch U. The infratemporal fossa approach for nasopharyngeal tumors. Laryngoscope 1983; 93: 36–44

[6] Sekhar LN, Janecka IP. Intracranial extension of cranial base tumors and combined resection. In: Jackson CG, ed. The Neurosurgical Perspective in Surgery at Skull Base Tumors. New York, NY: Churchill Livingstone; 1991:222–224

[7] Magnano M, gervasio CF, Cravero L et al. Treatment of malignant neoplasms of the parotid gland. Otolaryngol Head Neck Surg 1999; 121: 627–632

[8] Friedman O, Neff BA, Willcox TO, Kenyon LC, Sataloff RT. Temporal bone hemangiomas involving the facial nerve. Otol Neurotol 2002; 23: 760–766

[9] Pensak ML, Gleich LL, Gluckman JL, Shumrick KA. Temporal bone carcinoma: contemporary perspectives in the skull base surgical era. Laryngoscope 1996; 106: 1234–1237

[10] Gidley PW, Gantz BJ, Rubinstein JT. Facial nerve grafts: from cerebellopontine angle and beyond. Am J Otol 1999; 20: 781–788

[11] Guntinas-Lichius O, Streppel M, Stennert E. Postoperative functional evaluation of different reanimation techniques for facial nerve repair. Am J Surg 2006; 191: 61–67

[12] Terzis JK, Olivares FS. Long-term outcomes of free-muscle transfer for smile restoration in adults. Plast Reconstr Surg 2009; 123: 877–888

[13] Frey M, Michaelidou M, Tzou CH et al. Three dimensional video analysis of the paralyzed face reanimated by cross-face nerve grafting and free gracilis muscle transplantation. Plast Reconstr Surg 2008; 122: 1709–1722

[14] Symon L, Cheesman AD, Kawauchi M, Bordi L. Neuromas of the facial nerve: a report of 12 cases. Br J Neurosurg 1993; 7: 13–22

[15] Sherman JD, Dagnew E, Pensak ML, van Loveren HR, Tew JM, Jr. Facial nerve neuromas: report of 10 cases and review of the literature. Neurosurgery 2002; 50: 450–456

[16] Madhok R, Kondziolka D, Flickinger JC, Lunsford LD. Gamma knife radiosurgery for facial schwannomas. Neurosurgery 2009; 64: 1102–1105, discussion 1105

[17] Jobe RP. A technique for lid loading in the management of the lagophthalmos of facial palsy. Plast Reconstr Surg 1974; 53: 29–32

[18] Guntinas-Lichius O, Straesser A, Streppel M. Quality of life after facial nerve repair. Laryngoscope 2007; 117: 421–426

17 The Facial Nerve in Otologic Infection and Iatrogenic Injury

Jacob Seth McAfee and Barry E. Hirsch

17.1 Introduction

The facial nerve is afflicted by paralysis more frequently than any other nerve in the body,[1] most commonly in its peripheral segment as it courses through the temporal bone. Facial paralysis markedly affects a patient's social life and may potentially cause significant psychological damage.[2] The gravity of such a morbidity was well communicated by a poll conducted in 1991, which revealed that the level of discomfort Americans felt upon meeting those with facial abnormalities was second only to that associated with interacting with the mentally ill, and it far exceeded anxiety about encountering the senile, mentally retarded, deaf, blind, and those confined to a wheelchair.[3] Encountering and managing facial paralysis is inevitable in the career of surgeons managing otologic pathology, especially among those whose focus is narrowed to maladies of the ear. Sources of otologic facial paralysis are widespread. This chapter focuses on inflammatory etiologies of facial palsy to include acute and chronic otitis media and malignant otitis externa, as well as a discussion of iatrogenic injury.

17.2 Structural Considerations

The anatomic complexity of the facial nerve is greater than that of any other nerve in the body; details on anatomy are given in Chapter 1. The tortuous course of the nerve through the temporal bone, in addition to the variety of important, closely adjacent structures, yields great potential for hazard both in otologic surgery and in diseases primary to the ear. A sound understanding of facial nerve anatomy is a cornerstone in managing associated pathology. These anatomic concepts were unknown until the 1550s when the intricate course of the facial nerve was described by Gabriel Fallopius. His early anatomic discoveries were followed by the physiologic work of Charles Bell in the 1800s, outlining the separation of sensory and motor function of the face.[4]

The facial nerve courses through the temporal bone within the bony confines of the fallopian canal (▶ Fig. 17.1). The fallopian canal originates as a deep sulcus within the primordial, cartilaginous otic capsule. The remainder of the cartilaginous circumference of the labyrinthine and tympanic segments is derived from

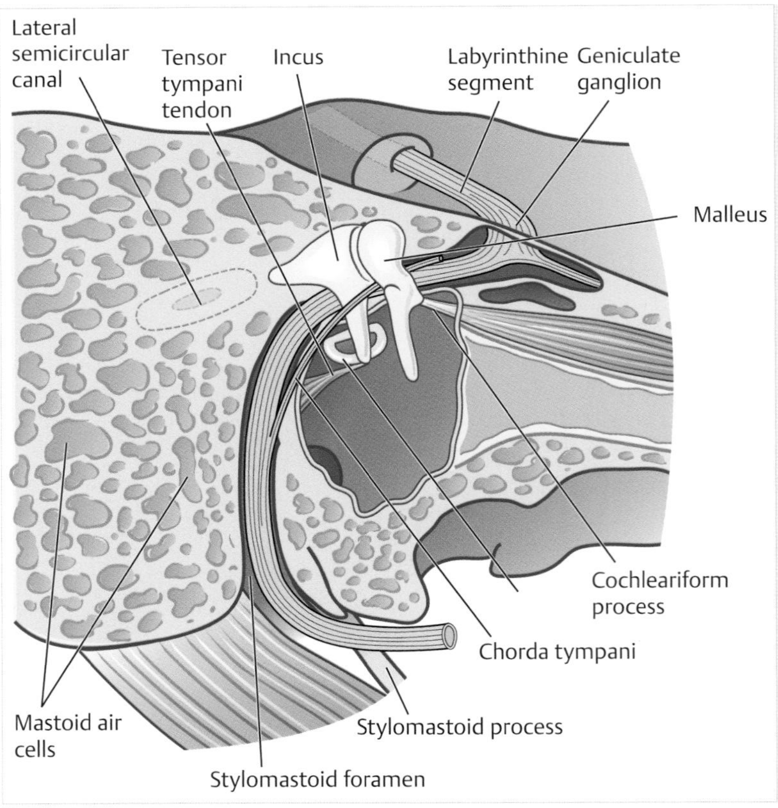

Fig. 17.1 The course of the facial nerve from the fundus of the internal auditory canal to the stylomastoid foramen.

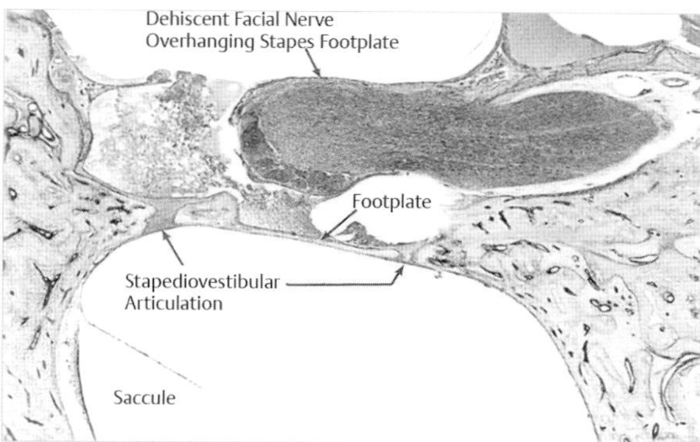

Fig. 17.2 The facial nerve, dehiscent at the oval window. (Reproduced with permission from Gulya AJ, Schuknecht HF. Anatomy of the temporal bone with surgical implications. 2nd ed. Pear River, NY: Parthenon Press; 1995.)

Reichert's cartilage, with origin from mesoderm. Ossification of the canal begins at an embryologic age of 10 weeks, progressing to completion by the end of the first postnatal year.[5] This process is punctuated by segments of incomplete bony coverage, most commonly in the tympanic course above the oval window (▶ Fig. 17.2). Baxter reported a study of 535 temporal bones in which 294 (55%) contained a total of 369 dehiscences.[6] Similar findings were noted by Dietzel, demonstrating an incidence of fallopian canal dehiscence of 57% in a sample of 211 temporal bones.[7] The commonality of bony dehiscence along the course of the fallopian canal is not surprising, given the dual embryologic origin described above.[5] As the nerve of the second branchial arch, the facial nerve maintains an intimacy with the middle ear and mastoid cavity. These structures, as constituents of the upper respiratory tract, are inherently liable to compromise by infection. Due to the dehiscent segments of the fallopian canal, the facial nerve is in potential jeopardy from exposure to adjacent pathology.[1]

Bony dehiscences along the course of the fallopian canal are common and should be considered to be present in every surgical patient.

The facial nerve begins its intratemporal course as it exits the cerebellopontine cistern and enters the porus of the internal auditory canal. It is here that it embarks on a longer journey through bone than any neural structure in the body. Exiting the internal auditory canal at its fundus, it enters the confines of the fallopian canal through the meatal foramen, coursing a distance of approximately 26 mm, where it acutely alters its course at two locations (the first and second genu) before exiting the stylomastoid foramen (▶ Fig. 17.3). Its tortuous passage through

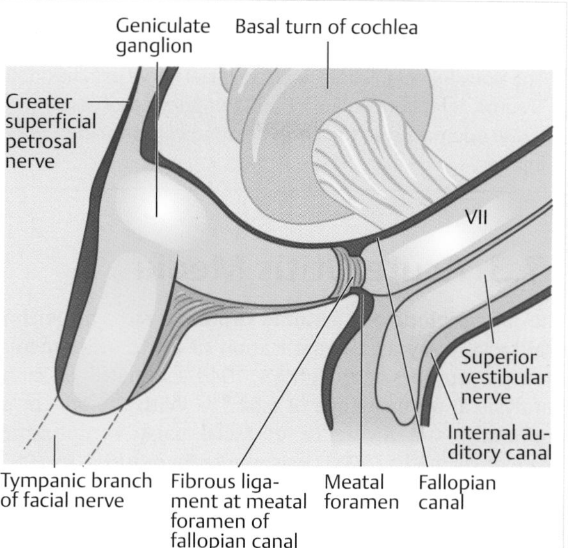

Fig. 17.3 The intratemporal course of the facial nerve. (Adapted with permission from May M, Schaitkin BM, eds. The Facial Nerve. New York, Stuttgart: Thieme; 2000.)

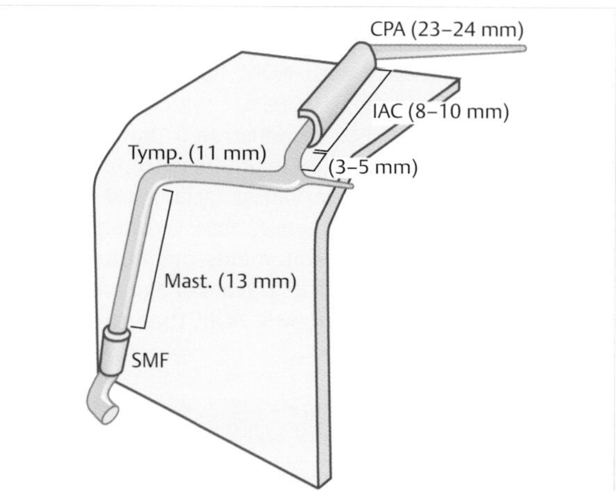

Fig. 17.4 Surgical anatomy of the lateral internal auditory canal, meatal foramen, and first genu of the facial nerve. Left ear, superior view. IAC, internal auditory canal; CPA, cerebellopontine angle; Mast., mastoid segment; SMF, stylomastoid foramen; Tymp., tympanic segment.

such a long bony conduit, further surrounded by additional bone of the petrous apex and mastoid, renders the facial nerve vulnerable to injury by a variety of pathologic mechanisms. The noncompliance of the fallopian canal limits the tolerance of the nerve to trauma, infection, and other inflammatory processes. This is especially true at the meatal foramen, where the nerve occupies 83% of the available diameter of the fallopian canal, a mere 0.68 mm (▶ Fig. 17.4).

> !
>
> The bony fallopian canal restricts facial nerve expansion. Trauma, infection, and other inflammatory processes cause edema inside the canal creating compression injuries.

17.3 Acute Otitis Media

The preantibiotic era featured dramatic rates of peripheral facial palsy as a complication of acute otitis media. Multiple authors cite Kettle's 1943 estimate[8] of facial paralysis at an incidence of 0.6%.[9–11] With the advent of antibiotics, the incidence of facial palsy complicating acute otitis media (AOM) was markedly reduced. In 1982, Pollock[9] reported a series of 1,250 patients with otitis media, only 2 of whom sustained peripheral facial palsy. This represents an incidence of 0.16%, a fourfold decrease compared with that of the preantibiotic era. Similar findings were reported by Kangsanarak and colleagues[12] with an estimated incidence of 0.2%. Neither of these studies drew a distinction between patients with acute and chronic disease, suggesting that even these significantly decreased numbers may represent inflated estimates. More contemporary reports evaluating facial paralysis exclusively in patients with AOM have suggested incidence estimates as low as 0.005%,[13] which is a 100-fold decrease. Ellefson further demonstrated that the risk of facial palsy complicating AOM in adults is 10 times that of children.[13] Despite this observation, facial paralysis in the setting of AOM is a phenomenon observed nearly exclusively in children.[1] These statements are influenced by the fact that children less than 2 years of age are at a 200 times greater risk for developing AOM than the remainder of the population.[13,14]

> Facial nerve palsy caused by acute bacterial otitis media is very rare in the postantibiotic era. Adults who get acute otitis media (AOM) have a greater rate of associated facial paralysis, but, because AOM is of much greater incidence in children, most practitioners see more children with this condition.

17.3.1 Pathophysiology

The pathophysiology of facial paralysis secondary to AOM has long been debated. Several proposed hypotheses are reported in the literature, suggesting a lack of consensus. However, authors agree that paralysis results from inflammatory changes to the nerve. The method by which neuritis develops, however, remains speculative. Facial nerve paralysis occurring in the context of a middle ear infection invariably results from direct extension of the inflammatory process into the fallopian canal.[1,10,15] Exposure of the facial nerve within its fallopian canal by way of congenital dehiscence has been well documented.[5,6,16] In addition, Tschiassny[17] implicates physiologic canaliculi for the stapedial and chorda tympani nerves as well as vascular connections between the fallopian canal and mastoid air cells. These anatomic passages provide potential access to the facial nerve by pathologic processes occupying the mastoid cavity and tympanum. However, given the prominence of fallopian canal dehiscence and frequency of AOM, and the relative infrequency of associated facial paralysis, it is unlikely that this hypothesis alone adequately explains the pathogenesis of peripheral facial palsy. In consideration of this point, the facial nerve sheath and middle ear mucosa appear to impose a resistant barrier to the spread of bacteria from the middle ear space to the intraperiosteal lining of the facial nerve.[18]

Other authors propose alternative mechanisms in the etiology of facial nerve palsy that include bacteria-liberated toxins instigating inflammatory edema and myelin injury. The pathogens common to AOM including *Streptococcus pneumoniae*, *Haemophilus influenzae*, *Moraxella catarrhalis*, group A streptococcus, and *Staphylococcus aureus* have also been identified in cases of AOM complicated by facial paralysis. This has been corroborated by multiple authors. Both Yonamine[19] and Ellefson[13] reported culture results in patients with AOM complicated by facial paralysis that mirrored the flora of AOM without other complications. Bacteriological research has yet to support the contention that these pathogens release toxins that provoke an acute, inflammatory neuritis.[9,20] Furthermore, fulminant, systemic, immunological responses to liberated toxins would be expected, and such responses have been observed rarely. Despite this, some authors suggest that neurotoxicity is likely to be an etiology, via previously unrecognized cellular mediators or activation of latent viruses.[21,22] Hyden[22] proposed that simultaneous involvement of bacteria and viruses in AOM worsens clinical outcomes, and increases the risk for complications.

Multiple authors have proposed that facial paralysis results from neural compression and ischemia due to inflammatory edema.[1,18] Candela presumed that acute neuritis, and subsequent paresis, was the result of a progressive process of hyperemia, cellular infiltration, microhemorrhage, venous thrombosis, and consequent ischemia.[1] Alteration of the blood supply within the fallopian canal may compromise the nerve, such that paralysis results. Studies have demonstrated that the damaging effect of pressure on a peripheral nerve is related more to occlusion of its vascular supply than to actual compression.[1] Similar concepts were supported by Telischi,[15] proposing that venous congestion and eventual arterial obstruction were causes for nerve hypoxia, and ultimately degeneration.

The role of osteitis in facial paralysis complicating AOM has also been proposed. Persistent infection in the middle ear space may yield suppuration that obstructs the aditus and yields a coalescing mastoid infection. Subsequent osteitis and bony resorption of the fallopian canal may also result in neural injury.[21] However, the short lag time seen between onset of infection and development of facial paralysis points away from osteitis as a likely mechanism, as such a process typically requires 2 to 3 weeks to develop.[9,11,21]

> !
>
> The pathophysiology of facial palsy in case of acute otitis media is unclear. Neuritis due to extension of the inflammatory process, a reaction to bacterial toxins, neural compression and ischemia due to inflammatory edema, and/or neural injury resulting from osteitis and bony resorption of the fallopian canal are possible mechanisms. A multifactorial mechanism is likely.

17.3.2 Electrophysiologic Diagnostics

The role of electrophysiologic testing in management of patients with facial palsy secondary to AOM remains debated; details of the electrophysiologic tests are given in Chapter 6. While some advocate use of electrophysiologic testing to delineate which candidates will benefit from operative intervention,[19,23,24] others strictly oppose this point of view.[10,25] Goldstein[21] points out that electrophysiologic testing may be of value in patients with complete paralysis. All patients in Goldstein's study with incomplete paralysis recovered to a House-Brackmann grade I with a myringotomy and tube, as did patients with complete paralysis that demonstrated electrical activity on electromyography (EMG). The timing of electrical testing was not indicated. Of two patients with complete paralysis and no electrical activity on EMG, one experienced full recovery of the nerve after mastoidectomy, while the other remained at a House–Brackmann grade V. While no definitive statements can be made based on the results of these facts, there is suggestion that electrical testing may be of value in patients with complete paralysis, to identify those patients with no electrical response, who might benefit from surgical intervention. Similarly, Yonamine[19] reports a cohort of patients who were treated with mastoidectomy and facial nerve decompression due to poor prognosis on electrical testing. Despite a longer duration to nerve recovery, final nerve recovery was comparable with that of the patients with good prognosis on electrical testing who were managed without mastoid surgery. Further studies are necessary to define the utility of electrical testing in this patient population.

> !
>
> As is true for facial palsy due to other etiologies, for patients with facial palsy caused by acute otitis media it can be stated: incomplete paralysis has a good prognosis, and in the context of complete palsy, electromyography may help to assess the severity of the nerve lesion.

17.3.3 Treatment

The care of patients with facial nerve paralysis secondary to AOM should be considered urgent. ▶ Table 17.1 provides an overview of the most important treatment options. A review of the literature demonstrates unanimity in the aggressive use of antimicrobial therapy against routinely found AOM pathogens.[11,19,21,23–25] Similarly, in

Table 17.1 Therapy options for facial palsy caused by acute otitis media

Measure	Comment
Antibiotic treatment	Empiric antibiotic treatment should be started immediately. Effectiveness of the selected antimicrobial should be based on culture data
Myringotomy	In case of absence of spontaneous tympanic membrane rupture, use myringotomy to take a bacterial culture
Placement of tympanostomy tube	Matter of debate. Tympanostomy tube should be considered in patients with a history of recurrent otitis. Some authors advocate tube placement regardless of the presence or absence of prior middle ear disease in all cases of facial palsy in relation to acute otitis media
Corticosteroid therapy	Corticosteroid therapy is controversial, widely used but therapy effectiveness has not yet been proven
Mastoidectomy	Matter of debate. Proponents see an indication in cases of complete facial paralysis exceeding 3 weeks duration, progression of paralysis while on medical therapy, if the acute otitis media is refractory to antimicrobial therapy, coalescent mastoiditis, or in cases of late-onset of paralysis 2 weeks after onset of acute otitis media, and in cases of poor prognosis due to electrophysiologic testing
Facial nerve decompression	Cannot be recommended, no evidence for effectiveness, quite contrary results are not satisfactory

the absence of spontaneous tympanic membrane rupture, myringotomy is a well supported and commonly considered standard of care.[21] Placement of a tympanostomy tube should be considered in patients with a history of recurrent otitis. Joseph[21] reported on two patients failing initial myringotomy who returned with persistent facial paralysis, a healed tympanic membrane, and an opacified middle ear space requiring repeat myringotomy and tube placement. Consequently, some authors advocate tube placement regardless of the presence or absence of prior middle ear disease to prevent premature closure of the tympanic membrane and to permit ongoing surveillance of the middle ear.[21] Although commonly sterile, bacterial cultures should be taken at the time of myringotomy to confirm the efficacy of the selected antimicrobial regimen. This also facilitates rare identification of a resistant strain.[25]

!

All patients should receive systemic antibiotics and a myringotomy with or without tube in the absence of spontaneous tympanic membrane rupture.

In contrast to the widespread support for myringotomy and antibiotics, no such consensus exists regarding the role of other treatment options. Prescribing systemic steroids for patients with facial nerve paralysis secondary to AOM is common practice. Steroids are touted as the most effective treatment for inflammatory, virally induced, immune-mediated disease.[21] However, no conclusive data exist to establish their clear benefit. Popovtzer[11] reported on a cohort of 7 of 13 patients with facial paralysis secondary to AOM. All 13 were treated with myringotomy and parenteral antibiotics, but only 5 received adjunctive steroid therapy. All 13 patients fully recovered, irrespective of the use of steroids. De Zinis[25] authored a case series of 11 patients with identical pathology, all of whom demonstrated complete recovery to a House–Brackmann grade[26] I without steroid treatment. Finally, Makeham[10] reports full recovery to House–Brackmann grade I in six patients with complete facial paralysis treated only with tube placement and antimicrobial therapy. Although the use of steroid therapy is controversial, it is likely that it will continue to be widely supported until its role has been refuted with scientific evidence.

!

Many patients with facial paralysis complicating acute otitis media also receive systemic corticosteroids, but the effectiveness of such a treatment is not proven.

Perhaps of greatest controversy among treatment options is the role of mastoid surgery in treatment of facial paralysis complicating AOM. Furthermore, if surgery is thought to be therapeutic, the otologic surgeon must then ask, "What surgery should be performed?" The literature demonstrates considerable variety in the decision of when and how to implement mastoid surgery for these patients. The following are proposed indications for cortical mastoidectomy for patients sustaining facial paralysis as a complication of AOM:

- Complete facial paralysis exceeding 3 weeks duration.[11,13,25]
- Progression of paralysis while on medical therapy.[11,13,21,25]
- AOM refractory to antimicrobial therapy.[11,13,25]
- Coalescent mastoiditis.[25]
- Onset of paralysis 2 weeks after onset of AOM.[18]
- Poor prognosis on electrical testing.[19,23,24]

Makeham[10] reported on 10 patients with facial palsy associated with AOM, half of whom had complete paralysis. Paralysis was 3 weeks in duration in multiple patients. All patients recovered to House–Brackmann grade I (except for one House–Brackmann grade 2), without mastoid surgery. Goldstein[24] recommended mastoidectomy without facial nerve decompression for patients who failed to respond to conservative measures. In contrast to surgical management of facial paralysis secondary to chronic otitis media, facial nerve decompression is generally not recommended because the potential for damage to the nerve in an acutely inflamed and friable state is elevated.[21] Poor recovery has been demonstrated in patients undergoing facial nerve decompression in AOM.[27] Goldstein[21] reported on two patients with complete paralysis. The patient who underwent mastoidectomy alone improved to a House–Brackmann grade I, while the patient who underwent mastoidectomy and nerve decompression failed to recover better than grade V.

!

The role of mastoidectomy in patients with facial palsy due to acute otitis media is a matter of debate. The consensus indicates that facial nerve decompression cannot be recommended.

17.3.4 Prognosis

The prognosis of facial palsy caused by AOM is favorable in both children and adults, and multiple authors assert that complete remission should be the rule by which outcomes are compared.[10,13,25] Although younger patients have been shown to be more likely to sustain paralysis (due to greater prevalence of disease), no correlation has been proven regarding age and subsequent potential for nerve recovery. Greater variability in degree of recovery has been shown among patients with complete paralysis[24]; however, full recovery even in this patient population is common.[13,15,21] Recovery should be expected to be of longer duration for patients with complete paralysis as opposed to those with facial nerve paresis.

> !
>
> If treated appropriately most cases of facial palsy caused by acute otitis media have a very good prognosis and show a complete recovery.

17.4 Chronic Otitis Media

Paralysis of the facial nerve due to chronic otitis media (COM) is a known complication of advanced disease. Fortunately, facial palsy is seldom encountered in the clinical setting. Despite its infrequency, the morbidity of chronic otitis of such severity is debilitating. Facial paralysis secondary to otitis media occurs more frequently in children and is a more common complication of AOM.[28,29] In 52 cases of otitic facial paralysis, May[29] found 36 cases attributable to AOM, 13 cases attributable to COM with cholesteatoma, and 3 cases attributable to COM without cholesteatoma. A review of the literature provides a reported incidence of facial nerve paralysis in COM ranging from 0.16% to 5.1%.[9,12,30] In 2012, Kim et al[31] reported on a series of 3,435 patients with COM over a period of 20 years, of which only 46 (1.33%) presented with facial paralysis. Similarly, Quaranta[32] reports an incidence of facial paralysis in 1.2% of 1,400 patients with cholesteatoma over a period of 30 years.

> !
>
> Facial palsy due to chronic otitis media, with or without the presence of cholesteatoma, is very rare, even rarer than in cases of acute otitis media.

17.4.1 Pathophysiology

Numerous authors have proposed various mechanisms by which the function of the facial nerve becomes compromised in COM.[1,2,15,18,23,31–34] Hypotheses remain largely conjectural, given the lack of histopathologic confirmation during a window of active disease. Nonetheless, external compression, neural ischemia, osteitis, bone erosion, nerve edema, inflammation, and neurotoxic cellular mediators all have been proposed as potential culprits.

It is well documented that suppurative disease of the middle ear space has multiple routes by which it can access the facial nerve. As mentioned previously, Baxter[6] demonstrated the frequency of nonpathologic dehiscence in a study of temporal bones from the Massachusetts Eye and Ear Infirmary. Additionally, the chorda tympani and stapedial muscle each provide a portal of potential entry to the fallopian canal. Despite this, chronic suppuration of the mesotympanum and mastoid rarely is associated with facial palsy.[18,33] To this end, Graham[18] postulated that natural or acquired dehiscences do not appear to significantly predispose to facial palsy. Furthermore, facial palsy does not appear to be correlated with the degree of fallopian canal involvement. Yetiser[33] reported a series of 24 patients with facial palsy due to COM. Four of these patients presented with varying degrees of paralysis, each of whom demonstrated an intact fallopian canal at the time of surgery. Similarly, multiple cases have been documented in which there was massive exposure of the facial nerve in a bed of inspissated debris, with intact nerve function.[18,33] Both the vertical and the horizontal segments may be involved, but disruption of the nerve is most common in its horizontal course,[23,31–33] likely owing to its inherently thin bony covering. Furthermore, this reflects the commonality by which cholesteatoma exits the posterior epitympanum and mesotympanum, affecting the facial nerve as it transitions from its tympanic segment through the second genu to the vertical segment within the mastoid.

> !
>
> In case of facial palsy caused by chronic otitis media, the nerve damage is most often located in the tympanic segment through the second genu.

Facial palsy in COM may occur with abrupt or gradual onset. A palsy of abrupt onset is commonly due to acute infection superimposed on the presence of cholesteatoma. Such an occurrence should serve as a reminder that not all facial paralysis of acute onset is due to Bell's palsy. Multiple authors hypothesize that gradual, progressive pressure on the facial nerve by adjacent cholesteatoma is the primary mechanism by which facial palsy occurs.[1,2,31] Further neural degeneration and bony resorption are thought to result from the concomitant inflammatory response, facilitated by release of neurotoxic mediators, proteolytic enzymes (collagenases), and osteoclast activity.[1,31,33] Despite the intimate contact of cholesteatoma with the facial nerve, cholesteatoma does not commonly cause abrupt or progressive paresis, and cholesteatoma can often be dissected away from the nerve without violation of neural function.[18] In a population of patients with COM and facial paralysis, the reported range of patients also having cholesteatoma was from 59% to 80%.[30,31,33,35] This suggests that an additional mechanism of action must be present in provoking facial palsy in COM, as a substantial fraction of patients in these studies lacked cholesteatoma. Quaranta,[32] in accordance with other authors,[33] suggests that the primary mechanism by which palsy develops is spread of infection along the course of the facial nerve rather than compression and subsequent ischemia. This theory is supported by the fact that facial nerve dysfunction caused by compression can be expected only after blockage of > 50% of nerve fibers.[36] The likelihood of developing infection in a field of cholesteatoma before such compression could occur is high. Furthermore, Quaranta[32] points out that surgical management of COM without cholesteatoma has demonstrated similar rates of nerve recovery compared with COM with cholesteatoma, affirming the notion that infection plays the more paramount role in the process of facial paralysis.

!

Facial palsy in chronic otitis media with cholesteatoma is often caused by the spread of infection and not primarily by infiltration by cholesteatoma.

It is well known that cholesteatoma of the petrous apex poses greater risk for facial palsy than cholesteatoma of the middle ear and mastoid.[2,33,37–39] Bartels[40] reviewed the literature pertaining to middle ear cholesteatoma extending medially to the petrous bone and reported that 46.2% of cases involved facial paralysis. Atlas[41] et al found facial nerve dysfunction in 7 of 14 patients with cholesteatoma of the same distribution. Similar findings have been found in cholesteatoma extending to the anterior epitympanum.[42] Chu and Jackler[42] report on a series of five patients with anterior epitympanic cholesteatoma and failed facial nerve recovery despite early surgical intervention.

Cholesteatoma of the petrous apex and of the anterior epitympanum have a higher risk for facial palsy and worse facial nerve recovery.

It is likely that the etiology of facial palsy in COM is multifactorial. Despite numerous publications and hypotheses, the pathogenesis of facial palsy in COM remains unclear. An improved understanding, supported by histopathologic evidence, is necessary to develop sound treatment strategies and improved clinical outcomes.

17.4.2 Treatment

There is little controversy regarding treatment for facial paralysis associated with COM. An outline of treatment considerations is presented in ▶ Table 17.2. Careful management with early surgical intervention has proven its efficacy in supporting neural recovery and facial reanimation. Antibiotics and steroids are considered adjunctive measures. The outcomes of surgical intervention in context of facial nerve paralysis due to cholesteatoma are variable. Quaranta[32] reported on a series of 13 patients with cholesteatoma and facial paralysis in which 70% experienced restoration of function to a House–Brackmann grade I or II status after surgical intervention. Restoration of facial function to a grade II paresis was reported to be between 57.2 and 82% by two other authors.[2,33] Harker[34] reported restoration to at least grade II in all patients, while Yetiser[33] asserts that facial paralysis in context of cholesteatoma is uniformly associated with a poor prognosis. However, the clinical utility of such broad statements is difficult to interpret without further case-by-case analysis of the details of clinical presentation and management. It is unclear whether the presence of cholesteatoma affects prognosis of neural recovery. Kim[31] demonstrated greater surgical gain in patients with facial paralysis in absence of cholesteatoma, yet no such result could be reproduced by other authors.[33] The grade of paralysis has not been shown to have significant impact on potential for recovery.[32,34] It has been found that the prognosis of facial paralysis caused by COM is worse than the spontaneous course of Bell's palsy and conductive blockage of the axonal flow seen in traumatic paralysis.[33]

The timing of surgery in relation to the onset of facial palsy is paramount. Patients should be taken to the

Table 17.2 Therapy options for facial palsy caused by chronic otitis media

Measure	Comment
Antibiotic treatment	Antibiotics are considered an adjunctive measure. For chronic suppurative disease or for patients with acute infection superimposed on cholesteatoma, empiric antimicrobial therapy should be initiated and tailored based on culture data
Corticosteroid therapy	The utility of corticosteroid therapy in chronic otitis media with facial palsy is limited
Tympanomastoidectomy	Urgent surgical intervention is imperative in supporting early neural recovery and facial reanimation. Regardless of the exact surgical methodology, complete eradication of cholesteatoma and infection in a single procedure is the goal
Facial nerve decompression	Exploration and potentially decompression of the facial nerve is a secondary goal to eradication of disease. No consensus exists regarding specific surgical methodology in facial nerve management

operating room without delay, regardless of the extent of paralysis, the duration of time since onset of paralysis, the presence or absence of cholesteatoma, age, or history of prior otologic surgery.[31,33] Quaranta[32] demonstrated complete return of function in all patients managed surgically within 7 days of paralysis onset. Similarly, Telischi[15] reported on 10 patients who were managed surgically within 10 days of paralysis onset, all of whom experienced complete recovery. This principle is supported by other authors who report that poor or no recovery of the facial nerve was restricted to a fraction of patients in whom paralysis was not managed with surgical urgency.[2,31] Despite this rule, multiple reports exist documenting complete recovery in the occasional individual with long-standing paralysis prior to surgical intervention.[33] This affirms that notion that these patients should be approached with surgical urgency regardless of the duration of facial paralysis.

!

Facial palsy secondary to chronic otitis media (COM) is a clear indication for immediate surgery. The degree of paralysis is not prognostic, but the duration of paralysis seems to be. Regardless, all patients with facial paralysis resulting from COM are considered for immediate surgery.

The goals of surgery are to eradicate all cholesteatoma and infection and to explore the facial nerve.[15,18,33] Under most circumstances, this involves modified radical mastoidectomy and facial nerve decompression.[15] However, such pathology has been managed alternatively with both intact canal wall and canal wall down operations, and studies have failed to document statistically significant differences in nerve recovery from one technique to the next.[33] No consensus has been reached regarding management of the facial nerve at the time of surgical intervention.

!

Facial palsy in a patient with cholesteatoma requires immediate surgery, but there is controversy over the ideal surgical procedure chosen to eradicate the cholesteatoma.

Management strategies range from decompressing the facial nerve with neurolysis, to decompression without neurolysis, to partial and complete preservation of the fallopian canal. Cawthorne[43] suggested lysis of the epineurial sheath in only those patients with complete paralysis, while Kim[31] proposes conservative opening of the epineurial sheath in areas clearly involved in the inflammatory process. Others report decompression from the geniculate to stylomastoid foramen with complete preservation of the nerve sheath.[33] Still more conservative, some authors explore the nerve but maintain the fallopian canal, removing bone in only the areas of significant erythema and neural edema.[2] Further evidence is needed to definitively support or refute one method over another. Regardless of the specifics of surgical methodology, the complete eradication of disease in a single procedure should be the operative goal for patients with facial paralysis caused by COM.[31] The presence of extensive and erosive cholesteatoma may preclude total removal when it is adherent to an exposed nerve at the region of the horizontal segment and oval window niche.

!

Optimal management of the facial nerve when performing middle ear surgery in a patient with facial palsy and chronic otitis media is not yet clear. Most important is the eradication of the underlying disease. There is currently no evidence that a more aggressive approach to the facial nerve (complete decompression or lysis of the epineurial sheath) results in better facial nerve outcome.

17.5 Necrotizing Otitis Externa

Early reports of necrotizing otitic infections date back to 1959 when Meltzer and Kelemen[44] reported osteomyelitis involving the temporal bone, mandible, and zygoma. Initial publications documented mortality rates exceeding 50%.[45,46] Chandler soon coined the term "malignant otitis externa" in a comprehensive description of the disease process, owing to uniformly grim outcomes.[47] More recently, authors have favored the term necrotizing otitis externa (NOE), given the absence of an invasive neoplastic process. NOE was quickly identified as a disease occurring almost exclusively among diabetic patients, especially those of advanced age.[24,46–52] Reviews have quoted the prevalence of diabetes in NOE at 90 to 100%.[49,51] Growing experience further disclosed the commonality of NOE in patients of immunocompromised status, irrespective of etiology, to include HIV, AIDS, neoplasia, splenectomy, post-transplant immunosuppression, and steroid-induced immunosuppression, among others. In the rare instance that NOE occurs in the pediatric population, it usually is diagnosed in context of malnutrition or malignancy.[49] The symptomatic hallmark is deep, intense otalgia, commonly out of proportion to clinical examination findings.[15] Pain has been described as excruciating, and is commonly most intense at night-time. Patients typically have failed multiple courses of outpatient therapy and experience persistent otorrhea.[49]

> ⚠
>
> If a patient has persistent otorrhea despite multiple courses of therapy, severe otalgia, and reason for immunosuppression, with or without facial palsy, one should consider necrotizing otitis externa.

NOE is known to involve multiple cranial nerves, the most common of which is the facial nerve.[51–53] This is the result of its proximity to the external acoustic meatus and the stylomastoid foramen. Authors have reported rates of facial palsy among patients with NOE up to 70%.[48,50,54] Chandler's early publications (1974) asserted that facial palsy was an ominous prognostic finding[55] that conferred a greater risk of mortality.[56,57] More recent studies have clarified this point, demonstrating that indeed facial palsy does correlate with aggressive disease[46] and disease progression,[50] but that it is not prognostic of adverse outcomes[50–52,54] or worsened survival.[46,51] The majority of patients treated appropriately should expect good recovery of facial function.[15,52] Permanent paralysis presumably indicates necrosis of the nerve, and reanimation procedures should be considered.

> !
>
> Up to 70% of patients with necrotizing otitis externa develop a facial palsy.

17.5.1 Pathophysiology

It is proposed that self-inflicted or iatrogenic trauma to the external auditory canal, albeit minor, is the mechanism by which acute otitis externa develops.[15,58] Cerumen in healthy patients is known to provide protective benefit in controlling the pH of the external auditory canal, yielding an environment that prevents maceration and excessive bacterial colonization. It is proposed that these protective features of cerumen are absent among patients with diabetes, permitting bacterial overgrowth and increased susceptibility to tissue invasion.[59] Microvascular disease, common to diabetics and the elderly,[15,49] is paramount in the pathophysiology of NOE. Diabetic microangiopathy results in ischemic, nutritionally deficient, devitalized tissue. Associated neuronal dysfunction dulls the perception of pain, allowing "silent" disease to remain subclinical and flourish. Chronic hyperglycemia interferes with polymorphonuclear phagocytic function and cell-mediated immunity, and host resistance becomes impaired.[60] Impaired local and systemic immune systems lack the ability to control local infection, permitting progression of uncomplicated otitis externa to a fulminate, systemic invasive infection. Pathogens access the skull base at the most vulnerable portion of the external canal,[15] the osseocartilaginous junction, and proceed to infiltrate the parotid gland and facial nerve by way of the fissures of Santorini. Traversing the tympanomastoid suture and fissures of Santorini provides access to the infratemporal fossa and jugular foramen, placing cranial nerves IX, X, and XI at risk for injury.[51,53] Venous channels and fascial planes provide a scaffold by which pathogens reach the marrow spaces of the skull and eventually the petrous apex, placing cranial nerves V and VI at risk.[51,53] Further extension through the petro-occipital fissure carries the infection intracranially and may result in subperiosteal abscesses or epidural/subdural empyema.[53]

Infection reaches the facial nerve by one of several routes. Proximal injury results from involvement of the main trunk at the stylomastoid foramen via direct extension from the external auditory canal or by direct extension into the pneumatized spaces of the mastoid, where the vertical segment is at risk. A suppurative, granulomatous osteitis may interfere with neuronal depolarization or even transect the nerve.[48] Alternatively, distal involvement may result from extension into the parotid gland and suppurative sialoadenitis.

17.5.2 Diagnostic Work-Up

NOE is diagnosed based upon data gathered from three parameters: clinical examination, serum inflammatory markers, and radiographic studies. It goes without saying that the clinical history commonly proves invaluable in offering clues to narrow the differential. To that end, all diabetic patients with presumed acute otitis externa refractory to standard therapy should be suspected of harboring an invasive pseudomonal infection.[15] Classically, manipulation of the pinna generates far less pain than would be expected for uncomplicated acute otitis externa. Granulation tissue at the junction of the cartilaginous and osseous external auditory canal is said to be a pathognomonic finding in diagnosis of NOE.[15,47,51] However, multiple reports have documented the absence of this finding in patients with concomitant HIV and NOE.[49,61] Alternatively, otomicroscopic examination may demonstrate bone exposure, dehiscence, and adjacent soft tissue changes at the osseocartilaginous junction. External auditory canal skin is routinely edematous and erythematous, and otorrhea is common. The tympanic membrane is typically spared, and commonly the middle ear and mastoid lack the severe inflammatory changes involving the external canal and skull base.[15,48,53] In contrast, fungal otitis externa has been seen to originate more often in the mastoid or middle ear space.[49] Fever, leukocytosis, and other signs of systemic toxicity are typically absent on initial presentation.[15,51]

Despite the clues afforded by the history and physical examination, differentiating NOE from alternative otologic maladies may be difficult. Other pathologies in the differential diagnosis should include otitis externa, cholesteatoma, malignancy, and chronic otomastoiditis. Information provided by an imaging work-up can help to establish a conclusive diagnosis, and a variety of radiographic studies may be of value. Among the most effective studies is computed tomography (CT). CT scanning is readily available and can be obtained quickly. In general, CT illustrates its strength in assessing bony architecture, to include the middle ear space, mastoid cavity, petrous apex, fallopian canal, and carotid canal. Fine anatomic detail provided by CT imaging facilitates identification of the site of facial nerve involvement.

> !
>
> CT is the imaging of first choice when necrotizing otitis externa is suspected.

CT provides early identification of subtle bony erosion and decreased skull base density (▶ Fig. 17.5), but it should be noted that such findings might be absent early in the course of osteomyelitis.[49,52] It has been estimated that 30 to 50% demineralization is necessary before lytic lesions become manifest.[62] Additionally, CT facilitates assessment of the parapharyngeal and subtemporal spaces, the infratemporal fossa, and the nasopharynx. Soudry[46] reported on 57 patients with severe NOE, finding that temporomandibular joint destruction and soft tissue involvement of the infratemporal fossa or nasopharynx were prognostic of aggressive and recalcitrant disease. In the context of NOE, the strength of CT exists in establishing an initial diagnosis and determining the anatomic extent of disease. Contrast-enhanced images may also be effective in demonstrating persistence or resolution of soft tissue changes. However, CT is thought to have limited capacity in following the course of disease, given the rarity at which erosive changes reverse. An end-of-treatment scan may be of value in assessing the bony architecture of the skull base and establishing a new "anatomic baseline" by which future scans may be compared if disease recurs.[63] Magnetic resonance imaging (MRI) provides the added benefit of assessment of the meninges (▶ Fig. 17.6) and medullary bone spaces.[49] It is sensitive in evaluating mucosal changes of the middle ear and mastoid, as well as soft tissue of the external auditory canal and central skull base.[49,63] Fat-suppressed T-1 sequences provide value in marrow-rich regions of the skull base, for the purpose of demonstrating contrast uptake by bone. MRI is thought to be among the most sensitive of radiographic studies for detecting skull base osteomyelitis, especially when bone marrow is present[63] and is a complimentary study to CT in assessing the initial extent of disease. CT and MRI are distinguished from nuclear modalities of imaging in their ability to provide exquisite anatomic detail.

> !
>
> Magnetic resonance imaging can be complimentary to computed tomography in evaluating the skull base for osteomyelitis in patients with necrotizing otitis externa.

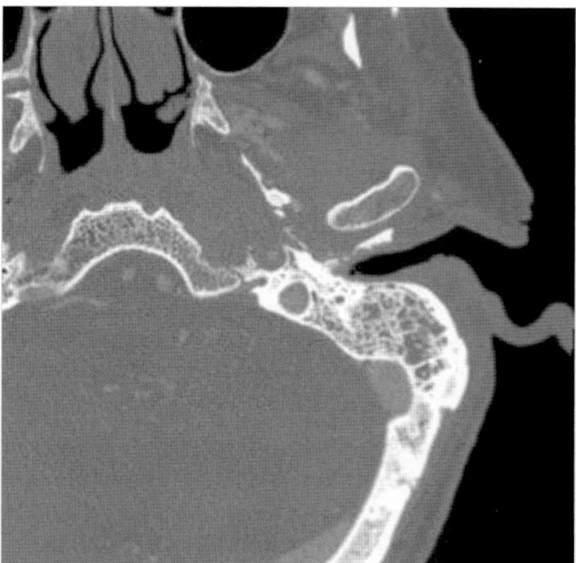

Fig. 17.5 CT demonstrating bony erosion of the anterior external auditory canal in a case of necrotizing otitis externa.

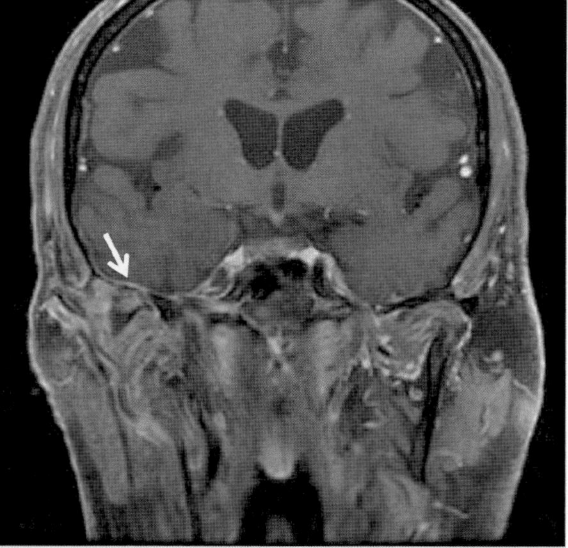

Fig. 17.6 MRI demonstrating dural enhancement (*arrow*) and septic arthritis of the adjacent temporomandibular joint in necrotizing otitis externa.

Table 17.3 Therapy options for facial palsy caused by necrotizing otitis externa

Measure	Comment
Aural toilet	Standard treatment to remove necrotic material and clean the external meatus
Glycemic control	Standard treatment, as most patients are diabetic
Antipseudomonal therapy	Ciprofloxacin is the drug of choice in a dose of 750 mg twice daily for a duration of 6 weeks and until all signs of inflammation have disappeared. For patients that fail on first-line therapy or grow resistant strains of *Pseudomonas*, intravenous cefotaxime in combination with aminoglycoside should be used. A microbiological diagnosis with corresponding sensitivities is mandatory in such cases, and a fungal pathogen should be suspected
Surgery	For abscess drainage, removal of necrotic sequestra, debridement, and biopsy to exclude malignancy or to harvest material for microbiological diagnosis

Various nuclear medicine techniques have been utilized in management of NOE, including technetium, indium, and gallium. Despite the sensitivity of these studies, they are entirely nonspecific and anatomically imprecise. Technetium Tc99 m methylene diphosphonate scintigraphy (bone scanning) provides a sensitive, rapid, and inexpensive method of identifying osteomyelitis. Technetium accumulates in sites of osteoblastic activity, and bone scanning may be positive as early as 24 hours after the onset of infection.[15,49,63] Hence, the value of bone scanning is in early identification of disease. However, as osteogenic activity lacks specificity for infection, bone scanning lacks specificity for NOE. Any of a variety of other pathologies may produce similar results on bone scan. Furthermore, although symptoms subside and clinical evidence of infection resolves, osteoblastic activity may persist indefinitely on technetium imaging, as osteoneogenesis is an ongoing process. This limits the ability of technetium to assess the response to therapy.[15,49,63] Similarly, indium-labeled autologous white blood cells have been shown to be a sensitive marker for infection, and, in contrast to bone scanning, abnormal uptake with indium scanning resolves with resolution of the disease process.[15] However, use of indium is laborious, expensive, and fraught with false positives and false negatives.[15,49] Finally, gallium 67 citrate is a radionuclide bound by granulocytes that accumulates in areas of active inflammation. Similar to other nuclear imaging modalities, it is sensitive and nonspecific, and provides poor anatomic resolution. It is distinguished, however, in that gallium scans quickly revert to normal as infection subsides, providing application for assessing the response to therapy. Despite this feature, gallium scanning is expensive and time intensive, as imaging does not occur until 24 to 48 hours after injection of the radionuclide.[63] Additionally, it delivers a considerably higher dose of radiation to the patient compared with technetium and indium scanning.[49] The anatomic imprecision and nonspecific nature of nuclear imaging prevent the widespread use of nuclear medicine techniques,[15] leaving MRI and CT as the primary imaging modalities in NOE.[53]

!

Technetium Tc99 m scintigraphy can detect osteoblastic activity in the affected bony areas, but it is not specific for necrotizing otitis externa. Gallium is sometimes used to monitor the course and resolution of the disease under therapy.

17.5.3 Treatment

Evolving treatment strategies combined with timely, aggressive management have reduced mortality rates from greater than 50% to between 10 and 20%.[52] The key features of the treatment of NOE with facial palsy are listed in ▶ Table 17.3. Early reports promoted radical surgical debridement as the mainstay of treatment,[49] yet this philosophy has been superseded by a primarily nonsurgical approach, implementing systemic antibiotic therapy as the first-line intervention.[51,53] Key management strategies among patients with NOE include close monitoring with regular aural toilet, systemic antipseudomonal therapy, and tight glycemic control.[49] It is well known that *Pseudomonas aeruginosa*, an aerobic, gram-negative coccobacillus, is universally the most common pathogen in NOE. Typically it is of low virulence and rapidly eliminated by local measures such as canal cleaning and ototopical therapy.[15] However, once established, it has the capacity for angioinvasion with subsequent thrombotic consequences and eventual coagulative necrosis of involved tissues.[49] Treatment should be guided by culture-based antimicrobial therapy in all cases, and cultures should be taken regularly throughout the course of treatment to confirm adequacy of the antimicrobial regimen in the context of increasing prevalence of resistant strains.[49]

!

Standard therapy for necrotizing otitis externa includes regular aural toilet, systemic antipseudomonal therapy (based on confirmatory culture), and tight glycemic control.

Given the commonality with which patients have had multiple prior courses of oral and topical therapy, culture results may show no growth. Empiric treatment with antipseudomonal therapy should then be started. Initially, NOE was managed with a combination of a semisynthetic penicillin (carbenicillin, piperacillin, ticarcillin) and parenteral aminoglycoside (gentamicin, tobramycin, amikacin). The advent of oral antipseudomonal quinolones eliminated the need for parenteral therapy. Oral quinolones have been shown to effectively penetrate bone with a lesser toxicity profile,[64] although dose adjustment is necessary in patients with renal impairment and creatinine clearance rates of less than 30 mL/min.[65] Ciprofloxacin is suggested as the drug of choice for NOE.[49,66] Of concern, use of other oral fluoroquinolones such as levofloxacin, has been shown to predispose patients to infection by resistance pathogens, especially in the context of multiple prior courses of antibiotic therapy before a diagnosis of NOE was established. In the presence of incomplete control from a single agent, authors have suggested that optimal antibiotic therapy consists of ciprofloxacin in combination with a third-generation or fourth-generation cephalosporin.[51] Treatment should not end until symptoms have regressed, systemic inflammatory markers have fallen into normal range, and pathologic examination findings have resolved.

!

Necrotizing otitis externa with facial palsy is treated until symptoms resolve, serum inflammatory markers fall into normal range, and aberrant physical findings regress.

There is growing concern regarding the prevalence of *Pseudomonas* resistance to ciprofloxacin in the context of NOE.[67] Subtherapeutic dosing,[68] treatment of inadequate duration,[49] widespread community use for upper respiratory tract infections,[69] and routine topical use for ear infections have all been shown to promote resistance.[49,51] It should be noted that topical antimicrobials may promote bacterial overgrowth without otherwise affecting the course of disease.[15] The role of ototopical therapy is limited.

⚠

Topical antibiotic treatment with ear drops cannot be recommended. It can promote bacterial overgrowth and does otherwise not affect the course of necrotizing otitis externa.

Oral ciprofloxacin should be prescribed at a dose of 750 mg twice daily for a duration of 6 weeks and until all signs of inflammation have disappeared.[15] For patients that fail to demonstrate improvement on first-line therapy or grow resistant strains of *Pseudomonas*, intravenous cefotaxime in combination with an aminoglycoside should be used. A microbiological diagnosis with corresponding sensitivities is of even greater value in this population, and a fungal pathogen should be suspected. Despite the overall rarity of fungal NOE, fungi are isolated with relative frequency among nondiabetic, immunosuppressed patients, particularly those with HIV AIDS.[15] *Aspergillus* sp. is the most common fungal pathogen. Finally, consensus in the literature describes the application of surgery when necessary for abscess drainage, removal of necrotic sequestra, debridement, and biopsy, the latter of which is for the purpose of excluding malignancy from the differential diagnosis and guiding antimicrobial therapy.[15,49,51] There is extremely infrequent indication for full facial nerve decompression, given the commonality of responsible pathology at the stylomastoid foramen. More aggressive surgery is indicated only in the context of recalcitrant disease as a last resort.[15]

!

Inpatients with necrotizing otitis externa and facial palsy, surgery may be necessary for drainage of abscess or debridement of sequestration, but directly approaching the facial nerve, for instance for decompression, should be reserved as a last resort when all other treatment options have failed.

17.6 Perioperative Management of Acute Facial Palsy during Middle Ear and Mastoid Surgery

During the early days of mastoid surgery, the mallet and chisel, gouge, or curette were used without magnification, and the resulting incidence of iatrogenic facial palsy was as high as 15%.[70] This number was dramatically reduced with the advent of the operating microscope, the high-speed otologic drill, and suction/irrigation. More current reports have estimated iatrogenic facial nerve injury to occur in 1 of 100 cases.[71] In 1997 Nilssen[72] reported an incidence of iatrogenic facial paralysis in 1.7% from a series of 1,024 mastoidectomies. Factors which predispose a patient to iatrogenic injury are numerous and challenge even the most accomplished of surgeons. Among the more common of these are distorted anatomic landmarks and tissue planes in revision surgery, inflammatory disease obscuring or altering the normal course of the nerve, congenital structural anomalies, and aberrant microsurgical technique.[73–76]

!

Although rare, most cases of iatrogenic facial nerve injury during ear surgery are seen during mastoidectomy; see Chapter 9.

Multiple authors have published reports discussing the incidence of facial palsy in mastoid surgery.[72,73,77] Green et al[73] reported on 22 patients with facial palsy over a period of 27 years, 57% of which occurred during mastoidectomy. Nilssen and Wormald[72] reported on 17 patients with facial paralysis, all of which occurred during radical or modified radical mastoidectomy. Removal of bony exostoses is also commonly implicated in iatrogenic facial paralysis and is a more difficult procedure than is generally accepted. This is due to the challenge of identifying facial nerve along the posterior inferior canal wall in a transcanal approach.[77]

During excision of exostosis, the facial nerve is at risk during a transcanal approach to the posterior inferior canal wall region.

It is said that no otologic surgeon, despite the extent of his experience or skill, will complete his career without encountering the dreaded complication of iatrogenic facial paralysis.[71–73,76] No other nerve draws the immediate attention of the public as does the facial nerve. While various deficits such a hearing loss and taste aberrations are subtle, the absent motility of half the face is easily noticed from across a room.[71] Such a complication is devastating to all parties involved,[73,78] which, unfortunately, commonly results in litigation. Second to hearing loss, facial paralysis is the second most common reason for malpractice lawsuits in otologic surgery today; see Chapter 28.[74,79] Any surgeon managing pathology intimately associated with the facial nerve should be well versed in the diagnosis, work-up, and management of facial palsy. The full breadth of this topic is beyond the scope of this chapter; however, the aim of the following discussion is to outline the management of acute facial palsy in the immediate postoperative period following otologic surgery in the authors' practice.

17.6.1 Immediate, Complete Paralysis

All patients undergoing otologic surgery should be examined immediately afterwards to confirm normal functional activity of the facial nerve. Evidence of an intact nerve may be elicited during emergence from anesthesia with nasal alar flaring or symmetric animation of the face in response to a painful stimulus.[76] It should be noted that eye closure as a means of confirming an intact nerve lacks the reliability of full facial mobility. The effect of gravity in a supine position, postoperative facial edema, or restricted tissue mobility from application of a head dressing may augment or impair normal eye closure, conveying inaccurate information regarding neural integrity.[76] Furthermore, young patients with good skin turgor, especially those of Asian descent, may have a completely transected facial nerve and still have adequate eye closure and normal facial tone immediately postoperatively.[77]

!

All patients with surgery near the facial nerve should have an immediate postoperative clinical assessment of function.

If, upon the patient waking, the surgeon is confronted with an immediate, complete paralysis, there are several issues that deserve consideration. The concern for such an event should be shaped by the surgeon's impression of the status of the facial nerve over the duration of the procedure; more details on decision-making in cases of iatrogenic facial nerve lesions are given in Chapter 9. Typically, injury is unlikely if the nerve was intentionally identified.[77] Use of a local anesthetic is a known source of temporary paralysis that causes alarm and anxiety to the surgeon, patient, and family.[74,75,77,78] If the surgeon identified the nerve and is confident of its integrity, patience should be all that is necessary for return of facial function as the effects of local anesthesia subside. This process may take as long as 12 hours, depending upon the duration of action of the chosen anesthetic.[76] Similarly, use of packing material may inflict undue stress and compression of the facial nerve, resulting in loss of function.[74,80] Prior to consideration of more invasive management options, packing material should be carefully removed to facilitate return of function. Further management decisions begin when palsy persists despite removal of packing and the waning effects of local anesthesia have passed. Many otologic surgeons would agree that this scenario warrants surgical exploration.[73,74,78] However, others contend that the decision to explore at this point in time should be based upon the documented status of the facial nerve, or lack thereof, at the time of surgery.[72,77] Green et al[77] suggest that if the status of the facial nerve is unknown, the most experienced surgeon for such a case should proceed with exploration in an expeditious fashion. Similarly, if the nerve was aggressively instrumented, the ear should be explored.[72] However, if the surgeon is confident the nerve is intact despite gentle manipulation, observation with electrophysiologic testing may be appropriate.[72,77]

!

In the case of facial palsy after otologic surgery, the site should be re-explored if there are any doubts after any possible effect of local anesthetic or packing have been ruled out. Electrophysiologic testing can be very helpful to evaluate nerve continuity with intact voluntary motor unit action potentials.

Electromyography (EMG) may serve as a diagnostic adjunct in the acute setting, for aiding in the decision to explore or observe; see Chapter 6 and Chapter 9. Recall that EMG is capable of demonstrating the presence of volitional motor unit action potentials (VMUAPs) even when no movement can be detected visually.[76] If the nerve is transected, EMG will immediately show loss of VMUAPs. However, it should be noted that loss of VMUAPs is not necessarily indicative of a transected nerve. Similar findings may occur as a result of neuropraxia.[81] Therefore, in context of acute facial paralysis on waking from surgery, demonstration of VMUAPs via EMG is helpful to the surgeon in that it indicates that the nerve is intact, eliminating the immediate need for exploration. Loss of VMUAPs in this setting is less helpful, as limited information regarding the extent of injury is provided to the surgeon. If palsy is complete and early exploration is deferred, serial electrophysiologic testing with electroneurography (ENoG) is indicated after 48 to 72 hours have passed. Reduction in the ENoG response to less than 10% of the normal side within 5 days of injury is indicative of severe injury and potentially transection.[76,80] At this point EMG should be utilized to survey for VMUAPs. If no volitional activity is noted on EMG, the patient should be taken for re-exploration.[76,78,80] Exploration should be performed as soon as possible to avoid the complexities of developing inflammatory changes, scar, and granulation tissue.[74,76] Consideration should be given to enlisting the evaluation and opinion of a second, seasoned otologic surgeon.[72,74,76] The quality of the outcome declines dramatically when surgery is delayed beyond 30 days postinjury. When repair is delayed past 1 year, results are uniformly poor.[76,78] No return of function should be anticipated sooner than 4 months after repair, and at least some recovery should begin by 8 months. Function may continue to return upwards of 2 years.[76]

!

In case of a complete postoperative palsy after otologic surgery, mainly electromyography, but also electroneurography, is helpful for the surgeon for further decision-making if exploration by a seasoned otologic surgeon might be necessary.

For cases that do not meet initial electrophysiologic criteria for exploration, the nerve is presumed to be intact. Still, the ENoG may be significantly reduced or even disappear during the first 14 to 21 days. This indicates damage to the axons sufficient to block neural transmission. Delayed recovery is likely over several months. There is no evidence that exploration, resection, grafting, or nerve repair is beneficial under these circumstances.[80] VMUAPs on EMG are indicative of a favorable prognosis, and they may appear as early as 3 to 6 weeks. Despite the appearance of polyphasic potentials, however, recovery will be incomplete, and surgical intervention at this time is not likely to improve outcomes.[76]

17.6.2 Delayed-Onset, Incomplete Palsy

Recovery outcomes for patients with incomplete palsy are generally favorable. Full, spontaneous recovery should be anticipated in this scenario.[82] In the context of delayed-onset facial palsy, the integrity of the nerve is maintained, and the prognosis ultimately is good (House–Brackmann grade I or II).[72,77] Nilssen and Wormald[72] suggest that the pathophysiology behind delayed paralysis in patients with canal wall down cavities is likely to be due to infection of the cavity, compression from packing in the mastoid, or a combination of both. In turn, they advocate removal of packing and painting of the mastoid and tympanic cavity with an antibiotic/steroid cream. Delayed facial palsy that progresses to become complete should be managed similar to Bell's palsy, in that serial electrophysiologic testing with ENoG should be performed until 10 days have transpired since the injury.[72] Exploration should be performed if the nerve degenerates to 10% or less of the normal side within the first week.[73,74,77,78] Patients with delayed-onset facial palsy, even when it progresses to a complete palsy, generally achieve satisfactory recovery.[76]

!

As in other cases of traumatic facial palsy, most patients with incomplete or delayed facial palsy after otologic surgery generally achieve a good facial nerve recovery and do not require surgery.

Undoubtedly, the best way avoid the consequences and emotionally exhaustive sequelae of iatrogenic palsy is to avoid injury in the first place. Imperative to the effort of prevention is a thorough knowledge of the anatomy of the facial nerve as it appears in the operative field, meticulous surgical technique, and the ability to identify cases at risk.[76] Adequate, preoperative counseling is paramount, especially in patients with disease or structural features that heighten risk to the nerve. Due to changing socioeconomic conditions, diseases requiring mastoid surgery are becoming less common, which reduces the opportunity of training residents to develop proficiency in this type of surgery. Despite the rarity of available postmortem histopathologic mastoid specimens, the importance of ongoing temporal bone dissection, to master the anatomy and avoid facial nerve injury, cannot be overstated.[77]

17.7 Key Points

- The intimate structural relationship between the facial nerve, temporal bone, and adjacent otologic organ creates potential for injury by a variety of mechanisms.
- Suppurative infection, neural compression, ischemia, and neurotoxins all may play a role.
- Microsurgery, as a means of solving these inflammatory problems, also poses risk to the facial nerve.
- Facial palsy carries a heavy morbidity that extends beyond concerns of cosmetic outcomes and may be evident of life-threatening infection.
- Recognition and timely management of facial nerve dysfunction is critical to avert the potential morbidity incurred by these inflammatory processes.

References

[1] Antoli-Candela F, Jr, Stewart TJ. The pathophysiology of otologic facial paralysis. Otolaryngol Clin North Am 1974; 7: 309–330

[2] Ikeda M, Nakazato H, Onoda K, Hirai R, Kida A. Facial nerve paralysis caused by middle ear cholesteatoma and effects of surgical intervention. Acta Otolaryngol 2006; 126: 95–100

[3] Taylor H, Wurf N. Public Attitudes Toward People with Disabilities. Study no. 912028. New York: Louis Harris and Associates; 1991

[4] LaRouere MJ, Lundy LB. Anatomy and physiology of the facial nerve. In: Jackler RK, Brackmann DE, eds. Neurotology. Mosby; 2005:1199–1211

[5] Nager GT, Proctor B. Anatomic variations and anomalies involving the facial canal. Otolaryngol Clin North Am 1991; 24: 531–553

[6] Baxter A. Dehiscence of the fallopian canal. An anatomical study. J Laryngol Otol 1971; 85: 587–594

[7] Dietzel K. On dehiscence of the facial nerve canal [in German] Z Laryngol Rhinol Otol 1961; 40: 366–379

[8] Kettel K. Facial palsy of otitic origin: With special regard to its prognosis under conservative treatment and the possibilities of improving results by active surgical intervention: An account of 264 cases subjected to reexamination. Arch Otolaryngol 1943; 37: 303–348

[9] Pollock RA, Brown LA. Facial paralysis in otitis media. In: Graham MD, House WF, eds. Disorders of the Facial Nerve: Anatomy, Diagnosis, and Management. New York: Raven Press; 1982:221–224

[10] Makeham TP, Croxson GR, Coulson S. Infective causes of facial nerve paralysis. Otol Neurotol 2007; 28: 100–103

[11] Popovtzer A, Raveh E, Bahar G, Oestreicher-Kedem Y, Feinmesser R, Nageris BI. Facial palsy associated with acute otitis media. Otolaryngol Head Neck Surg 2005; 132: 327–329

[12] Kangsanarak J, Fooanant S, Ruckphaopunt K, Navacharoen N, Teotrakul S. Extracranial and intracranial complications of suppurative otitis media. Report of 102 cases. J Laryngol Otol 1993; 107: 999–1004

[13] Ellefsen B, Bonding P. Facial palsy in acute otitis media. Clin Otolaryngol Allied Sci 1996; 21: 393–395

[14] Pukander J, Luotonen J, Sipilä M, Timonen M, Karma P. Incidence of acute otitis media. Acta Otolaryngol 1982; 93: 447–453

[15] Telischi FF, Chandler JR, May M, Schaitkin BM. Infection: otitis media, cholesteatoma, necrotizing external otitis, and other inflammatory disorders. In: May M, Schaitkin BM, eds. The Facial Nerve. New York: Thieme; 2000:383–392

[16] Yetiser S. The dehiscent facial nerve canal. Int J Otolaryngol 2012; 2012: 679708

[17] Tschiassny K. Is facial palsy, when complicating a case of acute otitis media, indicative for immediate operation. Cincinnati J Med 1944; 25: 262–266

[18] Graham MD. Facial palsy in acute bacterial infections of the ear. In: Fisch U, ed. Facial nerve surgery: Proceedings of the third International Symposium on Facial Nerve Surgery. Zurich, Switzerland: Kugler Medical Publications; 1976:409–413

[19] Yonamine FK, Tuma J, Silva RF, Soares MC, Testa JR. Facial paralysis associated with acute otitis media. Braz J Otorhinolaryngol 2009; 75: 228–230

[20] Elliott CA, Zalzal GH, Gottlieb WR. Acute otitis media and facial paralysis in children. Ann Otol Rhinol Laryngol 1996; 105: 58–62

[21] Joseph EM, Sperling NM. Facial nerve paralysis in acute otitis media: cause and management revisited. Otolaryngol Head Neck Surg 1998; 118: 694–696

[22] Hydén D, Akerlind B, Peebo M. Inner ear and facial nerve complications of acute otitis media with focus on bacteriology and virology. Acta Otolaryngol 2006; 126: 460–466

[23] Orobello P. Congenital and acquired facial nerve paralysis in children. Otolaryngol Clin North Am 1991; 24: 647–652

[24] Goldstein NA, Casselbrant ML, Bluestone CD, Kurs-Lasky M. Intratemporal complications of acute otitis media in infants and children. Otolaryngol Head Neck Surg 1998; 119: 444–454

[25] Redaelli de Zinis LO, Gamba P, Balzanelli C. Acute otitis media and facial nerve paralysis in adults. Otol Neurotol 2003; 24: 113–117

[26] House JW, Brackmann DE. Facial nerve grading system. Otolaryngol Head Neck Surg 1985; 93: 146–147

[27] Chandler JR, May M. Infection: malignant external otitis and other inflammatory disorders. In: May M, ed. The Facial Nerve. New York: Thieme; 1986

[28] Hof E. Facial palsy of infectious origin in children. In: Fisch U, ed. Facial Nerve Surgery. Birmingham, AL: Aesculapius; 1977

[29] May M, Fria TJ, Blumenthal F, Curtin H. Facial paralysis in children: differential diagnosis. Otolaryngol Head Neck Surg 1981; 89: 841–848

[30] Savić DL, Djerić DR. Facial paralysis in chronic suppurative otitis media. Clin Otolaryngol Allied Sci 1989; 14: 515–517

[31] Kim J, Jung GH, Park SY, Lee WS. Facial nerve paralysis due to chronic otitis media: prognosis in restoration of facial function after surgical intervention. Yonsei Med J 2012; 53: 642–648

[32] Quaranta N, Cassano M, Quaranta A. Facial paralysis associated with cholesteatoma: a review of 13 cases. Otol Neurotol 2007; 28: 405–407

[33] Yetiser S, Tosun F, Kazkayasi M. Facial nerve paralysis due to chronic otitis media. Otol Neurotol 2002; 23: 580–588

[34] Harker LA, Pignatari SS. Facial nerve paralysis secondary to chronic otitis media without cholesteatoma. Am J Otol 1992; 13: 372–374

[35] Altuntas A, Unal A, Aslan A, Ozcan M, Kurkcuoglu S, Nalca Y. Facial nerve paralysis in chronic suppurative otitis media: Ankara Numune Hospital experience. Auris Nasus Larynx 1998; 25: 169–172

[36] Selesnick S, Jackler RK. Facial paralysis in suppurative ear disease: Management considerations. Oper Tech Otolaryngol–Head Neck Surg 1992; 3: 61–68

[37] Yanagihara N, Matsumoto Y. Cholesteatoma in the petrous apex. Laryngoscope 1981; 91: 272–278

[38] Axon PR, Fergie N, Saeed SR, Temple RH, Ramsden RT. Petrosal cholesteatoma: management considerations for minimizing morbidity. Am J Otol 1999; 20: 505–510

[39] Grayeli AB, Mosnier I, El Garem H, Bouccara D, Sterkers O. Extensive intratemporal cholesteatoma: surgical strategy. Am J Otol 2000; 21: 774–781

[40] Bartels LJ. Facial nerve and medially invasive petrous bone cholesteatomas. Ann Otol Rhinol Laryngol 1991; 100: 308–316

[41] Atlas MD, Moffat DA, Hardy DG. Petrous apex cholesteatoma: diagnostic and treatment dilemmas. Laryngoscope 1992; 102: 1363–1368
[42] Chu FW, Jackler RK. Anterior epitympanic cholesteatoma with facial paralysis: a characteristic growth pattern. Laryngoscope 1988; 98: 274–279
[43] Cawthorne T. Intratemporal facial palsy. Arch Otolaryngol 1969; 90: 789–799
[44] Meltzer P, Kelemen G. Pyocyaneus osteomyelitis of the temporal bone, mandible and zygoma Laryngoscope 1959; 69: 1300–1316
[45] Bhandary S, Karki P, Sinha BK. Malignant otitis externa: a review. Pac Health Dialog 2002; 9: 64–67
[46] Soudry E, Hamzany Y, Preis M, Joshua B, Hadar T, Nageris BI. Malignant external otitis: analysis of severe cases. Otolaryngol Head Neck Surg 2011; 144: 758–762
[47] Chandler JR. Malignant external otitis. Laryngoscope 1968; 78: 1257–1294
[48] Chandler JR. Pathogenesis and treatment of facial paralysis due to malignant external otitis. Ann Otol Rhinol Laryngol 1972; 81: 648–658
[49] Hollis S, Evans K. Management of malignant (necrotising) otitis externa. J Laryngol Otol 2011; 125: 1212–1217
[50] Soudry E, Joshua BZ, Sulkes J, Nageris BI. Characteristics and prognosis of malignant external otitis with facial paralysis. Arch Otolaryngol Head Neck Surg 2007; 133: 1002–1004
[51] Mani N, Sudhoff H, Rajagopal S, Moffat D, Axon PR. Cranial nerve involvement in malignant external otitis: implications for clinical outcome. Laryngoscope 2007; 117: 907–910
[52] Mehrotra P, Elbadawey MR, Zammit-Maempel I. Spectrum of radiological appearances of necrotising external otitis: a pictorial review. J Laryngol Otol 2011; 125: 1109–1115
[53] Nawas MT, Daruwalla VJ, Spirer D, Micco AG, Nemeth AJ. Complicated necrotizing otitis externa. Am J Otolaryngol 2013; 34: 706–709
[54] Corey JP, Levandowski RA, Panwalker AP. Prognostic implications of therapy for necrotizing external otitis. Am J Otol 1985; 6: 353–358
[55] Chandler JR. Malignant external otitis and facial paralysis. Otolaryngol Clin North Am 1974; 7: 375–383
[56] Rubin Grandis J, Branstetter BF, IV, Yu VL. The changing face of malignant (necrotising) external otitis: clinical, radiological, and anatomic correlations. Lancet Infect Dis 2004; 4: 34–39
[57] Sreepada GS, Kwartler JA. Skull base osteomyelitis secondary to malignant otitis externa. Curr Opin Otolaryngol Head Neck Surg 2003; 11: 316–323
[58] Rubin J, Yu VL, Kamerer DB, Wagener M. Aural irrigation with water: a potential pathogenic mechanism for inducing malignant external otitis? Ann Otol Rhinol Laryngol 1990; 99: 117–119
[59] Driscoll PV, Ramachandrula A, Drezner DA, Hicks TA, Schaffer SR. Characteristics of cerumen in diabetic patients: a key to understanding malignant external otitis? Otolaryngol Head Neck Surg 1993; 109: 676–679
[60] Kontras SB, Bodenbender JG. Studies of the inflammatory cycle in juvenile diabetes. Am J Dis Child 1968; 116: 130–134
[61] Ress BD, Luntz M, Telischi FF, Balkany TJ, Whiteman ML. Necrotizing external otitis in patients with AIDS. Laryngoscope 1997; 107: 456–460
[62] Noyek AM. Bone scanning in otolaryngology. Laryngoscope 1979; 89 Suppl 18: 1–87
[63] Hirsch BE. Otogenic skull base osteomyelitis. In: Jackler RK, Brackmann DE, eds. Neurotology. Philadelphia: Elsevier; 2005:1096–1106
[64] Barza M. Pharmacokinetics and efficacy of the new quinolones in infections of the eye, ear, nose, and throat. Rev Infect Dis 1988; 10 Suppl 1: S241–S247
[65] Flor S, Guay D, Opsahl J, Tack K, Matzke G. Pharmacokinetics of ofloxacin in healthy subjects and patients with varying degrees of renal impairment. Int J Clin Pharmacol Res 1991; 11: 115–121
[66] Lee YJ, Liu HY, Lin YC, Sun KL, Chun CL, Hsueh PR. Fluoroquinolone resistance of Pseudomonas aeruginosa isolates causing nosocomial infection is correlated with levofloxacin but not ciprofloxacin use. Int J Antimicrob Agents 2010; 35: 261–264
[67] Berenholz L, Katzenell U, Harell M. Evolving resistant pseudomonas to ciprofloxacin in malignant otitis externa. Laryngoscope 2002; 112: 1619–1622
[68] Levenson MJ, Parisier SC, Dolitsky J, Bindra G. Ciprofloxacin: drug of choice in the treatment of malignant external otitis (MEO). Laryngoscope 1991; 101: 821–824
[69] Grossman RF. The role of fluoroquinolones in respiratory tract infections. J Antimicrob Chemother 1997; 40 Suppl A: 59–62
[70] Shambaugh G. Facial nerve decompression and repair. In: Shambaugh G, ed. Surgery of the Ear. Philadelphia: Saunders; 1959:546
[71] Schuring AG. Iatrogenic facial nerve injury. Am J Otol 1988; 9: 432–433
[72] Nilssen EL, Wormald PJ. Facial nerve palsy in mastoid surgery. J Laryngol Otol 1997; 111: 113–116
[73] Green JD, Jr, Shelton C, Brackmann DE. Iatrogenic facial nerve injury during otologic surgery. Laryngoscope 1994; 104: 922–926
[74] Wiet RJ. Iatrogenic facial paralysis. Otolaryngol Clin North Am 1982; 15: 773–780
[75] Long YT, bin Sabir Husin Athar PP, Mahmud R, Saim L. Management of iatrogenic facial nerve palsy and labyrinthine fistula in mastoid surgery. Asian J Surg 2004; 27: 176–179
[76] May M, Schaitkin BM, Wiet RJ, Gupta P. Trauma to the facial nerve: external, surgical, and iatrogenic. In: May M, Schaitkin BM, eds. The Facial Nerve. New York: Thieme; 2000:367–382
[77] Green JD, Jr, Shelton C, Brackmann DE. Surgical management of iatrogenic facial nerve injuries. Otolaryngol Head Neck Surg 1994; 111: 606–610
[78] House JW. Iatrogenic facial paralysis. Ear Nose Throat J 1996; 75: 720–723, 723
[79] Blake DM, Svider PF, Carniol ET, Mauro AC, Eloy JA, Jyung RW. Malpractice in otology. Otolaryngol Head Neck Surg 2013; 149: 554–561
[80] May M. Nerve repair. In: May M, Schaitkin BM, eds. The Facial Nerve. New York: Thieme; 2000:571–609
[81] Schaitkin BM, May M, Klein SR. Topognostic, otovestibular, and electrical testing: diagnosis and prognosis. In: May M, Schaitkin BM, eds. The Facial Nerve. New York: Thieme; 2000:213–230
[82] Graham MD. Prevention and management of iatrogenic facial palsy. Am J Otol 1984; 5: 513

18 Facial Nerve and Vestibular Schwannoma

John C. Goddard, Courtney C. J. Voelker, and Derald E. Brackmann

18.1 Introduction

The evolution of surgery for vestibular schwannoma over the past 60 years has led to improved facial nerve outcomes.[1] Developments in microsurgical techniques and facial nerve monitoring capabilities combined with a growing surgical experience, particularly at high-volume centers, has served as the foundation for this functional improvement.[2] Although facial nerve anatomy within the temporal bone is fairly consistent, the presence of vestibular schwannoma may distort the location, caliber, and course of the facial nerve within the internal auditory canal (IAC) and cerebellopontine angle (CPA). As a consequence, a sound understanding of facial nerve anatomy as it relates to the various approaches for vestibular schwannoma surgery is of vital importance.

18.2 General Considerations in Vestibular Schwannoma Surgery

18.2.1 Indications and Patient Selection

A complete discussion of the management of vestibular schwannoma is beyond the scope of this chapter. However, it is imperative to recognize that the three main treatment options for sporadic vestibular schwannoma are observation with serial imaging, radiation, and surgical resection. Patient preference, tumor characteristics, and experience of the treatment team are just a few of the relevant factors that help guide a treatment decision (▸ Table 18.1). Patients undergoing surgical resection are treated with one of three main approaches: retrosigmoid, middle fossa, or translabyrinthine. In each approach, the facial nerve must be safely navigated by both the neurotologist and the neurosurgeon. While absolute tumor size is the key factor in determining the risk of facial palsy, any situation in which the facial nerve is between the surgeon's line of sight and the tumor will invariably increase this risk as well. The aforementioned anatomical situation is more commonly encountered in the middle fossa approach, which leads to a slightly higher risk of facial palsy, in general, than in either the retrosigmoid or the translabyrinthine approach. Various methods of stereotactic radiation therapy are also available to treat vestibular schwannomas. Regardless of the exact method of radiation employed, the treating physicians must be knowledgeable of facial nerve anatomy in the setting of vestibular schwannoma.

> **!**
>
> Detailed knowledge of facial nerve topography is highly relevant for each approach to the vestibular schwannoma, be it the retrosigmoid, middle fossa, or translabyrinthine approach.

18.2.2 Patient Information and Consent: Surgical

Irrespective of surgical approach, patients undergoing vestibular schwannoma surgery must be fully informed of the potential risks and complications, particularly as they relate to the facial nerve. Facial paresis or paralysis (temporary or permanent, immediate onset or delayed) may occur with any type of treatment for vestibular schwannoma. The prevalence of long-term facial nerve paresis is highly dependent on tumor size as well as the experience of the treatment team. Consequently, discussions about the percentage risks to the facial nerve must

Table 18.1 Considerations when choosing a treatment plan for vestibular schwannoma

Patient factors	Tumor factors	Other factors
Age	Size	Cerebral venous anatomy
Prior treatment experience	Location	Auditory brainstem response data
Occupation	Characteristics (cystic versus solid)	Videonystagmography results
Medical comorbidities	Rate of growth	Treatment center and team experience
Hearing ability	Degree of brainstem compression	
Symptom severity		
Personal preference		

be individualized to both patient and treatment center. The possibility that the tumor may arise from the facial nerve, though rare, should be discussed with the patient. Additionally, the possibility of facial nerve transection and the subsequent need for direct neural repair should also be discussed. Taste disturbances, eye dryness, decreased saliva, aberrant reinnervation, and the need for additional procedures are discussed. Injury to the fifth cranial nerve is another potential complication that is reviewed with the patient preoperatively, as concomitant trigeminal and facial nerve injuries can lead to an increased risk of vision loss in the affected eye.

18.2.3 Patient Information and Consent: Stereotactic Radiation

Patients undergoing stereotactic radiation treatment of their vestibular schwannoma must be fully informed of all potential risks and complications. Although there are a number of risks and complications associated with stereotactic radiation, the present discussion will focus on the facial nerve. Facial paralysis and paresis (temporary or permanent) are possible complications that are explained to the patient before treatment. While facial weakness is most commonly noted immediately or very soon after surgery, facial weakness is often delayed for several weeks following stereotactic radiation. Associated eye dryness, taste disturbance, and nervus intermedius dysfunction are also discussed. Trigeminal nerve dysfunction, particularly as it relates to decreased corneal sensation, is mentioned as this could have more significant consequences in the setting of an associated facial weakness.

18.3 Stereotactic Radiation

18.3.1 Patient Selection

There remains some degree of variability in the indications for stereotactic radiation treatment among practitioners. While a full discussion of this topic is beyond the scope of this chapter, some basic principles of patient selection are applicable. Vestibular schwannoma patients with brainstem compression, hydrocephalus, fifth nerve compression, or lower cranial nerve symptoms are *not* offered stereotactic radiation treatment as a first-line therapy. Patients with tumors less than 2.5 cm within the CPA would be considered potential candidates for stereotactic radiation, while patients with larger tumors would typically be offered surgery. Radiation may be offered to patients with and without serviceable hearing. (Hearing is typically considered serviceable when the pure-tone average [PTA] is 50 dB or less, and the word recognition score [WRS] is 50% or more.)

!

Tumors less than 2.5 cm within the cerebellopontine angle *without* brainstem compression, hydrocephalus, fifth nerve compression, or lower cranial nerve symptoms are potential candidates for stereotactic radiation therapy.

18.3.2 Treatment Steps

A basic principle of stereotactic radiation therapy is to maximize dose to the lesion while minimizing delivery to any surrounding "normal" structures. Motor nerves are felt to be fairly resistant to radiation effects, though efforts to protect the facial nerve are warranted. The course of the facial nerve within the temporal bone is quite consistent and the location of the labyrinthine segment of the facial nerve should be kept in mind during treatment planning. Although high-resolution T2-weighted magnetic resonance imaging (MRI) has been extremely useful in delineating cranial nerves within cerebrospinal fluid spaces, the presence of a vestibular schwannoma usually limits accurate identification of the complete course of the facial nerve; see Chapter 5. Nevertheless, these sequences can help identify the medial aspect of the facial nerve as it leaves the brainstem when the tumor has a small cisternal component. Consequently, treatment planning should minimize radiation to this area to help protect the facial nerve as well as the motor nuclei within the brainstem. Computed tomography (CT) provides a more detailed and accurate view of the labyrinthine segment of the facial nerve than MRI and may be used by some practitioners to better delineate the cochlea as well. However, the authors do not routinely use CT in treatment planning except for cases of suspected facial nerve schwannomas, which often involve the labyrinthine facial nerve and geniculate ganglion.

!

In cases of suspected facial nerve schwannomas, computed tomography, in addition to magnetic resonance imaging, may be helpful to determine if the tumor involves the labyrinthine facial nerve and/or geniculate ganglion.

- Always document facial nerve function before and after therapy
- Treatment planning should be designed to minimize radiation to both the labyrinthine segment and root entry zone of the facial nerve.

18.4 Microsurgery

18.4.1 Retrosigmoid Approach

Patient Selection

The retrosigmoid approach is typically reserved for patients with serviceable hearing (PTA better than 50 dB and WRS greater than 50%) and medially placed tumors, desiring an attempt to preserve hearing. Tumors that extend to the fundus of the IAC may be treated via the retrosigmoid approach, but visualization of the lateral-most aspect of the tumor is often not possible without violating the inner ear. In these cases, if the inner ear is not violated, dissection of the fundal region of the IAC must often be done "blindly" below a bony ridge. Visualization can be aided with the use of angled endoscopes, but it still might be limited. In many centers, the retrosigmoid approach may be used for various sized tumors in patients with or without serviceable hearing. The authors' preference, however, is to use the translabyrinthine approach for any patient (with tumors of any size) electing surgical excision when the hearing is not serviceable. On rare occasions, the retrosigmoid approach may be used in place of the translabyrinthine approach, such as with a prior mastoid cavity (i.e., in a patient with chronic ear disease or previous mastoid cavity) or in a patient with a very anteriorly located sigmoid sinus.

The retrosigmoid approach is generally reserved for medially based tumors in patients with serviceable hearing, *but* visualization of the lateral-most aspect of the tumor, and its relationship to the facial nerve in this area, is limited.

Anesthesia and Positioning

General anesthesia is required in all cases. A head holder with three-point fixation of the skull is used. The patient may be positioned either supine with the head turned away or placed in a lateral decubitus position with the nontumor ear down. Great care is taken during positioning to minimize pressure points and traction injuries. When the patient is placed in the lateral decubitus position, an axillary roll is used to help prevent brachial plexus injury. Somatosensory evoked potentials are often monitored when the patient's head is in three-point fixation. Lumbar puncture with placement of a lumbar drain is performed prior to beginning the case to assist with cerebellar relaxation and wound closure. Facial nerve monitoring (four channels) is used in all cases and requires the presence of a neurophysiologist throughout the case; see Chapter 15.

!

Facial nerve monitoring is recommended in any case of vestibular schwannoma surgery.

Surgical Steps

The scalp incision, soft tissue dissection, and bone flap craniotomy (or craniectomy) are performed in a standard fashion and have little relationship to the facial nerve. Once the sigmoid and transverse sinuses are well delineated and an adequate craniotomy has been performed, the dural opening is made. Identification of the cisterna magna and the release of cerebrospinal fluid prior to cerebellar retraction (facilitated by the lumbar drain) are critical to prevent cerebellar edema and possible herniation through the wound. Once the tumor is identified within the CPA (▶ Fig. 18.1), the facial nerve stimulator should be used to scan for the possibility of an irregularly positioned facial nerve or to identify the tumor as a facial nerve schwannoma.

!

Stimulation with the probe is typically begun at 0.3 mA and decreased incrementally if a positive response is obtained. Positive responses over the posterior aspect of the tumor or the entire tumor surface are suggestive of a posteriorly displaced facial nerve or a facial nerve schwannoma, respectively.

If responses are not obtained along the visualized tumor surface, surgical debulking is performed. Continued use of the facial nerve stimulator is recommended with each subsequent "step" in dissection as no assumptions can be made regarding the course of the facial nerve (▶ Fig. 18.2). It is not uncommon for the facial nerve to take a circuitous course, particularly near the porous acusticus. Severe splaying of the facial nerve is often seen in larger tumors, with fibers of the nerve spread out over a large portion of the tumor. Depending on tumor size, the facial nerve may be identified at the level of the brainstem.

Use of the facial nerve stimulator is recommended with each subsequent step in tumor dissection because of the unpredictability of the facial nerve course.

Once adequate tumor debulking has occurred within the CPA, drilling of the superior, posterior, and inferior

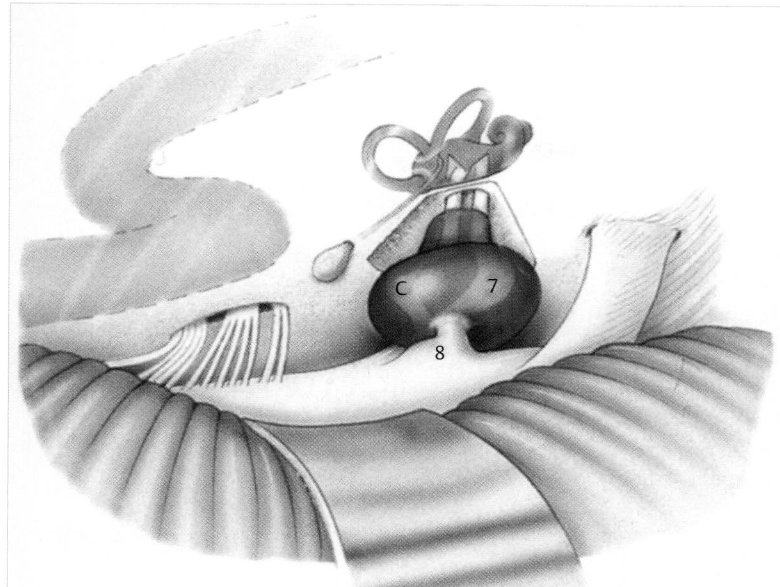

Fig. 18.1 Schematic view obtained through a retrosigmoid approach (left side). A tumor that extends into the internal auditory canal is visualized after bone removal. C, cochlear nerve; 7, facial nerve; 8, eighth cranial nerve. (Reproduced with permission from Jackler R. Atlas of Skull Base Surgery and Neurotology. New York, NY: Thieme Publishing Group; 2009.)

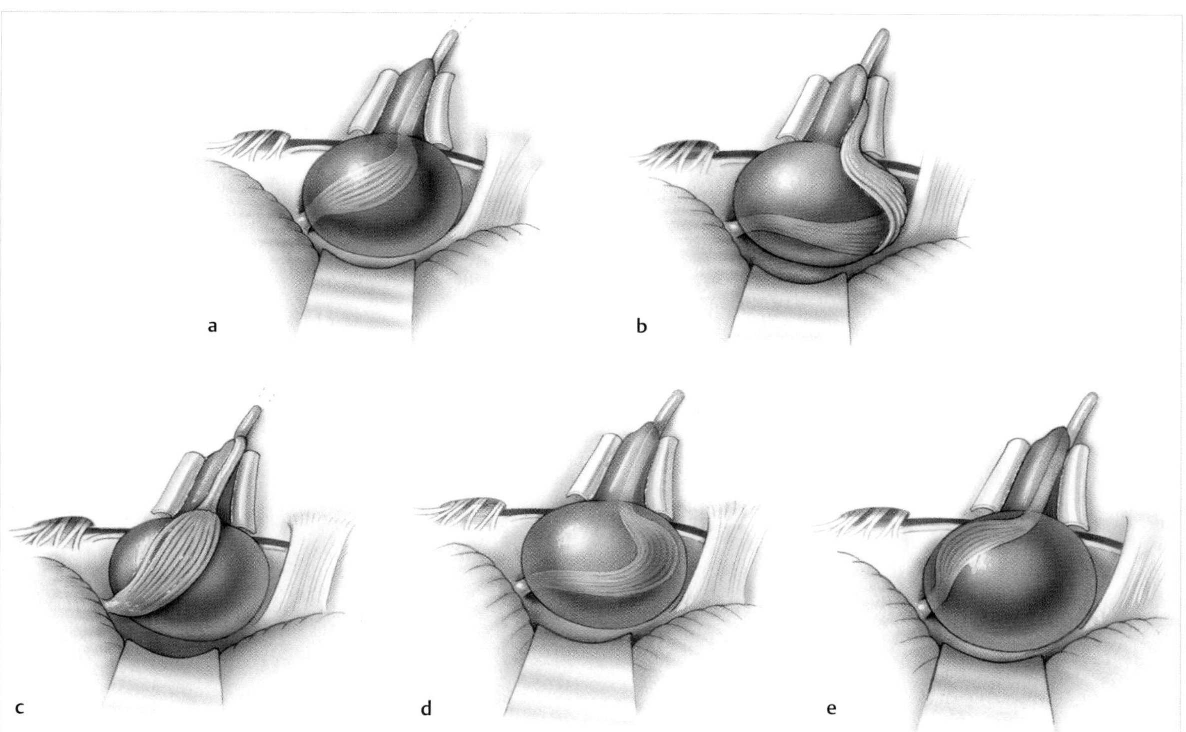

Fig. 18.2 (a–e) Schematic view showing various courses of the facial nerve in relation to a large vestibular schwannoma (left side). (Reproduced with permission from Jackler R. Atlas of Skull Base Surgery and Neurotology. New York, NY: Thieme Publishing Group; 2009.)

aspects of the IAC is required to improve exposure of the lateral extent of the tumor and the tumor–facial nerve interface within the IAC. During bone removal, copious irrigation is used to improve visualization and minimize heat production, which can lead to facial nerve injury. Adequate bone removal around the IAC is critical to optimize visualization of the lateral extent of the tumor. The authors use the facial nerve stimulator to try and "map" the expected course of the facial nerve during bony removal around the IAC. By doing so, one can determine where bone removal can be performed more extensively. As the facial nerve often lies more superiorly within the IAC, bone removal along the superior aspect of the IAC must be done cautiously and with great attention to help minimize any trauma to the underlying dura. The facial nerve monitor will often display an electromyographic burst if the nerve is close to the upper aspect of the IAC dura during bone removal in this region. Identification of the facial nerve laterally within the IAC will often allow for demarcation of the tumor–nerve interface. However, minimizing traction is an important consideration and consequently, tumor debulking should be continued before dissecting the lateral tumor too aggressively. In essence, the dissection of the tumor–facial nerve interface, particularly as it relates to the porous, should be one of the last portions of the tumor dissection.

!

Tumor debulking may be performed with a variety of instruments. At the authors' center, a combination of sharp dissection, handheld ultrasonic aspiration, and laser excision are used. The authors emphasize tumor debulking throughout the case and advocate maximal tumor debulking before dissecting the tumor–facial nerve interface to any significant extent.

Identification of the cochleovestibular nerve at the brainstem is an important anatomical landmark. If at all possible, the cochlear nerve should be maintained during dissection to provide support and minimize unwanted traction on the facial nerve. As the authors typically perform the retrosigmoid approach when attempting hearing preservation, maintaining the integrity of the cochlear division of the eighth cranial nerve is an important goal in every case. However, even when the nerve cannot be salvaged secondary to tumor involvement, an attempt is made to maintain the nerve for the purpose of stability during dissection. Adherence of the tumor to the facial nerve may necessitate leaving a small layer of tumor capsule to protect the integrity of the facial nerve. While many factors are involved and each case must be handled individually, preservation of facial nerve function has significantly improved by using this principle.

- Frequent use of the facial nerve stimulator helps identify the facial nerve course
- Copious irrigation during drilling is necessary to improve visualization and minimize thermal energy production within the internal auditory canal and intracranial cavity
- Tumor adherence to the facial nerve may necessitate leaving a cuff of tumor to protect the integrity of the facial nerve.

18.4.2 Middle Fossa Approach

Patient Selection

The middle fossa approach is ideally suited for patients with serviceable hearing and small- to medium-sized lesions (up to 1.8 cm in total transverse diameter) found within the IAC and CPA (▶ Fig. 18.3). Tumors with a small cisternal component may also be approached via middle fossa craniotomy, but further medial extension generally precludes the use of this approach.

Favorable candidates for middle fossa surgery are patients with small- to medium-sized tumors found within the internal auditory canal (with minimal cerebellopontine angle extension) and serviceable hearing.

Division of the superior petrosal sinus can improve medial access within the posterior fossa, although this technique is typically reserved for superiorly placed IAC/CPA meningiomas, which are often based along the tentorium. The middle fossa approach may also be used as a means of decompressing the contents of the IAC in selected

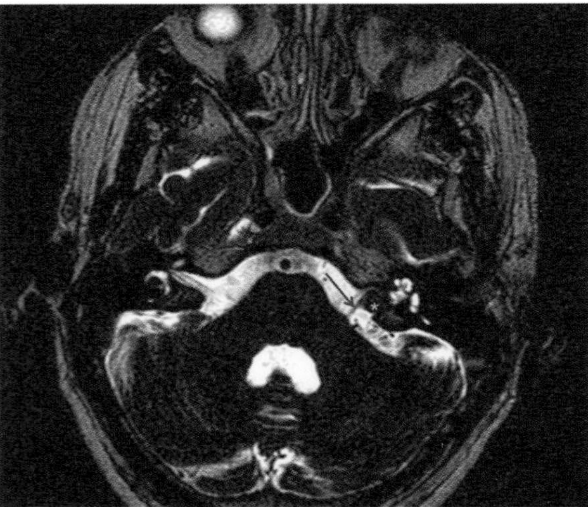

Fig. 18.3 Axial, high-resolution T2-weighted image demonstrating a left internal auditory canal filling defect (*asterisk*). Cerebrospinal fluid is seen between the tumor and the fundus, indicating that the tumor has not impacted the cochlear aperture. The facial nerve can be seen running anteriorly along the tumor (*blue arrow*).

cases.[3] Poor preoperative auditory brainstem response (ABR) waveform morphology and a lack of cerebrospinal fluid lateral to the tumor portend a lower chance of hearing preservation with the middle fossa approach.[4–6] Preoperative videonystagmography and vestibular evoked myogenic potential testing may provide information about the status of the superior and inferior vestibular nerves and thus provide some information as to the expected nerve of origin. In combination with preoperative ABR data and MRI characteristics, this information assists in counseling patients regarding the likelihood of hearing preservation.

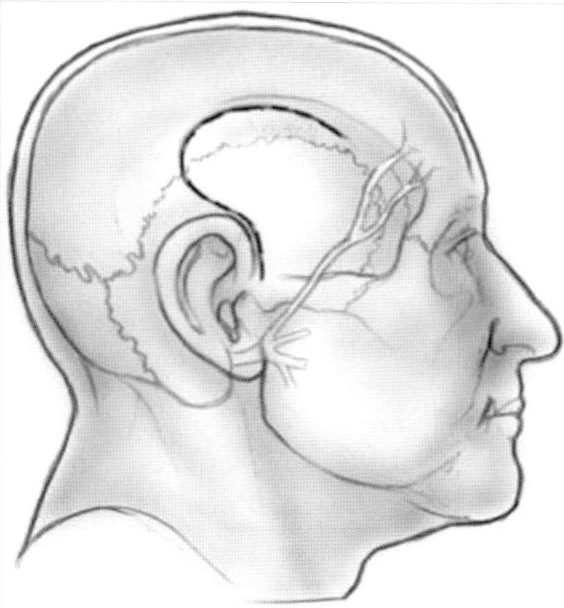

Fig. 18.4 The "reverse question mark" incision for a right middle fossa approach is marked in the temporal region. (Reproduced with permission from Brackmann D, Shelton C, Arriaga M, eds. Otologic Surgery. 3rd ed. Philadelphia, PA: Saunders Elsevier; 2010.)

Anesthesia and Positioning

General anesthesia and four-channel facial nerve monitoring are used in all cases. Long-acting muscle relaxants are strictly avoided and a neurophysiologist is present throughout the case to assist with facial nerve monitoring. The patient is placed in a supine position with the head turned away from the affected side. The surgeon is seated at the head of the bed with the scrub nurse positioned on the patient's left side and the microscope positioned on the right side.

Surgical Steps

A reverse-question mark incision is outlined in the temporal area, beginning in the pretragal region and extending toward the hairline (▶ Fig. 18.4). Local anesthesia should not be infiltrated near the mastoid tip or at the level of the zygomatic arch to avoid neuropraxia of the facial nerve. The scalp and temporalis muscle are incised and elevated anteriorly. Soft tissue dissection continues inferiorly to the root of the zygomatic arch. To avoid injury to the temporal branch of the facial nerve, care is taken to remain near the junction between the bony ear canal and the zygomatic root.

Local anesthesia should *not* be used near the mastoid tip or at the level of the zygomatic arch to avoid neuropraxia of the facial nerve!

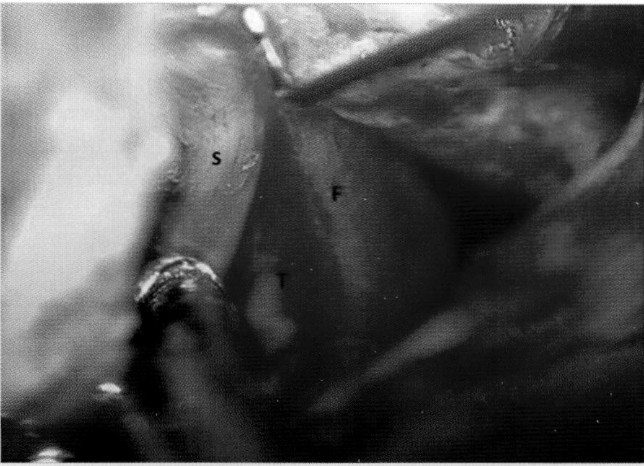

Fig. 18.5 Intraoperative photograph of a left-sided vestibular schwannoma arising from the inferior vestibular nerve. The superior vestibular nerve (S) and facial nerve (F) are seen coursing over the top of the tumor (T).

A bone flap craniotomy (approximately 5 × 5 cm) is performed to expose the temporal lobe dura. Elevation of the temporal lobe dura proceeds from posterior to anterior, thereby minimizing the potential for avulsion injury of an exposed geniculate ganglion and greater superficial petrosal nerve within the floor of the middle cranial fossa. Drilling of the bony IAC commences medially until the IAC is well delineated. While the typical course of the facial nerve is anterior to the tumor in the middle fossa approach, one must be prepared for an irregularly positioned facial nerve. The nerve of origin of the tumor (inferior versus superior vestibular nerve) will often dictate the precise location of the facial nerve (▶ Fig. 18.5).

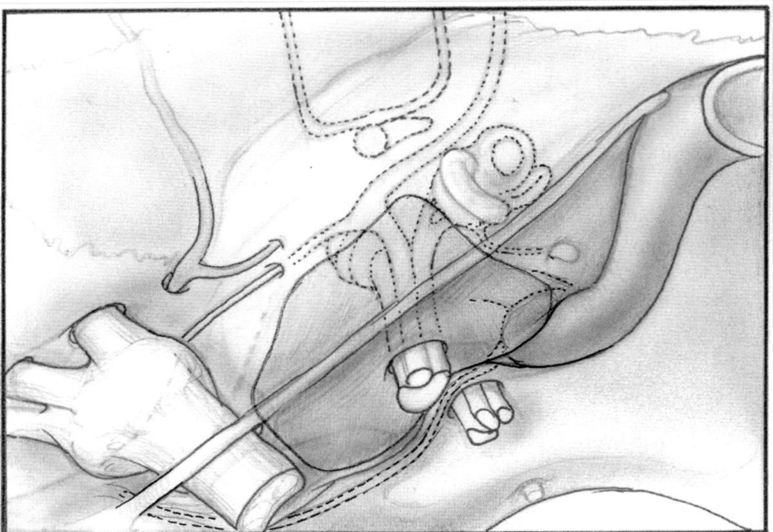

Fig. 18.6 Diagram demonstrating the labyrinthine segment of the facial nerve as visualized in the middle fossa approach (right side). Bill's bar is a vertical crest of bone that separates the facial nerve from the superior vestibular nerve. (Reproduced with permission from Brackmann D, Shelton C, Arriaga M, eds. Otologic Surgery. 3rd ed. Philadelphia, PA: Saunders Elsevier; 2010.)

!

Vestibular schwannomas arise from either the superior or inferior vestibular nerve. The arrangement of the vestibular, cochlear, and facial nerves within the "normal" internal auditory canal is quite consistent: the vestibular nerves are found posteriorly and the facial and cochlear nerves are found anteriorly. Consequently, an inferior vestibular nerve tumor will often have the facial nerve on its superior surface, requiring that the surgeon work "around" the nerve to remove the tumor. A superior vestibular nerve tumor may push the facial nerve anteriorly and inferiorly, typically allowing for less manipulation of the facial nerve during tumor removal. Although these relationships may not be discernible preoperatively, it is important to keep these potential variations of facial nerve position in mind during both bone removal and tumor dissection.

The facial nerve stimulator should be used to map the course of the facial nerve during removal of the bone around the IAC. The facial nerve will often stimulate through the thin dura of the IAC. Continuous irrigation and avoidance of direct trauma to the dura and its contents are important principles. Bone removal over the labyrinthine segment of the facial nerve is performed as one of the final steps in the bony dissection. Following medial identification of the IAC, the surgeon must proceed laterally by staying directly superior to the IAC. Great care must be taken to avoid violating the cochlear lumen during lateral IAC dissection, but adequate bone removal must occur in this region to improve visualization along the anterior aspect of the lateral IAC. Palpation of the lateral aspect of the IAC can be performed using a blunt right-angle hook and may help delineate the expected takeoff point of the labyrinthine facial nerve. High-power magnification and copious irrigation are required when removing bone over the labyrinthine facial nerve (▶ Fig. 18.6). It is imperative that the bone over the lateral-most aspect of the IAC be removed to allow for adequate exposure near the fundus, thereby minimizing the need for "blind" tumor dissection in this region.

→•

Facial nerve outcomes are enhanced by the use of the facial nerve stimulator, high-power magnification, and copious irrigation.

The geniculate ganglion and greater superficial petrosal nerve, which may be exposed secondary to dehiscence of the overlying petrous bone, serve as additional landmarks for identification of the labyrinthine facial nerve. The dural opening is typically performed in the posterior half of the IAC to help avoid direct injury to the facial nerve. The facial nerve stimulator is used to help identify the nerve course prior to and throughout the dural opening process. When the facial nerve is splayed superiorly over the tumor, dissection is particularly challenging. In these instances, the surgeon must work with the facial nerve directly between their line of sight and the tumor. Adequate bone removal around the IAC both anteriorly (medially, within the petrous apex just deep to the cochlea) and posteriorly (toward the semicircular canals) is essential to create working space so

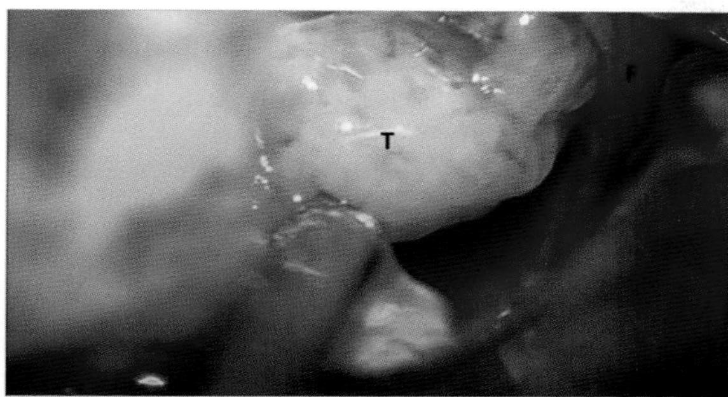

Fig. 18.7 Intraoperative photograph demonstrating vestibular schwannoma removal through a left middle fossa approach. The facial nerve (F) is visualized (anteriorly) as the tumor (T) is manipulated.

that the tumor is easier to manipulate during extirpation (▶ Fig. 18.7).

Middle Fossa Decompression of Vestibular Schwannoma

- The temporal branch of the facial nerve crosses near the middle third of the zygomatic arch and is at risk during dissection and retraction of the scalp and muscle flaps during the middle fossa approach.
- Use the facial nerve stimulator to help confirm the expected location of the geniculate ganglion as the bone over the geniculate ganglion may be dehiscent.
- Reduce the revolutions per minute of the drill to minimize thermal energy production and use the forward and reverse features to help direct any drill skips away from the facial nerve and contents of the internal auditory canal (IAC). If operating on a right-sided tumor, when drilling the posterior (rear) portion of the IAC, the drill is placed in reverse ("right, rear, reverse"). The drill is kept in forward position when drilling the bone anterior to the IAC. For a left-sided tumor, the drill is kept in forward for the posterior dissection, while it is placed in reverse for the anterior dissection.

In certain situations, the middle fossa approach may be used to decompress the contents of the IAC by removing the bone around the IAC and opening the dural sheath. This technique, known as middle fossa decompression, involves the same steps as the standard middle fossa approach described earlier and has similar considerations for handling the facial nerve. This technique may be used in patients with neurofibromatosis type 2 who have a growing tumor in their only hearing ear or who have had a recent decline in the quality of hearing in an only hearing ear. Alternatively, patients with sporadic vestibular schwannoma whose tumor is in the only hearing ear may also be candidates for this approach. Finally, patients with facial nerve schwannomas within the IAC may also benefit from middle fossa decompression. Because of the limited intradural dissection with this approach, the risk to the facial nerve is lower than in cases involving tumor removal.

18.4.3 Translabyrinthine Approach

Patient Selection

The translabyrinthine approach may be used for CPA tumors of any size. Patients with nonserviceable hearing, regardless of tumor size, or large tumors, for which hearing preservation is unlikely, are typical candidates for this approach. The translabyrinthine approach provides excellent exposure of the CPA and does not require brain retraction. In addition, it allows for early identification of the facial nerve.

The translabyrinthine approach is a good choice for patients with nonserviceable hearing, regardless of tumor size, or large tumors for which hearing preservation is unlikely.

Anesthesia and Positioning

General anesthesia and facial nerve monitoring are required in all cases. Long-acting muscle relaxants are avoided. A neurophysiologist is present to assist with facial nerve monitoring. The patient is placed in a supine position with the head turned away from the affected side.

Surgical Steps

A C-shaped incision is marked approximately two fingerbreadths posterior to the postauricular crease. A wide mastoidectomy is performed with decompression of the tegmen mastoideum, posterior fossa dura, and sigmoid sinus. It is important to identify the location of the vertical segment of the facial nerve in order to maximize exposure of the IAC (▶ Fig. 18.8). Removal of bone overlying the vertical facial nerve requires copious irrigation and use of a medium-sized diamond bur. The facial nerve stimulator may be used to confirm the location of the facial nerve throughout this process. It is important to leave bone over the facial nerve to protect it from inadvertent injury during the remainder of the procedure.

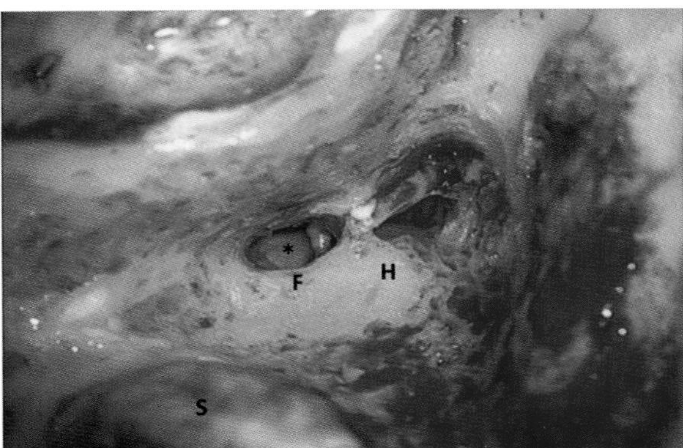

Fig. 18.8 Intraoperative photograph of the vertical facial nerve (F) during a left translabyrinthine craniotomy. The horizontal semicircular canal (H), facial recess (*asterisk*), and sigmoid sinus (S) are helpful landmarks during surgery.

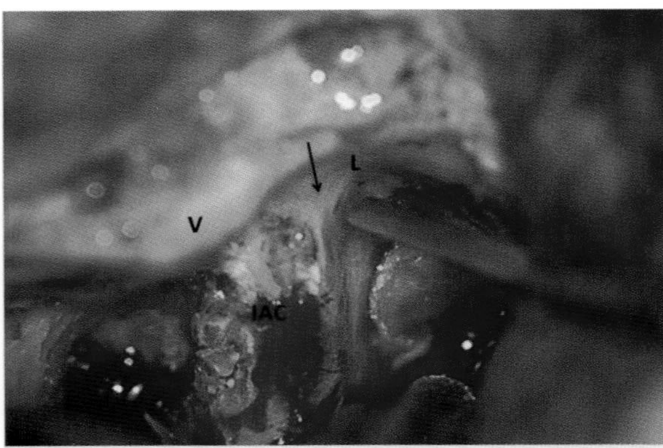

Fig. 18.9 Intraoperative photograph of the labyrinthine facial nerve (L) during a left translabyrinthine craniotomy. The *arrow* shows the location of the vertical crest (Bill's bar); the vertical facial nerve (V) and internal auditory canal (IAC) are also identified.

!

In many cases, the tympanic segment of the facial nerve is visualized through the antrum and facial recess. The recess is typically opened and the incus removed to allow for packing of the eustachian tube and middle ear space in an effort to reduce the chance of postoperative cerebrospinal fluid leakage and associated rhinorrhea. Care must be taken to avoid injury to the facial nerve during this step as the bone overlying the tympanic segment of the nerve can often be dehiscent.

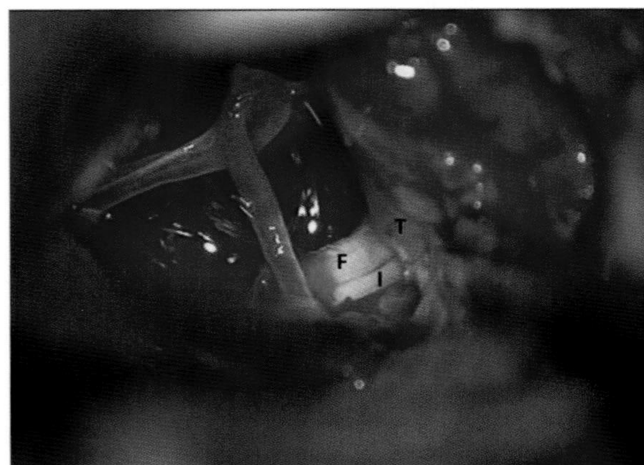

Fig. 18.10 Intraoperative photograph of the interface of the facial nerve (F) and the tumor (T) at the brainstem during a left translabyrinthine approach. The nervus intermedius (I) is also seen.

After the labyrinthectomy has been performed, the IAC dura is skeletonized. As bone is removed and the dura is exposed, the facial nerve stimulator should be used to probe the dura superiorly and inferiorly to identify the course of the facial nerve. This technique can aid the surgeon in identifying where bone can safely be removed. Avoidance of heat production by copious irrigation is particularly important while drilling superior to the IAC as the facial nerve is often located along the superior margin of the tumor. Bone removal must continue until the entire IAC is decompressed, preferably nearly 300 degrees circumferentially and along its entire length. The expected location of the labyrinthine segment of the facial nerve is fairly consistent and identification of the nerve is performed by carefully skeletonizing the bone over the nerve (▶ Fig. 18.9). Identification of the labyrinthine facial nerve as it interfaces with the tumor is performed laterally within the IAC. Once the dura is opened, the facial nerve stimulator should again be used to confirm that the entire tumor surface does not stimulate, which would be suggestive of a facial schwannoma. (In cases of unexpected facial nerve schwannoma, with normal preoperative facial nerve function, the authors typically perform a complete bony decompression of the IAC and avoid tumor removal. If the tumor is causing severe brainstem compression, tumor resection would be indicated and a nerve graft should be performed if possible.) Laterally, the superior vestibular nerve is identified and the vertical crest (Bill's bar) is palpated with a small right-angle hook. The facial nerve stimulator is used to confirm the identification of the facial nerve, which lies just on the other side of Bill's bar. The superior vestibular nerve is then sharply transected, providing visualization of the facial nerve. The lateral tumor-facial nerve interface is not typically dissected at this point. Rather, tumor dissection begins from a more medial and posterior aspect, debulking the tumor and attempting to identify the facial nerve near the brainstem (▶ Fig. 18.10).

!

Leaving the facial nerve–tumor interface "intact" laterally within the internal auditory canal (IAC) provides stability during tumor dissection more medially. Although early identification of the facial nerve at the level of Bill's bar is important, lateral-to-medial tumor dissection should be delayed until late in the extirpative process. By preserving the interface between the tumor and the lateral contents of the IAC, the surgeon minimizes potential stretch injury of the facial nerve that might otherwise occur during medial tumor dissection and debulking if the nerve were not stabilized by attachments to the tumor and eighth nerve fibers.

As the tumor is progressively debulked, the interface between the entire length of the facial nerve and the tumor is more clearly defined. Once medial dissection and tumor extirpation have been performed as much as possible, the lateral facial nerve–tumor interface is dissected and continued medially toward the porous acusticus. The facial nerve is often most adherent to tumor at the level of the porous acusticus and thus great care and patience must be displayed in this region. The facial nerve stimulator should be used during this dissection to help map the location of the facial nerve. Dissection techniques or maneuvers that lead to long-standing facial nerve activity ("train" activity) should be modified to minimize traction on the nerve. Additionally, it is important to maintain a moist working environment (through copious and frequent irrigation) to prevent drying of the facial nerve within the CPA. The degree of tumor adherence to the brainstem or facial nerve will dictate whether tumor tissue will be left in place or not. In many cases, total removal of the tumor is possible, but if there is any concern that continued dissection could compromise neural function, then dissection is stopped and a small layer of tumor capsule is left behind.

→•

- Excellent exposure can be achieved with a properly performed translabyrinthine approach. Adequate bone removal around the internal auditory canal (IAC) significantly improves visualization during tumor dissection and helps with the ability to more safely dissect tumor from the facial nerve.
- Be sure to monitor the heat production of the microscope light source. High-powered, high-intensity light microscopes can cause excessive heat production, leading to dessication of tissue. Frequent irrigation should be used to help prevent this.
- Identification of the vertical segment of the facial nerve is necessary as it allows for safer and more complete bone removal medially, thereby improving overall exposure.
- Look for the possibility of an exposed tympanic segment of the facial nerve, particularly during middle ear packing, and recognize this as another site of potential facial nerve injury.
- During bone removal near the porous acusticus and IAC, use the facial nerve stimulator probe to try and determine the course of the cisternal and IAC portions of the facial nerve.

18.5 Postoperative Considerations

It is important to assess facial nerve function of the vestibular schwannoma patient after awakening from surgery. Normal facial nerve function upon awakening is more likely to result in a favorable long-term outcome than when immediate facial nerve dysfunction is noted. Correlation of facial nerve function, short or long term, with electrical stimulation values at the end of a surgical case is quite unreliable in the authors' experience. Nevertheless, strong electrical responses at low amperage levels combined with normal facial nerve function on awakening will usually portend an excellent long-term prognosis. The authors routinely use postoperative corticosteroids as well as antiviral medications in an effort to reduce edema associated with facial nerve dissection and prevent delayed facial weakness.[7] Careful and frequent assessment of facial function is necessary in the postoperative period as gradual facial nerve paresis and a more delayed facial nerve weakness may both occur. In cases of delayed facial nerve paralysis occurring 2 or more weeks after surgery, the patient is often re-dosed with corticosteroids. Regardless of the timing of facial weakness in the postoperative period, emphasis on proper and continuous eye protection is stressed to the patient and family members. Ophthalmology consultation is obtained for the small number of patients with facial nerve paralysis that may be prolonged or whose cornea demonstrates a potential for dryness and irritation.

18.6 Complications

Facial nerve injury, including stretch, crush, or thermal injury, and partial or complete transection, can occur in all approaches. Larger tumors are often associated with greater risk to the facial nerve, generally as a consequence of the splaying of the facial nerve fibers, which makes it more susceptible to injury. Trigeminal nerve injury, although rare, may also affect corneal sensation, which can compound a facial nerve paresis or paralysis.

18.6.1 Measures for Specific Complications

Facial nerve paralysis in the setting of an intact facial nerve is managed conservatively. Eye care is of critical importance and diligent lubrication of the eye is required. Progressive or delayed facial weakness after an initial period of normal facial nerve function postoperatively will almost always improve over time. Facial nerve grafting is useful in cases of transection when a nerve stump is available at the brainstem. Facial–hypoglossal nerve grafts and cross-facial nerve grafts with free tissue transfer may be employed when direct anastomosis is not possible; see also Chapter 20.

18.7 Key Points

- Facial nerve injury and associated dysfunction are possible with all treatments for vestibular schwannomas.
- A fully informed consent, with particular emphasis on the potential for facial nerve paresis or paralysis, is required before a patient undergoes treatment for vestibular schwannoma.
- Stereotactic radiation treatment should minimize radiation delivery to the facial nerve, when possible.
- The facial nerve stimulator should always be used during surgery for vestibular schwannoma, regardless of approach and tumor size.
- The facial nerve may be injured at various sites *other* than the cerebellopontine angle/internal auditory canal section of the nerve during vestibular schwannoma surgery.
- Tumor debulking is critical to successful vestibular schwannoma surgery with minimization of facial nerve injury.
- A thorough understanding of facial nerve anatomy and acknowledgement of the potential variability of the course of the facial nerve in cases of vestibular schwannoma is required.
- Tumor debulking, use of the facial nerve stimulator, frequent and copious irrigation, and minimization of traumatic facial nerve dissection are important aspects for achieving optimal facial nerve outcomes.

References

[1] Brackmann DE, Cullen RD, Fisher LM. Facial nerve function after translabyrinthine vestibular schwannoma surgery. Otolaryngol Head Neck Surg 2007; 136: 773–777

[2] Slattery WH, Schwartz MS, Fisher LM, Oppenheimer M. Acoustic neuroma surgical cost and outcome by hospital volume in California. Otolaryngol Head Neck Surg 2004; 130: 726–735

[3] Slattery WH, Hoa M, Bonne N et al. Middle fossa decompression for hearing preservation: a review of institutional results and indications. Otol Neurotol 2011; 32: 1017–1024

[4] Goddard JC, Schwartz MS, Friedman RA. Fundal fluid as a predictor of hearing preservation in the middle cranial fossa approach for vestibular schwannoma. Otol Neurotol 2010; 31: 1128–1134

[5] Phillips DJ, Kobylarz EJ, De Peralta ET, Stieg PE, Selesnick SH. Predictive factors of hearing preservation after surgical resection of small vestibular schwannomas. Otol Neurotol 2010; 31: 1463–1468

[6] Kutz JW, Jr, Scoresby T, Isaacson B et al. Hearing preservation using the middle fossa approach for the treatment of vestibular schwannoma. Neurosurgery 2012; 70: 334–340, discussion 340–341

[7] Brackmann DE, Fisher LM, Hansen M, Halim A, Slattery WH. The effect of famciclovir on delayed facial paralysis after acoustic tumor resection. Laryngoscope 2008; 118: 1617–1620

19 The Facial Nerve and Parotid Surgery

Orlando Guntinas-Lichius and Mira Finkensieper

19.1 Introduction

Parotid surgery often also means facial nerve surgery. When using a classical parotidectomy approach in parotid tumor surgery, the surgery is mainly directed by the dissection of the facial nerve and its peripheral branches. By doing this, the tumor resection is advanced and finally the tumor can be extirpated. When performing an extracapsular dissection approach for a small mobile parotid tumor, the facial nerve is not explored. Even then, or perhaps especially in this situation, the surgeon has to think about the facial nerve, as facial nerve monitoring in some countries, for instance in Germany, is recommended as a mandatory prerequisite for extracapsular dissection to decrease the risk of unwanted facial nerve injury.[1,2] Depending on the underlying disease, patients undergoing parotid surgery have a risk for transient and even permanent paresis of the facial nerve. Therefore, the facial nerve and its functions are an important topic in the presurgical consultation and the patient's informed consent. The surgeon has to consider all possible measures before and during parotid surgery to avoid facial palsy. Furthermore, one has to be prepared to manage a facial nerve lesion during parotid surgery and in follow-up.

19.2 Definition

Parotid surgery ranges from a small biopsy to radical parotidectomy and includes surgery of the accessory parotid gland. A facial palsy occurring during or after parotid surgery is the result of a special form of a trauma to the facial nerve; see Chapter 9. It can occur intentionally as part of the surgical plan, for instance in cases of malignant parotid tumors with facial nerve infiltration, but most frequently it occurs unintentionally and is detected after surgery when the patient awakens. The facial palsy can be incomplete (paresis) or complete (paralysis). This differentiation is important as it has an important impact on the management of the palsy.

19.3 Epidemiology and Etiology

The incidence of temporary deficits after lateral and total parotidectomy varies in literature reports from 18% to approximately 65%, depending on the method used to assess facial nerve function.[3–6] Using more limited approaches to the parotid gland, such as extracapsular dissection, the reported incidence varies from 10 to 24%.[2,7] A permanent facial paresis rate from 2 to 8% is reported. The possible types of injury are listed in ▶ Table 19.1. Many cases of litigation for medical malpractice related to parotid surgery are about facial nerve palsy.[8] Most cases pertaining to facial nerve injury are cited for improper performance of the operation. To date there are no cases cited for not using a facial nerve monitor as grounds for the suit, at least in Germany or the United States; see Chapter 15.

19.4 Risk Factors for Postoperative Facial Palsy After Parotid Surgery

Risk factors for transient and permanent facial palsy are listed in ▶ Table 19.2. Data on risk factors for permanent palsy are rare as long follow-up intervals are needed to verify a permanent palsy. Furthermore, most of our knowledge on risk factors for postoperative facial palsy

Table 19.1 Etiology of facial palsy after parotid surgery

Etiology	Comment
Compression	Compression, for instance by a retractor on the marginal mandibular branch against the mandible, can lead to facial palsy of the target area of this nerve branch; compression by postoperative hemorrhage after parotidectomy does not normally lead to facial palsy
Crush	Special type of compression: force from two opposite sides diminishes the possibility of the nerve avoiding the traumatic force, e.g., unwanted grasp with forceps, clamp, or coagulation probe
Stretch	Stretch injuries typically occur when nerve branches are already elongated and under tension from a tumor displacing the nerve and are then they are relieved of the stretch resulting from the tumor
Transection	Planned or unwanted sectioning of the nerve
Thermal injury	Use of the coagulation probe next to nerve branches or mistaking a nerve branch for a vessel can lead to thermal damage; this can be a minor injury or equal to a complete transection
Electrical injury	Electrical injury produced by excessive nerve stimulation can induce a facial palsy

Table 19.2 Risk factors for postoperative facial palsy after parotid surgery

Factor	Comment
Transient palsy	
Diabetes mellitus	No hard data, but shown in a few retrospective studies
Extent of surgery	Has been proven in general in several studies, independent of the exact type of parotid surgery
Extracapsular dissection < partial < lateral < total parotidectomy	Has been shown at least for benign tumors in several studies and a meta-analysis. Be aware of a selection bias, larger tumors need more extended surgery (how is this different than extent of surgery)
Older age (> 70 years)	Revealed in one large retrospective study,
Surgery time	Correlates with extent of surgery, definitive higher risk in parotid surgery > 4 hours
Specimen volume (> 70 cm^3)	Larger tumors normally involve more extensive surgery
Sialadenitis	Acute and chronic inflammation of the parotid tissue is an independent risk factor
Parotid duct ligation	Zygomatic and buccal branches are at higher risk for damage
Warthin's tumor	Probably due the frequent finding of such a tumor at the lower pole of the gland; the cervical branch of the nerve is at risk
Malignant tumor	Relevant risk factor even when the surgeon tries to protect the nerve; shown in several retrospective studies
Contact of the parotid tumor to the nerve	If a nerve branch has direct contact with the tumor, the risk of postoperative palsy is increased
Permanent	
Total parotidectomy	Has the highest risk for permanent palsy in several retrospective studies
Revision surgery	Proven risk factor in many studies
Probably no risk factor	
Nerve stimulation	Frequent stimulation with standard parameters seems to be riskless (but: using a electric current beyond standard limits can cause electrical injury!)
No nerve monitoring	No proof even in prospective studies that nerve monitoring definitively decreases the risk
Nonspecialized center	Without increased risk, at least for benign tumors
Learning curve	Without increased risk when included in a standardized training program supervised by an experienced parotid surgeon
Children	Facial palsy rate not higher than in adults
Facial nerve preparation technique	Controversial results, so far no evidence that retrograde preparation technique includes higher risk; again be aware of a selection bias: retrograde technique is more often chosen for large tumors

after parotid surgery is based on monocenter and retrospective studies. Most of these studies include a selection bias in which tumor gets which operation, and the procedures in these reports are generally performed by surgeons who perform a high volume of these operations. This is quite important considering the influence of the extent of surgery on the risk of postoperative facial palsy. The selection of the surgical technique is primarily dependent on the histology, size, and localization of the tumor. Extracapsular dissection or partial parotidectomy techniques are not feasible for large tumors or tumors of the deep parotid lobe. Vice versa, total parotidectomy is typically not chosen for small superficial tumors. The facial nerve is at greater risk in patients with congenital anomalies, presence of inflammatory disease, trauma surgery with parotid involvement, malignant tumor surgery, and previous surgical interventions in the parotid region.[9–11] Proven risks factors for a permanent palsy are extent of surgery and revision surgery.[3,12,13] On the other hand, it should be known that facial nerve stimulation during surgery is not associated with a higher risk. Parotid gland surgery in children, when done in a specialized center, is not associated with a higher risk for the facial nerve.[14] There is an ongoing debate on the role of facial nerve monitoring, which is covered in detail in Chapter 15. Briefly, facial nerve monitoring can be helpful to identify the facial nerve and especially thin peripheral branches. It might help to avoid accidental facial nerve lesions during surgery but to date there is no proof, even by prospective clinical studies, that nerve monitoring definitively decreases the risk.[9,15–17]

!

Facial nerve monitoring during parotid surgery is a matter of debate because it is still not proven that electric facial nerve monitoring prevents postoperative facial palsy. It is not recommended to use monitoring with the view that it might prevent medicolegal arguments in cases of postoperative facial palsy!

19.5 Preoperative Assessment and Measures to Avoid Postoperative Facial Palsy

Methods and actions to evaluate the risk to the facial nerve preoperatively are listed in Box 19.1 (p. 252). It is important to be aware of the individual risk factors of your patient. If it is a revision case, it is obligatory to ask the patient if they had any facial palsy, even transiently, after the first operation. If yes, this is a clear sign that the facial nerve was exposed during the first surgery. Do not be deceived into thinking that a small scar means that a minor surgery was performed previously. New imaging of the parotid should always be obtained. Ultrasound should be complemented with magnetic resonance imaging (MRI) in larger tumors or in cases with risk of deep lobe extension or malignancy. When faced with these situations, the patient should be advised about the increased risk for, at least, a transient facial palsy is possible. ▸ Table 19.3 gives an overview of the most frequent types

Table 19.3 Frequent types of parotid surgery

Type of parotid surgery	Comment
Incision and drainage	Acute suppurative parotitis is managed by drainage. Exposure of the facial nerve is not usually necessary. To avoid a facial lesion it is most important to choose the correct type of skin incision; see ▸ Fig. 19.2.
Biopsy	Fine-needle aspiration is without risk for the facial nerve. To avoid an unintentional facial nerve lesion, the incision should be orientated to the course of the facial plexus and the peripheral end branches. Postaspiration infection is rare
Extracapsular dissection	The dissection of a small mobile lump with surrounding normal parotid tissue. By definition, the facial nerve is not exposed during extracapsular dissection; otherwise, the surgery is not extracapsular dissection. Therefore, some surgeons recommend always using electrical monitoring when performing extracapsular dissection. Very important: the final decision of whether an extracapsular dissection is feasible is made during surgery. It might be necessary to switch over to a more extended type of parotid surgery and the patient should be informed
Partial superficial parotidectomy	The dissection of a part of the superficial lobe, including dissection of parts of the facial plexus. Parts of the facial fan are exposed. This type of surgery is performed mostly for lesions in the lower third of the gland. A lesion of the marginal mandibular branch needs to be prevented when separating the specimen. This nerve branch should be dissected beyond the planned excision line
Superficial parotidectomy	The complete removal of the superficial parotid lobe. At the end of the procedure, the lateral parotid is removed exposing the complete facial fan. In surgery for benign disease, some surgeons recommend covering the facial fan with a local muscle or fascia flap to avoid the nerve branches lying directly under the skin. In contrast, other surgeons recommend never using a local cover so that they have control of the former tumor region during follow-up
Total parotidectomy	This is the complete removal of the parotid gland. To resect the deep parotid lobe, the facial nerve fan needs to be mobilized
Radical parotidectomy	At least one end branch of the facial nerve is resected in a radical parotidectomy. Immediate repair is recommended if feasible
Accessory parotid excision	The buccal branch located next to Stensen's duct is at risk during accessory parotid excision

of parotid surgery and associated factors relevant for the facial nerve, and the preoperative assessment and interview with the patient.

Box 19.1 Check list: Measures that help to avoid facial palsy during/after parotid surgery

- Deep lobe tumor? Check imaging results: is it possible or even clear that the tumor is located in the deep lobe?
- Malignant tumor? Check complete diagnostic work-up: are there hints for a malignant process?
- Use optical monitoring—leave the ipsilateral face exposed or use a transparent drape
- Use electrical monitoring—in combination with electrical stimulation, but be aware: the monitoring is observing only the muscles and related nerve branches where the surgeon places the recording electrodes (▶ Table 19.3 indicates that monitoring does not help)
- Use magnification—loupes or operating microscope when preparing the nerve
- In case of revision surgery—it should be in the hands of a high-volume surgeon, it should be planned with enough time for revision surgery, and the surgeon should be capable of using retrograde techniques
- Preparation techniques—the surgeon should be trained in anterograde and retrograde facial nerve identification
- Preparation techniques—if a retrograde approach is used, avoid trauma to the branching points of the nerve
- In case of bleeding, even for minor bleeding, take a suction device to locate the source of bleeding, as the source might be a vessel directly next to the facial nerve. The surgeon should avoid overuse of the coagulation probe with risk of damaging the facial nerve
- If electrical stimulation is used: if you are in doubt as to whether you are dissecting a facial nerve branch or a small vessel, use electrical stimulation. In complex and unclear situations, such as in revision surgery with scar tissue, some surgeons use electrical stimulation to screen an area where you expect the facial nerve or one of its branches to be. However, there are no studies confirming that electrical stimulation is helpful

In case of revision surgery, ask the patient if he had a facial palsy after the previous parotid surgery. If yes, the risk of a new facial palsy is increased.

19.6 Intraoperative Measures to Prevent a Facial Nerve Lesion

Intraoperative measures to prevent a facial nerve lesion are also listed in Box 19.1. In some countries, routine use of electrical monitoring is recommended; details are given in Chapter 15. This rationale of its advocates is that routine use increases the likelihood that it will be used and interpreted expertly. Be aware that electrical monitoring gives only information of the facial areas recorded. If, for instance, two-channel monitoring of the orbicularis oculi and the orbicularis oris muscle is performed, the monitoring does not give any information of the facial muscle areas in between. Therefore, it is recommended to combine electrical monitoring with optical monitoring (▶ Fig. 19.1a). The hemiface is covered with a transparent drape allowing the surgical assistant and the nurse to observe even small movements of the face during surgery. This is important as the surgeon might have a restricted visual field using loupes or a surgical microscope. When starting the preparation of the facial nerve or during extracapsular dissection of small facial nerve branches, a loupe or microscope is extremely helpful. The authors prefer a microscope, but the surgeon should use the device on which he or she has been trained (▶ Fig. 19.1b). During dissection of the facial nerve it is suggested that scissors with a blunt tip to avoid injuring the facial nerve are used (▶ Fig. 19.1c). The appropriate incision line has to be chosen depending on the type of surgery, not only for aesthetic reasons but also to diminish the risk of facial nerve trauma (▶ Fig. 19.2).

If a surgeon decides to use electrical monitoring—electrical monitoring observes some but not all facial muscles and related peripheral nerve branches. It will not detect facial nerve trauma in nonobserved facial regions.

19.6.1 Identification of the Extratemporal Portion of the Facial Nerve and Its End Branches

The facial nerve exits the skull base at the stylomastoid foramen of the temporal bone (▶ Fig. 19.3). The nerve lies about 9 mm superior to the posterior belly of the digastric muscle and 11 mm from the bony external meatus. The facial nerve trunk then passes downward and forward over the styloid process and the associated muscles for about 13 mm before entering the substance of the parotid gland. The first part of the facial nerve gives off the posterior auricular nerve supplying the auricular muscles and also branches to the posterior belly of the digastric and stylohyoid muscles. The extratemporal facial nerve trunk can be identified proximally using an anterograde technique, which is most commonly taught, or with a retrograde technique (▸ Table 19.4); also see the anatomy descriptions in Chapter 1.

The two most reliable surgical landmarks used to identify the facial nerve trunk are the tympanomastoid suture line and the posterior belly of the digastric muscle.

Sometimes the main trunk is not identifiable proximally at the stylomastoid foramen or cannot be safely approached because the tumor is located in this region and is displacing the main trunk. Alternative means of identifying the trunk must then be used. One approach is to locate a branch of the facial nerve distally using a retrograde technique. The marginal mandibular branch usually passes superficial to the posterior facial vein, which has been encountered and divided when elevating the parotid off the sternocleidomastoid muscle. The buccal branch can be identified at the anterior border of the parotid gland, at a point horizontal from the nasal alar rim to the inferior rim of the external auditory canal. The zygomatic branches can be identified as the nerve crosses the zygomatic arch, usually at its midportion, between the outer canthus of the eye and the temporomandibular joint. If all of the above approaches fail, the transmastoid approach can be used, drilling down the mastoid to identify the facial nerve in

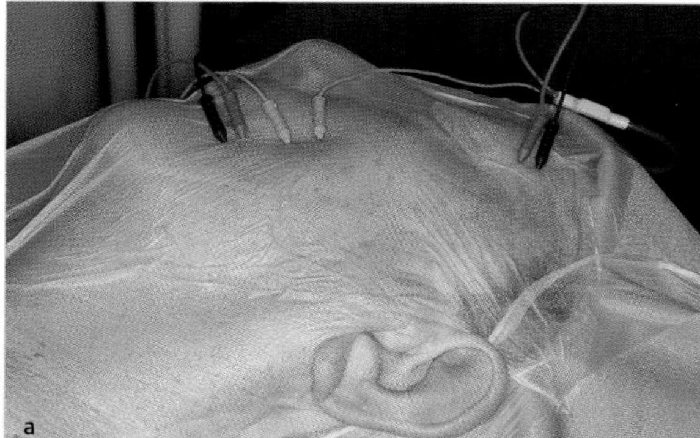

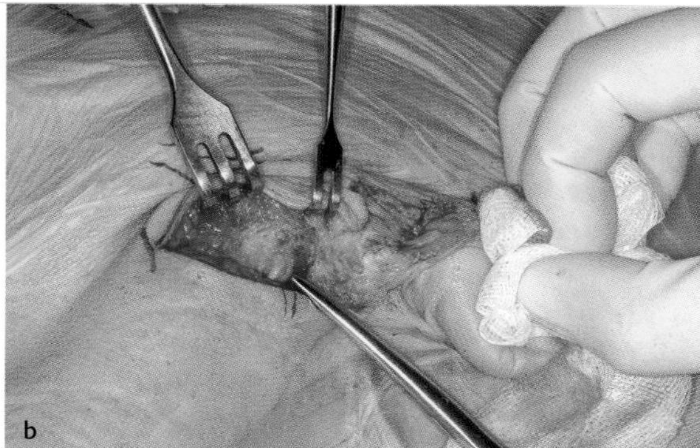

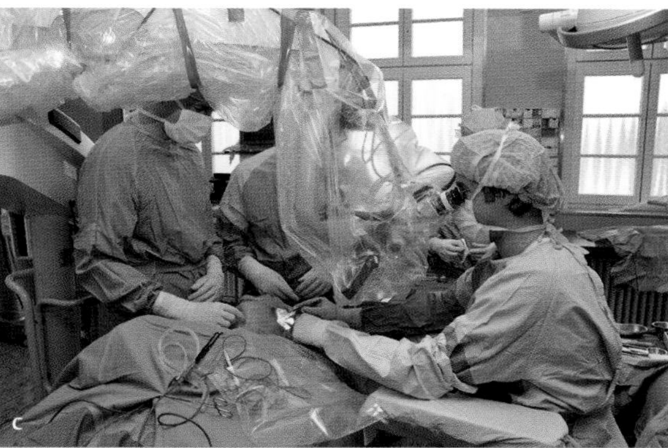

Fig. 19.1 Intraoperative setting of typical parotid surgery and measures to prevent facial nerve lesion. **(a)** Use a transparent drape to cover the face to allow easy visual monitoring. In this case the surgeon elected to use facial nerve monitoring. **(b)** For atraumatic preparation of the facial nerve, use of scissors with a rounded tip is recommended. **(c)** Use loupes or an operating microscope, as shown, when preparing the facial nerve.

the middle ear and following it inferiorly to reach the tympanomastoid suture.

On entering the parotid gland, the facial nerve separates into two divisions: the temporofacial and cervicofacial trunks. The division of the nerve is known as the pes anserinus. From these two divisions, the facial nerve further divides into five named branches: the temporal and zygomatic branches, usually from the upper division; and the buccal, mandibular, and cervical branches from the lower division, but the exact configuration is extremely variable. The peripheral branches of the facial nerve form anastomoses between adjacent branches to form the parotid plexus. Six main patterns have been described, as shown in ▸ Fig. 1.4. In fewer than 6% of cases there are no anastomoses between the mandibular branch and the adjacent branches. The frontal branch also often lacks anastomoses to adjacent branches. Therefore, the mandibular branch and the frontal branch are extremely vulnerable to any trauma.

> **!**
>
> Be extremely careful with the marginal mandibular branch, because often it has no anastomoses with other branches, leading to a lack of possible compensation after cases of trauma.

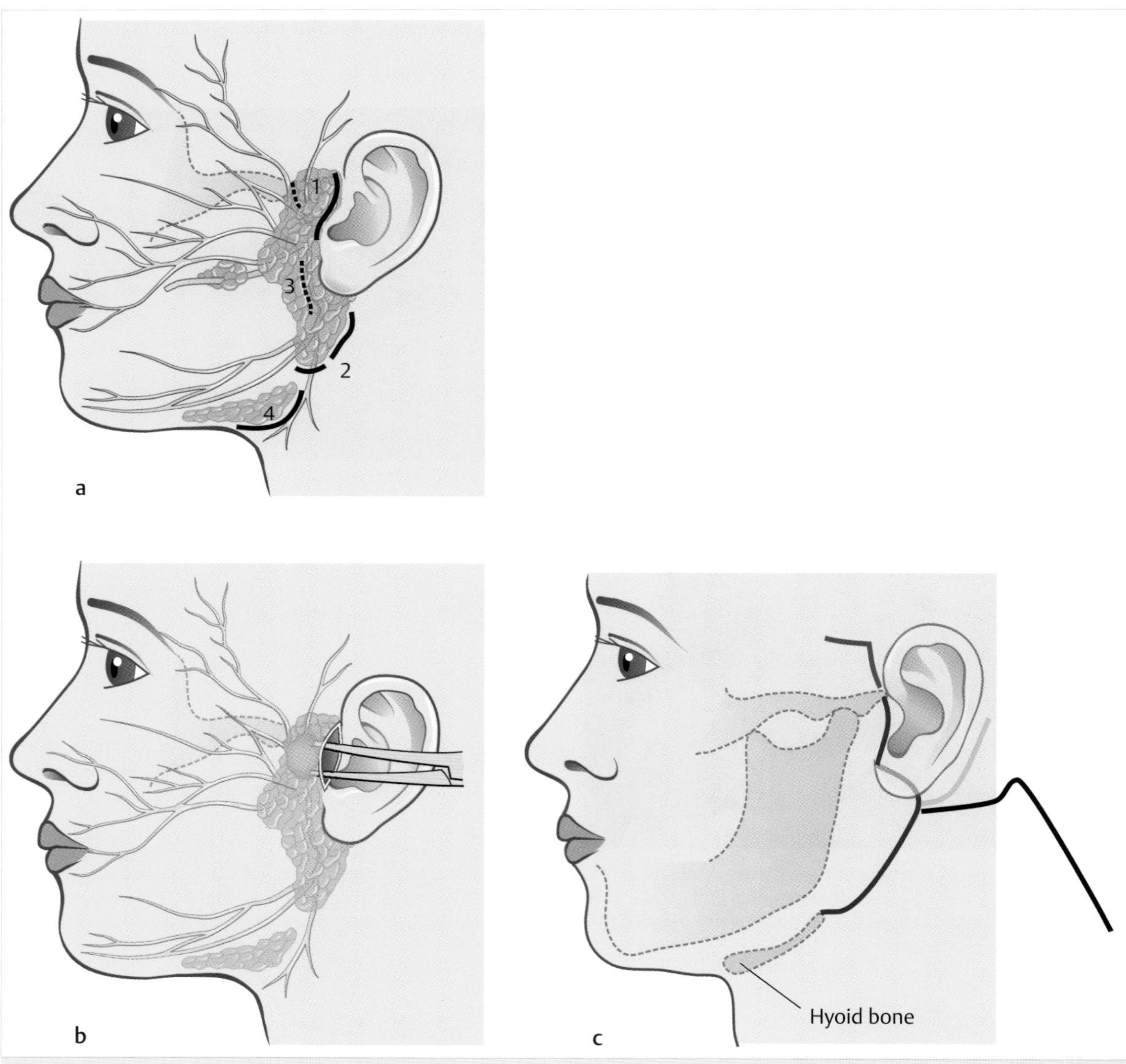

Fig. 19.2 Recommended skin incision line(s) for: **(a)** parotid incisions, **(b)** biopsies, and **(c)** parotidectomy.

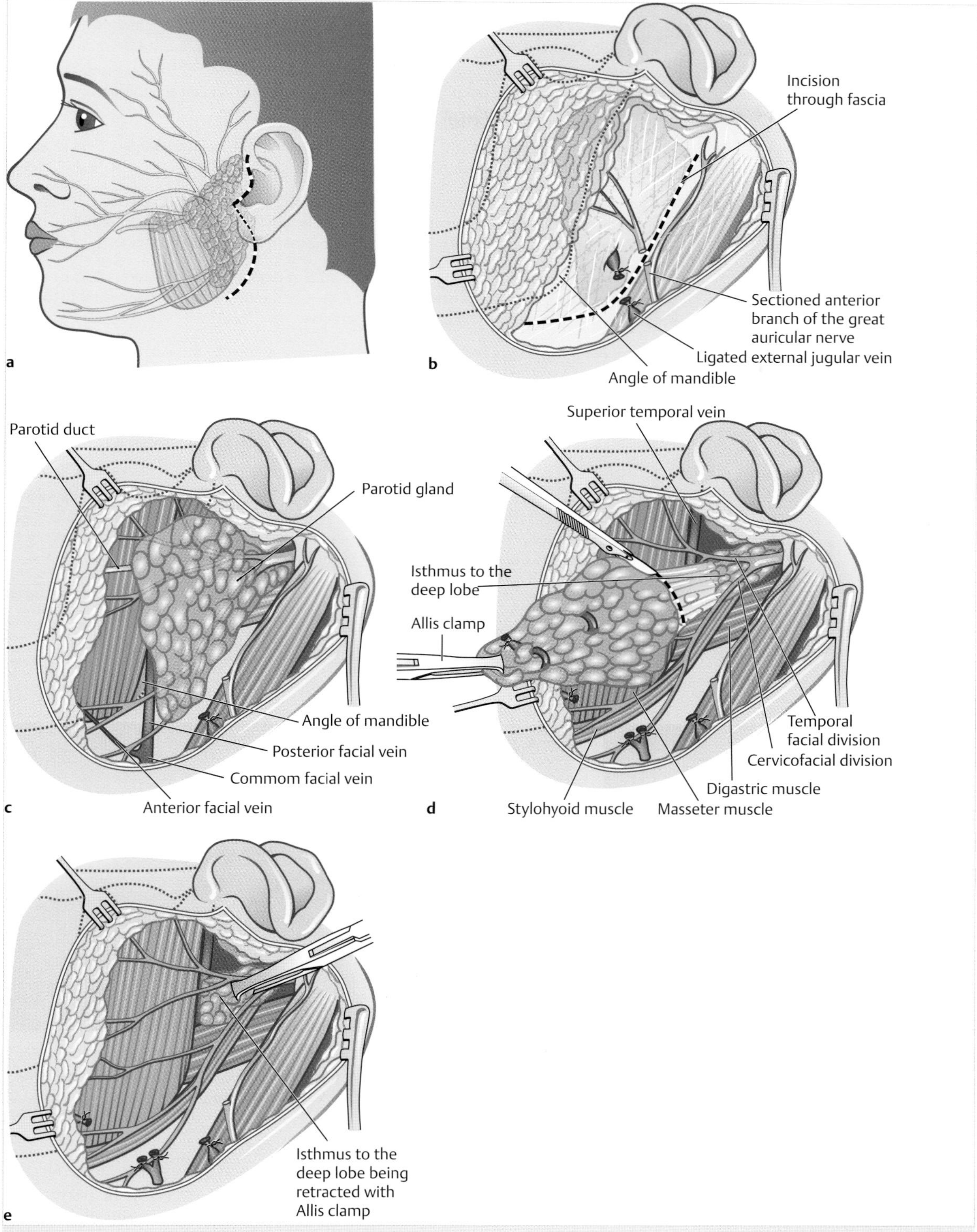

Fig. 19.3 (a–e) Topographic anatomy of the facial nerve. The most important landmarks are shown to identify the facial nerve via anterograde or retrograde approach.

Table 19.4 Landmarks for localization of the facial nerve during parotid surgery[a]

Technique	Landmark
Anterograde preparation (localization of the main trunk)	The tragal pointer: the facial nerve trunk is located approximately 1–2 cm deep and slightly anteroinferiorly. The tragal pointer has a blunt and variable tip that can change with retraction. It is probably the least consistent landmark to use
	The posterior belly of the digastric muscle: the facial nerve trunk is located 0.5–1.5 cm deep at the same level as the muscle as it attaches to the digastric groove
	The tympanomastoid suture line: the facial nerve trunk is usually located 2–4 mm deep to the inferior end of the tympanomastoid suture line. This landmark may not be visualized and can be detected only on palpation. Follow the tympanomastoid suture with your finger
	The styloid process: the facial nerve trunk is located in the inferior and superficial soft tissue. But be careful: if the styloid process is used to identify the nerve, the surgeon is likely to become lost and there is a risk of injury to the nerve
Retrograde preparation (starting with a peripheral end branch)	Stensen's duct: the buccal branch is located cranial and parallel to the duct
	Zygomatic arch: the buccal branch is located 1 cm caudal to the arch
	Zygomatic arch: the frontal branch crosses the arch and is very vulnerable at this superficial location
Vascular approach	Posterior facial vein: tunneling the vein from the caudal area into the substance of the lower parotid pole will lead to the cervical and marginal mandibular branch. But be careful: although for the vast majority of time the nerve is lateral to the vein, sometimes it passes medially or it splits and sends branches lateral and medial to the vein.
Mastoid approach	After mastoidectomy the mastoid segment of the facial nerve is dissected and the mastoid tip is removed.

[a]See ▶ Fig. 19.3.

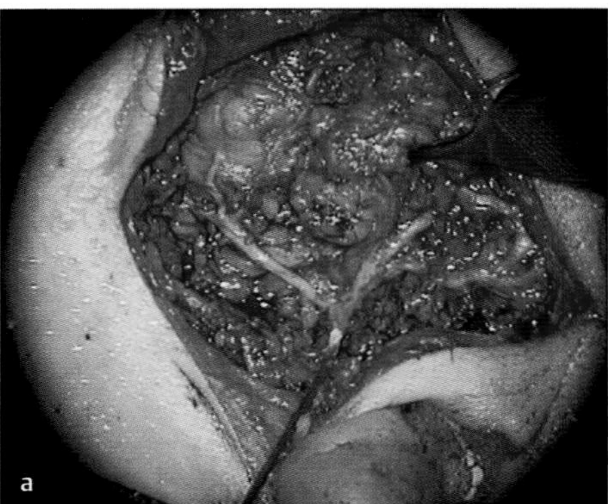

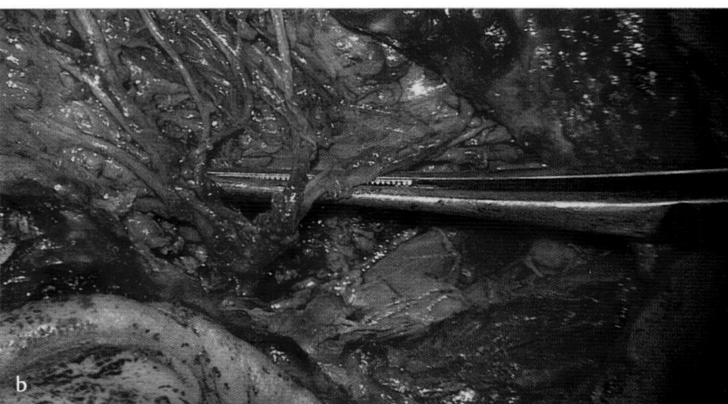

Fig. 19.4 Typical intraoperative appearance on the left side after superficial parotidectomy. **(a)** The complete facial plexus with its five end branches and some interconnections are visible. **(b)** For total parotidectomy, the complete facial plexus is mobilized to resect the deep parotid lobe. At the end the facial plexus is lying directly on the mandible and the masseter muscle.

19.6.2 Management of the Facial Nerve Depending on the Type of Surgery

The typical uncovering of the facial nerve when completing a superficial or total parotidectomy is shown in ▶ Fig. 19.4. It is mandatory that any patient being considered for surgery in the vicinity of the facial nerve is informed that there is a risk of transient or permanent facial palsy, no matter how carefully or skillfully the surgery is done and regardless of the final diagnosis. If surgery is started as an extracapsular dissection, the surgeon must be prepared to switch to a more extensive surgery if necessary.

When performing a superficial parotidectomy, the surgeon should establish a surgical model for the procedure:

1. Start with anterograde preparation of the main trunk, using the landmarks described in Identification of the Extratemporal Portion of the Facial Nerve and its End Branches. Alternatively, or additionally, use the mastoid tip as landmark: if the surgeon lays his finger on the mastoid tip, the nerve will be directly anterior to the midpoint of the finger at the level of the digastric muscle.
2. If the tumor is located cranial to the main trunk, start the anterograde preparation of the facial nerve from caudal, i.e., dissecting cervical branches and the marginal mandibular branch.
3. Then, systematically proceed step-by-step more cranially, i.e., identify the next branch lying more proximally starting by going back to the initial point at the main trunk. By doing so, the complete plexus is prepared from caudal to cranial, ideally without seeing or touching the tumor. However, frequently the capsule of the tumor will abut one or more nerve branches.
4. Alternatively, if the tumor is located caudal to the main trunk, use the other direction from cranial to caudal in the same manner.
5. If the main trunk is not accessible because the tumor is located on the main trunk or due to changes made by previous surgery, start with retrograde preparation of an end branch distant to the tumor until the main trunk is identified, and then finally switch back to an anterograde preparation.

In case of total parotidectomy:

1. Start with a superficial parotidectomy, as described in the previous list.
2. Gently lift the facial nerve branches lying lateral to the tumor.
3. Often these branches have to be freed step-by–step, changing back and forth between anterograde and retrograde preparation.
4. Finally remove the deep lobe tumor and parotid tissue.
5. Some benign deep tumors allow for the superficial lobe, which has been pedicled anteriorly, to be preserved and replaced at the end of the procedure, protecting the nerve and enhancing cosmesis.

In patients undergoing radical parotidectomy try to minimize the facial nerve resection to the areas that are infiltrated by the malignant tumor. If the patient has a malignant tumor but the facial nerve is not infiltrated, it is worthwhile and oncologically safe to preserve the facial nerve. Sometimes, in cases of revision surgery of pleomorphic adenoma, one or more of the benign nodules can only be reached if a branch is transected. If preoperative consent for such a strategy has been obtained, restrict the resection to this area, and reconstruct the nerve.

> **!**
>
> If the face is paralyzed preoperatively it is likely that the nerve is involved and will be resected and if possible reconstructed. If the nerve is functioning normally preoperatively, effort should be made to dissect the nerve away from the tumor if at all possible.

19.7 Management of Intraoperative Facial Nerve Lesions

If the facial nerve is injured intraoperatively unintentionally or intentionally, direct facial nerve reconstruction gives the best functional results. The principals of facial nerve reconstruction in case of iatrogenic trauma are presented in Chapter 9. The primary tenet is that the best result, where possible, is to reestablish continuity between the facial nerve nucleus and facial musculature. All relevant surgical techniques for facial nerve reanimation are presented in detail in Section VI, Rehabilitation Techniques for Chronic Facial Palsy. The facial nerve reconstruction techniques presented in Chapter 20 are relevant for the management of facial nerve lesions occurring during parotid surgery. If the facial nerve or one of its branches is cut sharply, tension-free end-to-end nerve suture is the method of choice (▶ Fig. 19.5). If there are doubts that a tension-free resuture is possible, or if a gap of > 1 cm is obvious, use a small nerve graft. Even if the surgeon believes that the nerve is cut only incompletely and it looks like it is gaping, most often a complete transection and resuture is the best choice for optimal alignment of the nerve stumps. In cases of large and complex lesions of the facial plexus, then nerve grafts, a hypoglossal-facial jump nerve suture, or a combination of both should be considered depending on patient factors, tumor resection factors, and timing. If possible cover the suture sites with remnants of the parotid gland, small local muscle flaps, or subcutaneous tissue. Rarely, the situation might arise that a primary facial nerve repair is not wanted. In such cases mark the nerve stumps with clips or permanent sutures to facilitate finding the nerve ends later when performing a secondary repair.

In addition, surgery for improvement of eye closure, for instance with upper lid loading, can be performed in the same surgical session; details are given in Chapter 24. Some surgeons prefer to wait with lid loading and perform it in a second session: If so, the patients will have the paralysis for a couple weeks, and they present then for measurement of the size of gold weight to be implanted. This strategy might help to better define the optimal lid weight in the individual situation.

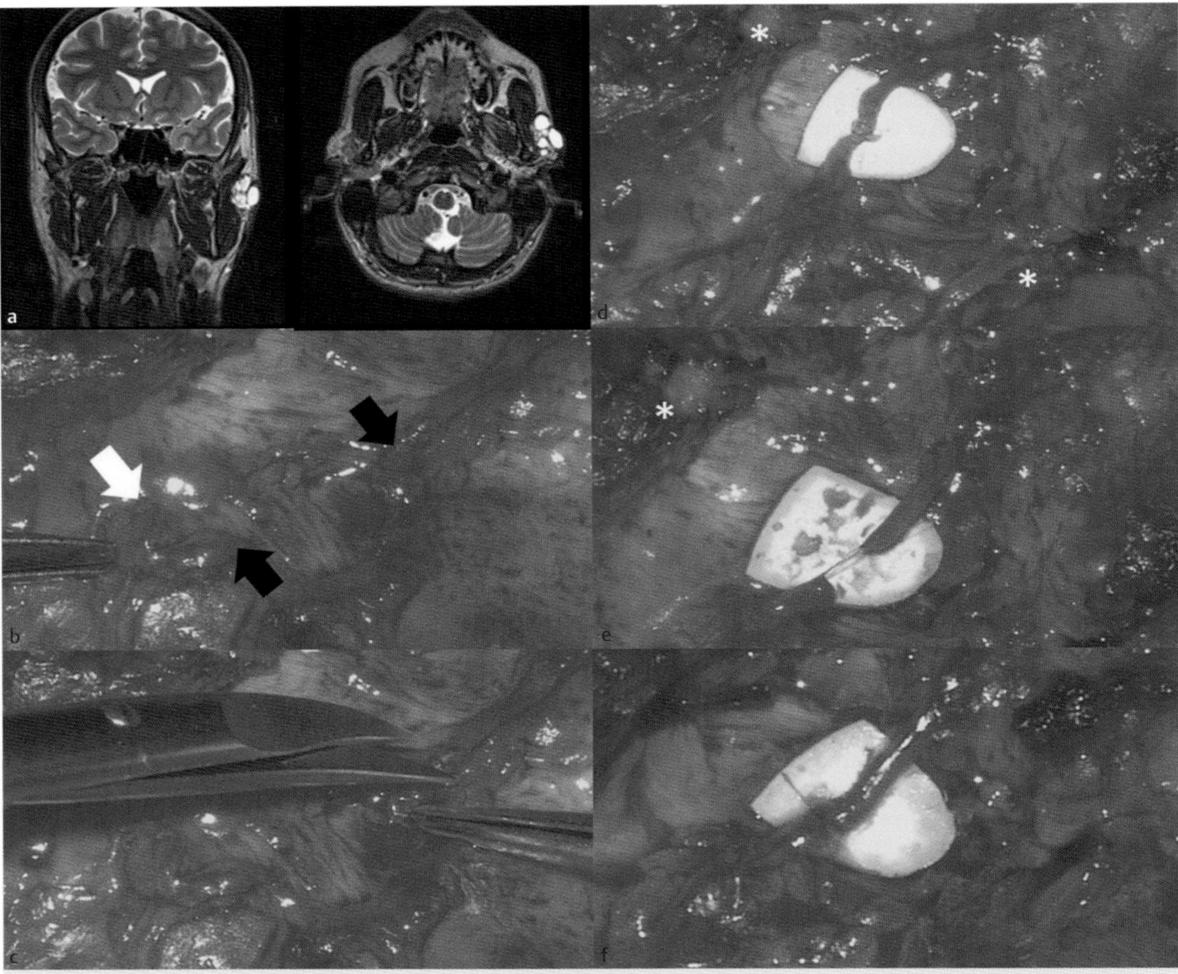

Fig. 19.5 Management of a planned transection and repair of the lower branch of the zygomatic branch of the facial nerve during parotid revision surgery. **(a)** MRI showing a multinodular third recurrence of a pleomorphic adenoma of the left parotid gland. It was agreed with the patient during the presurgical consultation that a peripheral branch could be transected and immediately repaired if needed for complete tumor removal. **(b)** Situation after transection of the peripheral facial nerve branch with the two nerve stumps (*arrows*) and tumor removal. **(c)** Trimming of the nerve stumps. **(d)** A platform is used to prepare the direct nerve suture. **(e)** End-to-end nerve suture with monofilament suture 10–0. **(f)** Situation after tightening the suture.

19.8 Management of Postoperative Facial Palsy

Four different situations need to be distinguished:

1. A facial nerve lesion occurs during parotid surgery and is recognized.
2. The patient wakes up after parotid surgery and has a complete facial palsy on the side of surgery.
3. The patient wakes up after parotid surgery and has an incomplete facial palsy.
4. The patient develops a delayed facial palsy.

19.8.1 A Facial Nerve Lesion Occurs During Parotid Surgery and Is Recognized

If the facial nerve was repaired at surgery, the patient is monitored using clinical examination and electromyography (EMG). If the repaired branch is quite distal, the first regeneration potentials might occur after 2 months. In cases of repair of the main trunk or the proximal facial plexus, the first regeneration potentials occur after 4 to 6 months. If facial nerve neuromuscular training is planned, it can begin when the patient shows first regeneration potentials; see Chapter 26. Before then, such training can result in only frustration for the patient. First synkinetic movement typically occurs 2 to 3 months after first regeneration potentials. The final result, including defective healing, is reached 12 to 18 months after surgery. The patient is seen postoperatively, for instance every 3 months, until the final result is achieved. If available, EMG helps to objectify the improvement and final result. When no further improvement is noticed, adjuvant measures such as small surgical procedures, for instance to improve facial symmetry at rest, or adjuvant treatment with botulinum toxin should be considered; see Chapter 25. There is no evidence that corticosteroids, used routinely in Bell's palsy, improve the final result of facial nerve repair.

19.8.2 The Patient Wakes Up After Parotid Surgery and Has a Complete Facial Palsy on the Side of Surgery

At the conclusion of all parotid surgery the nerve should be stimulated at its most proximal point of dissection. If the nerve stimulates the entire face, then waking up with a complete facial palsy does not require further investigation. The patient should be told that there has been an injury from either dissection or traction but that the nerve is intact because it stimulated. This does not mean that the patient will have a perfect result. It means that no additional tests are needed and nothing can be done to improve the final result. Steroids are generally employed in these cases but no data exist that they change the outcome.

If the surgeon did not stimulate the nerve at the end of the parotidectomy, a diagnostic work-up has to be performed, as presented in Chapter 9. The algorithm in ▶ Fig. 19.6 shows the different scenarios and their management. A paresis, i.e., a weakness of voluntary movement, partial loss of voluntary movement, or impaired movement, has to be differentiated from a paralysis in which all voluntary movement is lost. In the clinical setting, we often speak synonymously of complete palsy as a paralysis and of incomplete palsy in cases of paresis. A clinical examination of all facial regions gives information of the patient's situation. Local anesthesia used in the region of the main trunk can affect facial nerve function but should be gone in 6 hours. Voluntary EMG is used to evaluate an acute postoperative paralysis. Immediate presence of voluntary motor unit action potentials (VMUAPs) indicates that the nerve is intact and no re-exploration is needed. It does not mean that the final result will be normal. The absence of VMUAPs does not indicate that the nerve is severed, but the status of the nerve is unknown. If the facial nerve was not identified during parotid surgery, for instance in biopsy cases or during extracapsular dissection, the facial nerve should be re-explored if the EMG does not show VMUAPs. In all other situations, i.e., when the facial nerve was explored but a degenerative lesion could not be explained, the facial nerve should be re-explored and also if the EMG suggests transection. If a lesion of the nerve is detected, a primary repair is performed. If the EMG shows a reduced to full interference pattern, this is an indirect sign for a nondegenerative lesion and a wait-and-see policy is indicated. This finding should be confirmed by at least one follow-up EMG. If there is deterioration of facial function over time, EMG is immediately repeated. If there are any doubts or controversial findings, an EMG should be performed 10 to 14 days after surgery, because from then on it will be possible to detect pathological spontaneous activity (fibrillation potentials and positive sharp waves) if the facial nerve has been severely damaged. Follow-up examinations are scheduled until recovery or defective healing is complete.

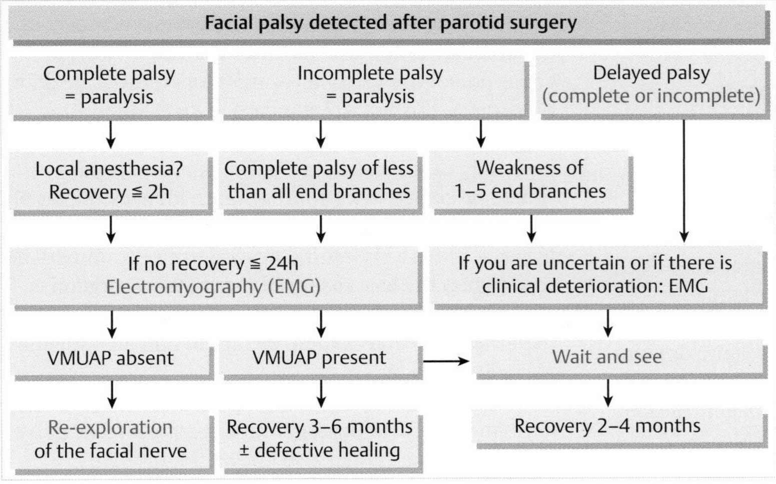

Fig. 19.6 Algorithm for the management of facial palsy detected after parotid surgery when the patient is awake. If there is only weakness of some facial nerve-end branches or in cases of delayed palsy, EMG control is not usually necessary. EMG is recommended if there is deterioration of facial nerve function or if the surgeon is uncertain whether the palsy was delayed or immediate. VMUAP, voluntary motor unit action potential.

> **!**
>
> If the integrity of the nerve is preserved, recovery is usually noted between 1 and 6 months after surgery. Recovery noted within the first 3 to 6 weeks of injury portends a favorable final result, while loss of voluntary motor unit action potentials on electromyography and detection of spontaneous pathological fibrillations or positive sharp waves indicate a more severe injury. Even in such cases, an intact nerve will usually begin a spontaneous recovery within 3 to 6 months. The patients with delayed recovery will normally have a recovery level of House–Brackmann grade II or worse.

19.8.3 The Patient Wakes Up After Parotid Surgery and has an Incomplete Facial Palsy

As described in The Patient Wakes Up After Parotid Surgery and has a Complete Facial Palsy on the Side of Surgery, EMG can also help to confirm an incomplete facial palsy, although this is generally obvious and is not usually performed. Two situations need to be differentiated. The surgeon should document if there is global weakness of the entire face or if this is a weakness of a single branch or branches. In cases with a global but incomplete facial weakness, a wait-and-see policy is indicated. In the second scenario of a patient with a partial paralysis that is caused by complete paralysis of one or more branches, the branches in question should be treated identically to that described in The Patient Wakes Up After Parotid Surgery and has a Complete Facial Palsy on the Side of Surgery where the entire nerve is cut out after surgery. EMG must be performed and documented for both affected and nonaffected branches. Using the same EMG criteria the surgeon can decide if this nerve branch should be reexplored. Re-exploring an isolated frontal branch injury rarely gives a satisfactory result even after repair and a brow lift is often preferred.

19.8.4 The Patient Develops a Delayed Facial Palsy

If the patient develops a delayed complete or incomplete facial palsy, i.e., later than 2 to 3 days after parotid surgery, the severity is recorded by clinical examination, clinical grading, and EMG or electroneurography (ENoG) examination. An exact description is important to recognize deterioration during the further follow-up. Photo and video documentation is helpful for serial examinations. If no deterioration occurs the palsy will recover within 2 to 4 months. The sooner recovery begins the better the final result. Even in patients with EMG signs of a degenerative lesion, there is in principle no indication for surgical exploration, because exploration does not lead to better results than a wait-and-see strategy. Therefore, in such a situation, the role of EMG should not be overestimated. The exact cause of the delayed palsy will remain unclear. Late secondary ischemia caused by edema surrounding the nerve, as typically seen in traumatic facial palsy in patients with temporal bone fracture, is unlikely to occur to the extratemporal facial nerve. Even severe hematoma formation due to secondary bleeding or local infection in the parotid gland does not in practice lead to a facial palsy because the nerve is not compressed in a bony canal. Delayed facial palsy can theoretically also result from reactivation of herpes simplex virus type 1 within the geniculate ganglion and occurs 3 to 14 days after a traumatic injury, i.e., is not directly related to the parotid surgery. But there is no clear-cut serologic testing for herpes simplex virus reinfection is such a situation. Facial palsy due to herpes simplex virus type 1 virus reactivation can be treated with virostatic drugs and prednisolone theoretically; for details see Chapter 10. Otherwise, and this is the rule for most situations, there is no evidence that postoperative adjuvant therapy with corticosteroids will improve the final result of recovery after delayed facial palsy.[18]

19.9 Key Points

- Well-documented risk factors for facial palsy after parotid surgery are extent of surgery and revision surgery. This should be emphasized in the presurgical consultation with the patient.
- The differentiation between immediate, delayed, incomplete, and complete postoperative facial palsy is important for the management after parotid surgery.
- The nerve should always be stimulated proximally at the end of the procedure to avoid ambiguity about the nerve status. All areas of the face should be observed.
- Electrical facial nerve monitoring can be helpful for the surgeon to find the facial nerve and to be informed when the operation reaches the nerve. However, there is no evidence that monitoring improves any aspect of the procedure. In most countries the majority of surgeons do not use facial nerve monitors for routine parotid surgery. It is not the standard of care. Monitoring is no guarantee that a facial nerve injury will not occur, especially in revision surgery. The parotid surgeon should be skilled in all approaches to identify the facial nerve during parotid surgery.
- If the facial nerve is injured intraoperatively, immediate repair gives the best results. If the primary surgeon is not capable of making an excellent microscopic repair, then the nerve ends should be tagged and an immediate referral made.
- Electromyography plays a key role in decision-making for management of postoperative complete facial palsy, but the surgeon should also know its limitations.

References

[1] Klintworth N, Zenk J, Koch M, Iro H. Postoperative complications after extracapsular dissection of benign parotid lesions with particular reference to facial nerve function. Laryngoscope 2010; 120: 484–490

[2] Iro H, Zenk J, Koch M, Klintworth N. Follow-up of parotid pleomorphic adenomas treated by extracapsular dissection. Head Neck 2013; 35: 788–793

[3] Guntinas-Lichius O, Gabriel B, Klussmann JP. Risk of facial palsy and severe Frey's syndrome after conservative parotidectomy for benign disease: analysis of 610 operations. Acta Otolaryngol 2006; 126: 1104–1109

[4] Guntinas-Lichius O, Klussmann JP, Wittekindt C, Stennert E. Parotidectomy for benign parotid disease at a university teaching hospital: outcome of 963 operations. Laryngoscope 2006; 116: 534–540

[5] Nouraei SA, Ismail Y, Ferguson MS et al. Analysis of complications following surgical treatment of benign parotid disease. ANZ J Surg 2008; 78: 134–138

[6] Koch M, Zenk J, Iro H. Long-term results of morbidity after parotid gland surgery in benign disease. Laryngoscope 2010; 120: 724–730

[7] Albergotti WG, Nguyen SA, Zenk J, Gillespie MB. Extracapsular dissection for benign parotid tumors: a meta-analysis. Laryngoscope 2012; 122: 1954–1960

[8] Hong SS, Yheulon CG, Sniezek JC. Salivary gland surgery and medical malpractice. Otolaryngol Head Neck Surg 2013; 148: 589–594

[9] Dulguerov P, Marchal F, Lehmann W. Postparotidectomy facial nerve paralysis: possible etiologic factors and results with routine facial nerve monitoring. Laryngoscope 1999; 109: 754–762

[10] Ellingson TW, Cohen JI, Andersen P. The impact of malignant disease on facial nerve function after parotidectomy. Laryngoscope 2003; 113: 1299–1303

[11] Gaillard C, Périé S, Susini B, St Guily JL. Facial nerve dysfunction after parotidectomy: the role of local factors. Laryngoscope 2005; 115: 287–291

[12] Umapathy N, Holmes R, Basavaraj S, Roux R, Cable HR. Performance of parotidectomy in nonspecialist centers. Arch Otolaryngol Head Neck Surg 2003; 129: 925–928, discussion 928

[13] Yuan X, Gao Z, Jiang H et al. Predictors of facial palsy after surgery for benign parotid disease: multivariate analysis of 626 operations. Head Neck 2009; 31: 1588–1592

[14] Owusu JA, Parker NP, Rimell FL. Postoperative facial nerve function in pediatric parotidectomy: a 12-year review. Otolaryngol Head Neck Surg 2013; 148: 249–252

[15] Witt RL. Facial nerve monitoring in parotid surgery: the standard of care? Otolaryngol Head Neck Surg 1998; 119: 468–470

[16] Grosheva M, Klussmann JP, Grimminger C et al. Electromyographic facial nerve monitoring during parotidectomy for benign lesions does not improve the outcome of postoperative facial nerve function: a prospective two-center trial. Laryngoscope 2009; 119: 2299–2305

[17] Eisele DW, Wang SJ, Orloff LA. Electrophysiologic facial nerve monitoring during parotidectomy. Head Neck 2010; 32: 399–405

[18] Roh JL, Park CI. A prospective, randomized trial for use of prednisolone in patients with facial nerve paralysis after parotidectomy. Am J Surg 2008; 196: 746–750

Part VI

Rehabilitation Techniques for Chronic Facial Palsy

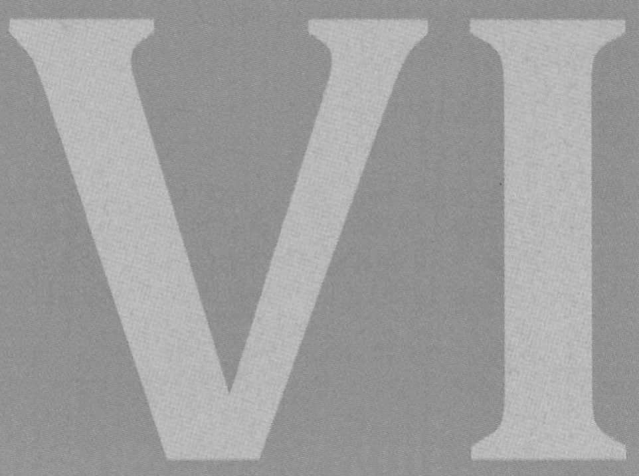

20 Facial Nerve Reconstruction

Orlando Guntinas-Lichius and Mira Finkensieper

20.1 Introduction

To receive optimal functional results after surgical repair of the facial nerve, it is necessary to be experienced in a variety of nerve repair techniques.[1–3] Decision-making depends on many factors including site of the lesion, extent of the lesion, viability of the proximal facial nerve stump, sensory function of the trigeminal nerve, etiology of the lesion, diagnosis, age of the patient, comorbidities, denervation time, life expectancy, and the patient's wishes (► Table 20.1). The better the diagnostic assessment of these factors, the easier it is to select the best repair technique and to achieve satisfactory facial nerve function for the patient.

> **!**
>
> The time between nerve injury and repair is the most significant factor in determining which procedures are most appropriate and whether the surgery is successful.[4]

> **⚠**
>
> If the trigeminal nerve or one of the three afferent branches is also sacrificed, the results of facial nerve reconstruction are significantly worse. Even an optimally reconstructed efferent facial nerve is dependent on an intact afferent trigeminal system.[5]

20.2 Definition

Facial nerve reconstruction includes all kinds of surgical nerve repair after disruption of the facial nerve, using the intact distal facial nerve stump or several intact more distal facial nerve branches (► Table 20.2 and ► Table 20.3; ► Fig. 20.1, ► Fig. 20.2 and ► Fig. 20.3). The intact facial nerve has a physiological normal connection to the different mimetic facial muscles via its distal end branches. This means that direct facial nerve reconstruction via nerve suture leads to reanimation via nerve regeneration

Table 20.1 Factors influencing the selection of the optimal surgical technique

Factor	Comment
Lesion site	The more proximal the lesion, the more elaborate is the reconstruction. The more proximal the lesion, the longer the regeneration time. When a patient has a central facial nerve defect, the best possible result is connecting the facial nerve nucleus to the periphery. However, nerve substitution may be selected to avoid repeat craniotomy
Extent of the facial nerve lesion	A complex lesion of the facial nerve fan needs forward-thinking planning of the nerve grafts needed. A possible alternative to selecting one technique is to combine techniques (combined approach)
Viability of the proximal facial nerve stump	Intraoperative biopsy via frozen section is often an unreliable examination on the viability of the proximal stump. In case of a denervation time longer than 3–6 months, it is better to directly plan a nerve substitution procedure such as a hypoglossal–facial jump nerve suture
Sensory function of the trigeminal nerve	Intact trigeminal nerve function is important to obtain optimal facial function and to support postsurgical physical rehabilitation
Etiology of the lesion	Traumatic lesions and iatrogenic lesions are cases for immediate and early repair, respectively, with high probability of a satisfactory functional result. In cases of malignant tumor infiltration, life expectancy is an important factor (see below). The need for postoperative radiotherapy is not a contraindication for facial nerve repair
Age of the patient	Beyond the age of 60 years, the result is often worse than in a younger patient. This is of course not an exclusion criterion, but needs to be considered when informing the patient
Denervation time	Best results are obtained within 30 days of injury, and there is a significant decline in good results beyond 2 years of injury
Life expectancy	Recovery after facial nerve reconstruction needs time. Depending on the lesion site and distance to the mimic muscles, the first clinical signs of reinnervation cannot be seen before 6–9 months after surgery and the final result needs 12–15 months. If life expectancy is far shorter, alternatives for faster facial reanimation should be chosen
Patient's wishes	The patient needs to exercise the patience to wait 12–15 months for the best results. If a faster solution is preferred, alternatives such as muscle transposition and sling plasties should be considered

Table 20.2 Surgical techniques for facial nerve reanimation

Dynamic procedures	Static procedures
Facial nerve plasties • Facial–facial nerve suture • Facial nerve interpositional graft • Hypoglossal–facial nerve suture • Hypoglossal–facial jump nerve suture • Cross-face facial nerve suture • Other cross-nerve sutures • Combined approach	Eye; see Chapter 24 • Upper lid loading • Palpebral spring • Canthoplasty • Tarsorrhaphy
Muscle plasties; see Chapter 21 • Temporal muscle transposition • Masseter muscle transposition • Digastric muscle transposition	Angle of the mouth; see Chapter 21 • Fascia lata sling • Palmaris longus sling
Combined nerve and muscle plasties; see Chapter 22 • Nerve substitution to free muscle transplantation with hypoglossal nerve, masseteric nerve or cross-face facial nerve suture	Other techniques • Facelift • Forehead lift (brow plasty)
Face transplantation; see Chapter 23	

Table 20.3 Overview of facial nerve reconstruction techniques

Technique	Indication criteria
Direct facial–facial end-to-end nerve suture	Peripheral lesion ≤ 1 cm, avoid any tension
Facial–facial nerve interpositional graft	Peripheral lesions > 1 cm, simple segmental defect
Hypoglossal–facial nerve suture and hypoglossal–facial jump nerve suture	Proximal facial nerve stump not available Proximal facial nerve stump available but peripheral lesions > 1 cm, complex segmental defect Chronic facial palsy (> 3–6 months)
Cross-face facial nerve suture	Complex segmental defect Chronic facial palsy (> 3–6 months)
Other cross-nerve sutures	If ipsilateral hypoglossal nerve or contralateral facial nerve not available but hypoglossal–facial (jump) nerve suture or cross-face facial nerve suture indicated
Combined approach	Complex segmental defect Chronic facial palsy (> 3–6 months)

of the original target muscles in the face connected to the facial nerve nucleus. A direct facial nerve repair is when the proximal stump is directly reconnected to the distal facial nerve stump with or without an interpositional graft allowing the nerve fibers of the proximal facial nerve stump to regrow in the distal nerve stump. An indirect or cross-nerve facial nerve reconstruction involves cases where the proximal nerve stump belongs to a peripheral nerve other than the facial nerve, i.e., the nerve fibers of another nerve regrow into the distal facial nerve to reinnervate the facial musculature. The aim of all facial nerve reconstruction techniques is to restore function by reinnervation of the original musculature, i.e., to obtain facial muscle movement (see the results of different techniques in ▶ Fig. 20.4, ▶ Fig. 20.5 and ▶ Fig. 20.6). These facts differentiate facial nerve reconstruction techniques from muscle transposition techniques. When using a muscle transposition technique, another nerve and other muscles take over part of the facial muscle functions. The two techniques, facial nerve reconstruction and muscle transposition, are called dynamic techniques because they allow the patient active facial movements. In contrast, static techniques aim to improve the appearance and symmetry of the face at rest but cannot restore movement.

> **!**
>
> The best results in facial nerve reconstruction are achieved when the proximal facial nerve stump can be reconnected to the peripheral facial nerve stump within 30 days of injury.

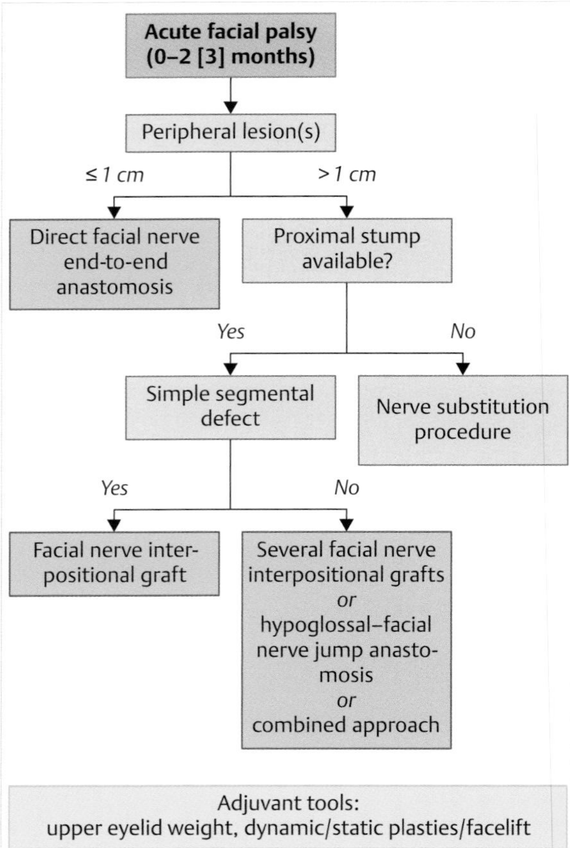

Fig. 20.1 Algorithm showing the possibilities for facial nerve reconstruction in patients with an acute facial nerve lesion. (Reproduced with permission from Bradley PJ, Guntinas-Lichius O, eds. Salivary Gland Disorders and Diseases: Diagnosis and Management. New York, Stuttgart: Thieme; 2011.)

20.3 Direct Facial–Facial Nerve Reconstruction

20.3.1 Indications

Direct nerve repair by end-to-end nerve suture is only possible if the defect is smaller than 1 cm. The nerve stumps must be definitely tumor-free. This is common in traumatic or iatrogenic sharp lesions of a nerve branch or the main trunk. Direct nerve repair results in good functional recovery only if it is a tension-free primary repair and if it is performed as soon as possible, preferably within 6 months from the time of injury.

20.3.2 Patient Information, Consent

The patient has to be informed about functional outcome failure, and the possible need for revision surgery. The patient must be told that it takes 6 to 18 months (depending on the site of the lesion) to complete nerve regeneration.

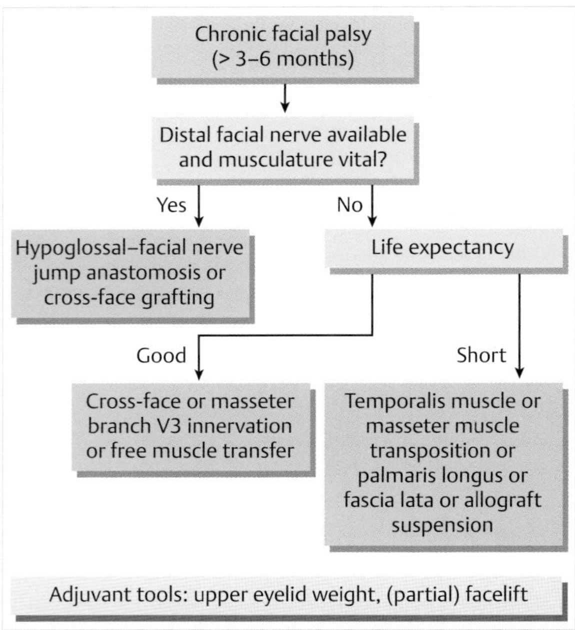

Fig. 20.2 Algorithm showing the possibilities for facial nerve reconstruction in patients with a chronic facial nerve lesion.

20.3.3 Anesthesia and Positioning

General anesthesia is mandatory. The patient lies in the supine position with rotation of the head to the opposite side of the lesion.

20.3.4 Surgical Steps

1. Wide exposure of the lesion site is imperative and the use of magnification is mandatory. The authors' center prefers to use the operating microscope to identify the facial nerve and its branches. In trauma cases, meticulous wound rinsing is mandatory. In tumor cases, tumor-free nerve stumps have to be confirmed by frozen section or definitive histology.
2. The affected nerve endings are freshened and the epineurium is cut back a little bit before nerve suture (▶ Fig. 20.7).
3. The peripheral facial nerve is a monofascicular nerve, i.e., an epineurial nerve suture is performed using individual stitches with nonabsorbable monofilament 8–0 to 11–0 suture material depending on the nerve caliber. The repair requires enough sutures to provide for apposition without tension or bulging (usually 3–6 are used).

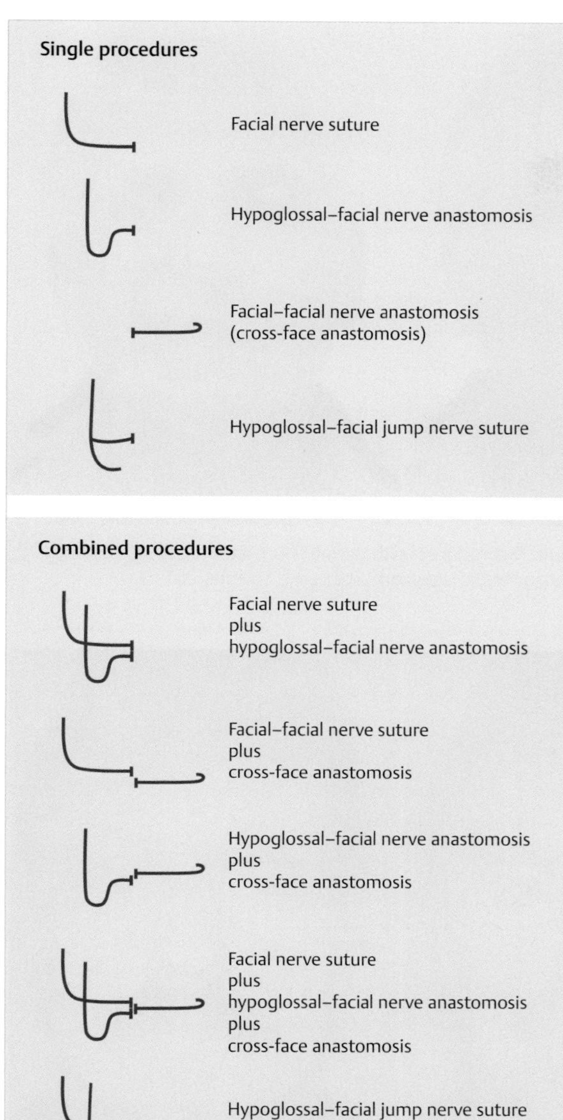

Fig. 20.3 Schematic overview of all types and combinations of facial nerve reconstruction.

- Gentle mobilization of the nerve stumps will reduce tension on the suture site.
- Soft tissue in the proximity of nerve suture site should be placed so as not to place tension on the repair. Because of the mobility of the neck tissue, nerve suture is preferred over fibrin glue.
- In trauma cases with salivary gland laceration or foreign debris, the suture ends, proximal and distal, should be marked with metallic clips of long permanent-colored suture to facilitate later surgery.
- As a general rule for nerve microsurgery: make a colored background, such as a round 1 cm piece of the suture package, and place it under the suture site to provide stability. Prevent drying-out of the nerve stumps by regularly sprinkling them with saline.

20.3.5 Complications

If correct surgical case selection is employed and meticulous microsurgical nerve reconstruction is practiced, then success rate of the procedure is extremely high. The best tool for monitoring nerve regeneration is electromyography (EMG) starting 3 months after surgery. EMG will detect axon regeneration into the facial musculature and an increase in regeneration about 3 months earlier than clinical movements can be seen. Therefore, EMG will also reveal failing regeneration much earlier than clinical examination. In such cases a re-exploration of the suture site and alternative choices for facial rehabilitation may need to be discussed with the patient.

20.3.6 Postoperative Care

There is no current evidence that electrostimulation of the musculature has a positive influence on the degree of reinnervation. In addition, it hinders EMG interpretation during follow-up because it produces long-term electrical artifacts in the musculature. At the moment when the first signs of muscle reinnervation become obvious, mimic training can start, as described in Chapter 26; commencing mimic training before this only causes frustration for the patient.

20.3.7 Outcomes

Direct facial nerve repair gives the best results compared with all other rehabilitation procedures. The patient should achieve good resting tone and good-to-satisfactory voluntary movements. All patients develop permanent sequelae; the most difficult are synkinesis and hyperkinesis.

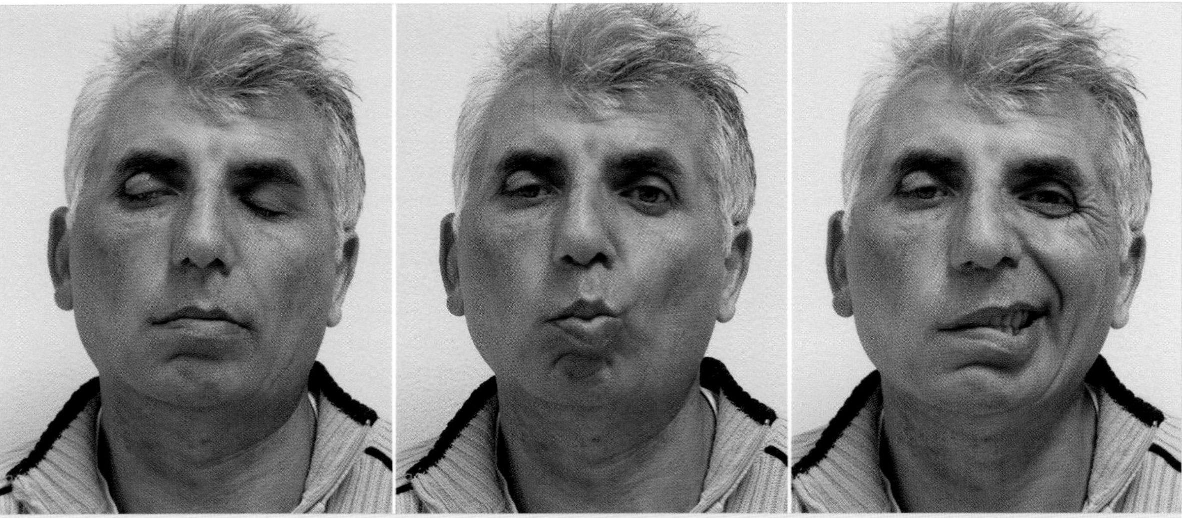

Fig. 20.4 Facial–facial interpositional graft, 1 year after the reconstruction. (Reproduced with permission from Bradley PJ, Guntinas-Lichius O, eds. Salivary Gland Disorders and Diseases: Diagnosis and Management. New York, Stuttgart: Thieme; 2011.)

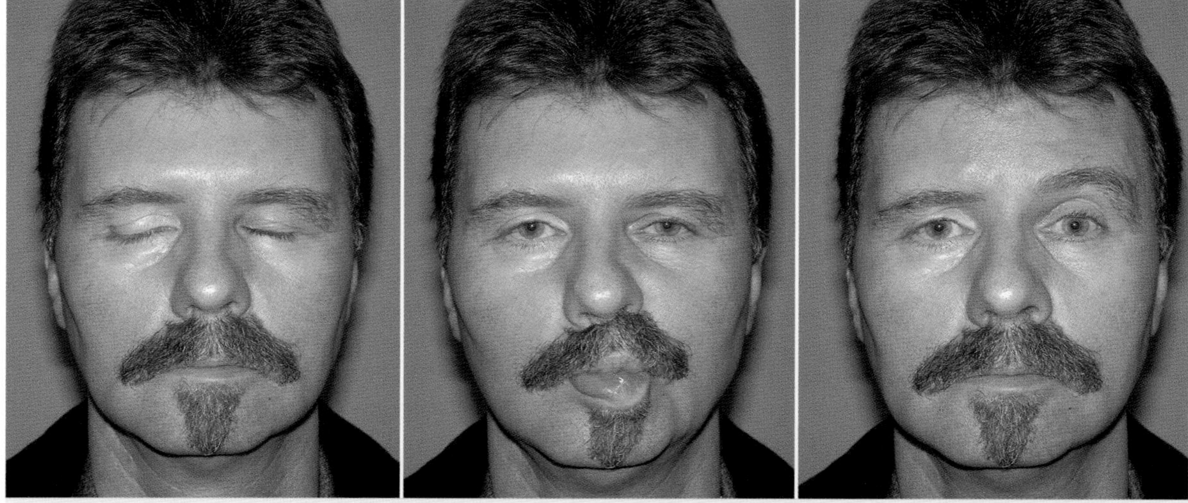

Fig. 20.5 Hypoglossal–facial jump nerve suture, 1 year after the reconstruction. (Reproduced with permission from Bradley PJ, Guntinas-Lichius O, eds. Salivary Gland Disorders and Diseases: Diagnosis and Management. New York, Stuttgart: Thieme; 2011.)

20.4 Facial–Facial Nerve Interposition Graft

20.4.1 Indications

If the peripheral facial nerve defect is larger than 1 cm or in patients with a segmental defect in the facial nerve, a facial–facial nerve interposition graft provides a good functional result (► Fig. 20.8).

20.4.2 Patient Information, Consent

Patient information and consent are the same as for direct end-to-end-anastomosis: the patient has to be informed about functional outcome failure and revision surgery. The patient must be told that it takes 6 to 18 months (depending on the site of the lesion, and time postinjury) to complete nerve regeneration. In addition, the harvest of the graft will lead to deficient sensitivity in the target area of the donor nerve, i.e., numbness in the ear region (for the greater auricular nerve, or of the dorsal lower leg and lateral foot for the sural nerve).

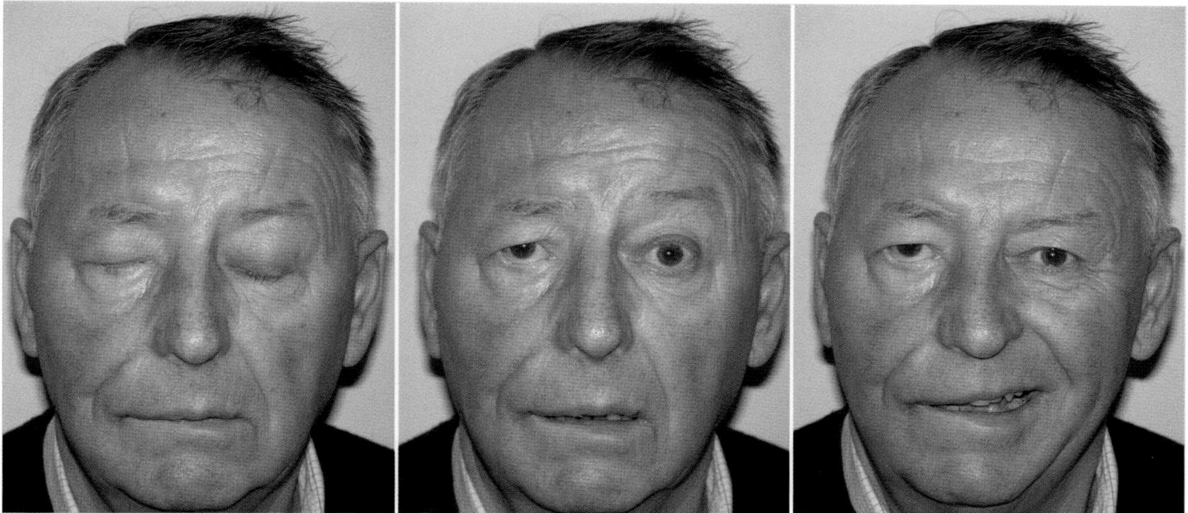

Fig. 20.6 Static reconstruction with a sling using the palmaris longus tendon, 1 year after the reconstruction. (Reproduced with permission from Bradley PJ, Guntinas-Lichius O, eds. Salivary Gland Disorders and Diseases: Diagnosis and Management. New York, Stuttgart: Thieme; 2011.)

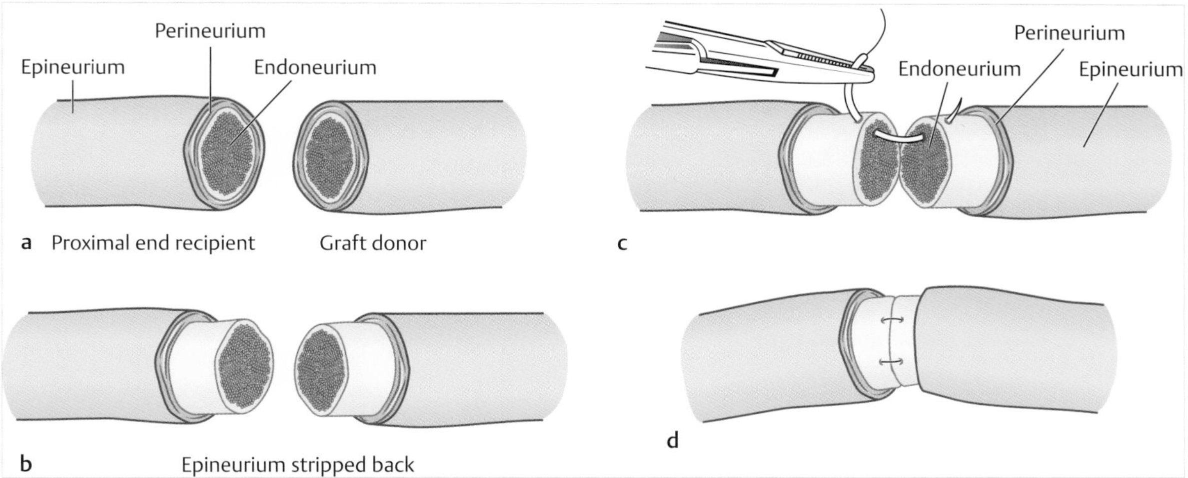

Fig. 20.7 Principles of facial nerve suture technique. **(a,b)** If possible, the epineurium is peeled back to expose the protruding endoneurial surface. **(c)** The ends of the nerve are placed over a work platform. **(d)** The ends are brought together without tension. The surfaces of the nerve stump should be matched. Monofilament suture material (8–0 to 11–0 depending on the nerve diameter) is used.

Postoperative infection and wound dehiscence are rare if the surgeon uses a meticulous technique and multilayered closure.

20.4.3 Anesthesia and Positioning

General anesthesia is mandatory. The patient is supine with rotation of the head to the opposite side of the lesion during the reconstruction. If harvest of the contralateral greater auricular nerve is necessary, the head has to be rotated for this part of surgery.

20.4.4 Surgical Steps

1. The first steps of preparation are the same as for direct nerve suture; see Direct Facial–Facial Nerve Reconstruction, Surgical Steps, steps 1 to 3.
2. Preparation of the nerve graft.
   (a) The greater auricular nerve is identified at the posterior border of the sternocleidomastoidal muscle crossing the muscle in direction of the parotid gland and the preauricular crest (▶ Fig. 20.9). The nerve is cut as distally as possible. If necessary the branching into the anterior and posterior ramus

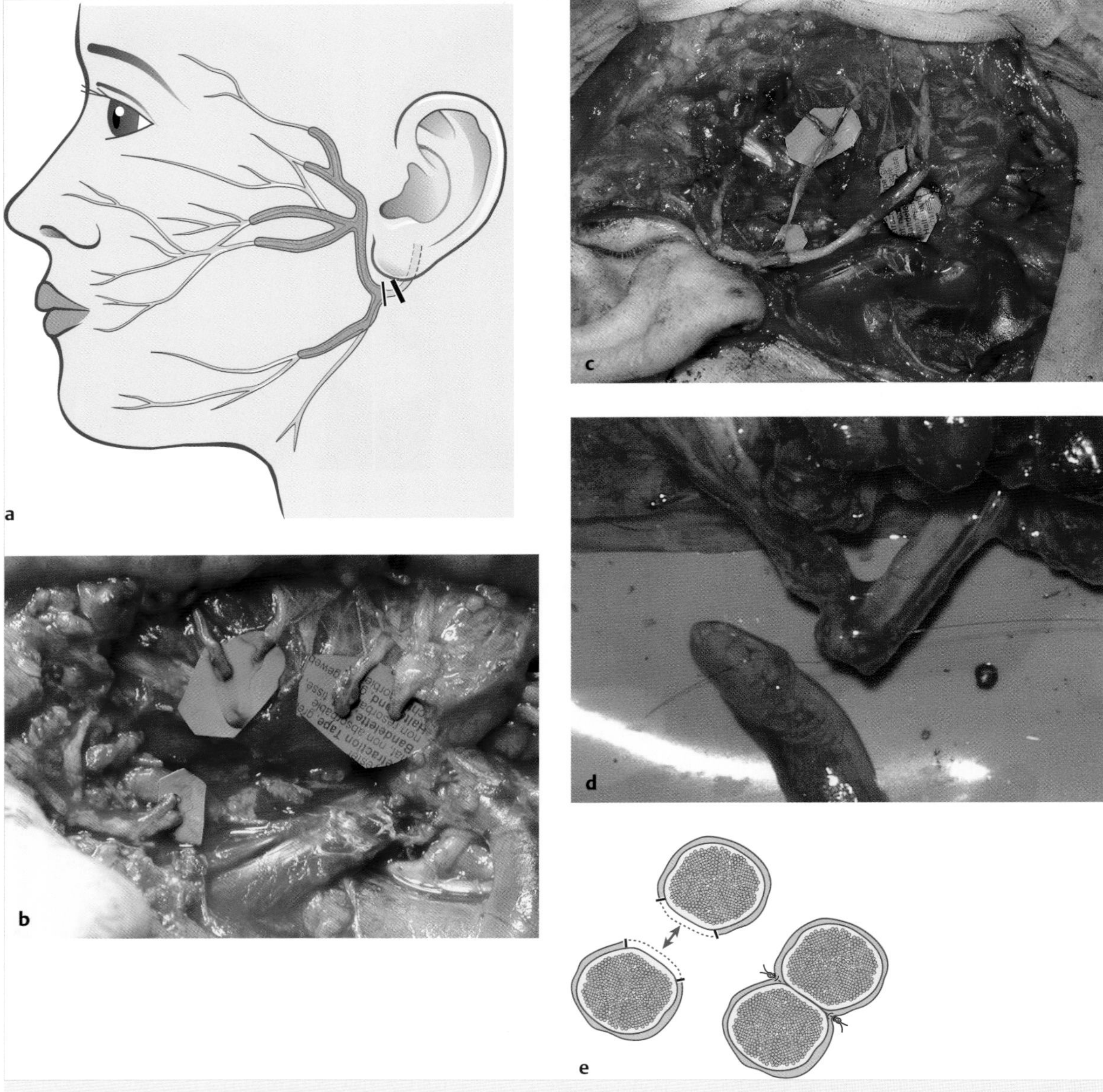

Fig. 20.8 Reconstruction of a segmental facial nerve defect. **(a)** A typical surgical segmental defect in the facial nerve plexus is shown. **(b)** The proximal and distal nerve endings are pooled and trimmed for the nerve suture. **(c)** Reconstruction with several branches of the greater auricular nerve. **(d)** Peripheral thin branches are pooled and sutured together to increase the nerve diameter. **(e)** The epineurium is peeled off in the attachment zone. (Reproduced with permission from Bradley PJ, Guntinas-Lichius O, eds. Salivary Gland Disorders and Diseases: Diagnosis and Management. New York, Stuttgart: Thieme; 2011.)

can be dissected if this branching is useful for the reconstruction. Then, the nerve graft is followed down the dorsal neck as distally as possible. The nerve graft should be handled gently and placed in a moist environment until needed for reconstruction.

(b) If the ipsilateral greater auricular nerve is not available (for instance, because of tumor infiltration in the neck in patients with parotid cancer) the nerve can be harvested on the contralateral side.

(c) The sural nerve is harvested with several transverse 1 cm incisions at the back of the lower leg (▸ Fig. 20.9 and ▸ Fig. 20.10). The sural nerve can be found between the lateral malleolus and Achilles tendon, lying posterior to the lesser saphenous vein. The nerve lies superior to the deep fascia. Using blunt dissection or a stripper the nerve can be followed cranially. Near the two heads of the gastrocnemius muscle a communicating

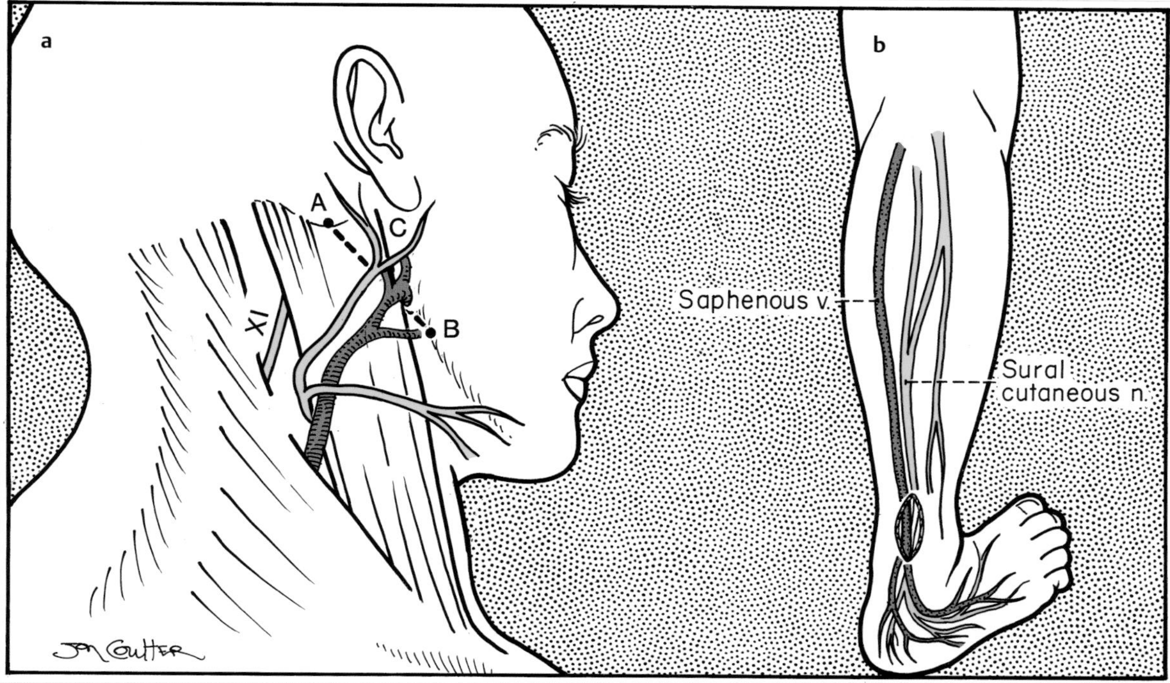

Fig. 20.9 Donor nerves for facial nerve grafts. (a) The ipsilateral cervical plexus is the preferred area to harvest the greater auricular nerve. Usually a 7 to 10 cm graft can be obtained with a main trunk and if necessary with up to four to five branches. (b) The sural nerve is the alternative for long grafts as lengths of up to 30 to 40 cm can be obtained. (Reproduced with permission from May M, Schaitkin BM, eds. The Facial Nerve. New York, Stuttgart: Thieme; 2000.)

branch to the peroneal nerve can block the stripper. Endoscopic nerve harvest of the sural nerve can be performed in a similar way to saphenous vein harvest for cardiac surgery.[6]

3. The graft or several graft pieces are positioned end-to-end in the segmental defect(s). Multiple nonabsorbable monofilament 8–0 to 11–0 sutures, depending on the nerve caliber, are used to perform an end-to-end tension-free anastomosis.

- In larger segmental defects a discrepancy in caliber size between the thick proximal facial nerve stump and thinner distal stumps, and a discrepancy in the number of nerve branches, can be overcome by pooling of peripheral branches, and/or by diversification of the interpositioned nerve graft. For pooling, the branches are sutured together side-by-side (▶ Fig. 20.8). Alternatively an additional measure to enlarge the diameter is to cut the stump diagonally, and/or double grafts can be used (▶ Fig. 20.11).
- A small caliber discrepancy is not a problem.
- For most extratemporal defects, one greater auricular nerve is usually sufficient if the maximal amount of nerve is harvested.
- Ligating the proximal stump of the donor nerve or burying it in muscle may prevent neuroma formation.

20.4.5 Complications

If the rules of patient selection are followed, the only important complication, i.e., that of no nerve regeneration, is very rare. In such cases re-exploration of the suture site and an alternative of facial rehabilitation should be discussed with the patient. The time course of regeneration is monitored after direct nerve suture to decide if re-exploration is necessary; see Direct Facial–Facial Nerve Reconstruction, Complications.

20.4.6 Postoperative Care

Postoperative care is similar to that described in Direct Facial–Facial Nerve Reconstruction, Postoperative Care.

20.4.7 Outcomes

The outcome of facial nerve grafting is in good resting tone on the paralytic side and satisfactory movements with aberrant regeneration.

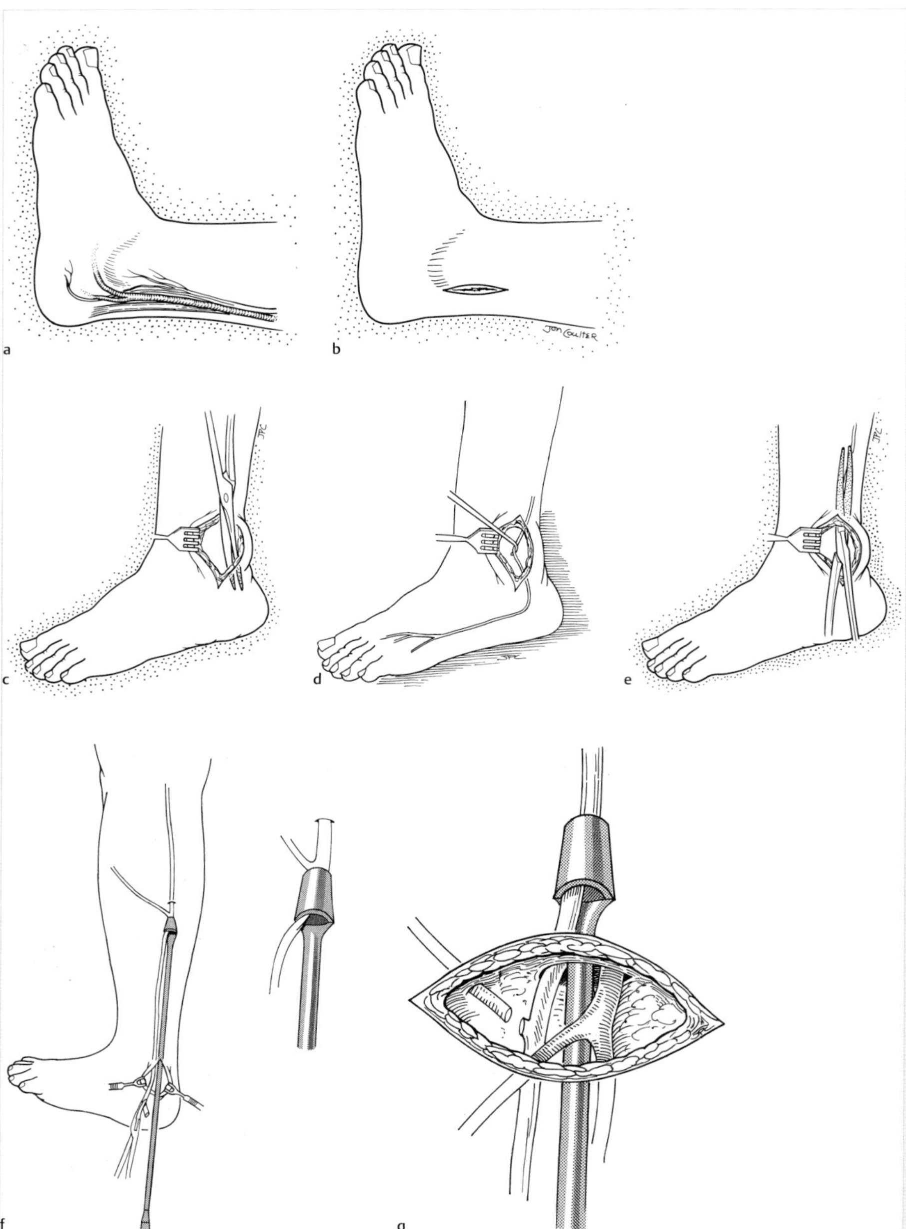

Fig. 20.10 Harvesting the sural nerve graft. **(a)** The sural nerve is identified between the Achilles tendon and the lateral malleolus. **(b)** An incision is made behind and above the lateral malleolus. **(c)** The nerve is freed up distally. **(d)** A nerve hook places the nerve kindly on stretch as it is cut with scissors. **(e)** The nerve is dissected superiorly with a blunt scissor. **(f)** The fascia stripper is then placed in the wound. The distal end of the nerve is brought through the opening of the stripper. The stripper is finally inserted up to the leg until it reaches resistance of the lateral communicating branch. **(g)** A counter incision is made. The lateral branch is divided. The stripper is advanced further up to the gastrocnemius muscle and the popliteal fossa. The nerve is finally divided and removed. If needed, 40 cm of nerve can be obtained in this way. (Reproduced with permission from May M, Schaitkin BM, eds. The Facial Nerve. New York, Stuttgart: Thieme; 2000.)

20.5 Hypoglossal–Facial Nerve Suture and Hypoglossal–Facial Jump Nerve Suture

20.5.1 Indications

This type of reconstruction is the best choice if the proximal facial nerve is damaged irreversibly, or in cases of delayed reconstruction between 6 months and 2 years.[7,8] In addition, although it is always best when possible to reconnect the facial nerve nucleus to the facial musculature, some patients may refuse to have an additional craniotomy and elect for nerve substitution. The characteristics of the classical hypoglossal–facial cross-nerve suture and the jump technique are juxtaposed in ▶ Table 20.4.

20.5.2 Patient Information, Consent

When using the classic hypoglossal–facial nerve suture, the patient will develop atrophy of the ipsilateral tongue. This can lead to swallowing and speech problems.[9] When performing a hypoglossal–facial jump nerve suture, a nerve graft is needed; for details see Direct Facial–Facial Nerve Reconstruction and Facial–Facial Nerve Interposition Graft. In most cases the greater auricular nerve is sufficient for the nerve graft. When performing a hypoglossal–facial jump nerve suture, there is a theoretical risk of ipsilateral tongue palsy if too much or the complete hypoglossal nerve is transected accidentally, but the incidence is very low.[7] Then, the patient would complain of swallowing and speech problems. The patient should be informed that cross-nerve anastomoses with other nerves, as described in Other Cross-Nerve Sutures, such as the spinal accessory or the phrenic nerve, result in a much poorer function. Cross-face facial nerve grafting, as described in Cross-Face Facial Nerve Suture, is an alternative, and is mostly used in combination with free-muscle transfer, as described in Chapter 22. Follow-up for at least 18 months is necessary to monitor facial recovery. The motor branch of the third division of the trigeminal nerve is increasingly being employed as alternative for a motor nerve to reanimate the face.[10]

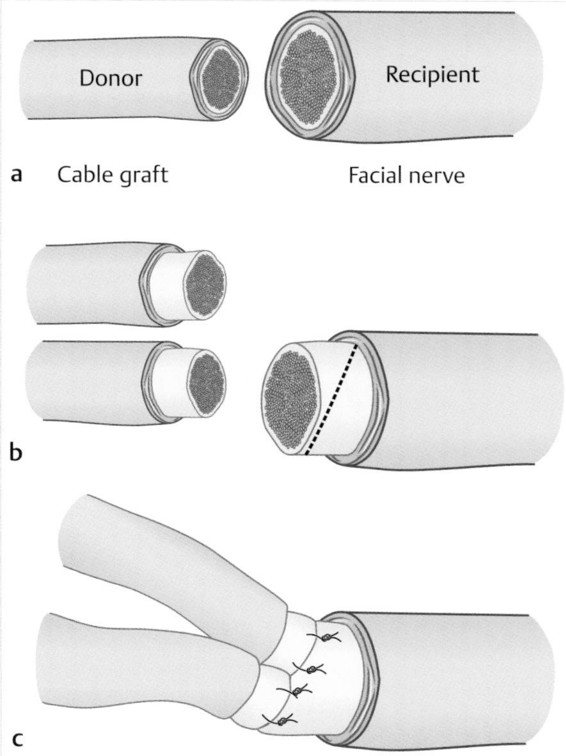

Fig. 20.11 (a–c) To overcome a discrepancy between the diameter of the donor nerve graft and the recipient facial nerve, double nerve grafts are useful. The diameter of the facial nerve stump or the donor nerve can be enlarged by resection of a vertical segment.

20.5.3 Anesthesia and Positioning

General anesthesia is mandatory. The patient is lying in supine position with rotation of the head to the opposite side during the reconstruction. The ipsilateral neck must be exposed to allow the approach to the hypoglossal nerve.

20.5.4 Surgical Steps

1. The first steps of the preparation of the distal facial nerve stump or branches are the same as for direct nerve suture, as described in Direct Facial–Facial Nerve Reconstruction, Surgical Steps, steps 1 to 3.
2. To identify the hypoglossal nerve, the posterior belly of the digastric muscle is retracted superiorly and the jugular vein posteriorly (▶ Fig. 20.12 and ▶ Fig. 20.13). The nerve is isolated on the undersurface of the digastric muscle about 1 to 2 cm distal to the descendens hypoglossi branch. The next steps for classic hypoglossal–facial nerve suture are different to those described for direct nerve suture (5–8) and the jump technique (3–4).
3. Hypoglossal–facial jump nerve suture. About 1 cm distal to this branch the hypoglossal nerve is incised to accommodate the caliber of the greater auricular graft and the incision is never greater than one-third of the diameter of the hypoglossal.

Table 20.4 Comparison of classical hypoglossal–facial nerve suture and hypoglossal–facial jump nerve suture

Advantage/disadvantage	Classical hypoglossal–facial nerve suture	Hypoglossal–facial jump nerve suture
Advantages	Established procedure applied to many patients. There is much more experience with this than with the jump technique Proven high rate of success	More frequently used than the classic technique Less synkinesis and no mass movements Even possible in cases of contralateral palsy of the hypoglossal nerve Can be performed on both sides
Disadvantages	Palsy of the ipsilateral tongue Chronic dysphagia possible Speech problems possible Strong synkinesis and sometime mass movements Strong resting tonus of the face Cannot be performed if the patient also has a vagal nerve palsy	Less stronger voluntary activity than classic technique A graft is needed

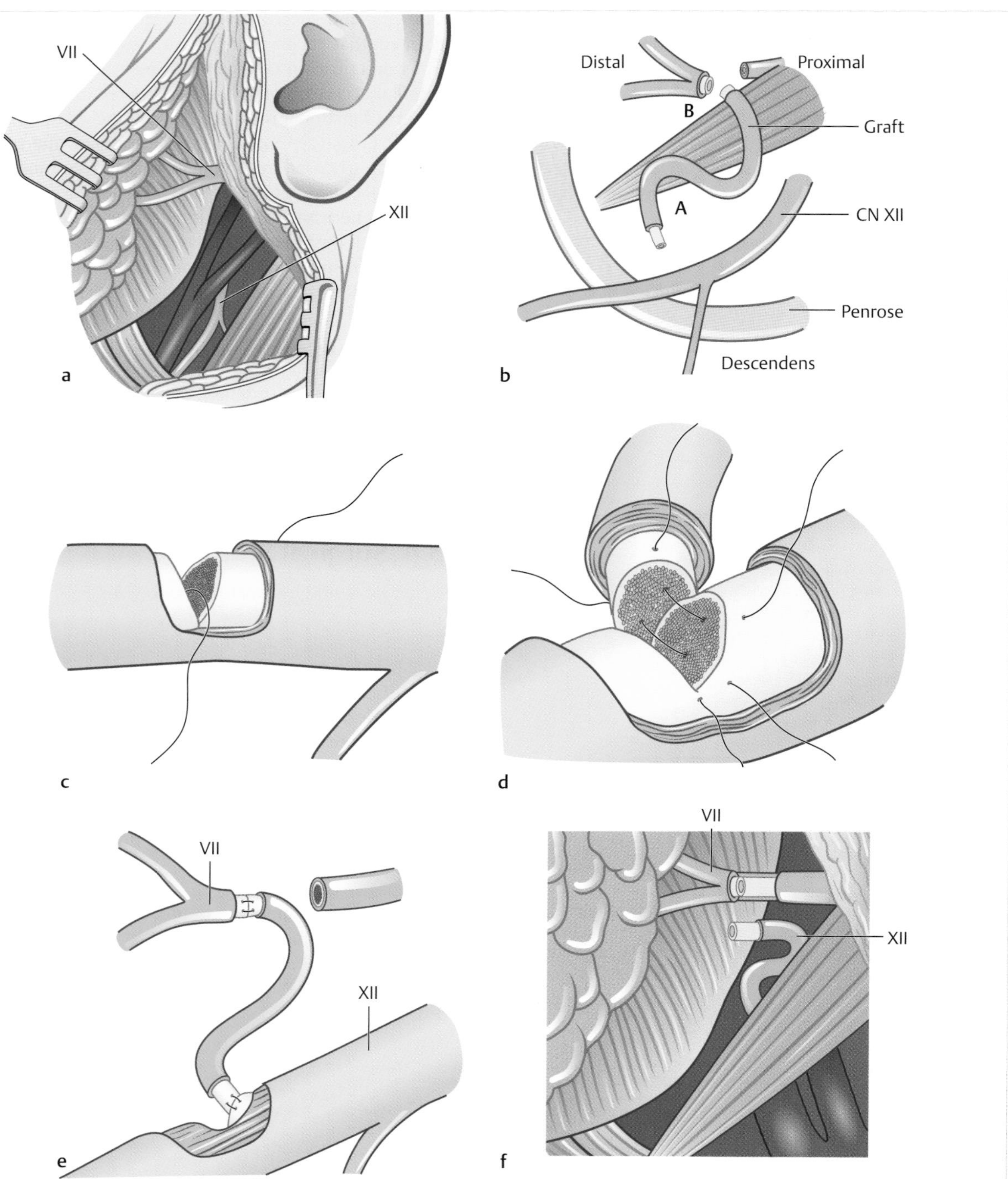

Fig. 20.12 **(a–f)** Hypoglossal–facial jump nerve suture, and **(f)** classical hypoglossal–facial nerve suture. **(a)** Preauricular parotidectomy incision. The facial nerve trunk is freed at its exit out of the stylomastoid foramen. The facial nerve is followed to just past the pes anserinus. A parotidectomy is not necessary. The hypoglossal nerve is isolated as it courses between the jugular vein and carotid vessels just on the undersurface of the digastric muscle. **(b)** An end-to-side nerve suture to the hypoglossal nerve and an end-to-end nerve suture to the distal facial nerve stump are planned after trimming of the epineurium of the graft and the facial nerve stump. **(c)** The hypoglossal nerve is incised about by about one-third. Due to the elastic forces in the nerve, it will gape automatically. **(d)** Proximally, the end-to-side nerve suture is performed from the graft to the hypoglossal nerve. **(e)** Distally, the end-to-end nerve suture is performed to the distal facial nerve. **(f)** For a classic hypoglossal–facial nerve suture, the hypoglossal nerve is transected completely. The proximal stump of the nerve is turned up and then resutured end-to-end directly to the distal facial nerve stump.

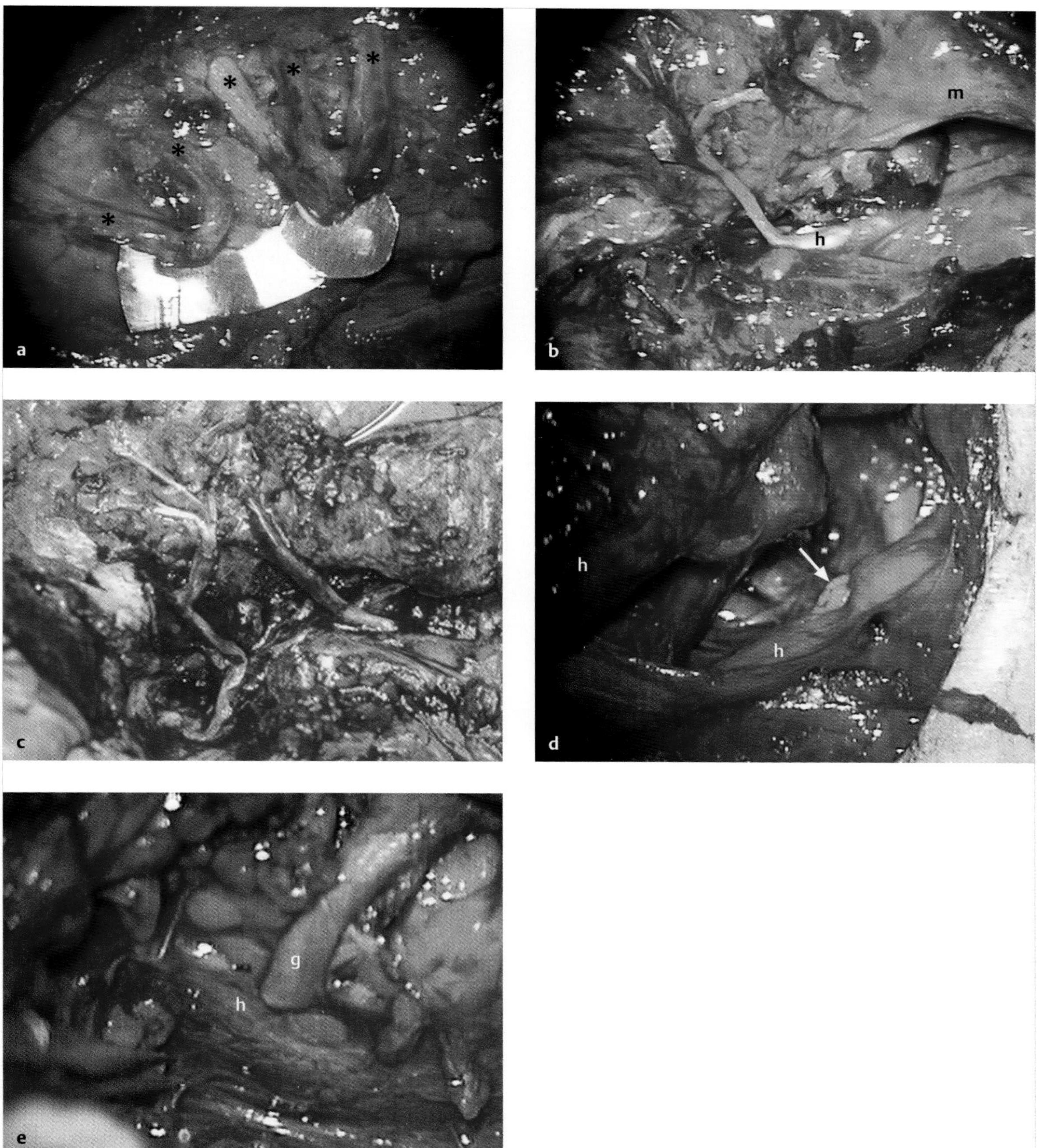

Fig. 20.13 **(a,b,d,e)** Reconstruction with hypoglossal–facial jump nerve suture, and **(c)** a combined approach. **(a)** A large defect of the facial fan after surgery for malignancy, resulting in a separate grouping of the peripheral stumps (*asterisks*) related to the upper and lower face. **(b)** If the proximal facial stump is not identifiable, the reconstruction can be performed by using a hypoglossal–facial nerve jump anastomosis.**(c)** Alternatively, if the proximal stump is available, repair can be completed using a combined approach: The upper face is reanimated by a facial nerve interpositional graft and the lower face by using a hypoglossal–facial nerve jump anastomosis. For hypoglossal–facial nerve jump anastomosis, **(d)** the hypoglossal nerve (h) is for one-third of the defect, and **(e)** a graft (g) is jumped with an end-to-side anastomosis to the proximal cut surface. g, graft; h, hypoglossal nerve; m, mandible; s, sternocleidomastoid muscle. (Reproduced with permission from Bradley PJ, Guntinas-Lichius O, eds. Salivary Gland Disorders and Diseases: Diagnosis and Management. New York, Stuttgart: Thieme; 2011.)

4. The greater auricular nerve is prepared as described in 20.4 Facial–Facial Nerve Interposition Graft, Surgical Steps (see ▶ Fig. 20.9). A graft of at least 5 cm is needed and the nerve should be placed with redundancy to allow for free neck excursion without producing graft tension.
5. Classic hypoglossal–facial nerve suture (▶ Fig. 20.12 f). The hypoglossal nerve is isolated as it courses between the jugular vein and carotid vessels just on the undersurface of the digastric muscle. In contrast to the jump technique, it is necessary to divide the descendens hypoglossi nerve. Otherwise, it is not possible to mobilize the proximal stump of the hypoglossal nerve as needed.
6. After the epineurium is trimmed proximally and distally, exposing the perineurium containing endoneurial material, scissors are used to divide the hypoglossal nerve in this zone distal to the descendens hypoglossi nerve.
7. The main trunk of the facial nerve is exposed. The epineurium is trimmed back proximally and distally over the facial nerve. The perineurial and endoneurial content is exposed. If possible, the deep surface of the epineurium is not divided, thus holding the facial nerve in position.
8. The proximal stump of the hypoglossal nerve is brought medial to the digastric muscle and significant length is achieved with this maneuver.
9. A microsurgical tension-free repair is performed with two to four sutures (nonabsorbable monofilament 8–0 to 11–0).

→•

- Some authors have described a jump anastomosis without interposition graft by placing the hypoglossal nerve directly to the facial nerve by "turning down" the proximal facial nerve to meet the hypoglossal nerve.[11,12] If the mastoid segment of the facial nerve and thereof all distal parts of the nerve are intact, it is possible to decompress the nerve via mastoidectomy. The facial nerve is cut as proximally as it can safely be done in the vertical segment. Even in cases when it is not anticipated that a graft is necessary, the surgical plan should always be prepared for the option of employing a graft.
- Identify the main trunk of the hypoglossal nerve clearly using electrostimulation and prepare the descendens hypoglossi branch. The point of using the nerve distally for jump graft is that this plugs only tongue motor fibers into the facial nerve so that tongue movement provides maximal stimulation.
- The anastomosis of the graft to the side of hypoglossal nerve can be facilitated by placing a penrose drain under the hypoglossal nerve and catching the ends of the penrose in a self-retaining retractor. This will gently elevate the nerve into the field of view for easier and less bloody exposure.
- Most cases can be reached easily with the greater auricular nerve passing over the digastric muscle.
- Optionally, a hypoglossal–facial jump anastomosis can be combined with a facial nerve interposition graft. This technique is described in more detail in Combined Approach. A combined approach is an optimal technique to reconstruct larger segmental defects when the proximal facial nerve stump is still available. In such cases, the upper face branches are reconstructed with a graft or grafts to the proximal facial nerve stump, and the lower face is reconstructed with a jump graft to the incised proximal hypoglossal nerve.

20.5.5 Complications

The hypoglossal nerve is a powerful motor nerve. If the rules of patient selection are followed, the only important complication, i.e., that no nerve regeneration takes place, is very rare. In such cases re-exploration of the suture site and alternative of facial rehabilitation should be discussed with the patient. If tongue atrophy occurs, the patient might need physiotherapy to improve swallowing and speech.

Measures For Specific Complications

The time course of regeneration is monitored with EMG, as described for after direct nerve suture in Direct Facial–Facial Nerve Reconstruction, Complications. At the start, it is important that the patient intentionally moves the tongue, for instance by pressing the tongue against the palate, to induce facial movements.

20.5.6 Postoperative Care

This is described in Direct Facial–Facial Nerve Reconstruction, Postoperative Care. In the moment when the first signs of muscle reinnervation become obvious, training can begin with a skilled physical therapist experienced in facial paralysis: the therapist and the patient will explore which tongue movement provides the best result. The younger the patient is, the faster the patient will induce facial movements without thinking about tongue movements.

20.5.7 Outcomes

Hypoglossal–facial nerve jump anastomosis results in good resting tone on the paralyzed side and a volitional smile with synkinesis. It is almost never possible to create a mimetic effect. The longer the delay between the onset of palsy and repair, then it is recommended to use jump anastomosis instead of a facial nerve interposition graft.

Rule of thumb:

- First 6 months: nerve graft
- 6 to 18 months: hypoglossal–facial nerve jump nerve suture with satisfactory results
- More than 18 months: hypoglossal–facial nerve classical nerve suture will still give a result, but the patient needs to understand the deficit is significant

20.6 Cross-Face Facial Nerve Suture

20.6.1 Indications

In patients with a complex segmental defect and/or a chronic facial palsy (> 3–6 months), a cross-face facial nerve suture is an alternative technique (▶ Fig. 20.14). It seems that cross-face nerve grafting is not suitable for use as a primary procedure, but that it might be valuable as an adjunct of other procedures; for example, a facial–facial nerve interposition graft, as described in Facial–Facial Nerve Interposition Graft, or a hypoglossal–facial jump nerve suture, as described in Hypoglossal–Facial Nerve Suture and Hypoglossal–Facial Jump Nerve Suture.[13] On the other hand the cross-face facial nerve suture is the basic procedure if a free muscle flap reconstruction of the paralyzed side is planned; see Chapter 22.[14] An alternative might be to use a temporalis or masseter muscle plasty; see Chapter 21.

20.6.2 Patient Information, Consent

This is the same as described for direct end-to-end-anastomosis and interposition graft: the patient should be informed about functional outcome failure, and revision surgery. The patient must be told that it takes 6 to 18 months (depending on the site of the lesion) to complete the nerve regeneration. For cross-face facial nerve suture, a graft from the sural nerve is necessary as the greater auricular nerve will not be long enough. The length of the greater auricular nerve is appropriate for a minifacial nerve cross-face graft, as described in section Surgical Steps. The harvest of the graft will lead to deficient sensitivity in the target area of the nerve, i.e., numbness in the region of the dorsal lower leg and lateral foot or the ear region. Postoperative infection and wound dehiscence in the leg is seldom if a meticulous layered suture is performed. Furthermore, the patient should be told that the procedure forfeits normal facial function on the healthy side for the potential benefit on the paralyzed side. The more distal the branches used on the normal side, the less the regenerative power provided. The more proximal the lesion site, the greater will be the relevant functional palsy or defective healing on the contralateral originally healthy side.

20.6.3 Anesthesia and Positioning

General anesthesia is mandatory. The patient lies in the supine position with alternating rotation of the head during the reconstruction.

20.6.4 Surgical Steps

1. To plan the skin incisions, the surgeon should decide which branches should be used on the healthy side to reanimate the paralyzed side. Furthermore, the surgeon should decide where on the paralyzed side the distal facial nerve branches should be reanimated. Peripheral branches in the zygomatic and buccal region can be reached via incision in the lip–cheek crease. For a more proximal access, a preauricular incision or a facelift incision is preferred.
2. With a lip–cheek crease incision: when the patient is still awake, a symmetrical lip–cheek crease is surgically marked on the paralyzed side mirroring that on the healthy side. Surgery then starts with incisions in the lip–cheek creases on both sides. Otherwise, a preauricular incision or a facelift incision is performed and the facial nerve branches are located anterior to the parotid gland.
3. Via the chosen incision, the plexus of facial nerve branches innervating the midface is dissected just deep to the facial muscles. A plastic marker is looped around these terminal branches as another loop is used to pull the facial artery laterally as it courses over these nerve endings.
4. Slight tension is placed on the twigs on the paralyzed side and the proximal portion of the nerve trunk is transected at a point away from their insertions into the undersurface of the facial muscles. The epineurium is stripped back as described previously.
5. The sural nerve is harvested as described in Facial–Facial Nerve Interposition Graft, Surgical Steps, step 2iii.
6. Using the binocular microscope, the nerve graft is sutured to the end of the facial nerve branch that will innervate the facial muscles. The number of axons available on the paralyzed side will vary depending upon the time postinjury.
7. Surgery is continued on the healthy side. Depending on which region of the facial nerve should be reanimated, the midface facial nerve plexus (most frequent case) on the normal side is found and sectioned in a

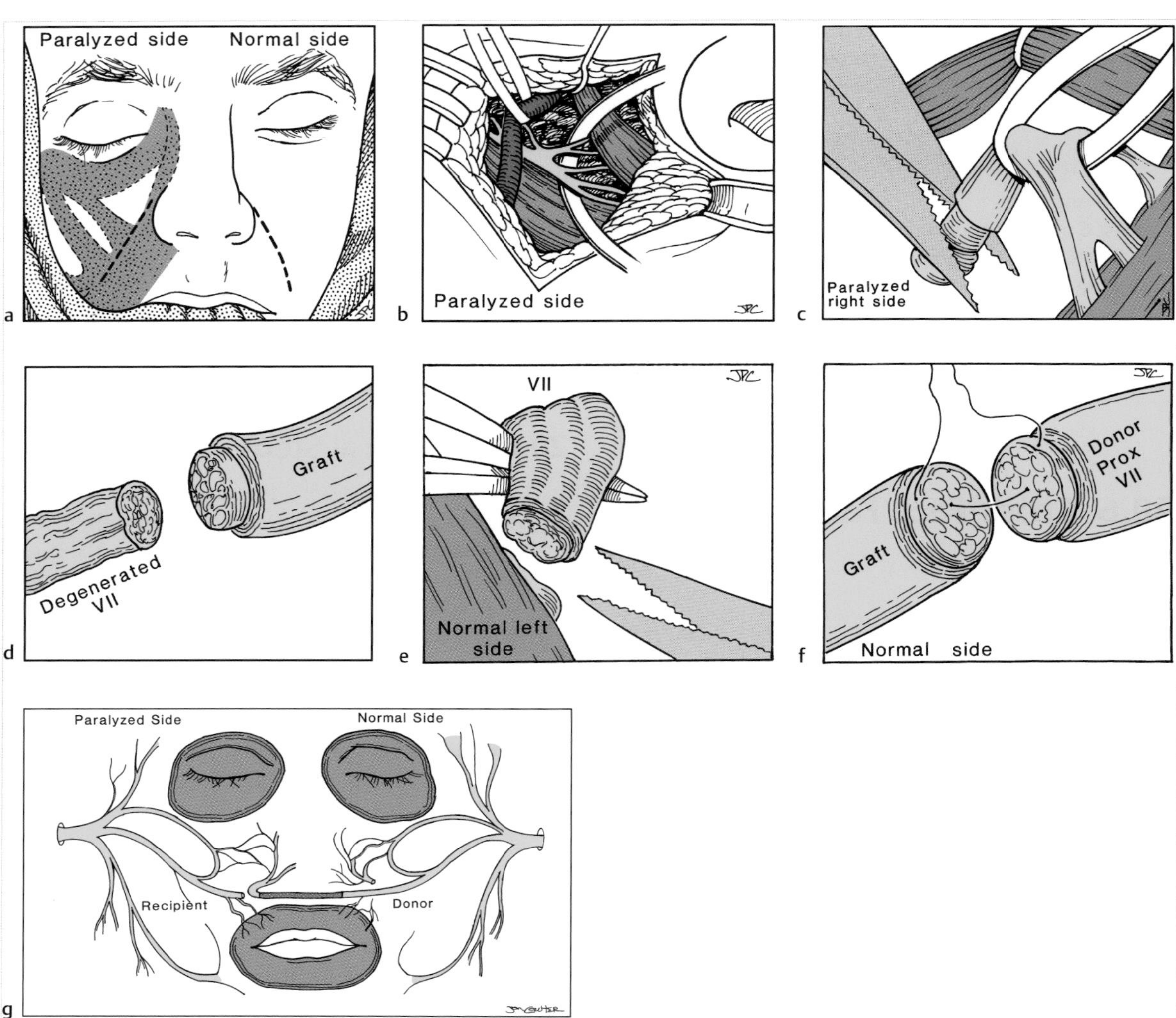

Fig. 20.14 Cross-face graft technique. As example the minifacial nerve cross-face graft technique is demonstrated. **(a)** Incisions are made in the lip–cheek crease on each side. **(b)** The plexus of facial nerve branches innervating the midface is found just deep to the facial muscles. A plastic marker is looped around these terminal branches and another loop is used to pull the facial artery laterally as it courses over these nerve endings. **(c)** Slight tension is applied to the twigs on the paralyzed side, and the proximal portion of the nerve trunk is transected at a point away from their insertions into the undersurface of the facial muscles. The epineurium is stripped back. **(d)** View through the binocular microscope of the degenerated facial nerve branch on the right paralyzed side. The graft is sutured to the end of the facial nerve branch that will innervate the facial muscles. Note that the number of axons available on the paralyzed side will vary depending upon the time postinjury. **(e)** The midface facial nerve plexus on the normal left side is found and sectioned in a similar fashion to that on the paralyzed side, except the facial nerve branch is divided as distally as possible to achieve maximum length for grafting. **(f)** Note that there usually is a good axon surface match on the normal side as opposed to the paralyzed side where the nerve is undergoing degeneration. The endoneurial surface provided by the graft is usually larger than the distal end of the seventh (the recipient) nerve. **(g)** This type of cross-face facial nerve reconstruction, as indicated by its title, is a mini procedure directed to reinnervate the oral sphincter region only. (Reproduced with permission from May M, Schaitkin BM, eds. The Facial Nerve. New York, Stuttgart: Thieme; 2000.)

similar fashion to that on the paralyzed side, except the facial nerve branch is divided as distally as possible to achieve maximum length for grafting.

8. There usually is a good axon surface match on the normal side as opposed to the paralyzed side where the nerve is undergoing degeneration.
9. When a minifacial cross-face graft is performed (typically via lip–cheek crease incisions; see ▶ Fig. 20.14), only a small graft is needed. The graft is passed over the upper lip from midface to midface. This procedure is indicated to reinnervate the oral sphincter region only.

10. Alternatively two grafts can be passed over the upper lip to reanimate branches of the upper and lower face on the paralyzed side separately (Fisch's technique).
11. When the surgeon is reanimating the lower face only, the graft can pass below the chin (Scaramella's technique); this can also be used when animating the complete main trunk (Conley's technique). Another route is also possible: via the frown, or a combination of tunnels in the upper and lower face (Anderl's technique).

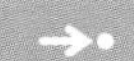

- Use a nerve stimulator when selecting the facial nerve branches to be forfeited for the cross-face innervation: With the help of a nerve stimulator, it can be easier to identify the branches supplying the mouth corner and upper lip as proximal as possible, and to identify "redundant" midface branches.
- The tunneling of the nerve graft from the paralyzed side to the healthy side can also be performed using a long hemostat or equivalent instrument that advances a sterile tube of approximately 18F from one side of the face to the other. The nerve graft is then attached to a heavy (1–0) suture with a stitch that, by its inherent firmness, is easily threaded through the tube, dragging the nerve graft behind.
- The minifacial cross-face graft provides good tone and symmetry in the midface and can be combined with other reanimation procedures.
- A special situation exists in incomplete recovery facial palsies, when the small amount of existing function should be preserved but the existing function alone is clinically insufficient. Whether surgery has a place in such a situation is a matter of debate: a few authors have described a cross-face nerve graft with distal end-to-side neurorrhaphy, which can be performed instead of end-to-end nerve sutures.[15] This policy is not accepted by others, as it has not been proven in larger series that surgery in such a situation produces better results that intensive physiotherapy.

20.6.5 Complications

If the facial nerve branches are transected too proximally on the healthy side, a relevant palsy or defective healing with synkinesis can occur on the previous healthy side.

Measure for Specific Complications

The time course of regeneration is monitored with EMG as for direct nerve suture, see Direct Facial–Facial Nerve Reconstruction, Complications. At the start, it is important that the patient intentionally moves the healthy side to induce facial movements.

20.6.6 Postoperative Care

This is described in Direct Facial–Facial Nerve Reconstruction, Postoperative Care. Facial nerve training can begin when first signs of muscle reinnervation become obvious. The patient and the therapist work together at this point to design exercises that maximize symmetrical facial expression.

20.6.7 Outcomes

Cross-face facial nerve sutures result in satisfying resting tone on the paralyzed side and satisfactory movements, especially when used for the midface.

20.7 Other Cross-Nerve Sutures

If a hypoglossal–facial (jump) nerve suture or cross-face facial nerve suture is indicated and the ipsilateral hypoglossal nerve or contralateral facial nerve is not available, a suboptimal alternative is to perform the cross-nerve suture with another motor nerve. There are a few case reports that describe using the spinal accessory or the phrenic nerve as an alternative. The functional results are much worse than after hypoglossal–facial (jump) nerve suture. A better alternative in such a special situation might be a dynamic muscle plasty, as described in Chapter 21.

20.8 Combined Approach

In patients with an acute facial palsy with a complex segmental defect, or chronic facial palsy (> 3–6 months), a combined approach is an alternative to a facial–facial nerve interposition graft, a hypoglossal–facial (jump) nerve suture, and/or a cross-facial nerve suture (▶ Fig. 20.13 c).[16,17] With a combined approach it is possible to resolve a complex situation that involves many thin far distal facial nerve stumps. It is possible to perform a combination of all the facial nerve reconstruction techniques, as described in Direct Facial–Facial Nerve Reconstruction, Facial–Facial Nerve Interposition Graft, Hypoglossal–Facial Nerve Suture and Hypoglossal–Facial Jump Nerve Suture, and Cross-Face Facial Nerve Suture (see ▶ Fig. 20.3). When combining a facial–facial nerve interposition graft to reconstruct peripheral facial nerve branches of the upper face with a reconstruction of the peripheral facial nerve branches of the lower face by a hypoglossal–facial jump nerve suture, it has the functional advantage that the upper face and lower face are separated to two different motor nerves. This reduces synkinetic activity between the upper and lower face. All of these nerve grafts techniques can be combined with static and eye reanimation procedures to improve the overall results.

20.9 Key Points

- From all factors influencing the outcome of facial nerve reconstruction, such as lesion site, extent of the facial nerve lesion, viability of the proximal facial nerve stump, sensory function of the trigeminal nerve, etiology of the lesion, and age of the patient, the time interval between nerve injury and repair is the most significant factor determining success.
- Facial nerve reconstruction techniques give better results than muscle transposition techniques and static sling procedures.
- Decision-making is a very individual for each patient, respecting the aforementioned factors, life expectancy, and the patient's wishes.
- The facial nerve surgeon should have knowledge of the whole repertoire of facial reconstruction techniques, i.e., direct nerve repair, interposition grafting, cross-nerve techniques, and cross-face grafting.
- To reduce synkinetic activity between the upper and lower face, a combined approach using two different techniques for upper and lower face reanimation is an interesting method.
- Successful surgery is only the first step of facial reanimation. The patient has to be accompanied through the process of nerve regeneration. Physiotherapy is necessary to support an optimal result when regeneration takes place. Adjuvant therapy is often helpful to improve and correct the final result.

References

[1] Guntinas-Lichius O. The facial nerve in the presence of a head and neck neoplasm: assessment and outcome after surgical management. Curr Opin Otolaryngol Head Neck Surg 2004; 12: 133–141

[2] Volk GF, Pantel M, Guntinas-Lichius O. Modern concepts in facial nerve reconstruction. Head Face Med 2010; 6: 25

[3] Chan JY, Byrne PJ. Management of facial paralysis in the 21st century. Facial Plast Surg 2011; 27: 346–357

[4] Guntinas-Lichius O, Straesser A, Streppel M. Quality of life after facial nerve repair. Laryngoscope 2007; 117: 421–426

[5] Guntinas-Lichius O, Streppel M, Stennert E. Postoperative functional evaluation of different reanimation techniques for facial nerve repair. Am J Surg 2006; 191: 61–67

[6] Hadlock TA, Cheney ML. Single-incision endoscopic sural nerve harvest for cross face nerve grafting. J Reconstr Microsurg 2008; 24: 519–523

[7] May M, Sobol SM, Mester SJ. Hypoglossal-facial nerve interpositional-jump graft for facial reanimation without tongue atrophy. Otolaryngol Head Neck Surg 1991; 104: 818–825

[8] Manni JJ, Beurskens CH, van de Velde C, Stokroos RJ. Reanimation of the paralyzed face by indirect hypoglossal-facial nerve anastomosis. Am J Surg 2001; 182: 268–273

[9] Schaitkin BM, Young T, III, Robertson JS, Fickel V, Wiegand DA. Facial reanimation after acoustic neuroma excision: the patient's perspective. Laryngoscope 1991; 101: 889–894

[10] Coyle M, Godden A, Brennan PA et al. Dynamic reanimation for facial palsy: an overview. Br J Oral Maxillofac Surg 2013; 51: 679–683

[11] Venail F, Sabatier P, Mondain M, Segniarbieux F, Leipp C, Uziel A. Outcomes and complications of direct end-to-side facial-hypoglossal nerve anastomosis according to the modified May technique. J Neurosurg 2009; 110: 786–791

[12] Beutner D, Luers JC, Grosheva M. Hypoglossal-facial-jump-anastomosis without an interposition nerve graft. Laryngoscope 2013; 123: 2392–2396

[13] Frey M, Michaelidou M, Tzou CH, Hold A, Pona I, Placheta E. Proven and innovative operative techniques for reanimation of the paralyzed face [in German] Handchir Mikrochir Plast Chir 2010; 42: 81–89

[14] Ghali S, MacQuillan A, Grobbelaar AO. Reanimation of the middle and lower face in facial paralysis: review of the literature and personal approach. J Plast Reconstr Aesthet Surg 2011; 64: 423–431

[15] Frey M, Giovanoli P, Michaelidou M. Functional upgrading of partially recovered facial palsy by cross-face nerve grafting with distal end-to-side neurorrhaphy. Plast Reconstr Surg 2006; 117: 597–608

[16] Stennert E. I. Hypoglossal facial anastomosis: its significance for modern facial surgery. II. Combined approach in extratemporal facial nerve reconstruction. Clin Plast Surg 1979; 6: 471–486

[17] Volk GF, Pantel M, Streppel M, Guntinas-Lichius O. Reconstruction of complex peripheral facial nerve defects by a combined approach using facial nerve interpositional graft and hypoglossal-facial jump nerve suture. Laryngoscope 2011; 121: 2402–2405

21 Muscle Flaps and Static Procedures

Markus Jungehülsing and Orlando Guntinas-Lichius

21.1 Introduction

To obtain optimal results after surgical repair to reanimate mimic function, it is necessary to be experienced in facial nerve reconstruction techniques, as described in Chapter 20, including muscle transfer (transposition) techniques and static procedures. Before the free muscle flap procedures emerged, as described in Chapter 22, muscle transfers were the gold standard when viable facial muscles no longer existed. When there is still a chance for reinnervating the native facial muscles, facial nerve repair is always the primary method offering the best possible outcome.[1,2] On the other hand, if there is no chance for facial muscle reinnervation, the first option to be considered in many centers is free muscle transfer for adults and especially in children.[3] Nevertheless, muscle transfer remains the main option for patients who are not candidates for the free flap procedures. If a muscle transfer is not indicated or feasible, static procedures using slings are another option, at least for the restoration of the midface and the lower face.[4] Static procedures can also be integrated with dynamic procedures to provide immediate support and improve the results.[5]

> **!**
>
> If the facial muscles are not available for reinnervation and free flap techniques are not feasible or available, regional muscle transfer is an option to reanimate the paralyzed hemiface. If a muscle transfer is not possible, a static procedure for the midface or lower face is a functionally limited but fast option with immediate result.

21.2 Definition

Muscle transfer for facial reanimation includes all regional muscle transposition techniques. The transposition is most frequently used to reanimate the corner of the mouth and a smile, but some techniques can also be used to reanimate the closure of the eye. Three regional muscles are currently used: the temporalis muscle, the masseter muscle, and the digastric muscle. The temporalis muscle is the most popular muscle because of its location and especially because of its vector to pull and restore the position of the corner of the mouth to create a lateral smile (▶ Fig. 21.1). The masseter muscle is

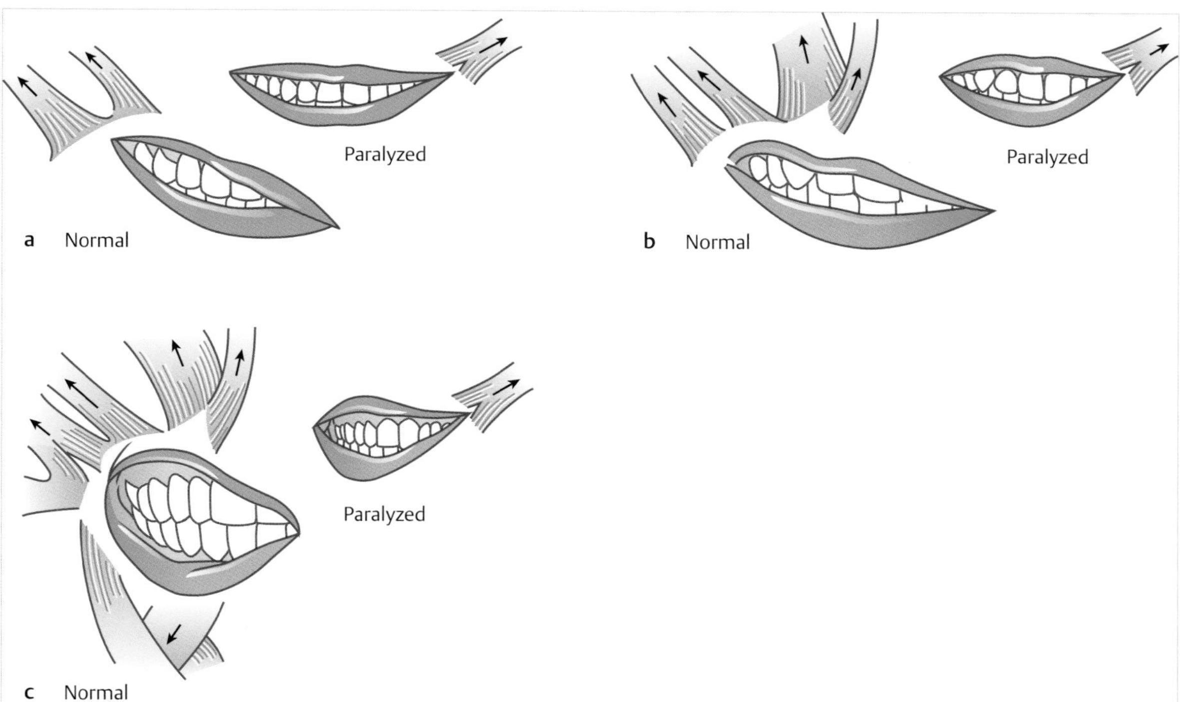

Fig. 21.1 The three different types of smiling: **(a)** lateral smile, **(b)** canine smile, and **(c)** full smile. The right side of the face is normal, and the effect of facial palsy is shown on the left side. Temporalis muscle transfer is ideal for reconstruction of the lateral smile. Reproduction of the canine smile or full smile is very difficult because of the complex interplay between several facial muscles. (Adapted with permission from May M, Schaitkin BM, eds. The Facial Nerve. New York, Stuttgart: Thieme; 2000.)

regarded by most surgeons as second choice if the temporalis muscle is not available. The masseter muscle cannot be used to reanimate the closure of the eye. The digastric muscle transposition is an adjunct procedure to partially restore the loss of the depressor effect on the lower lip on the paralyzed side. All muscle transfer procedures have in common that they are dynamic reconstruction techniques, i.e., the activation of the transposed muscle leads to an active movement in the direction of the vector of the transposed muscle. The movement is strictly limited to this vector. Other movements are not possible. In contrast, sling techniques are static procedures, i.e., the procedure leads to a suspension of the hemiface in the direction of the vectors of the two anchor points of the sling. At best, a sling improves the appearance of the face at rest, but will not improve movement of the face.

!

Muscle transposition is a dynamic reconstruction technique leading to a limited and specific movement in the face.

Sling procedures are static reconstruction techniques leading to a suspension of the face at rest in a specific direction.

21.3 Temporalis Muscle Transfer

21.3.1 Indications

Temporalis muscle transposition may be indicated if facial muscle paralysis persists for more than 1 to 2 years, if the facial muscles develop severe atrophy, if the peripheral facial nerve has been destroyed, or if a simple and rapid solution to facial weakness is desired, especially in patients with an anticipated short survival (▶ Fig. 21.2 and ▶ Fig. 21.3). In general, temporalis muscle transposition provides the best functional results of transposition, as the muscle has a better motion vector for elevating the angle of the mouth and is longer than the masseter muscle.

21.3.2 Patient Information, Consent

The patient should be aware that only one, or at best two, different directions of tension can be produced with the technique of regional muscle transplantation. During chewing, involuntary movements in the transposed part of the muscle may occur. The muscle that is transposed always leads to some degree of muscle bulging. The

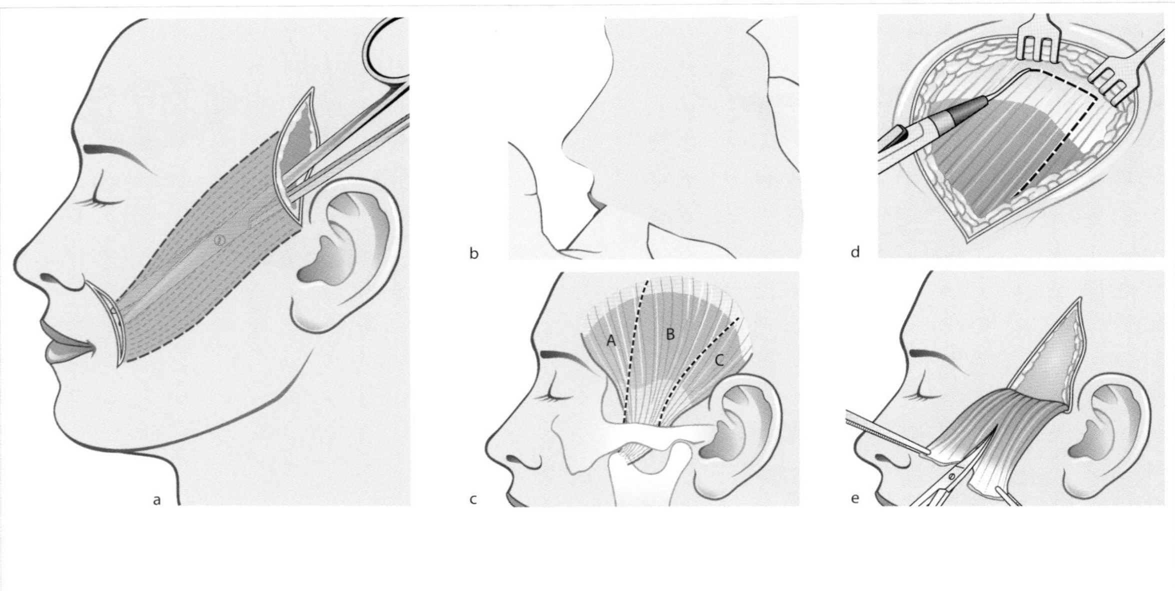

Fig. 21.2 Temporalis muscle transfer. The temporalis muscle is the best choice for muscle transposition, because of its vector to the angle of the mouth. **(a)** Preauricular and nasolabial fold incisions, and preparation of a tunnel for the muscle transfer. If the transfer is planned in combination with a facial nerve reconstruction technique, it is important not to damage the thin peripheral facial nerve branches during this step of surgery. **(b)** Completion of the blunt tunneling. **(c)** Location of the optimal muscle flap in the middle third of the temporalis muscle (B). **(d)** Harvest of the flap. **(e)** Splitting the caudal end of the flap for the reconstruction of the upper and lower edges of the angle of the mouth. (Adapted with permission from Bradley PJ, Guntinas-Lichius O, eds. Salivary Gland Disorders and Diseases: Diagnosis and Management. New York, Stuttgart: Thieme; 2011.)

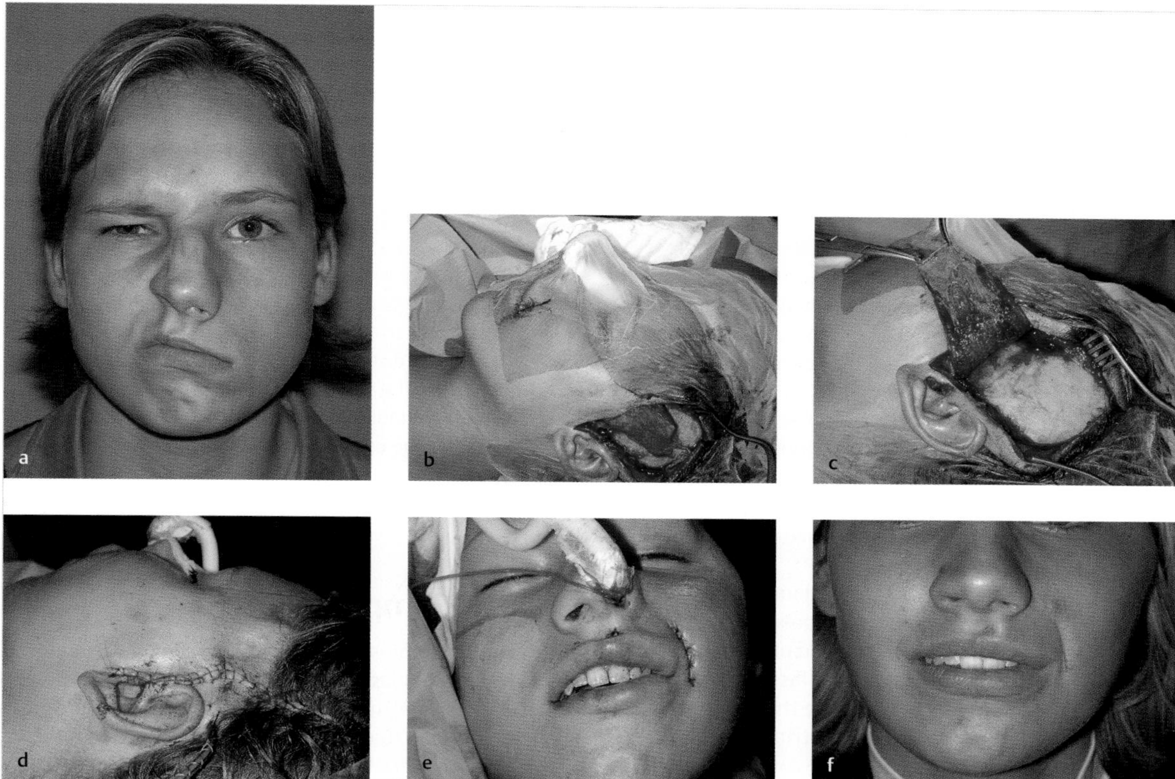

Fig. 21.3 Temporalis muscle transfer. A 19-year-old woman with congenital incomplete facial palsy of the left side of the lower face. (a) Preoperative. (b) Preparation of the temporalis muscle. Note the transnasal intubation to avoid displacement of the mouth. An incision in the new nasolabial fold has been already performed. (c) The muscle flap is detached at the cranial base and remains pedicled caudally. (d) Wound closure. (e) Slight overcorrection of the angle of the mouth at the end of surgery. (f) Angle of the mouth 1 year later.

temporalis muscle is used primarily for reanimation of the corner of the mouth, but it can also be used for reanimation of the eye. In such cases, involuntary closure of the eye can occur during chewing. At the corner of the mouth, the motion vector of the transposed muscle will produce a lateral smile. It should be stressed that this produces, as with masseter muscle transfer, only volitional but not emotional smiles.

21.3.3 Anesthesia and Positioning

General anesthesia is required. Nasal intubation is preferred. When the temporalis muscle is used to reanimate the eye only, some surgeons prefer local anesthesia. The patient is placed in a supine position. If the temporalis muscle is chosen, it may sometimes require lengthening using the fascia lata or palmaris longus tendon in order to reach the corner of the mouth. If autograft fascia is used, the thigh of the contralateral leg to the side of facial surgery, rotated slightly inwards, will provide good exposure of the fascia in the upper leg. If the palmaris longus tendon is preferred, its presence has to be confirmed before starting exploration; see Sling Technique for more details.

21.3.4 Surgical Steps

Surgical Steps for the Reanimation of the Corner of the Mouth

Several techniques have been described. The classic technique described by Gillies involves a transposition of the temporalis muscle over the zygomatic arch.[6] Alternatively, to avoid the contour defect and bulging over the zygomatic arch, a temporalis tendon transfer originally described by McLaughlin,[7] or a lengthening temporalis myoplasty developed by Labbe, or modified by several authors to be less invasive, can be performed.[8,9] The technique described as follows is based on Gillies' original technique.

1. To obtain a symmetrical nasolabial fold, it is important to mark the fold corresponding to it on the contralateral side preoperatively, before the patient is sedated or anesthetized. A finger is placed on the corner of the mouth, and upward and lateral pushing is used to find the best location for muscle insertion to create a nasolabial fold.
2. Four incisions are necessary:

- In the marked nasolabial fold.
- In the scalp, starting anterior to the helix and extending into the hair vertically in the parietal region, along the vermilion border of the upper lip in the lateral third.
- In the upper lips.
- In the lower lips.

3. After identification and blunt dissection of the superficial layer of the temporalis muscle, a tunnel is prepared, proceeding inferiorly in the direction of the corner of the mouth. This tunnel, created from above, is completed from below, i.e., from the side of the nasolabial fold. In addition, the fold is undermined to create a fold in the direction of the lip.
4. A sliver of muscle 4 cm wide from the midportion of the temporalis muscle is lifted from the lateral skull, then cut off with the underlying periosteum to develop it, and rotated caudally to act as a muscle flap. The neurovascular supply lies on the medial deep side of the flap.
5. The distal end of the flap is divided into two pedicles, each 2 cm wide, to allow accurate positioning. In most cases, an extension of the distal end of the muscle flap is needed. Strips (preferably of the fascia lata or palmaris longus tendon) of 1 cm wide are therefore sutured to the distal muscle pedicles. The strips have to be long enough to reach the incision in the corner of the mouth.
6. The flap is pulled through the tunnel. At the end of the suturing procedure, there should be a lateral smile with overcorrection, best created when the surgeon is able to visualize the first upper molar tooth. The flap or elongations are sutured to the upper and lower lip on the orbicularis oris muscle or, if muscles are not present, sutured into the submucosal layer under the skin of the angle of the mouth. A second layer of sutures is used to fix the muscle to the subdermal border of the cranial part of the incision at the nasolabial fold. These sutures will emphasize the nasolabial crease during smiling; 2–0 nonresorbable suture material is preferable.
7. The remaining lateral parts of the temporalis muscle are pulled together with 2–0 nonresorbable sutures. The wound is closed over one or two suction drainage tubes, and the skin is closed in two layers. The skin on the lip incisions can be closed with 5–0 nonresorbable suture material.
8. The ipsilateral hemiface is taped to support the overcorrection (see ▶ Fig. 21.9e), and the tape is left in place for 7 days.

Surgical Steps for the Reanimation of the Closure of the Eye

The dynamic reconstruction of the eyelid closure was originally described by Gillies and Millard,[10] and was further developed in the recent years by Frey. The technique is described in detail elsewhere.[11] However, since the introduction of upper lid weights, as described in Chapter 24, only a minority of surgeons still use this technique.

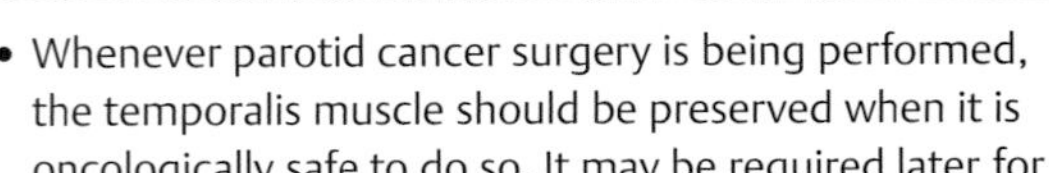

- Whenever parotid cancer surgery is being performed, the temporalis muscle should be preserved when it is oncologically safe to do so. It may be required later for facial reanimation.
- A rim of ear cartilage implanted into the nasolabial fold can help distribute the force of the transposed muscle over the whole area of the nasolabial fold.
- The mouth should be irrigated with disinfectant before and during the operation to reduce or prevent postoperative wound infection.

21.3.5 Complications

Infection is the most frequent complication encountered, especially if alloplastic or heterologous material has been used to lengthen the muscle flap. Seroma formation can be left, provided that no infection or reaction against heterologous material occurs. The risk of hematoma increases if suction drainage is removed too early. Dehiscence of the muscle from the limited available soft tissues is a major source of complication. Undercorrection of the corner of the mouth will lead to deterioration for the patient or it will leave the corner of the mouth unchanged from the preoperative situation. Massive overcorrection will lead to oral incompetence.

21.3.6 Postoperative Care

Suction drainage for at least 48 hours, perioperative antibiotics, and a soft diet for 3 weeks are recommended. After 6 weeks, the patient can begin physiotherapy to learn how to use the muscle transposition.

21.3.7 Outcomes

Following rehabilitation and learning of new movements intentionally and through concentration, most of patients develop a satisfactory lateral smile, although the functional results are far inferior to the facial nerve suture techniques described in Chapter 20.

21.4 Masseter Muscle Transfer

21.4.1 Indications

Masseter muscle transposition may be indicated if: the temporalis muscle is not available, facial muscle paralysis

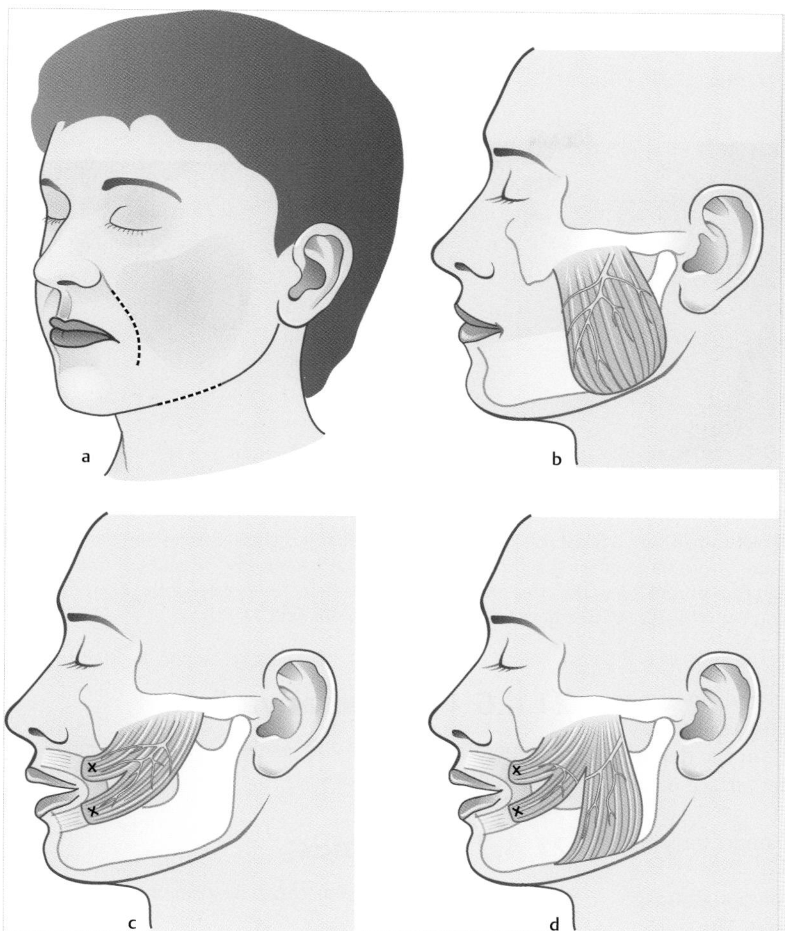

Fig. 21.4 Masseter muscle transfer. The vectors of the transposed masseter muscle are not as favorable as those of the temporalis muscle. **(a)** Incision lines required for this muscle transposition. **(b)** When lifting the muscle flap from the mandible, the nerve supply has to be preserved. **(c)** The masseter flap is attached to the lip–cheek crease and to the upper and lower corners of the angle of the mouth. **(d)** When splitting the caudal end of the muscle flap avoid lesions to the masseter motor nerve supply. (Adapted with permission from May M, Schaitkin BM, eds. The Facial Nerve. New York, Stuttgart: Thieme; 2000.)

persists for more than 1 to 2 years, the facial muscles develop severe atrophy, the peripheral facial nerve has been destroyed, or a simple and rapid solution to facial weakness is desired, especially in patients with an anticipated short survival (▶ Fig. 21.4 and ▶ Fig. 21.5).

21.4.2 Patient Information, Consent

This is the same as described for temporalis muscle transfer: briefly, the patient has to be informed about the limited functional outcome. The patient should be aware that normally only one direction of tension can be produced with this technique of regional muscle transplantation. During chewing, involuntary movements in the transposed part of the muscle may occur. The muscle that is transposed always leads to some degree of muscle bulging of the cheek. The aim is that the vector of the transposed masseter muscle produces a lateral smile at the corner of the mouth. It should be stressed that this produces, as with temporalis muscle transfer, only volitional but not emotional smiles.

21.4.3 Anesthesia and Positioning

These are same as those described for Temporalis Muscle Transfer: general anesthesia is required. Nasal intubation is preferred.

21.4.4 Surgical Steps

The technique presented here is an advancement of Lexer's technique.[12,13]

1. The surgical procedures, incisions, and sutures are basically the same as in temporalis muscle transposition. Only the identification and approach to the muscle are different.
2. The incision used to expose the masseter muscle runs along its attachment at the horizontal part of the ramus of the mandible.
3. Here, the muscle is elevated and separated from the mandible.
4. The muscle is transposed through a tunnel that has been created as far as the nasolabial fold.

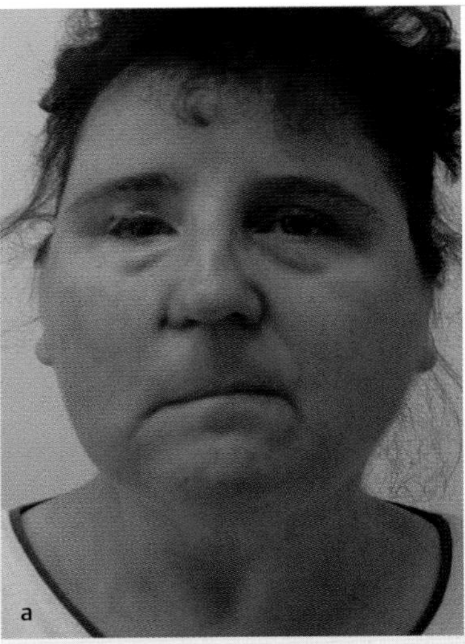
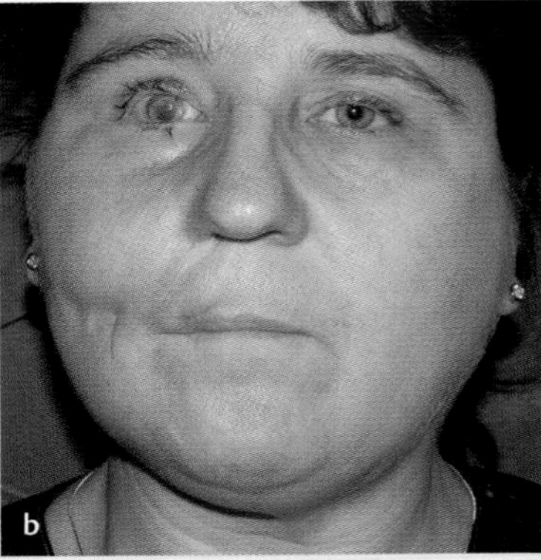
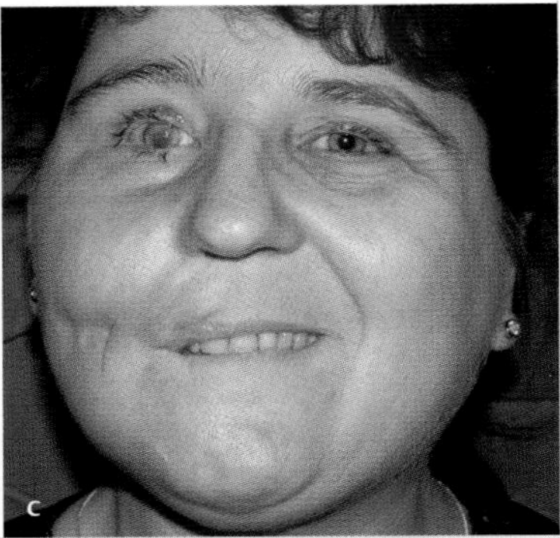

Fig. 21.5 Masseter muscle transfer. A 56-year-old woman with a facial palsy on the right side that has lasted 3 years since she underwent vestibular schwannoma surgery. Note severe xerophthalmia and corneal clouding. **(a)** Preoperative situation showing tarsorrhaphy with disturbed wound healing. **(b)** Face at rest 3 months after masseter muscle transfer, reopening of the tarsorrhaphy, and titanium chain lid implantation. **(c)** Face during activation of the masseter muscle on the right side.

5. As with the temporalis flap, the distal pedicle is split into two parts. Care should be taken to avoid injury to the neurovascular supply arising from the depth under the zygomatic arch to the undersurface of the muscle.
6. The masseter muscle is fixed with 2–0 nonresorbable sutures.
7. The wound is closed over one or two suction drainage tubes, and the skin is closed in two layers. The skin incisions can be closed with 5–0 nonresorbable suture material.
8. The ipsilateral hemiface is taped to support the overcorrection, and the tape is left in place for 7 days.

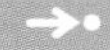

Alternatively, it has been advocated to perform masseter muscle transfer as a three-step procedure:

1. Place a hemioral fascia lata graft to act as an anchor reinforcement.
2. Transfer the split masseter muscle, suturing to the fascia lata reinforced oral commissure.
3. A reefing procedure is performed 6 to 10 months later under local anesthesia to reinforce attachment.[14]

21.4.5 Complications

Complications are the same as those described for Temporalis Muscle Transfer.

21.4.6 Postoperative Care

Postoperative care is the same as that described for Temporalis Muscle Transfer.

21.4.7 Outcomes

Outcomes are the same as those described for Temporalis Muscle Transfer.

21.5 Digastric Muscle Transfer

21.5.1 Indications

A developmental absence or injury to the mandibular branch of the facial nerve can be an indication for a digastric muscle transfer (▶ Fig. 21.6). An injury to the mandibular nerve creates a deformity of the lower lip, characterized by the inability to draw the lower lip downward and laterally. When the patients smiles, the lip on the paralyzed side remains in a neutral position and becomes inwardly rotated. A transposition of the temporalis muscle or the masseter muscle is incapable of treating this deformity.[15]

21.5.2 Patient Information, Consent

The goal of the operation is to create a normal depressor tension on the lip. Overcorrection might occur. The technique is ideal for patients with isolated injury of the marginal mandibular branch. If digastric muscle transfer is combined with a muscle transfer to elevate the corner of

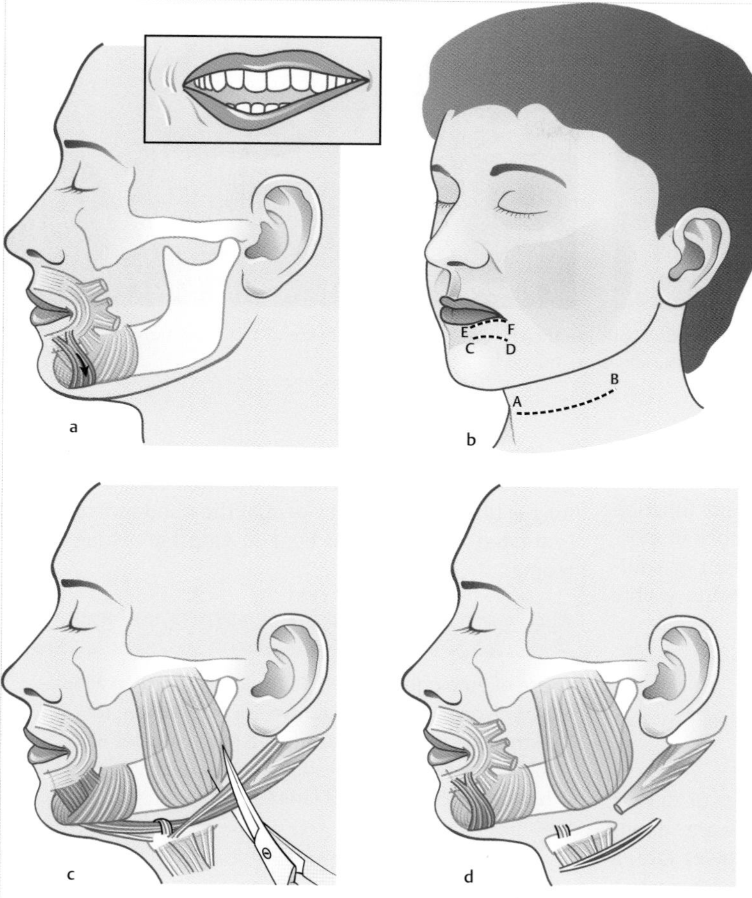

Fig. 21.6 Digastric muscle transfer. **(a)** The transposed anterior belly of the digastric muscle provides a vector that counters the lower lip defect. **(b)** Incisions in the region of the vermilion and in the chin–lip groove. **(c)** The facial bridge between the two bellies of the digastric muscle gives additional length for the muscle transfer. **(d)** Upward rotation of the anterior belly preserving the mylohyoid motor nerve supply. (Adapted with permission from May M, Schaitkin BM, eds. The Facial Nerve. New York, Stuttgart: Thieme; 2000.)

the mouth, as described in Temporalis Muscle Transfer and Masseter Muscle Transfer, there is a risk of oral incompetence.

21.5.3 Anesthesia and Positioning

General anesthesia is mandatory. Nasal intubation is preferred. The patient lies in a supine position with rotation of the head to the opposite side during the reconstruction.

21.5.4 Surgical Steps

1. The aim of the transposition of the anterior belly of the digastric muscle is to provide a vector that counters the lower lip defect. The technique presented here was developed by Conley.[15]
2. Three incisions are needed. The first is in the neck, and is a submandibular incision to free up and transpose the anterior belly of the digastric muscle. The second is a vermilion incision, and the third is a chin–lip groove incision. The latter two incisions are needed to fix the transferred muscle.
3. The fascial bridge is divided and additional length to the anterior belly of the digastrics muscle is obtained.
4. The digastric muscle is freed and rotated to the lower lip. The motor nerve supply by the mylohyoid nerve is preserved.
5. The muscle flap is fixed in two places at the chin-lip groove and in the vermilion area, so that the lower lip is retracted in a neutral position.
6. 2–0 nonresorbable suture material is preferable.
7. The skin on the lip incisions can be closed with 5–0 nonresorbable suture material.

21.5.5 Complications

Complications are the same as those described for Temporalis Muscle Transfer.

21.5.6 Postoperative Care

Postoperative care is the same as that described for Temporalis Muscle Transfer.

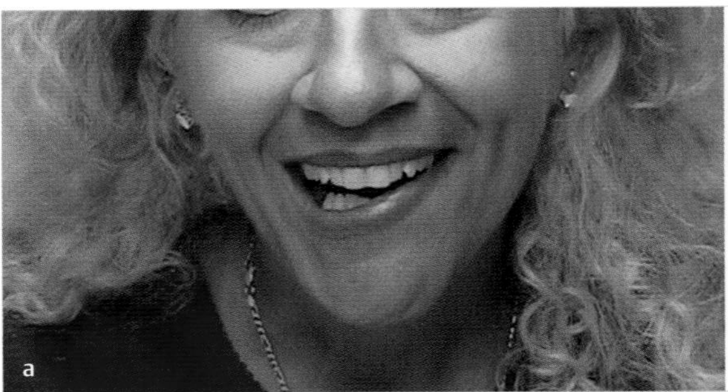

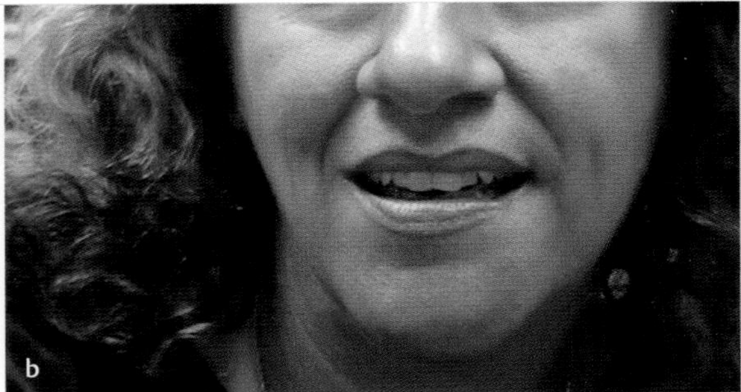

Fig. 21.7 Digastric muscle transfer. (a) Preoperative situation with insufficient depression of the angle of the mouth on the left side during smiling. (b) Improved symmetry during smiling after digastric muscle transfer.

21.5.7 Outcomes

The digastric muscle transfer has more of a static function than a dynamic function. Results are satisfactory in most cases.[15] However, during opening of the mouth or smiling, the lower lip deformity normally remains visible (► Fig. 21.7).

21.6 Sling Techniques

21.6.1 Indications

When nerve reconstruction, a free muscle flap, or muscle transposition is not possible, or if the patient wants a rapid solution to improve resting tone in the lower face, a static procedure with slings is a good alternative (► Fig. 21.8 and ► Fig. 21.9). There is also a preliminary report describing the placement of facial sling n selected cases of partially paralyzed hemifaces, with the aim of enhancing the facial movements.[16]

Static procedures with slings provide a fast solution for improvement of resting tone in the lower face.

21.6.2 Patient Information, Consent

Slings are only able to improve the appearance at rest; they do not allow active movement of the mouth or smiling.

21.6.3 Anesthesia and Positioning

General anesthesia is preferred. The patient is placed in a supine position. If the fascia lata or palmaris longus tendon is chosen, lengthening may sometimes be necessary. If autogenic fascia is used, the leg contralateral to the facial surgery side is slightly rotated internally to provide good exposure of the fascia at the upper leg. If palmaris longus tendon is used, the arm of the nondominant hand is rotated outwards and bent to ease harvesting of the tendon.

Use of autologous material is much better than alloplastic or lyophilized material. The risk of infection, the extrusion rate, and instability are much greater with alloplastic material. The additional morbidity related to harvesting of the sling is limited.

21.6.4 Surgical Steps

1. Four incisions are necessary in the paralyzed face (as described previously for dynamic procedures): a 1 cm incision in the upper lip and a 1 cm incision in the lower lip, along the vermilion; a 2 to 3 cm incision in the planned nasolabial fold (marked before surgery in the alert patient, symmetrical with the opposite side); and a 2 to 3 cm vertical incision in front of the ear to expose the zygomatic arch.
2. A tunnel is made between the subcutaneous tissue and the superficial musculoaponeurotic system, from the zygomatic arch to the nasolabial incision to the vermilion.
3. The distal end of the sling is bisected and then pulled through the tunnel. The sling is fixed in the vermilion region at the upper and lower lip submucosa with 4–0 nonresorbable sutures.
4. To emphasize the nasolabial fold, it is necessary to also fix the sling to the upper border of the nasolabial incision in the subcutaneous tissue .
5. The tendon is now pulled to create a lateral smile, and slightly overcorrected. The tissue will always lose some tension in the first weeks after surgery.

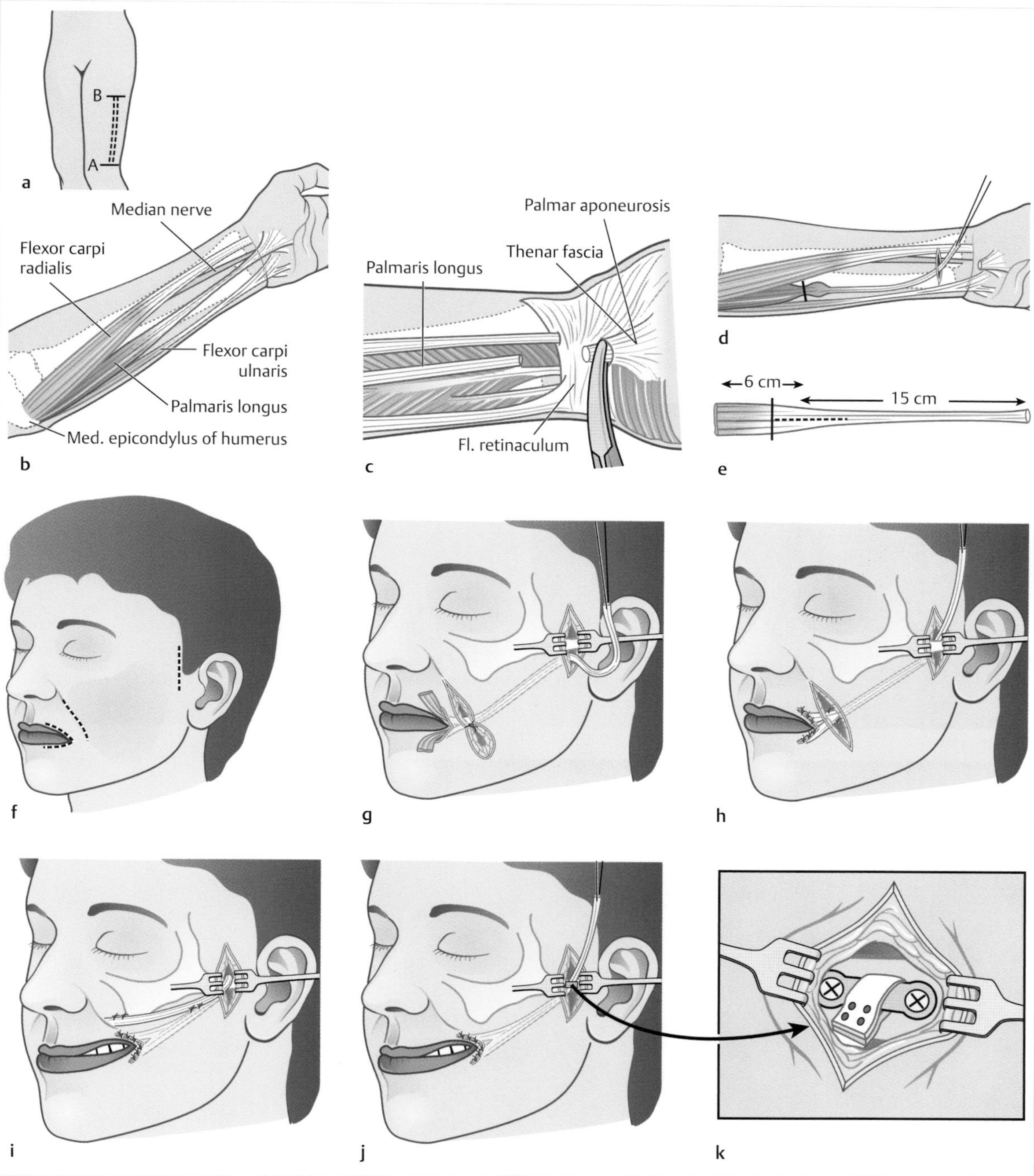

Fig. 21.8 Static sling techniques using the fascia lata or the palmaris longus tendon. **(a)** Optimal location of the fascia lata from the lateral thigh. **(b,c)** Landmarks for the dissection of the palmaris longus tendon. **(d)** Harvest of the tendon using two incisions in approximately the lower third of the forearm. A fascial stripper can facilitate the dissection of the tendon. **(e)** About 20 cm of muscle tendon can be harvested. **(f)** Three incisions are needed for the placement of the tendon: preauricular incision to expose the zygomatic arch, lip–cheek crease incision, and incision at the angle of the mouth. **(g–i)** Placement and fixation of the tendon with sutures. **(j,k)** Alternatively, a miniplate can be used to fix the tendon onto the zygomatic arch. (Adapted with permission from May M, Schaitkin BM, eds. The Facial Nerve. New York, Stuttgart: Thieme; 2000.)

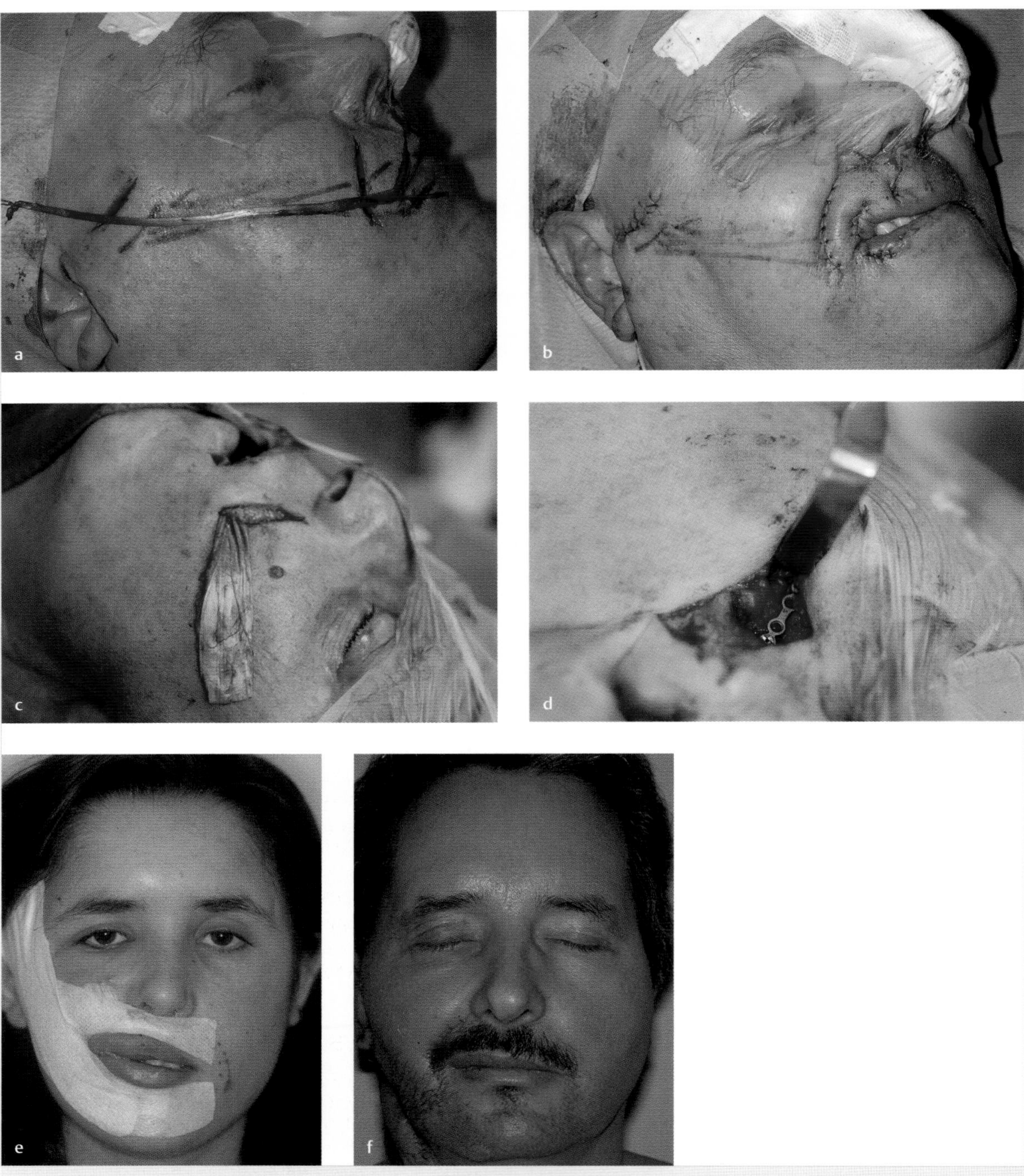

Fig. 21.9 Static sling techniques. **(a)** Placement of an autologous palmaris longus tendon on the right side. A preauricular incision, an incision in the planned plane of the nasolabial fold, and incisions in the upper and lower edges of the angle of the mouth are needed. **(b)** The patient is shown after wound closure, with overcorrection of the angle of the mouth. **(c)** Placement of a strip of autologous fascia lata from the upper lateral leg, using the technique described in **(a)** and **(b)**. **(d)** Cranial fixation of the strip on the zygomatic bone with an osteosynthesis plate to facilitate corrections in later years. **(e)** For 2 weeks the overcorrection is supported by external taping. This type of taping is also used for temporalis or masseter muscle transfers. **(f)** Patient with complete facial palsy on the right side after radical parotidectomy with complete resection of the peripheral facial fan because of parotid cancer. The patient is shown 3 weeks after reanimation with an upper lid weight and palmaris longus tendon sling plasty.

6. In this position, the sling is fixed around zygomatic arch or to the lateral aspect of the arch with the help of a miniplate. Excess sling is pulled back into the tunnel and can be used to tighten the nasolabial fold with additional 4–0 sutures.
7. The wound is drained and closed in two layers.

- Using a fascia stripper is not recommended. It is much easier to incise and remove a precisely sized rectangular piece of the fascia lata under direct vision.
- Using tissue infiltration with saline (hydrodissection) makes it easier to create a subcutaneous tunnel from the zygomatic arch to the nasolabial region.
- Using miniplates has the advantage that tunneling surgery in patients with loss of tension is made easier, as the sling can be retightened by loosening the plate and refixing it.
- A small sling can also be used for an isolated nasal lateralization. In such cases, only an incision in the nasolabial fold is necessary. The fascia is attached to the alar nasi on one side and to the maxilla on the other side.
- Some surgeons recommend use of the Mitek minianchor suture system (Mitek Products, Inc.) to fix the sling to bone in the nose–oral area.[17]

21.6.5 Complications

The possible complications are the same as those described for muscle transposition in Temporalis Muscle Transfer.

21.6.6 Postoperative Care

Postoperative care is the same as that described for Temporalis Muscle Transfer. When the first signs of muscle reinnervation become obvious, training can begin with a skilled physical therapist experienced in working with patients with facial paralysis: the therapist and the patient will explore which tongue movement provides the best result. The younger the patient is, the faster the patient will induce facial movements without thinking about tongue movements.

21.6.7 Outcomes

If the patients have been selected correctly, the outcome can be expected to be satisfactory, with low morbidity. Often the patients need revision surgery after some years, because the effect of the suspension weakens progressively over time.

21.7 Combining Procedures

A muscle transfer procedure, especially a temporalis muscle transfer, can also be combined with facial nerve reanimation surgery. This is the case especially when a hypoglossal–facial jump nerve suture in a patient with a denervation period between 12 and 18 months is planned, as described in Chapter 20. The muscle transfer in this case will give some immediate improvement. When combing nerve surgery with muscle transposition surgery, it is very important to preserve the thin peripheral facial branches when tunneling the face for the muscle transposition. Furthermore, if facial nerve reanimation surgery is not optimal after 2 to 3 years, an additional muscle transposition or a sling procedure, again preserving the facial nerve, might be indicated in individual situations.[18]

21.8 Key Points

- If the facial muscles are no longer viable and free-flap techniques are not feasible or available, regional muscle transfer is an option to reanimate the paralyzed hemiface.
- The temporalis muscle is first choice for most surgeons and the masseter muscle second choice for reanimation of the corner of the mouth.
- Some surgeons still use the temporalis muscle transfer to reanimate the closure of the eye, mainly in countries where upper lid weights are not available.
- A developmental absence or injury to the mandibular branch of the facial nerve can be an indication for a digastric muscle transfer.
- If a muscle transfer is not possible, a static procedure for the midface or lower face is a functionally limited but fast option, with an immediate result.
- The temporalis muscle transfer can also be combined with facial nerve reconstruction surgery, for instance together with a hypoglossal–facial jump nerve suture.

References

[1] Kecskes G, Herman P, Kania R et al. Lengthening temporalis myoplasty versus hypoglossal-facial nerve coaptation in the surgical rehabilitation of facial palsy: evaluation by medical and nonmedical juries and patient-assessed quality of life. Otol Neurotol 2009; 30: 217–222

[2] Faris C, Lindsay R. Current thoughts and developments in facial nerve reanimation. Curr Opin Otolaryngol Head Neck Surg 2013; 21: 346–352

[3] Barr JS, Katz KA, Hazen A. Surgical management of facial nerve paralysis in the pediatric population. J Pediatr Surg 2011; 46: 2168–2176

[4] Liu YM, Sherris DA. Static procedures for the management of the midface and lower face. Facial Plast Surg 2008; 24: 211–215

[5] Yoleri L, Güngör M, Usluer A, Celik D. Tension adjusted multivectorial static suspension with plantaris tendon in facial paralysis. J Craniofac Surg 2013; 24: 896–899

[6] Gillies H. Experiences with fascia lata grafts in the operative treatment of facial paralysis: (section of Otology and section of Laryngology). Proc R Soc Med 1934; 27: 1372–1382

[7] McLaughlin CR. Surgical support in permanent facial paralysis. Plast Reconstr Surg (1946) 1953; 11: 302–314

[8] Labbé D, Huault M. Lengthening temporalis myoplasty and lip reanimation. Plast Reconstr Surg 2000; 105: 1289–1297, discussion 1298

[9] Boahene KD. Principles and biomechanics of muscle tendon unit transfer: application in temporalis muscle tendon transposition for smile improvement in facial paralysis. Laryngoscope 2013; 123: 350–355

[10] Gillies H, Milllard DR. The Principles and Art of Plastic Surgery. London: Butterworths; 1957

[11] Frey M, Giovanoli P, Tzou CH, Kropf N, Friedl S. Dynamic reconstruction of eye closure by muscle transposition or functional muscle transplantation in facial palsy. Plast Reconstr Surg 2004; 114: 865–875

[12] Lexer E, Eden R. Über die chirurgische Behandlung der peripheren Facialislähmung. Beitr Klin Chir 1911; 73: 116

[13] Baker DC, Conley J. Regional muscle transposition for rehabilitation of the paralyzed face. Clin Plast Surg 1979; 6: 317–331

[14] Lesavoy MA, Fan KL, Goldberg AG, Dickinson BP, Herrera F. Facial reanimation by staged, split masseter muscle transfer. Ann Plast Surg 2014; 73: 33–38

[15] Conley J, Baker DC, Selfe RW. Paralysis of the mandibular branch of the facial nerve. Plast Reconstr Surg 1982; 70: 569–577

[16] Deleyiannis FW, Askari M, Schmidt KL, Henkelmann TC, VanSwearingen JM, Manders EK. Muscle activity in the partially paralyzed face after placement of a fascial sling: a preliminary report. Ann Plast Surg 2005; 55: 449–455

[17] Yu K, Kim AJ, Tadros M, Costantino PD. Mitek anchor-augmented static facial suspension. Arch Facial Plast Surg 2010; 12: 159–165

[18] Terzis JK, Olivares FS. Mini-temporalis transfer as an adjunct procedure for smile restoration. Plast Reconstr Surg 2009; 123: 533–542

22 Free Flaps

Caroline A. Banks and Tessa A. Hadlock

22.1 Introduction

The use of a free muscle graft for dynamic facial reanimation was first described in 1975 by Freilinger.[1] The following year, Harii et al performed the first gracilis free muscle transfer with microvascular anastomosis for facial rehabilitation.[2] Free flaps have since become the gold standard for treatment of prolonged facial paralysis, allowing for dynamic movement of the oral commissure following facial muscle atrophy or resection. Aviv et al described the ideal muscle for facial reanimation as having sufficient contractile force to produce midface movement, a reliable neurovascular pedicle, segmental innervation, minimal donor site morbidity, and ease of harvesting.[3] Based on these criteria, reconstructive surgeons have advocated multiple donor muscles for microneurovascular transfer including the abductor hallucis,[4] extensor digitorum brevis,[5] gracilis,[6] internal oblique,[7–9] latissimus dorsi,[10–15] pectorals minor,[16,17] rectus abdominis,[18] rectus femoris,[19] and serratus anterior.[20] The gracilis is the most frequently employed free muscle transfer, although the latissimus dorsi and pectorals minor are preferred by some institutions.

> **!**
>
> Reconstructive surgeons have advocated multiple donor muscles. The gracilis is the most frequently employed free muscle transfer. The latissimus dorsi and pectorals minor are other preferred donor muscles.

22.1.1 Two-Stage Procedures

Reanimation can be performed in one or two stages (▶ Table 22.1). The two-stage procedure is the standard technique in most centers and is accomplished by using a cross-face nerve graft coapted to facial nerve branches on the normal side, followed by free muscle transfer to the paralyzed side 6 to 12 months later. The sural nerve is frequently used for the cross-face nerve graft,[21] although other donor nerves including the lateral antebrachial cutaneous nerve, the anterior division of the medial antebrachial cutaneous nerve, the superficial radial nerve, and the lateral femoral cutaneous nerve have also been described.[3] The greatest advantage to the two-stage procedure is the ability to restore spontaneous, emotive

Table 22.1 Comparison of the two-stage procedure versus the one-stage procedure

	Two-stage procedure	One-stage procedure
Characteristics	Standard technique in most centers	When contralateral facial nerve is not available
	Neural input: facial nerve from the contralateral side	Neural input: masseteric nerve (mostly used), contralateral facial nerve
	First step: cross-face nerve graft	
	Second step: free muscle transfer to the paralyzed side 6–12 months later	
	Graft necessary: sural nerve most frequently used	
Advantages	Ability to restore spontaneous, emotive facial expression	Provides earlier results
	Preventing atrophy of the free flap while the cross-face nerve graft gains neural input	Reliably strong voluntary contraction
	Potential restoration of symmetry by partial denervation on the normal side of the face	
Disadvantages	Two neurorrhaphies necessary: risk of inadequate penetration across the suture sites	Lack involuntary mimetic facial expression
	Unsatisfactory smile excursion in approximately 20% of patients	If long donor nerve has to be used: loss of axons through the transected collateral branches and longer reinnervation times
		Longer reinnervation time leads to free flap muscle atrophy and poorer outcomes

facial expression, which is one of the most challenging goals of facial reanimation. Other advantages to this technique include preventing atrophy of the free flap while the cross-face nerve graft gains neural input and potential restoration of symmetry by partial denervation on the normal side of the face. The most distressing negative outcome of the two-stage technique is unsatisfactory smile excursion in approximately 20% of patients[22]; this is thought to result from inadequate penetration across the two neurorrhaphies.

!

The sural nerve is the most frequent used nerve supply for the cross-face nerve graft as the first step of the two-step procedure.

22.1.2 One-Stage Procedures

One-stage free flaps provide earlier results and are also options when the contralateral facial nerve is not available. One-stage procedures can be classified based on the innervation source. Classically, the masseteric nerve is used to innervate the flap. The masseteric nerve is favored because of its close proximity to the surgical site and a lack of donor site morbidity. When compared with flaps innervated by cross-face nerve grafts, masseteric-driven free flaps are more rapidly reinnervated and have higher success rates.[23] These flaps are characterized by reliably strong voluntary contraction; however, patients lack involuntary mimetic facial expression.

The contralateral facial nerve can also serve as a donor nerve in one-stage procedures by using free flaps with lengthy pedicles such as the latissimus dorsi and the serratus anterior muscles. An ultralong neural pedicle is harvested and connected to the contralateral facial nerve at the time of muscle inset. Disadvantages to this technique include loss of axons through the transected collateral branches and longer reinnervation times compared with the masseteric nerve, due to the long pedicle. Longer reinnervation time in turn leads to free flap muscle atrophy and poorer outcomes.[9,23]

!

The classical donor nerve for one-stage procedures is the masseteric nerve. An alternative for special situations is the contralateral facial nerve or ipsilateral proximal branches of the facial nerve.

Lastly, one-stage procedures may be performed using ipsilateral proximal branches of the facial nerve as the motor source for innervating the transferred muscle in select cases.[11,24,25] This approach may result in excessive muscle contraction when the entire facial nerve stump is used as the donor nerve; using isolated branches of the ipsilateral facial nerve produces more favorable results.[11]

The concept of "neural supercharging" free flaps, by introducing more than one neural input, is a recent development in the treatment of facial paralysis and aims to combine the spontaneity and symmetry of a cross-face nerve graft with the reliable, robust commissure excursion derived from the masseteric nerve. Based on neural augmentation techniques described by Yamamoto et al,[26] Biglioli et al were the first to describe a one-stage gracilis muscle flap with dual innervation to the obturator nerve from an end-to-end coaptation with the masseteric nerve and an end-to-side coaptation with the cross-face sural nerve graft.[27] All patients were reported to have recovered both voluntary and spontaneous smile. Those authors speculated that spontaneous smiling may occur directly from the axons of the cross-face nerve graft along with indirect activation of masseteric nerve fibers. Watanabe et al reported similar findings of voluntary and involuntary facial expression after a dually innervated latissimus dorsi flap.[28] More clinical assessment is needed to identify ideal candidates, to determine the long-term outcomes of dual innervation techniques, and to characterize which movements result from which neural sources.

There are multiple options available for the donor muscle and innervation source, and many variables are involved in performing successful facial reanimation using free flaps. Ultimately, surgeon familiarity and experience are critical factors in optimizing outcome.

!

The concept of "neural supercharging" free flaps describes the use of more than one donor nerve (end-to-end and end-to-side) to combine the spontaneity and symmetry of a cross-face nerve graft with the reliable, robust commissure excursion derived from the masseteric nerve. At best, this results in rehabilitation of voluntary and spontaneous smile.

22.2 Indications

In long-standing facial paralysis, frequently defined as paralysis for 12 months or more, facial muscles are atrophic and are not viable for reinnervation techniques. An exception to this arises in patients with severe synkinesis, in which the facial muscles have been autopreserved by aberrant innervation, as described in Chapter 3. Dynamic smile restoration in prolonged flaccid facial paralysis can only be accomplished through regional muscle transfer, as described in Chapter 21, or microneurovascular free tissue transfer. The choice of regional muscle transfer, usually temporalis muscle or temporalis tendon transfer, versus free tissue transfer, largely depends on surgeon preference or experience and patient factors. There are several benefits to free muscle transfer, including potential for a spontaneous emotive smile and greater excursion of the oral commissure.[22] Patients with recent-onset, irreversible flaccid facial paralysis, patients with congenital absence of facial muscles, those with long-standing nonflaccid facial paralysis who lack a meaningful smile, and patients who have had surgical resection of the midface musculature, are also candidates for smile reanimation with a free flap.

!

Patients with long-standing facial paralysis with atrophic nonviable facial muscles as well as patients with congenital lack of facial muscles are candidates for free muscle reinnervation techniques.

Free flaps should be performed in patients younger than 70 years old with a good prognosis. Older patients have longer reinnervation times[6] and poorer outcomes following cross-face nerve grafting. Though there is no strict age cut-off for performing a two-stage gracilis, the authors routinely offer this option to only healthy patients younger than 40 years of age. Indications for a one-stage gracilis include patients over 40 years old, those with bilateral facial paralysis (i.e., Möbius syndrome) or potential for disease of the contralateral facial nerve (i.e., neurofibromatosis type 2), patients who lack an adequate contralateral donor nerve for cross-face nerve graft, and patients with a previously failed cross-face nerve graft or gracilis.

!

Best results are observed with patients younger than 40 years of age. The functional results become worse in patients older than 70 years of age.

22.2.1 Gracilis Free Muscle Transfer in Special Populations

Möbius syndrome is a congenital disorder characterized by unilateral or bilateral facial paralysis and abducens palsy. These patients suffer from functional disabilities and lack of emotional expression, with sometimes profound psychosocial consequences. In unilateral cases, a cross-face nerve graft can serve as the motor nerve; bilateral facial paralysis can be successfully treated with bilateral gracilis muscle flaps innervated by the masseteric nerve.[29]

Neurofibromatosis type 2 (NF2), a genetic disorder defined by bilateral vestibular schwannomas, can lead to facial paralysis. Though devastating to patients, facial paralysis has historically been left untreated in this population. While facial paralysis is most frequently unilateral in patients with NF2, the contralateral nerve is at risk with progression of disease, and is therefore not an ideal option for facial reanimation procedures. Patients with NF2 can be successfully treated with one-stage gracilis free tissue transfer, driven by the masseteric nerve.[30]

Patients with bilateral Möbius syndrome and patients with bilateral neurofibromatosis type 2 (or at risk for bilateral neurofibromatosis) are typical candidates for gracilis free tissue transfer with the masseteric nerve as the donor.

Facial paralysis is especially challenging in the pediatric population. A study of pediatric patients undergoing gracilis free muscle transfer demonstrated fewer complete failures when compared with adult patients, as well as increased commissure excursion and improved quality of life.[31] Other studies report successful results following gracilis free muscle transfer in specific pediatric populations, including those with Möbius syndrome.[32] Based on these results, in the appropriately counseled family, patients do not need to wait until adulthood to undergo facial reanimation with a free flap. The gracilis free flap is recommended as a first-line treatment to restore a meaningful smile in children, as described in Chapter 12.

22.3 Patient Information and Consent

All patients undergo thorough preoperative medical clearance. Patients with vascular disease or other comorbidities who wish to proceed with surgery are informed of the higher likelihood of free flap failure from microvascular compromise. In addition to general surgical complications, patients are informed of the perioperative risks of face or leg hematoma and free flap failure, as well as the long-term risk of functional failure due to lack of neural input to the gracilis. Importantly, patients undergoing a two-stage gracilis transfer are counseled regarding the higher failure rate compared with one-stage procedures. They must be able to accept this risk and understand that in the case of failure, a salvage one-stage gracilis transfer remains an option. Facial movement is not expected from the free flap for 4 to 6 months after a one-stage procedure and 8 to 12 months after a two-stage free flap. Following first-stage cross-face nerve grafting, patients are informed that they will have numbness over a patch of skin on the lateral aspect of the foot and a 1.5 cm scar posterior to the lateral malleolus following endoscopic sural nerve harvest.

> !
>
> Facial movement is not expected from the free flap for 4 to 6 months after a one-stage procedure and 8 to 12 months after a two-stage free flap.

22.4 Anesthesia and Positioning

The patient is placed in a supine position on a split-leg operating table. Under general anesthesia, the patient is intubated with a nasotracheal tube in the contralateral nasal cavity. Nasal intubation prevents distortion of the mouth during gracilis muscle inset. The nasotracheal tube is sutured to the septum with 2.0 silk. The gracilis donor leg is abducted and flexed at the knee and then prepped from the knee to the hip 270 degrees with betadine solution. Steri-Strips are used to tape the eyes, and the planned facial incisions are injected with 1:100,000 solution of epinephrine. The entire face and the nasotracheal tube are prepped with alcohol to permit comparison of the paralyzed side with the nonparalyzed side, and sterile circuit tubing is connected. Ampicillin-sulbactam is given prophylactically, and the blood pressure is ideally maintained with systolic pressures of 100 to 120 mm Hg. The room temperature is kept close to 74 degrees Fahrenheit to promote vasodilatation.

22.5 Surgical Steps

22.5.1 First-Stage Cross-Face

A preauricular incision is made on the nonparalyzed side of the face, and a skin flap is raised on the parotideomasseteric fascia (PMF). Dissection is carried anteriorly to the masseteric fascia. Nerve branches are identified at the anterior border of the parotid gland and isolated with vessel loops. A Montgomery nerve stimulator (Boston Medical Products) is used to select donor branches of the facial nerve that are responsible for isolated smile movement. These branches are marked for later use. The sural nerve is harvested from the leg and transferred to the face. The nerve is tunneled subcutaneously from the nonparalyzed side, across the upper lip, to the gingivobuccal sulcus on the paralyzed side, using a Wright needle (▶ Fig. 22.1). Working under the operative microscope, the selected proximal end of the unaffected facial nerve branches are transected and sutured to the sural nerve with 10–0 nylon and fibrin glue. The tip of the nerve graft is marked with a 4–0 nylon suture and banked for later exposure during the second-stage free muscle transfer. The lip incision is closed with 4–0 chromic figure-of-eight suture under the microscope. Axon growth across the graft is followed clinically by tapping on the graft (the Tinel's sign); tingling in the zygomaticus muscle groups on the donor side indicates the presence of regenerating axons (▶ Fig. 22.2). In 6 to 9 months, the patient undergoes second-stage gracilis free muscle transfer.

22.5.2 Preparation of the Face and Neck for Free Flap

A no. 15 blade is used to perform an extended Blair incision, extending from the temporal region to 2 to 3 cm inferior to the angle of the mandible. Sharp dissection is continued through the skin, subcutaneous tissue, and superficial musculoaponeurotic system to the PMF. The PMF serves as the deep plane of dissection, and once identified, the dissection proceeds anteriorly along the PMF to the anterior border of the parotid gland using Colorado tip Bovie cautery or facelift scissors. A thick skin flap is critical to avoid tethering of the free flap muscle to the overlying skin. Facial nerve branches exit the parotid on the anterior surface of the gland, and care must be taken to avoid injury to any functional branches of the facial nerve (▶ Fig. 22.3). In cases of nonflaccid paralysis, a Montgomery nerve stimulator can be used to identify facial nerve branches. The masseter muscle is encountered directly anterior to the parotid gland.

Identification of the modiolus (▶ Fig. 22.4), defined as the chiasm of facial muscles involved in oral commissure movement, can be challenging in patients with prolonged facial paralysis and atrophic facial musculature. The superior surface of the zygomaticus major, traced anteroinferiorly, is used as a landmark to identify the oral commissure. The facial vessels also serve as landmarks for the modiolus. The facial artery and vein cross over the mandible at the anteroinferior border of the masseter muscle and course toward the oral commissure. Of note, the vein is more lateral and posterior and is encountered first. The facial vessels are dissected and isolated at this time.

The next objective is placement of inset sutures in the modiolus. Five 0-polyglactin sutures are placed in the muscles of the oral commissure from superficial to deep: two inferior to the oral commissure, one at the oral commissure, and two superior to the oral commissure. Careful placement is required to avoid tethering either the oral commissure mucosa or the overlying dermis.

The donor nerve is identified. For one-stage procedures, the masseteric branch of the trigeminal nerve is exposed by making a vertical incision in the soft tissue 3 cm anterior to the free edge of the tragus and 1 cm

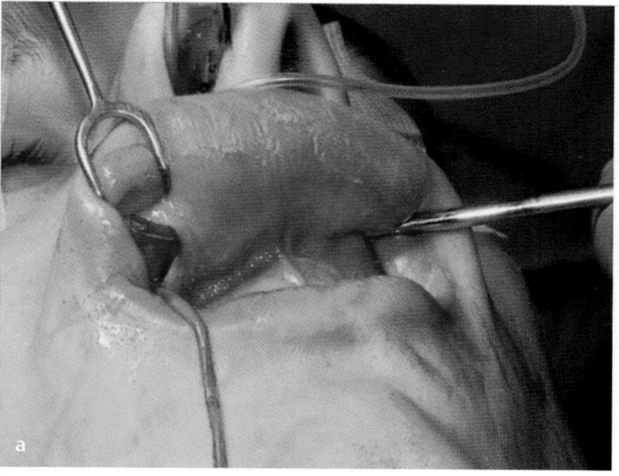

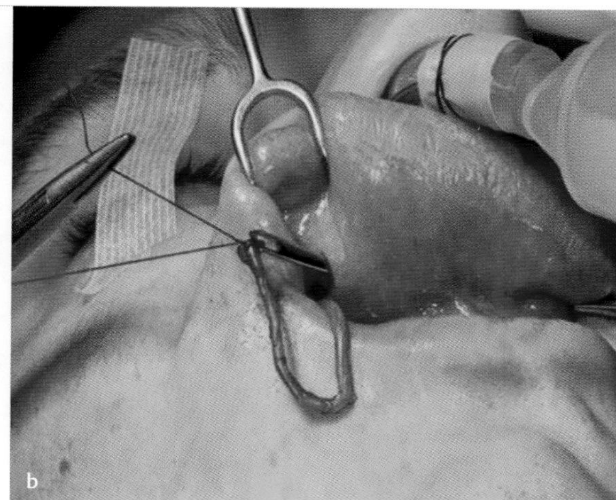

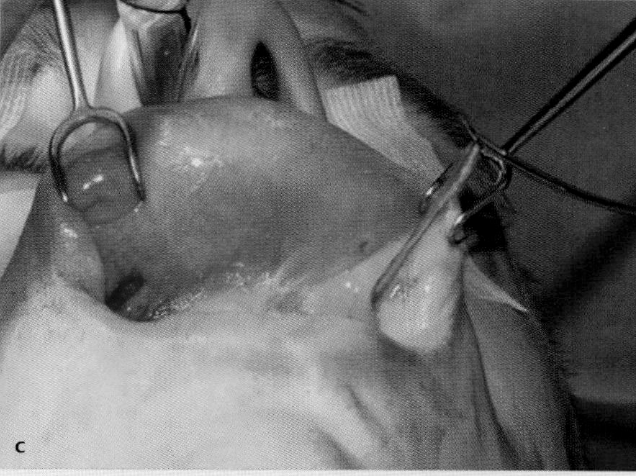

Fig. 22.1 Tunneling of the sural nerve graft. **(a)** The nerve is tunneled subcutaneously from the nonparalyzed side. **(b)** A Wright tissue needle is passed across the upper lip from the paralyzed side to the nonparalyzed side. **(c)** The tip of the nerve graft is brought to the gingivobuccal sulcus on the paralyzed side.

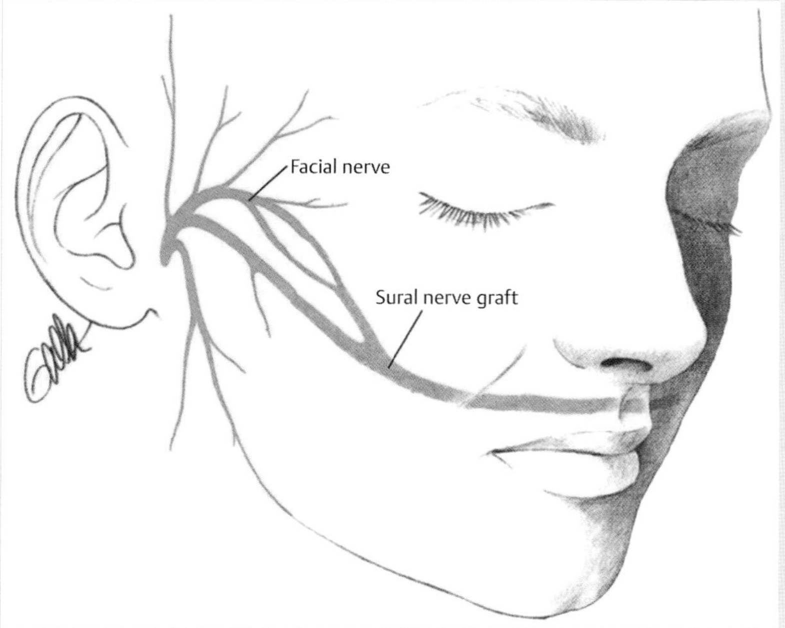

Fig. 22.2 Cross-face nerve graft connected to isolated smile branches of the nonparalyzed side.

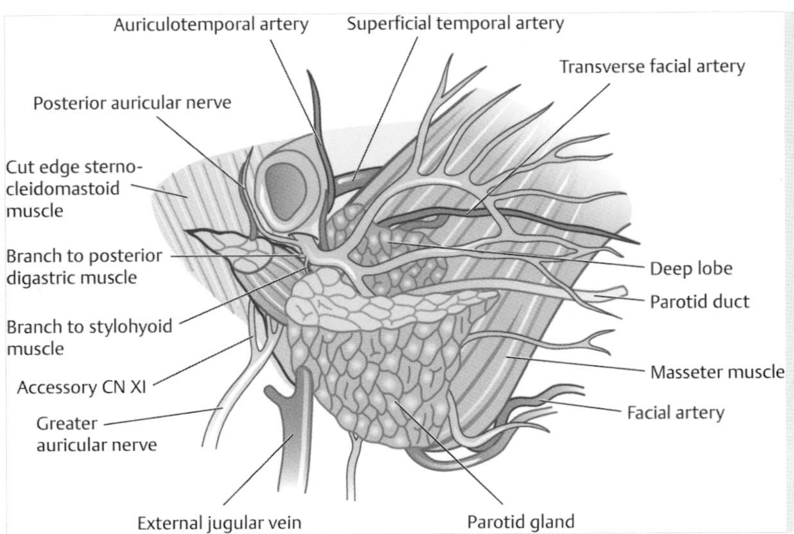

Fig. 22.3 Facial nerve branches along the anterior border of the parotid gland.

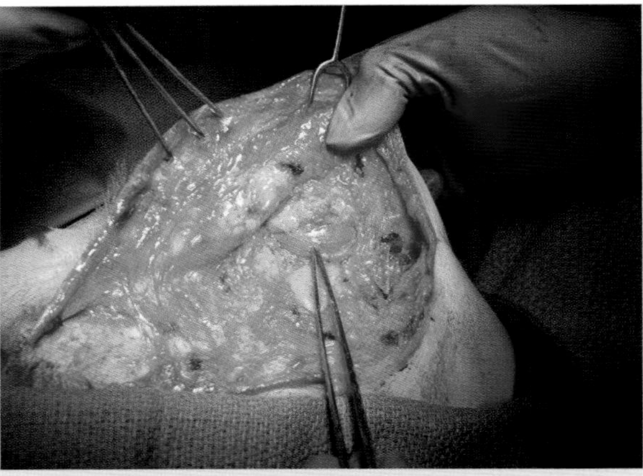

Fig. 22.4 Forceps point to the lateral border of the orbicularis oris muscle.

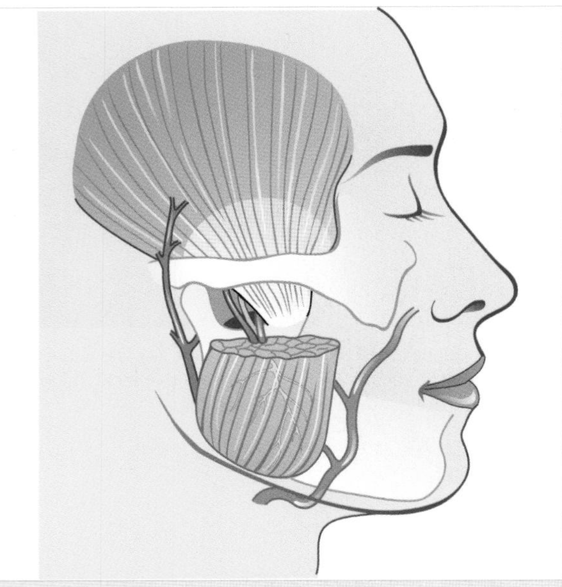

Fig. 22.5 The masseteric nerve running along the deep surface of the masseter muscle with accompanying artery and vein.

inferior to the zygoma.[33–35] In patients with preserved facial nerve function, care must be taken to identify the facial nerve branches running perpendicular to the incision. Dissection is executed bluntly in the direction of the masseter muscle fibers. The masseteric nerve runs from the infratemporal fossa, through the sigmoid notch between the mandibular condyle and coronoid process, and innervates the masseter muscles from the deep surface (▶ Fig. 22.5). A Montgomery nerve stimulator confirms identification of the nerve. An artery, vein, and multiple small perforating vessels accompany the masseteric nerve, and meticulous dissection is required to maintain hemostasis and adequate exposure. A vessel loop is placed around the nerve.

In two-stage gracilis muscle transfers, the tip of the cross-face nerve graft, previously marked with a 4.0 nylon suture, is identified in the gingivobuccal sulcus. The overlying mucosa is incised, the tip of the nerve graft is carefully dissected, and the distal portion of the nerve is transected to facilitate neurorrhaphy.

22.5.3 Gracilis Harvest

A dotted line is drawn between the pubic tubercle, which is readily palpable in all patients, and the medial condyle of the tibia. The planned incision is marked by drawing a parallel line 1.5 to 2 cm medial to the dotted line, approximately 12 to 15 cm in length (▶ Fig. 22.6). A no. 15 blade is used to incise the skin, and dissection is continued through the subcutaneous tissue using Bovie cautery. Large veins, including the great saphenous vein, run

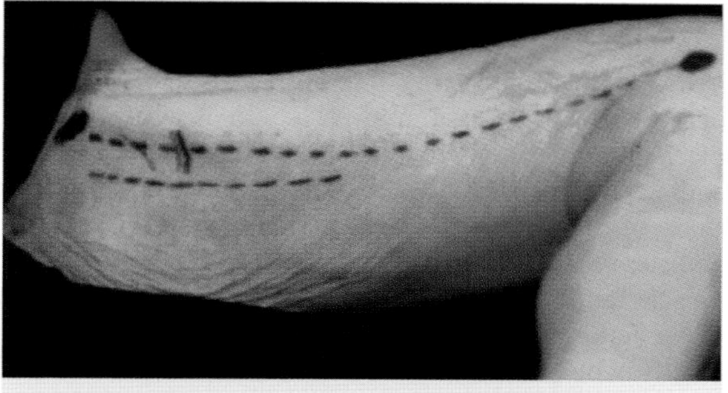

Fig. 22.6 The gracilis incision is planned by drawing a dashed line between the pubic tubercle and the medial condyle of the tibia. The incision is marked by drawing a parallel line 1.5 to 2 cm medial to the dashed line, approximately 12 to 15 cm in length.

within the tissue above the gracilis muscle and can be ligated and saved for possible vein grafts in the face.

The gracilis muscle is located in the medial thigh, deep to the subcutaneous tissue and superficial to the adductor longus, magnus, and brevis muscles (▶ Fig. 22.7). It is frequently the first muscle encountered after dissection through the subcutaneous tissue; however, it is sometimes difficult to distinguish the gracilis from the adductor longus or magnus, whose fibers run in the same direction. Identification of the pedicle entering the deep surface of the muscle is the best way to distinguish gracilis muscle from the other adductor muscles.

The gracilis is supplied by the adductor artery and two venae comitantes; the artery measures 1 to 1.5 mm in diameter, and the venae are 2 to 3 mm. The vessels enter the gracilis at a 90-degree angle, 8 to 10 cm inferior to the

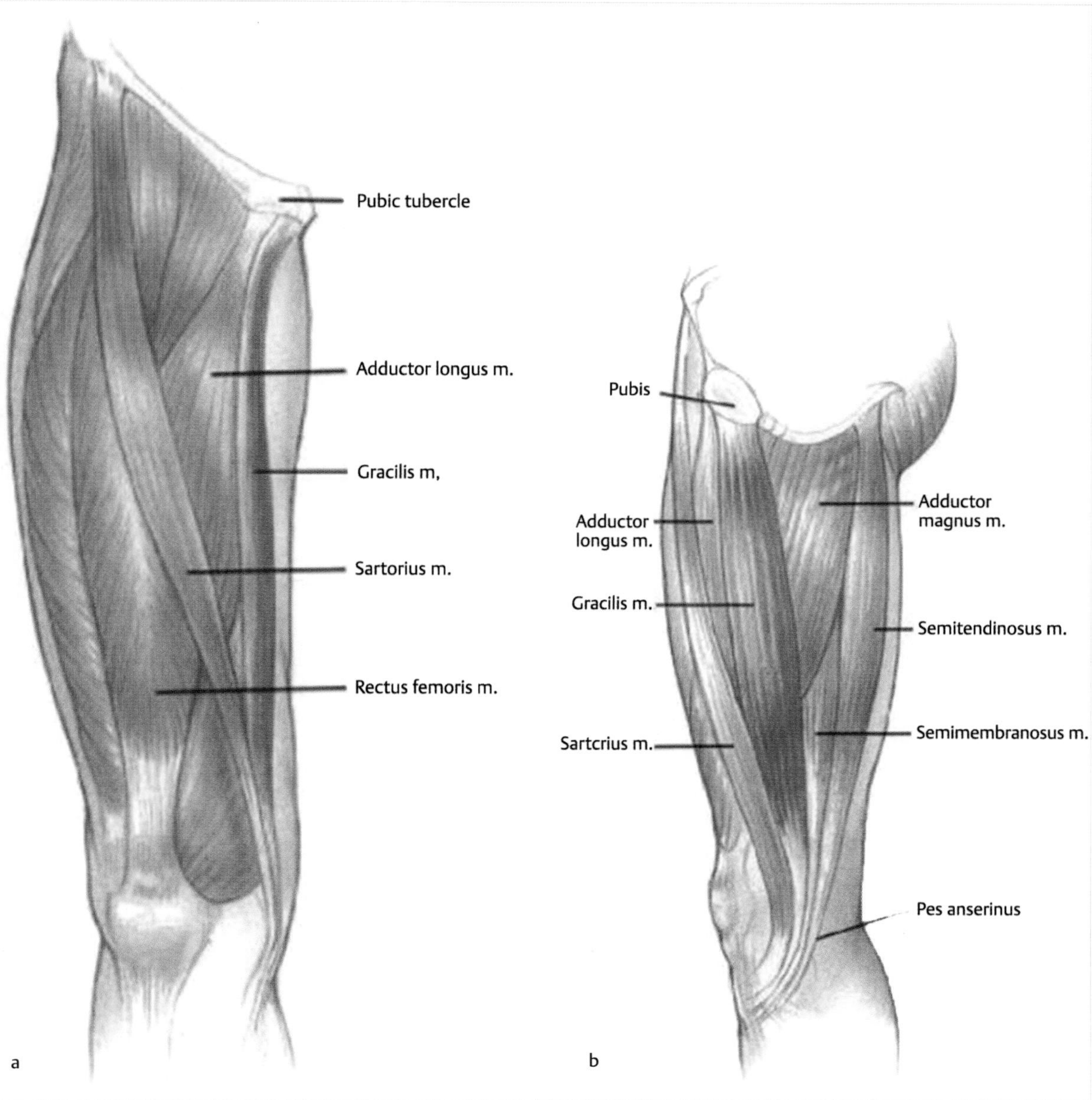

Fig. 22.7 (a,b) The gracilis muscle is located in the medial thigh, superficial to the adductor longus, magnus, and brevis muscles.

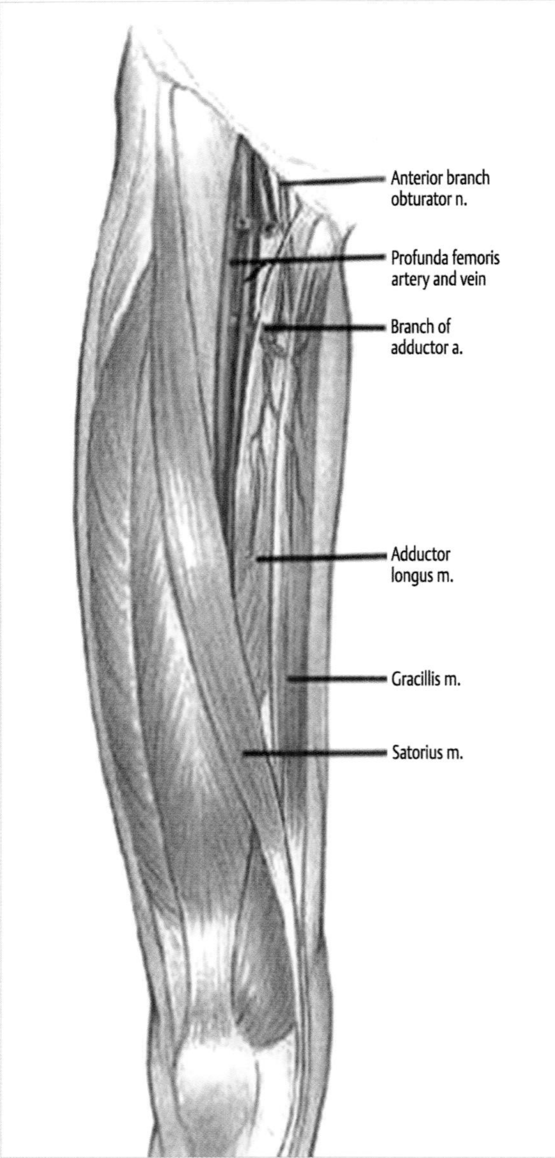

Fig. 22.8 The adductor artery and two venae comitantes enter the gracilis at a 90 degree angle, 8 to 10 cm inferior to the public tubercle. The gracilis is innervated by the anterior obturator nerve, which enters the muscle obliquely 1 to 2 cm superior to the vascular pedicle.

pubic tubercle. The adductor artery arises from the deep femoral or the medial circumflex femoral artery and travels between the adductor longus anteriorly and the adductor magnus posteriorly before entering the gracilis muscle. The gracilis is innervated by the anterior obturator nerve, which enters the muscle obliquely, 1 to 2 cm superior to the vascular pedicle (▶ Fig. 22.8). A nerve stimulator can be used to identify the approximate location of the nerve prior to dissection.

Once the pedicle is identified, the investing fascia surrounding the gracilis is dissected, and the muscle belly is freed of all attachments inferior and superior to the pedicle. The harvested muscle length is estimated by measuring from the tragus to the oral commissure and adding 2.5 cm. For contralateral muscle transfer, one-third of the muscle length is taken superior to the pedicle; for ipsilateral muscle transfer, two-thirds of the muscle length is taken superior to the pedicle, making dissection more challenging in the latter. The planned length is measured and marked with 2.0 silk sutures at the superior and inferior borders. Fifty percent of the width of the muscle is harvested with bipolar scissors (▶ Fig. 22.9), beginning with the inferior cut. A cut parallel to the long axis of the muscle is continued superiorly to the upper limit of the planned harvest, protecting the neurovascular pedicle. The final cut is made superiorly, and the gracilis remains attached only by the pedicle.

The obturator nerve is dissected superiorly and divided distal to branching of the nerve. The vascular pedicle is dissected. Adequate vascular pedicle length is achieved through ligation of the perforators to the adductor longus (▶ Fig. 22.10), and finally the pedicle is clamped and ligated.

The leg is placed back in a neutral position. The wound is irrigated and hemostasis is achieved. A suction drain is placed, and the wound is closed in multiple layers using 3–0 polyglactin sutures for the deep layers and 4–0 monofilament absorbable sutures in a running fashion intradermally for the superficial closure. Mastisol and Steri-Strips are placed over the incision, and the leg is wrapped with a gauze roll and elastic bandage.

22.5.4 Gracilis Preparation and Inset

The flap is prepared on the back table. Bipolar scissors are used to thin the flap down to 15 to 20 g, carefully protecting the pedicle (▶ Fig. 22.11). This step decreases excess bulk in the face after inset. To decrease muscle shearing during inset, a "neo-tendon" is created by placing 2–0 polyglactin sutures in a running interlocking fashion along the end of the flap that will attach to the oral commissure.

The gracilis muscle is oriented parallel to the direction of the zygomaticus major, with the pedicle positioned along the inferior edge of the muscle belly (▶ Fig. 22.12). If a cross-face nerve graft is the donor nerve, the obturator nerve is passed intraorally adjacent to the tip of the previously exposed sural nerve graft using a tissue passer, and is held in place with a bulldog clamp. The medial gracilis inset is executed by using the previously placed 0-polyglactin sutures and forming a figure-of-eight knot (▶ Fig. 22.13). Beginning with the superior suture, the stitch is passed through the gracilis from deep to superficial. The suture is then passed through the lateral border of the orbicularis oris muscle again, from superficial to deep, just inferior to the first suture, and finally is passed

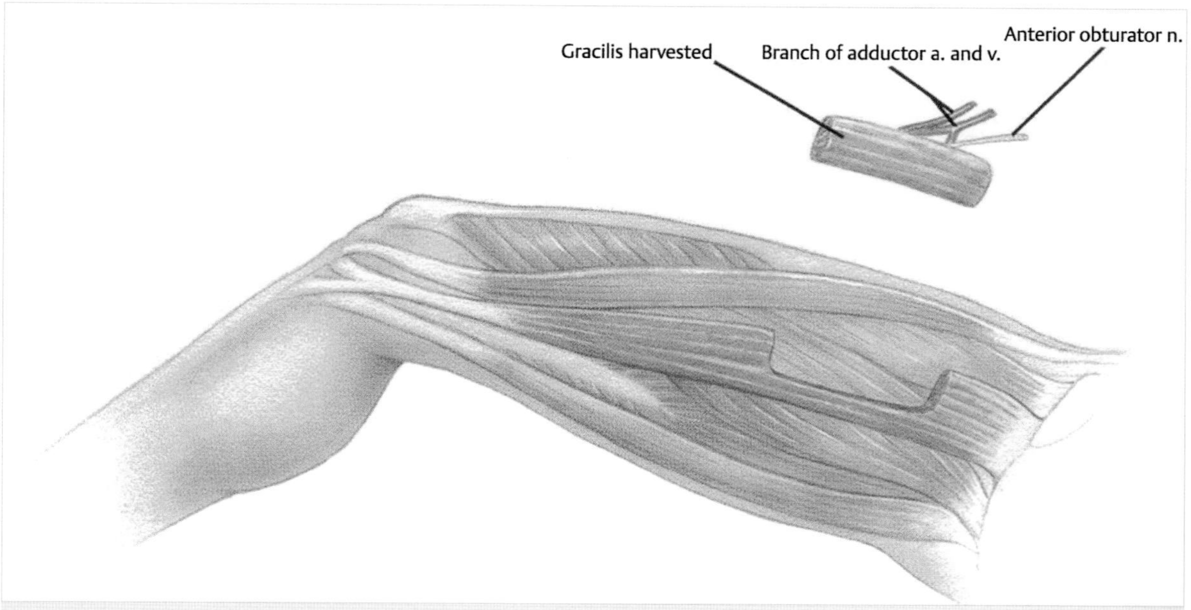

Fig. 22.9 Fifty percent of the width of the gracilis muscle is harvested with the neurovascular pedicle.

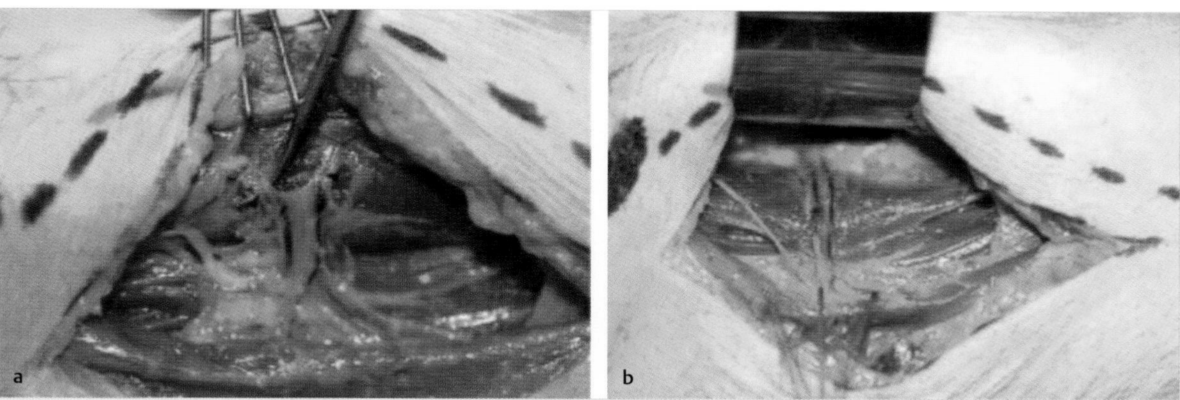

Fig. 22.10 (a,b) Dissection of the vascular pedicle. Adequate vascular pedicle length is achieved through ligation of the perforators to adductor longus.

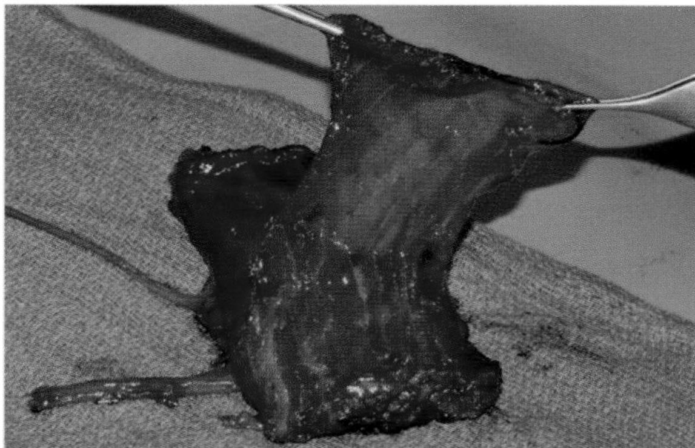

Fig. 22.11 Thinning of the gracilis flap on the back table.

through the gracilis again, running deep to superficial, inferior to the original suture. With each suture, the oral commissure is inspected to ensure that no dimpling arises. The remaining four sutures are evenly placed along the modiolus. Lastly, excess muscle along the inset sutures is trimmed.

Under the operating microscope, the arterial anastomosis is accomplished with 9–0 nylon sutures in an interrupted fashion. The dominant vena comitans is anastomosed to the facial vein with a venous coupling device (Ethicon Endo-Surgery). Once blood flow is established and perfusion is confirmed, the second vena comitans is clipped. The neurorrhaphy is completed using two or more 10–0 nylon epineural sutures, spaced 180 degrees apart. Fibrin glue is applied to the repair.

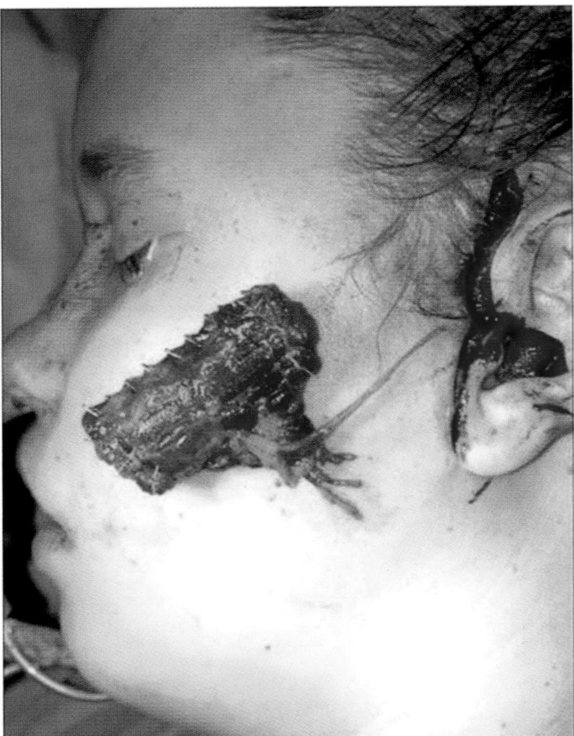

Fig. 22.12 The gracilis muscle is oriented along the direction of the zygomaticus major with the pedicle positioned along the inferior edge of the muscle belly.

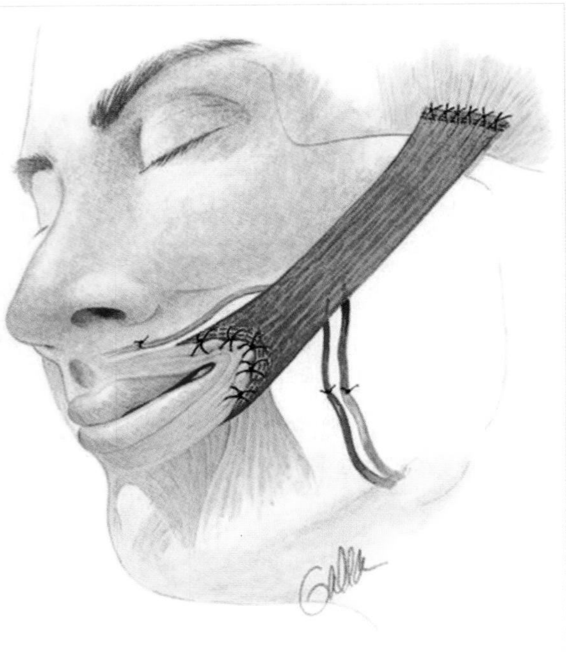

Fig. 22.13 Inset of the gracilis free muscle transfer. For a cross-face nerve graft, the obturator nerve is passed intraorally. The flap is sutured to the oral commissure using the previously placed 0-polyglactin sutures, forming a figure-of-eight knot.

Gracilis harvest, preparation, and inset:

- The leg must be abducted and flexed at the knee in "frog leg" position for ideal dissection.
- Subcutaneous veins running superficial to the gracilis can be ligated and saved for potential vein grafts.
- For contralateral muscle transfer, one-third of the muscle is taken superior to the pedicle; for ipsilateral muscle transfer, two-thirds of the muscle is taken superior to the pedicle.
- Several perforators from the vascular pedicle supply adductor longus. These must be ligated for adequate pedicle length.
- To avoid increased bulk in the face, the gracilis muscle is extensively thinned, taking care to protect the pedicle.
- A "neo-tendon" is created with suture on either end of the muscle flap, preventing shearing of the muscle fibers during inset.
- During inset, the oral commissure is inspected after each suture to ensure that there is no dimpling. The oral commissure should be slightly overcorrected after inset to the deep temporalis fascia.

A "neo-tendon" is placed along the superior edge of the flap using 2–0 polyglactin suture, and the flap is inset to the deep temporalis fascia with four 0-polyglactin sutures in a horizontal mattress fashion. The oral commissure should be slightly overcorrected (▶ Fig. 22.14 and ▶ Fig. 22.15). Excess muscle is trimmed from the suture line.

The face is irrigated with antibiotic-impregnated solution, and hemostasis is achieved. The wound is closed over a Penrose drain; a suction drain is employed if there is increased concern for postoperative hematoma. The incision is closed using 4–0 monofilament absorbable suture for the deep dermal layer and running 5.0 nylon suture for the skin.

22.6 Complications

Hematoma in the face is the most common complication after gracilis free muscle transfer. There is an increased risk of hematoma formation in the first 72 hours postoperatively. Frequent monitoring of the face ensures early detection of fluid accumulation, which is critical to avoid vascular compromise or disruption of the neurorrhaphy from the hematoma. Hematomas can be drained at the bedside or may require exploration in the operating room. Hematomas rarely occur in the thigh at the gracilis or fascia lata harvest site, although they are crucial to

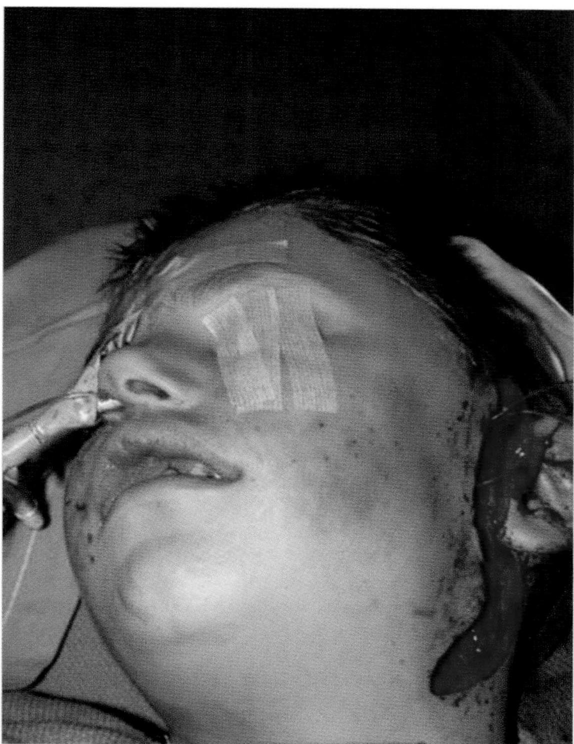

Fig. 22.14 Inset of the superior portion of the gracilis flap.

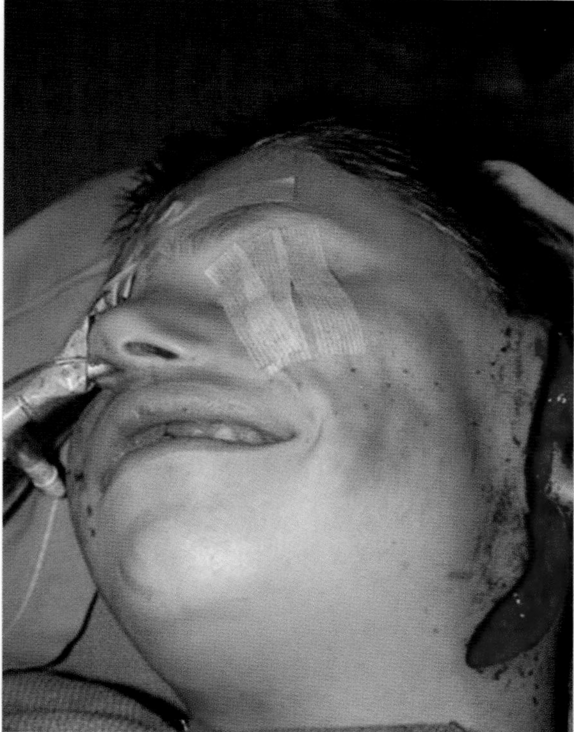

Fig. 22.15 The oral commissure is slightly overcorrected and then secured to the deep temporalis fascia.

identify as life-threatening amounts of blood can accumulate in the thigh with relatively few symptoms.

Rarely, vascular compromise occurs following free tissue transfer. Venous insufficiency is more common than arterial obstruction, especially in patients with vein grafts. Compromise in the venous system will present with palpable swelling and firmness of the gracilis, usually observed prior to a change in Doppler signal. Arterial insufficiency presents with a change in the Doppler signal and can be confirmed on duplex ultrasound. The most common cause of free flap failure is lack of neural input and manifests as the persistent inability to smile 4 to 12 months after the operation.

Unlike free flaps for reconstruction after cancer extirpation, gracilis free tissue transfer has a low rate of infection, occurring in fewer than 5% of patients.[36] Patients receive perioperative prophylaxis with ampicillin-sulbactam and are discharged home on oral antibiotics for 7 days.

!

The most important complications are, in descending order, hematoma formation, lack of neural input, and rarely vascular compromise or infection.

22.7 Postoperative Care

After surgery, the patient is kept warm with heated blankets to prevent vasospasm. Pain must be well controlled, and blood pressure is monitored closely, with the goal of 120 to 140/70 to 80 mm Hg to maintain adequate blood flow through the pedicle and to decrease the risk of postoperative bleeding. If using a Penrose drain, a dressing may be placed over the neck and held in place with a loose stockinet. Tight dressings that may compress the pedicle are avoided. The flap is monitored with a portable Doppler every 4 hours in the postoperative period. The Foley catheter is removed at midnight following surgery. On postoperative day 1, a duplex ultrasound is performed to verify appropriate muscle perfusion. The use of a vein graft, unfavorable vessel anatomy, and intraoperative low pulse pressure are indications for beginning low-dose aspirin on postoperative day 1. The thigh dressing is changed daily, and the patient may ambulate on postoperative day 1. On postoperative day 2, the Penrose drain is removed from the face, providing that there is no fluid accumulation. The thigh drain is removed on the day of discharge, which is usually postoperative day 3.

22.8 Key Points

- Multiple free muscle transfer options have been described to treat facial paralysis. The gracilis muscle is most commonly used.
- Gracilis muscle transfer can be performed as a single-stage procedure innervated by the masseteric nerve or by a two-stage procedure with innervation from a cross-face nerve graft.
- One-stage procedures have higher success rates, shorter times to reinnervation, and more robust smile excursion; however patients lack a spontaneous smile. Two-stage procedures restore spontaneous emotive expression, but have lower success rates due to the two neural coaptations.
- Dual innervation of the gracilis muscle is a recent development with promising preliminary results of combining reliable excursion from the masseteric nerve and spontaneous smile from the cross-face nerve graft.
- Gracilis free tissue transfer is effective in special populations, including pediatrics, bilateral facial paralysis, and neurofibromatosis type 2.
- The modiolus is atrophied in patients with long-standing facial paralysis. The zygomaticus major and facial vessels serve as landmarks for identification of the modiolus.
- The gracilis muscle is located in the medial thigh, deep to the subcutaneous tissue and superficial to the adductor longus, magnus, and brevis muscles.
- The adductor artery and two venae comitantes enter the gracilis at a 90 degree angle, 8 to 10 cm inferior to the public tubercle. The gracilis is innervated by the anterior obturator nerve, which enters the muscle obliquely 1 to 2 cm superior to the vascular pedicle.
- The most common complication of gracilis free muscle transfer is hematoma. Vascular compromise and infection are rare.

References

[1] Freilinger G. A new technique to correct facial paralysis. Plast Reconstr Surg 1975; 56: 44–48

[2] Harii K, Ohmori K, Torii S. Free gracilis muscle transplantation, with microneurovascular anastomoses for the treatment of facial paralysis. A preliminary report. Plast Reconstr Surg 1976; 57: 133–143

[3] Aviv JE, Urken ML. Management of the paralyzed face with microneurovascular free muscle transfer. Arch Otolaryngol Head Neck Surg 1992; 118: 909–912

[4] Liu AT, Lin Q, Jiang H et al. Facial reanimation by one-stage microneurovascular free abductor hallucis muscle transplantation: personal experience and long-term outcomes. Plast Reconstr Surg 2012; 130: 325–335

[5] Mayou BJ, Watson JS, Harrison DH, Parry CB. Free microvascular and microneural transfer of the extensor digitorum brevis muscle for the treatment of unilateral facial palsy. Br J Plast Surg 1981; 34: 362–367

[6] Bianchi B, Copelli C, Ferrari S, Ferri A, Bailleul C, Sesenna E. Facial animation with free-muscle transfer innervated by the masseter motor nerve in unilateral facial paralysis. J Oral Maxillofac Surg 2010; 68: 1524–1529

[7] Wang W, Qi Z, Lin X et al. Neurovascular musculus obliquus internus abdominis flap free transfer for facial reanimation in a single stage. Plast Reconstr Surg 2002; 110: 1430–1440

[8] Wei W, Zuoliang Q, Xiaoxi L et al. Free split and segmental latissimus dorsi muscle transfer in one stage for facial reanimation. Plast Reconstr Surg 1999; 103: 473–480, discussion 481–482

[9] Xu YB, Liu J, Li P, Donelan MB, Parrett BM, Winograd JM. The phrenic nerve as a motor nerve donor for facial reanimation with the free latissimus dorsi muscle. J Reconstr Microsurg 2009; 25: 457–463

[10] Takushima A, Harii K, Asato H, Kurita M, Shiraishi T. Fifteen-year survey of one-stage latissimus dorsi muscle transfer for treatment of longstanding facial paralysis. J Plast Reconstr Aesthet Surg 2013; 66: 29–36

[11] Takushima A, Harii K, Asato H, Ueda K, Yamada A. Neurovascular free-muscle transfer for the treatment of established facial paralysis following ablative surgery in the parotid region. Plast Reconstr Surg 2004; 113: 1563–1572

[12] Takushima A, Harii K, Asato H, Momosawa A, Okazaki M. One-stage reconstruction of facial paralysis associated with skin/soft tissue defects using latissimus dorsi compound flap. J Plast Reconstr Aesthet Surg 2006; 59: 465–473

[13] Biglioli F, Colombo V, Tarabbia F et al. Recovery of emotional smiling function in free-flap facial reanimation. J Oral Maxillofac Surg 2012; 70: 2413–2418

[14] Kurita M, Takushima A, Shiraishi T, Kinoshita M, Ozaki M, Harii K. Recycle of temporal muscle in combination with free muscle transfer in the treatment of facial paralysis. J Plast Reconstr Aesthet Surg 2013; 66: 991–995

[15] Ferguson LD, Paterson T, Ramsay F et al. Applied anatomy of the latissimus dorsi free flap for refinement in one-stage facial reanimation. J Plast Reconstr Aesthet Surg 2011; 64: 1417–1423

[16] Terzis JK. Pectoralis minor: a unique muscle for correction of facial palsy. Plast Reconstr Surg 1989; 83: 767–776

[17] Harrison DH, Grobbelaar AO. Pectoralis minor muscle transfer for unilateral facial palsy reanimation: an experience of 35 years and 637 cases. J Plast Reconstr Aesthet Surg 2012; 65: 845–850

[18] Sajjadian A, Song AY, Khorsandi CA et al. One-stage reanimation of the paralyzed face using the rectus abdominis neurovascular free flap. Plast Reconstr Surg 2006; 117: 1553–1559

[19] Yang D, Morris SF, Tang M, Geddes CR. A modified longitudinally split segmental rectus femoris muscle flap transfer for facial reanimation: anatomic basis and clinical applications. J Plast Reconstr Aesthet Surg 2006; 59: 807–814

[20] Krishnan KG, Schackert G, Seifert V. Outcomes of microneurovascular facial reanimation using masseteric innervation in patients with long-standing facial palsy resulting from cured brainstem lesions. Neurosurgery 2010; 67: 663–674, discussion 674

[21] Harrison DH. Current trends in the treatment of established unilateral facial palsy. Ann R Coll Surg Engl 1990; 72: 94–98

[22] Bhama P, Weinberg J, Lindsay R, Hohman M, Cheney M, Hadlock T. Objective outcomes analysis following microvascular gracilis transfer for facial reanimation: a 10-year experience at the Massachusetts Eye and Ear Infirmary/Harvard Medical School. JAMA Facial Plast Surg

[23] Faria JC, Scopel GP, Busnardo FF, Ferreira MC. Nerve sources for facial reanimation with muscle transplant in patients with unilateral facial palsy: clinical analysis of 3 techniques. Ann Plast Surg 2007; 59: 87–91

[24] Ueda K, Harii K, Asato H, Yoshimura K, Yamada A. Evaluation of muscle graft using facial nerve on the affected side as a motor source in the treatment of facial paralysis. Scand J Plast Reconstr Surg Hand Surg 1999; 33: 47–57

[25] Lin CH, Wallace C, Liao CT. Functioning free gracilis myocutaneous flap transfer provides a reliable single-stage facial reconstruction and reanimation following tumor ablation. Plast Reconstr Surg 2011; 128: 687–696

[26] Yamamoto Y, Sekido M, Furukawa H, Oyama A, Tsutsumida A, Sasaki S. Surgical rehabilitation of reversible facial palsy: facial–hypoglossal network system based on neural signal augmentation/neural supercharge concept. J Plast Reconstr Aesthet Surg 2007; 60: 223–231

[27] Biglioli F, Colombo V, Tarabbia F et al. Double innervation in free-flap surgery for long-standing facial paralysis. J Plast Reconstr Aesthet Surg 2012; 65: 1343–1349

[28] Watanabe Y, Akizuki T, Ozawa T, Yoshimura K, Agawa K, Ota T. Dual innervation method using one-stage reconstruction with free latissimus dorsi muscle transfer for re-animation of established facial paralysis: simultaneous reinnervation of the ipsilateral masseter motor nerve and the contralateral facial nerve to improve the quality of smile and emotional facial expressions. J Plast Reconstr Aesthet Surg 2009; 62: 1589–1597

[29] Bianchi B, Copelli C, Ferrari S, Ferri A, Sesenna E. Facial animation in patients with Möebius and Möebius-like syndromes. Int J Oral Maxillofac Surg 2010; 39: 1066–1073

[30] Vakharia KT, Henstrom D, Plotkin SR, Cheney M, Hadlock TA. Facial reanimation of patients with neurofibromatosis type 2. Neurosurgery 2012; 70 Suppl Operative: 237–243

[31] Hadlock TA, Malo JS, Cheney ML, Henstrom DK. Free gracilis transfer for smile in children: the Massachusetts Eye and Ear Infirmary Experience in excursion and quality-of-life changes. Arch Facial Plast Surg 2011; 13: 190–194

[32] Bianchi B, Copelli C, Ferrari S, Ferri A, Sesenna E. Facial animation in children with Möebius and Möebius-like syndromes. J Pediatr Surg 2009; 44: 2236–2242

[33] Collar RM, Byrne PJ, Boahene KD. The subzygomatic triangle: rapid, minimally invasive identification of the masseteric nerve for facial reanimation. Plast Reconstr Surg 2013; 132: 183–188

[34] Borschel GH, Kawamura DH, Kasukurthi R, Hunter DA, Zuker RM, Woo AS. The motor nerve to the masseter muscle: an anatomic and histomorphometric study to facilitate its use in facial reanimation. J Plast Reconstr Aesthet Surg 2012; 65: 363–366

[35] Urken ML. Atlas of Regional and Free Flaps for Head and Neck Reconstruction: Flap Harvest and Insetting. 2nd ed. Philadelphia: Wolters Kluwer Health/Lippincott Williams & Wilkins; 2012

[36] Lee LN, Susarla SM, Henstrom DK et al. Surgical site infections after gracilis free flap reconstruction for facial paralysis. Otolaryngol Head Neck Surg 2012; 147: 245–248

23 Functional Outcomes of Facial Nerve Repair following Face Transplantation

Maria Z. Siemionow and Bahar Bassiri Gharb

23.1 Introduction

In the past 8 years, with 30 face transplantations performed worldwide, many of the technical, logistic and ethical aspects of the procedure have been addressed and acceptable graft survival and functional outcomes have been achieved under the current immunosuppressive regimens.[1] No evidence of chronic rejection has been reported in face transplant cases, with the longest follow-up exceeding 8 years.[2] Therefore, face transplantation is playing an important role in the restoration of facial appearance and function in cases where conventional reconstructive techniques have failed or are at high risk of failure.

> **!**
> No evidence of chronic rejection has been reported in 30 face transplant cases performed worldwide so far.

Recovery of facial expression, restoration of oral continence, and return of eyelid closure following face transplantation are of the utmost importance to ensure the success of this innovative procedure (examples are shown in ▸ Fig. 23.1, ▸ Fig. 23.2 and ▸ Fig. 23.3). This chapter reviews the surgical approach to the facial nerve in face

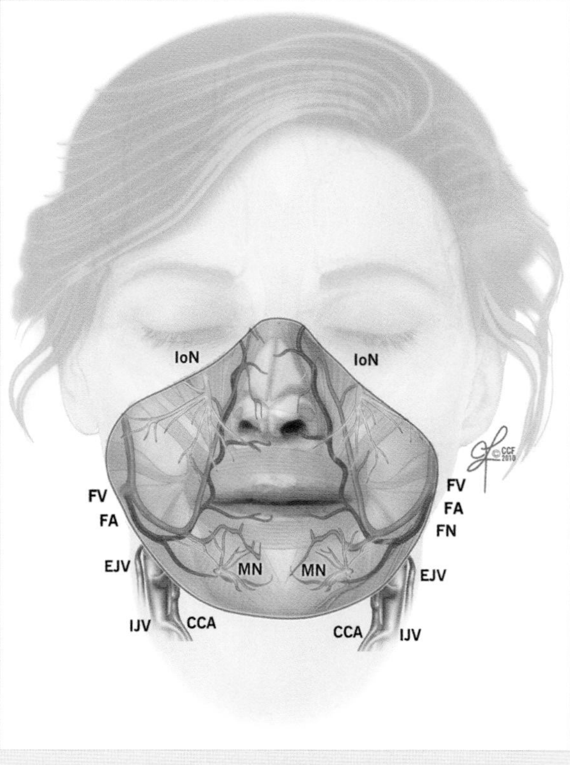

Fig. 23.1 Case no. 1 (▸ Table 23.1). The recipient was a 38-year-old woman with midface trauma after a dog bite. The patient underwent partial face transplantation, including nose, lips, chin, partial cheeks, and intraoral mucosa. The procedure took place in November 2005, in Amiens, France. CCA, common carotid artery; EJV, external jugular vein; FA, facial artery; FV, facial vein; FN, facial nerve; IJV, internal jugular vein; IoN, infraorbital nerve; MN, mental nerve.

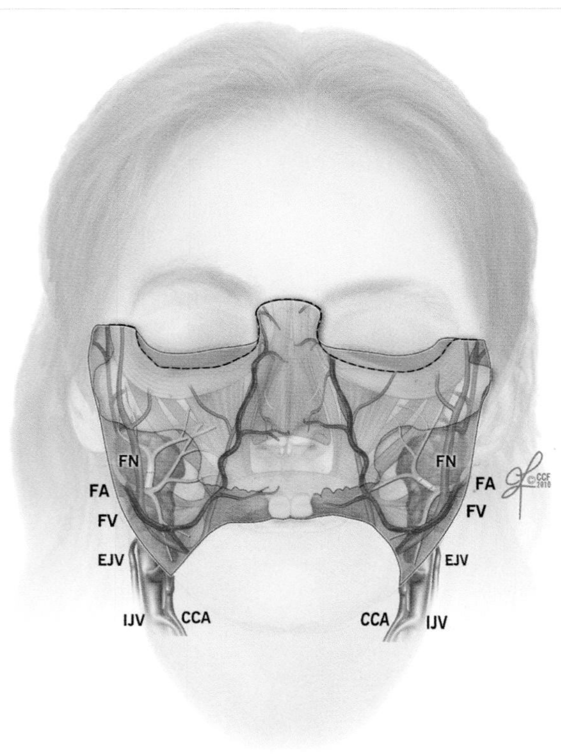

Fig. 23.2 Case no. 4 (▸ Table 23.1). The recipient was a 46-year-old woman who sustained a shotgun injury to the face. The patient underwent a near-total face transplantation, including composite Le Fort III midfacial skeleton, overlying skin, soft tissue, nose, lower eyelids, upper lip, total orbital floor, bilateral zygomas, bilateral parotid glands, anterior maxilla with central maxillary incisors, total alveolus, anterior hard palate, and intraoral mucosa. The procedure took place in December 2008 in Cleveland, Ohio, USA. CCA, common carotid artery; EJV, external jugular vein; FA, facial artery; FV, facial vein; FN, facial nerve; IJV, internal jugular vein.

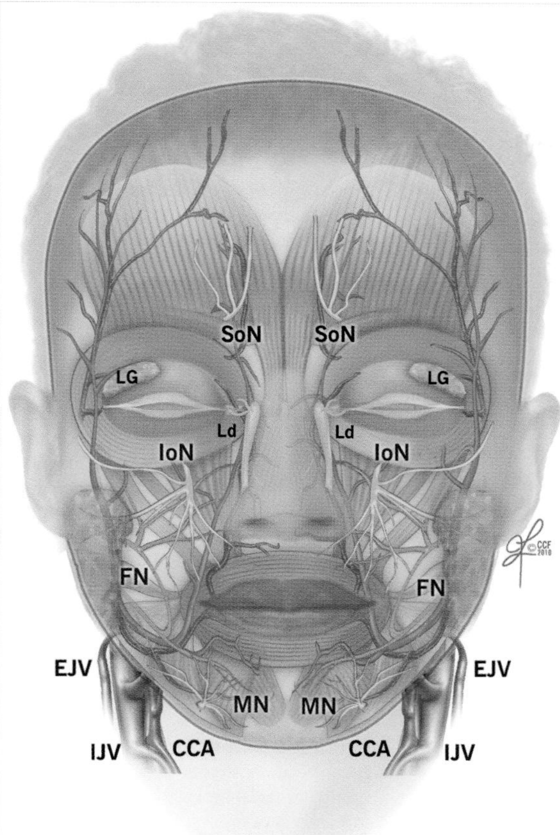

Fig. 23.3 Case no. 13 (▶ Table 23.1). The recipient was a 35-year-old man with neurofibromatosis. The patient underwent total facial transplantation, including overlying skin, soft tissue, ears, nose, lips, cheeks, eyelids, lacrimal glands and lacrimal ducts, and intraoral mucosa. The procedure took place in June 2010 in Paris, France. CCA, common carotid artery; EJV, external jugular vein; FA, facial artery; FN, facial nerve; IJV, internal jugular vein; IoN, infraorbital nerve; Ld, lacrimal duct; LG, lacrimal gland; MN, mental nerve; SoN, supraorbital nerve.

transplantation, followed by a discussion of the functional outcomes of facial nerve repair.

23.2 Surgical Approach to Facial Nerve Repair in Face Transplantation

Facial nerve repair in face transplantation follows skeletal fixation and vascular anastomosis. Often, due to the mismatch between the donor and recipient skeletal structures and facial allograft edema, which occurs following revascularization, the primary repair of the nerve has not been possible. Therefore, interpositional nerve grafts have been often used (vagus, ansa cervicalis, hypoglossal, greater auricular and thoracodorsal nerves; ▶ Table 23.1).

Two surgical approaches have been used for restoration of facial nerve continuity during face transplantation: (1) repair at the level of the main trunk/upper/lower divisions, and (2) repair of the terminal branches in the proximity of the target muscles.

1. Access to the facial nerve trunk and its principal divisions is accomplished through a preauricular incision via a parotidectomy approach. The main trunk of the facial nerve is found at the level of the tragal pointer and its exit from the stylomastoid foramen, between the posterior belly of the digastric muscle and the sternocleidomastoid muscle. Limited mastoidectomy can be performed to obtain an adequate length for the nerve repair. A superficial parotidectomy could be performed for the same purpose, as well as to improve access to the upper and lower divisions of the facial nerve and to decrease the bulk of the allograft in the preauricular area.[3,4]
2. For the targeted reinnervation of the effector muscles, the dissection starts from the preauricular incision, and is carried out in the lateral-to-medial direction in the sub-SMAS (superficial musculoaponeurotic system) layer. The facial nerve branches are identified at the level of their exit from the parotid gland and are tagged, elevated, and included as an integral part of the allograft.[5,6]

The first approach presents the advantage of repairing one of the large nerve trunks compared with the repair of the multiple smaller-sized nerve branches. However, the recovery time could be longer due to greater distance from the target muscles, and there is an increased risk of synkinesia. The second approach ensures fastest recovery due to the shorter distance to the effector muscles and the lower chance of developing synkinesia.[7]

!

When using long interpositional grafts for facial nerve reanimation in face transplantation patients, the patient can develop synkinesia as in other cases of facial nerve reconstruction.

23.3 Rehabilitation following Facial Nerve Repair in Face Transplantation

Facial nerve rehabilitation following face transplantation starts in the first postoperative week,[7] usually within the first 48 hours. Speech therapy, sensory reeducation, motor rehabilitation (both static and dynamic exercises),

Table 23.1 Summary of demographic data of face transplant patients, including the type of facial nerve repair and the available outcomes

Case no.	Date	Location age (years), gender, survival, sight	Type of facial nerve repair during face transplantation	Motor recovery
1	11/2005	Amiens, France 38, F, alive, normal sight	Left marginal mandibular direct repair	4months: started rapid and continuous improvement of muscle function. Chin–nose muscle contraction present. Complete mouth closure was achieved at 4 months and phonation still lacked labial occlusive phones 6 months: lip occlusion 18 months: symmetric smile 3 years: stable lip occlusion and muscle function 5 years: stable lip occlusion and muscle function. Normal mouth opening (36 mm), slight synkinesis on the left side. Orbicularis muscle recovery is incomplete. Blowing is normal. Patient chews and swallows. Pouting and kissing are still difficult. Patient can talk easily and intelligibly
2	4/2006	Xi'an, China 30, M, died, normal sight	Right facial nerve direct repair (the quality of repair was not satisfactory (stylomastoid foramen was avulsed and scarred, only the neural stem remained, which was difficult to dissect)	2 years: poor function (levator labii superioris, levator anguli oris); no function in buccal branches of facial nerve. Unable to smile symmetrically. Able to eat, drink, talk
3	1/2007	Paris, France 29, M, alive, normal vision right eye; blind left eye (glaucoma)	Bilateral direct facial nerve repair	3 months: EMG showed no evidence of reinnervation, except minor motor response to facial nerve stimulation in left orbicularis oculi 6 months: EMG activity detected during voluntary contraction in left orbicularis oculi and bilateral orbicularis oris 9 months: recovery of spontaneous mimicry. 12 months: EMG showed signs of motor reinnervation of facial territory. Bilateral zygomatic muscles voluntary contraction; bilateral orbicularis oris voluntary contraction with complete mouth closure. Blink response present in response to stimulation of supraorbital branches of trigeminal nerve (contraction of facial muscles)
4	12/2008	Cleveland, USA 46, F, alive, legally blind (right eye enucleated, left eye visual acuity 20/200)	Bilateral end-to-side facial nerve repair with interpositional nerve grafts between the upper trunk of recipient facial nerve and donor main trunk (hypoglossal graft on left; vagus on right) Lower division of facial nerve was damaged previously	6 months: slow motor recovery of facial muscles 8 months: progressive motor recovery. Upper lip occlusion. Facial mimicry present. Able to eat and drink, speak 12 months: almost full motor recovery
5	3/2009	Paris, France 27, M, alive, normal sight	Bilateral direct facial nerve repair	Fastest motor recovery in French experience 2 months: recovery of left orbicularis oris and left zygomatic muscles 3 months: recovery of right orbicularis oris and right zygomatic muscles 5 months: spontaneous mimicry 8 months: complete mouth closure 12 months: bilateral full recovery of zygomatic muscles

Table 23.1 continued

Case no.	Date	Location age (years), gender, survival, sight	Type of facial nerve repair during face transplantation	Motor recovery
6	4/2009	Boston, USA 59, M, alive, normal sight	Right: direct repair five facial nerve branches Left: direct repair six facial nerve branches	Progressive recovery over 12 months. Speech improved immediately postoperatively. Ability for oral intake by 3 days 12 months: symmetrical smile with 2–3 cm excursion of corners of mouth; motor control of transplanted upper lip. Unable to pucker or blow with lips. Absent synkinesia 3 years: functionally intact orbicularis oris and zygomaticus major contraction, bilaterally. Left levator anguli oris contracted weakly. Right levator anguli oris, buccinator, levator labii superioris, and levator labii superioris alaeque nasi were difficult to identify in contraction, or contraction was absent The degree of muscle excursion as measured by the Sunnybrook Facial Grading Scale demonstrated near normal and close to symmetric movements. The snarl on the right side was rated 1/5 (unable to initiate movement) and 2/5 on the left (initiates slight movement). Lip pucker was rated at 3/5 (initiated movement with mild excursion and moderate asymmetry)
7	4/2009	Paris, France (with bilateral hand transplantation) 37, M, died, normal sight	Bilateral direct facial nerve repair	Not reported
8	8/2009	Paris, France 33, M, alive, normal sight	Bilateral direct facial nerve repair Revision right facial nerve repair at 11 months	5 months: recovery of left zygomatic muscle and left orbicularis oris 9 months: asymmetry with a weaker right side (second side to be repaired) 12 months: absent complete mouth closure. Absent recovery of right zygomatic and right orbicularis oris muscles
9	9/2009	Valencia, Spain 42, M, died, normal sight	Bilateral lower facial nerve trunk repair: primary repair on the left; short interpositional nerve graft on the right	16 months: mouth opening 10 mm; swallowing and starting phonation
10	10/2009	Amiens, France 27, M, alive, normal sight	Bilateral direct facial nerve repair (6 months after face transplantation)	Not reported
11	1/2010	Seville, Spain 34, M, alive, normal sight	Bilateral direct facial nerve repair	6 months: motor recovery of levator labii superioris and buccinator muscles. Improved speech. Autonomous oral feedings
12	3/2010	Barcelona, Spain 30, M, alive, normal sight	Bilateral direct repair of the buccal, zygomatic, orbicularis oculi, and frontal branches of facial nerve	2.5 months: EMG showed no signs of reinnervation 4 months: EMG showed motor reinnervation at commissures of mouth. Active movement frontalis, lateral zygomatic muscles, upper orbicularis oculi. Unable to close eyes fully
13	6/2010	Paris, France 35, M, alive, not reported	Bilateral direct facial nerve repair	Not reported

Table 23.1 continued

Case no.	Date	Location age (years), gender, survival, sight	Type of facial nerve repair during face transplantation	Motor recovery
14	3/2011	Boston, USA, 25, M, alive, blind	Bilateral facial nerve repair Left: upper and lower divisions Right: frontal, zygomatic, buccal, marginal mandibular Both sides with interpositional thoracodorsal nerve grafts	4 months: movement of right-sided muscle groups and restoration of facial aesthetics. Left side: not reported
15	3/2011	Paris, France 45, M, alive, not reported	Not reported	Not reported
16	4/2011	Boston, USA 57, F, alive, blind (transplanted upper extremities were amputated)	Bilateral facial nerve repair: six branches including frontal, zygomatic, buccal, marginal mandibular Both sides with interpositional great auricular nerve grafts	3 months: no return of motor function
17	4/2011	Paris, France 41, M, alive, not reported	Not reported	Not reported
18	5/2011	Boston, USA 30, M, alive, normal sight	Bilateral direct facial nerve repair: bilateral buccal and marginal mandibular divisions	3 months: return of gross lip motion, along with restoration of facial aesthetics
19	1/2012	Antalya, Turkey 19, M, alive, normal sight	Not reported	Not reported
20	1/2012	Gent, Belgium M, alive, normal sight	Not reported	Not reported
21	2/2012	Ankara, Turkey 25, M, alive, not reported	Not reported	Not reported
22	3/2012	Baltimore, USA 37, M, alive, normal sight	Right direct facial nerve repair branches to upper lip, commissure and lower lip primary repair Left: repair same branches with interpositional nerve graft (ansa cervicalis graft); marginal mandibular repaired primarily	19 months: complete mouth closure
23	3/2012	Ankara, Turkey, 21, F, alive, normal sight	Not reported	Not reported
24	4/2012	Antalya, Turkey 27, M, alive, normal sight	Not reported	Not reported
25	2/2013	Boston, USA 44, F, alive, limited vision in left eye and blind in right eye	Bilateral facial nerve repair	4 months: cannot close mouth and left eye. No spontaneous facial expression
26	5/2013	Gliwice, Poland 33, M, alive, blind right eye and normal vision on left eye	Not reported	Not reported
27	7/2013	Antalya, Turkey 26, M, alive, normal sight	Not reported	Not reported
28	8/2013	Antalya, Turkey 54, M, alive, normal sight	Not reported	Not reported
29	12/2013	Gliwice, Poland 26, F, alive, not reported	Not reported	Not reported
30	12/2013	Antalya, Turkey 22, M, normal sight	Not reported	Not reported

and facial acceptance reeducation are performed daily during the first 3 months after transplantation.[8] The facial physical rehabilitation program includes: controlled movements, passive and active exercises, and the cortical reintegration protocol including imagery training.[9] The patient from Cleveland, who is legally blind, was instructed and guided by touching the points of facial muscle insertion to perform functional, isometric, as well as imagery movements.

23.4 Current Clinical Experience with Facial Nerve Repair in Face Transplantation

Thirty face transplantations have been performed in 23 men and 7 women (▶ Table 23.1). The average age was 34 years. After transplantation, 18 patients had normal vision, 2 patients lost vision in one eye, 2 patients were legally blind (lost vision in one eye and decreased visual acuity in the other eye), and 2 patients were totally blind. Detailed information on the facial nerve repair was available for 18 patients: in 16 patients the facial nerve was repaired bilaterally (32 hemifaces), and in 2 patients the repair was unilateral. In 16 hemifaces, the main trunk or the primary divisions of the facial nerve were repaired directly; in 8 hemifaces, a direct end-to-end repair was performed between the terminal branches of the recipient and donor facial nerves; in 2 hemifaces, a nerve graft was interposed between the donor and the recipient facial nerve trunks and in 2 cases, interpositional nerve grafts were repaired in an end-to-side fashion between the main trunk of the donor's facial nerve and the upper trunk of the recipient's facial nerve; in 4 hemifaces, interposition of the nerve grafts was necessary to bridge the gap between the terminal branches of the facial nerve.

> !
>
> The type of facial nerve repair in face transplantation has to be selected according to the individual.

23.5 Functional Outcomes of Facial Nerve Repair in Face Transplantation

Return of facial nerve function within the target muscles seemed to occur faster when the terminal branches of the facial nerve were repaired as opposed to main trunk repair: signs of reinnervation appeared between 2.5 and 4 months, with full functional recovery reported between 12 to 18 months after nerve repair during face transplantation. When the main trunk of the facial nerve was repaired the early signs of recovery or the electromyographic evidence of reinnervation were evident between 5 and 6 months, whereas progression of reinnervation was even slower when interpositional nerve grafts were used. In the group with a main trunk repair, the earliest report of full functional recovery was observed at 12 months. Tissue scarring and extensive facial nerve trauma prior to transplantation have a significant impact on facial nerve recovery and the functional outcomes.

> !
>
> In patients with face transplantation, signs of facial nerve reinnervation have been reported between 2 and 4 months, and full recovery between 12 and 18 months.

23.6 Key Points

- The results of facial nerve repair and facial reanimation following face transplantation are encouraging, since recovery of close to normal function could be expected with primary repair of the nerve, whereas faster recovery was observed when peripheral branches were selected over the main trunk.
- Immunosuppressive treatment with tacrolimus enhances nerve regeneration and promotes motor recovery, as has been shown in hand transplantation.[10–12]
- The presence of normal vision is deemed necessary, not only for the surveillance of the facial allograft, but also to ensure satisfactory motor rehabilitation and cortical integration of the recovered facial nerve function. However, the available data on the functional recovery in patients with decreased visual acuity or blindness are either underreported or controversial, and thus there is a need for more systematic evaluation.[1,13]

References

[1] Siemionow M, Gharb BB, Rampazzo A. Successes and lessons learned after more than a decade of upper extremity and face transplantation. Curr Opin Organ Transplant 2013; 18: 633–639

[2] Petruzzo P, Testelin S, Kanitakis J et al. First human face transplantation: 5 years outcomes. Transplantation 2012; 93: 236–240

[3] Alam DS, Papay F, Djohan R et al. The technical and anatomical aspects of the world's first near-total human face and maxilla transplant. Arch Facial Plast Surg 2009; 11: 369–377

[4] Meningaud JP, Hivelin M, Benjoar MD, Toure G, Hermeziu O, Lantieri L. The procurement of allotransplants for ballistic trauma: a preclinical study and a report of two clinical cases. Plast Reconstr Surg 2011; 127: 1892–1900

[5] Pomahac B, Pribaz JJ, Bueno EM et al. Novel surgical technique for full face transplantation. Plast Reconstr Surg 2012; 130: 549–555

[6] Dorafshar AH, Bojovic B, Christy MR et al. Total face, double jaw, and tongue transplantation: an evolutionary concept. Plast Reconstr Surg 2013; 131: 241–251

[7] Pomahac B, Pribaz J, Eriksson E et al. Three patients with full facial transplantation. N Engl J Med 2012; 366: 715–722
[8] Siemionow M, Papay F, Alam D et al. Near-total human face transplantation for a severely disfigured patient in the USA. Lancet 2009; 374: 203–209
[9] Devauchelle B, Badet L, Lengelé B et al. First human face allograft: early report. Lancet 2006; 368: 203–209
[10] Dubernard JM, Owen E, Herzberg G et al. Human hand allograft: report on first 6 months. Lancet 1999; 353: 1315–1320
[11] Owen ER, Dubernard JM, Lanzetta M et al. Peripheral nerve regeneration in human hand transplantation. Transplant Proc 2001; 33: 1720–1721
[12] Siemionow M, Gharb BB, Rampazzo A. Pathways of sensory recovery after face transplantation. Plast Reconstr Surg 2011; 127: 1875–1889
[13] Carty MJ, Bueno EM, Lehmann LS, Pomahac B. A position paper in support of face transplantation in the blind. Plast Reconstr Surg 2012; 130: 319–324

24 Surgery of the Periorbital Region

Kris S. Moe and Farhad Ardeshirpour

24.1 Introduction

Facial paralysis is a devastating condition, manifesting in quality of life–altering conditions that involve a myriad of fundamental functions from communication to mastication to visualization. Nowhere is this more apparent than in the periocular region where the inability to blink and convey emotion impacts all aspects of life. The underlying periorbital disorder in facial paralysis is loss of eyelid closure normally provided by the orbicularis oculi musculature (paralytic lagophthalmos). The third cranial nerve, which typically retains function, is then unopposed by the eye-closing function of the seventh cranial nerve. Thus the eye is able to open but not close.

> !
>
> In patients with complete facial palsy, the eye is unable to close but able to open, because this function is related to the normally unaffected oculomotor nerve.

Tear production and distribution are diminished as a consequence of facial paralysis. Furthermore, loss of tone in the lower eyelid results in additional exposure of the conjunctiva and cornea. These factors lead to increased evaporation of the tear film causing a dry, irritated eye (keratoconjunctivitis sicca or xerophthalmia; ▶ Fig. 24.1). Left untreated, particularly in patients with decreased corneal sensation, this condition can lead to loss of vision or blindness.[1] While Bell's phenomenon (upward rotation of the globe on attempted eye closure) may provide an element of protective moisturization, this is reflex is absent in 25% of the population, putting these patients at additional risk (▶ Fig. 24.2 and ▶ Fig. 24.3).

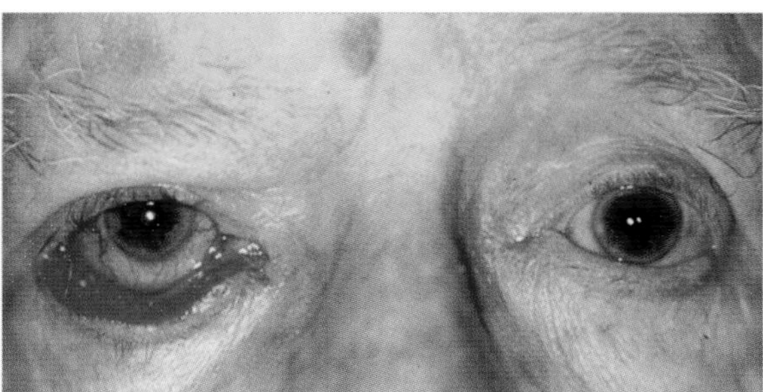

Fig. 24.1 Right upper and lower lid malposition from longstanding facial paralysis.

> Bell's phenomenon may provide an element of protective moisturization, but is absent in 25% of the population.

Further complicating the situation is that paralysis of the periocular musculature not only leads to failure of eye closure, but these muscles, which normally support the adjacent tissue and assist in maintaining proper eyelid position, become dependent on the medial and lateral canthi and tarsus for support. This further deforms these structures and interferes with eyelid position and function.[2,3] Patients with chronic paralysis may eventually develop soft tissue contraction, scarring, and a cicatricial component to the paralytic process.[2]

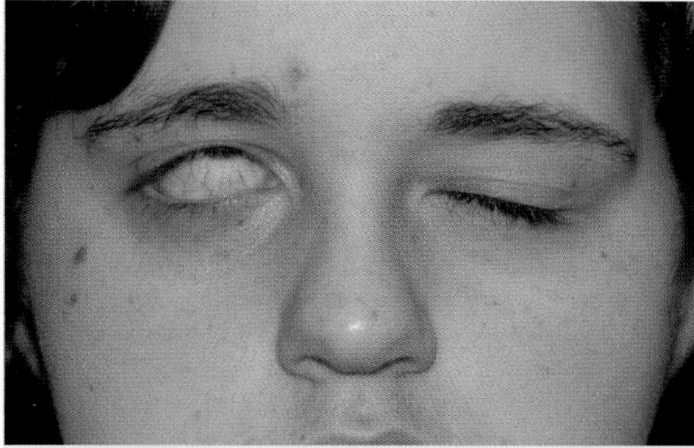

Fig. 24.2 Bell's phenomenon with right facial paralysis.

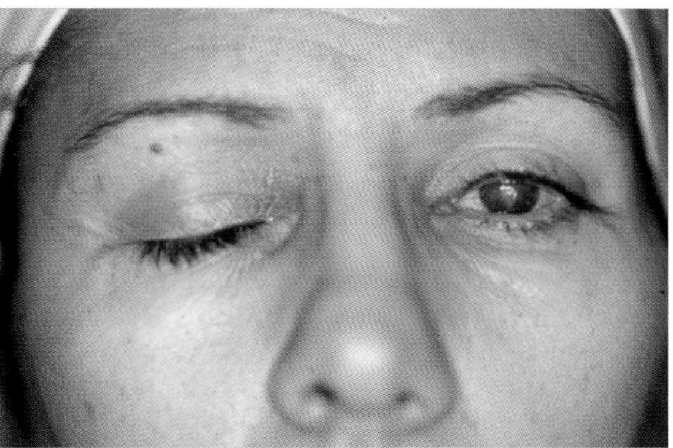

Fig. 24.3 Patient with left facial paralysis lacking Bell's phenomenon who developed left-sided blindness from corneal exposure damage.

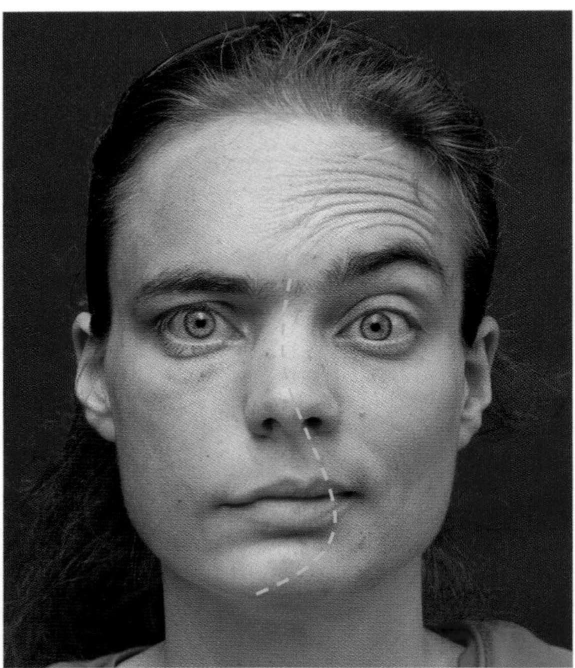

Fig. 24.4 “S”-shaped facial distortion with right facial paralysis.

It is important to realize that unilateral paralysis is a bilateral problem. Compensatory contralateral hypertonicity describes the state of hypercontraction of the normal side of the face that occurs when the contralateral side becomes paralyzed (▶ Fig. 24.4 and ▶ Fig. 24.5). This hypercontraction phenomenon may result from subconscious efforts to correct the position of the paralyzed side, thereby resulting in unintentional hypercontraction of the contralateral innervated musculature. Eventually the face takes the shape of an “S”.

!

Unilateral facial palsy can be a bilateral problem for the eyes. Compensatory contralateral hypertonicity can affect the facial muscles of the contralateral eye.

Fortunately, surgical technique has progressed to the point that much of the morbidity associated with paralysis of the periorbital tissue can be effectively treated.[4] Even in those cases where reinnervation is not possible, there are numerous procedures that can effectively be tailored to a patient's individual needs and provide a safe, nearly symptom-free eye. This chapter will describe the evaluation and treatment of malposition of the facial tissues impacting the periorbital region, including the eyelids, forehead, and midface, and provide a management protocol for the rehabilitation of these regions in facial paralysis.

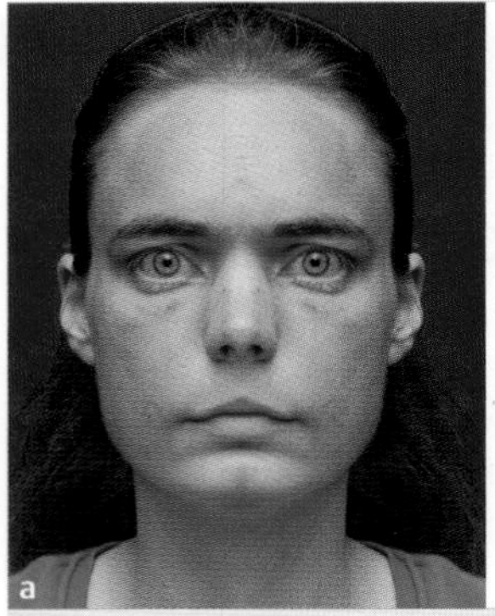

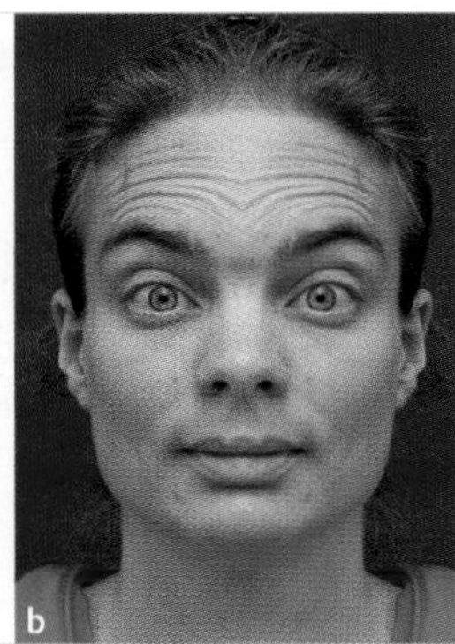

Fig. 24.5 The patient shown in ▶ Fig. 24.4. **(a)** Mirror-image duplication of paralyzed half of face. **(b)** Mirror-image duplication of nonparalyzed side of face.

24.2 Forehead and Brow

24.2.1 Browlift

Patient Selection

Paralysis of the frontal region may lead to descent of the forehead, brow, and the upper lid complex. The brow typically assumes a lower, flattened shape relative to the normal brow, often with accentuated lateral hooding. This process is more significant in elderly patients, unmasking the chronic soft tissue elevation that is provided by the underlying facial musculature. If the soft tissue descent is significant, it may cause obstruction of the superior visual fields.

The descent of the eyebrow complex frequently accentuates pre-existing blepharochalasis or dermatochalasis in the patient with facial paralysis. Visual field deficits represent one of several indications to elevate the brow complex. In addition, if the brow ptosis causes enough redundancy so that the upper eyelid skin superior to the eyelid crease coapts the inferior lid skin, it may adhere and worsen the lagophthalmos. This is particularly important to consider when performing a procedure such as placement of an upper eyelid weight, as the friction and adhesion from the blepharochalasis can lead to suboptimal function of the implant.

!

If you plan to perform upper lid loading make sure to examine the brow position. Brow ptosis can lead to suboptimal function of the lid loading if not addressed.

Another indication for correction of forehead or brow ptosis is hypercontraction of the contralateral side (▶ Fig. 24.4). As described previously, patients often develop excess contraction of the innervated brow, raising it well above the normal position at the superior orbital rim. This creates a significantly abnormal and highly asymmetric appearance and in theory could be a cause of frontal headaches.

It is important to consider that the innervated ptotic brow does not assume a static position; the height of the brow changes during the day beginning with an elevated position and descending in the evening with progressive fatigue. Thus, elevating the ptotic paralyzed brow to match the innervated brow cannot provide symmetry throughout the day. To achieve symmetry, the ptotic innervated brow should be corrected to a normal position, which will be maintained throughout the day, and the paralyzed brow should be restored to a matching position. Thus, as a general rule, if a patient would be a candidate for browlift due to ptosis from aging in the absence of facial paralysis, correction of the paralyzed brow is indicated, and a bilateral procedure will typically provide the optimal outcome.

Numerous techniques have been described for the repositioning of the forehead and the eyebrow, including coronal, pretrichial, mid forehead, direct brow, and endoscopic, or combined approaches.[1] The position of the hairline, the condition of the forehead skin, and the degree of soft tissue descent influence the choice of technique as all of these techniques have been demonstrated to be effective. It is recommended that the surgeon choose the approach that would be used in the absence of facial paralysis.

!

Choose the browlift technique you would use in the absence of facial palsy. If a browlift is also indicated for the contralateral side, it is best to treat both sides at the same time.

Patient Information and Consent

There is risk of injury to the frontal branch of the facial nerve, which has more consequences on the nonparalyzed side. Possible injury to the supraorbital and supratrochlear nerves will produce decreased or absent sensation to the forehead and scalp. Patients are at risk of noticeable scars especially in direct brow or mid forehead procedures and alopecia may occur along brow or scalp incisions. Coronal approaches may have greater risk than endoscopic approaches to raise the hairline.

Anesthesia and Positioning

General anesthesia is preferred in endoscopic and coronal browlifts unless the patient has medical contraindications. Direct browlifts can be performed under local anesthesia with or without sedation. Markings should be placed preoperatively because brow and lid positioning will change after the patient lies supine. Paralytic agents are avoided in order to prevent injury to frontal branches of the facial nerve on the normal side. Hair should be parted along the incisions and rubber bands may be used to tie off braided hair along the incision lines to improve visualization. Local anesthetic with epinephrine should be injected along the incision markings as well as in a ring around the forehead.

Surgical Steps

The following paragraphs describe the authors' endoscopic approach, as it is their preferred method. The nonparalyzed side is corrected first, thus creating a stable position to match on the paralyzed side. Five, 2-cm incisions are made 2 cm behind the hairline. Incisions include one vertical midline, a right and left intermediate incision (oriented in a vertical line between the lateral canthus and lateral limbus), and right and left temporal incisions (oriented obliquely, perpendicular to a diagonal line extending from the ipsilateral nasal ala through the lateral canthus; ▶ Fig. 24.6).[5]

The ideal brow position in a female patient lies at the supraorbital rim medially then arching as it runs laterally. The apex of the arch should be between the lateral limbus and the lateral canthus. The male brow should be less arched and lie at the level of the supraorbital rim.

⚠

Brow position and form is different in females and males.

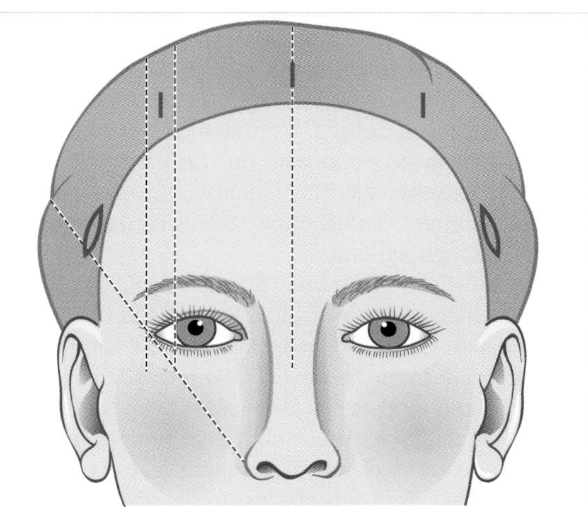

Fig. 24.6 Incision placement for endoscopic brow lifting. (Adapted with permission from Hartstein ME, Holds JB, Massry GG. Pearls and Pitfalls in Cosmetic Oculoplastic Surgery. New York: Springer; 2010.)

Care should be taken to avoid excessive raising of the medial head of the eyebrow, which creates an unnatural and operated appearance. Incisions in the hair-bearing scalp should be made parallel to the orientation of the hair follicles to avoid alopecia. The use of cautery should be minimized along the scalp incisions to avoid further injury to the follicles.

Medial to linea temporalis, the dissection is carried out in the subperiosteal plane. Laterally, the temporal fossa is dissected in a subtemporoparietal fascia plane. The lateral fossa dissection is joined with the medial subperiosteal plane by transecting the fascial condensation of linea temporalis. The zygomaticotemporal vein (sentinel vein) is identified endoscopically through the temporal incision, noting that the frontal branch of the facial nerve runs superficial to it in a perpendicular fashion. If injury to the sentinel vein occurs, it should be controlled with pressure rather than cautery to avoid injury to the frontal nerve. Medial to linea temporalis, the initial subperiosteal dissection can be undertaken blindly. From 2 cm above the superior orbital rim, endoscopic visualization is used to preserve the supraorbital neurovascular bundle. The periosteum must be transected along the arcus marginalis to adequately release the brow. To diminish central rhytids, the surgeon may choose to transect the corrugator supercilii and or the procerus muscles, although this should be done with caution due to the risk of widening the interbrow distance or overcorrecting the medial brow. Laterally, the dissection descends to the level of the lateral canthus along the bony rim. After the temporal lift is completed, an ellipse of scalp may be excised to aid in maintaining the lateral brow elevation.

The frontal periosteum is secured in the desired position by suturing it through the scalp incisions to the bone. There are numerous techniques to accomplish this, including the use of monocortical bone tunnels, titanium or bioabsorbable screws, and barb devices. The deficit in frontalis muscle function on the paralyzed side may require additional elevation beyond that needed on the innervated side. If desired, a simultaneous unilateral pretrichial lift can be performed on the paralyzed side to excise the excess tissue. The wounds are closed with deep dermal resorbable sutures and staples or nonresorbable sutures through the skin.

Alternatively, a subdermal pretrichial lift can be performed, which allows controlled resection of the forehead skin, hides the scar well, and can lower the hairline. Incisions adjacent to the hairline should be made in a trichophytic fashion by beveling the scalpel blade transversely to the hair follicles. After subdermal undermining, the resulting defect is closed in a supragaleal plane, which decreases the risk of sensory loss to the scalp. Direct and mid forehead lifts are performed in a similar fashion but have a greater risk of perceptible scars. Placing mid forehead lift incisions in skin creases at different levels on each side may aid in camouflaging the scars.

- Patients with unilateral facial paralysis should have the forehead addressed bilaterally so that symmetry can be obtained, given that brow position varies throughout the day.
- Cauterization should be avoided in the region of the sentinel vein to prevent injury to the frontal branch of the facial nerve. If bleeding occurs in this region, it is best to have an assistant apply pressure to the area, and work on the other side until the bleeding has stopped.

Complications

Complications from browlifting most commonly include asymmetry and temporary paresthesias. Inadequate arcus marginalis release, fixation, or positioning may result in abnormal brow position. Less common complications include permanent injury to the nonparalyzed facial nerve or sensory nerve injuries. There may be a foreign body reaction, pruritus, or intolerance of the fixation device. Infection, hematoma, hair loss, and noticeable scars are rare, especially in endoscopic approaches.[6]

Postoperative Care

A bland ointment is applied to the incisions and a light compressive dressing is wrapped around the forehead for 24 to 48 hours to eliminate the dead space. The patient can remove the dressing at home and a postoperative visit is scheduled 1 week later.

Outcomes

When performed on a suitable patient and with appropriate anatomic dissection, full arcus marginalis release, and bitemporal fixation, the brows should be safely returned to a normal, symmetric position. Aesthetic and functional outcomes are generally excellent.

24.3 Eyelids

It is critical to perform a detailed analysis of eyelid position and function as part of a comprehensive surgical plan. Analysis of lid position should be undertaken in a systematic fashion for each patient, and should be confirmed after the clinic visit by evaluation of photographs (► Fig. 24.7). The position of the upper lid relative to the pupil or light reflex (marginal reflex distance 1, MRD-1) is compared with the normal eye. In facial paralysis, the upper lid position when the eye is opened is typically unaffected, but the lid is often raised higher than the normal side due to loss of resting tone in the orbicularis

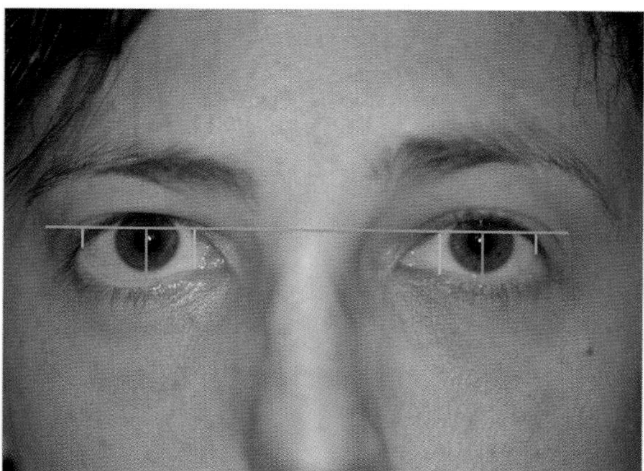

Fig. 24.7 Analysis of lid position in a patient with right facial paralysis. *Orange line*, lateral canthal height; *blue line*, marginal reflex distance 2; *yellow line*, medial canthal height.

muscle. The position of the lid on attempted closure is then checked, measuring the distance between the upper and lower lids (eyelid fissure), and noting the position on the upper lid of the point of maximum lagophthalmos. The latter is typically in the region of the midpupillary line or medial limbus.

To evaluate the position of the lower lid, the distance between the lower lid margin and the light reflex (MRD-2) is then compared with the contralateral side. The lid can be further analyzed on photographs, by drawing a line through the pupils, extending beyond the lateral orbital rims. From this horizontal line, the position of the medial canthus (medial canthal height, MCH), and lateral canthus (lateral canthal height, LCH), can be documented, demonstrating subtle changes in support and position relative to the contralateral lid. The position of the inferior lacrimal punctum relative to the caruncle should be noted. ▶ Fig. 24.7 demonstrates photographic analysis of lid position. The MRD-1 (not shown) is greater on the paralyzed side; the MCH is elevated, as is the MRD-2. The LCH is relatively symmetric, as is often the case in younger patients. Note that the affected eyebrow has also lowered.

24.3.1 Upper Lid

Weight Implantation

Patient Selection

All patients with facial paralysis must understand that their most important responsibility is to maintain ocular hydration. This typically requires the regular use of moisturizing eye drops during the day, and ophthalmic lubricant at night and possibly in the morning. During the night the eyelids may be taped shut, or other measures such as covering the eye with cellophane or a bandage containing a moisturizing bubble can be used. When outside, the use of dark glasses may ease the discomfort of bright light and offer protection from wind.

In assessing these patients, it is critical to check corneal sensation; those with diminished function of the fifth cranial nerve must be referred for evaluation and ongoing care by an ophthalmologist as they fail to sense the warning pain that accompanies a corneal ulcer.

Patients with symptoms attributable to paralytic lagophthalmos (dry eye, conjunctival erythema, pain, itching, photophobia, and wind intolerances) may be candidates for implantation of an upper eyelid weight to aid in eyelid closure and to restore a blink reflex. This is not the case for all patients with facial paralysis; those with Bell's phenomenon may be relatively asymptomatic, and therapy must be chosen on an individual basis.

Indications

Placement of a weight in the upper eyelid of a patient with paralytic lagophthalmos is indicated when symptoms occur that are refractory to therapy with moisturizing drops and ophthalmic lubricating ointment. The weight functions by replacing the function of the paralyzed facial nerve and orbicularis oculi muscle in active and spontaneous eye closure with passive gravitational closure. Given the persistent function of the third cranial nerve in opening the eye by elevation of the upper eyelid through the levator palpebrae muscle and aponeurosis, the patient is able to actively lift the eyelid and implanted weight to keep the eye open, and then relax the levator muscle to allow the eyelid to drop (▶ Fig. 24.8 and ▶ Fig. 24.9).

Temporary weights that are applied to the external lid with adhesive are available, and may be an option for patients who are unsuitable for a surgical procedure. In the authors' experience, these are not preferred by patients as a longer-term option.

> **!**
>
> If indicated as described, perform a surgical lid weight implantation. Temporary weights, fixed with adhesive to the external lid, offer a transient option or can be used longer term if the patient is unsuitable for a surgical procedure.

The timing of upper eyelid loading is often debated, and some experts advocate delayed implantation if recovery of facial nerve function is likely. The authors' practice is to implant the weight whenever it is needed. The weights are easily removed under local anesthetic should they no longer be needed, and rarely leave visible scars. It is important, however, to wait until evolution of the paralysis is complete to implant the weight. In some surgical cases involving resection of the facial nerve, the surgeon may elect to place a weight at the time of tumor

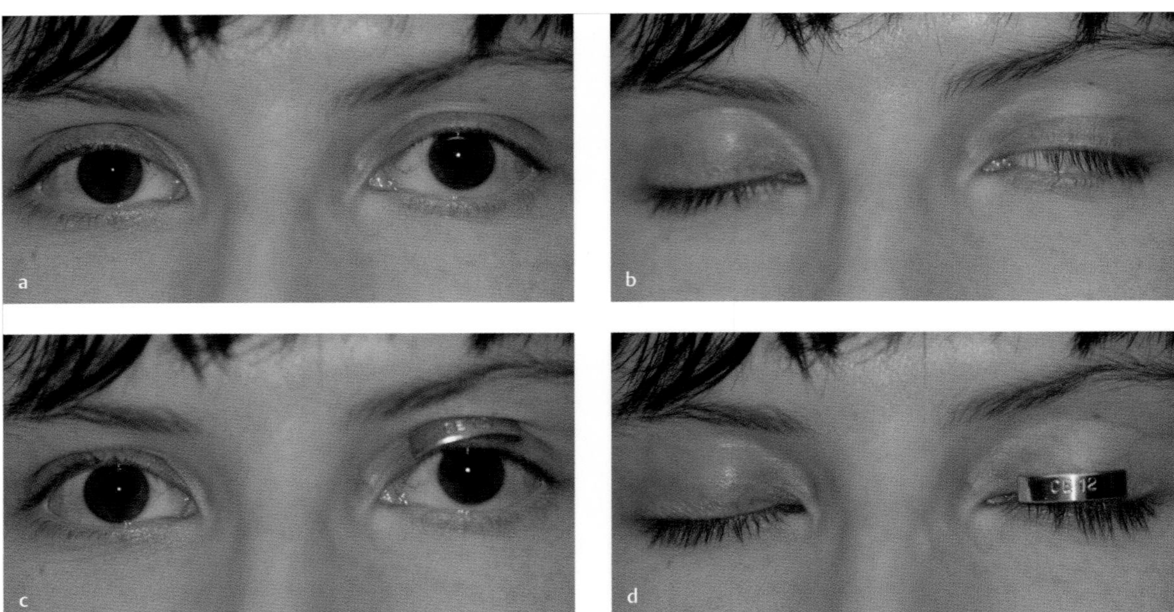

Fig. 24.8 Left facial paralysis. **(a)** Eyes open. **(b)** Attempted lid closure with marked lagophthalmos. Measuring the appropriate weight is demonstrated in **(c, d)**. **(c)** Eyes open (note minimal ptosis). **(d)** Eyes closed (note full closure).

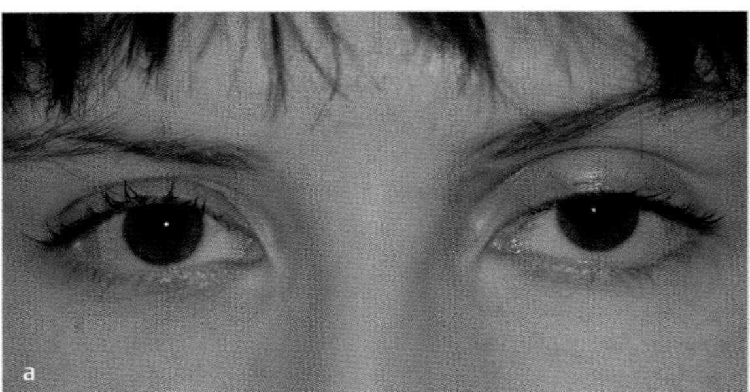

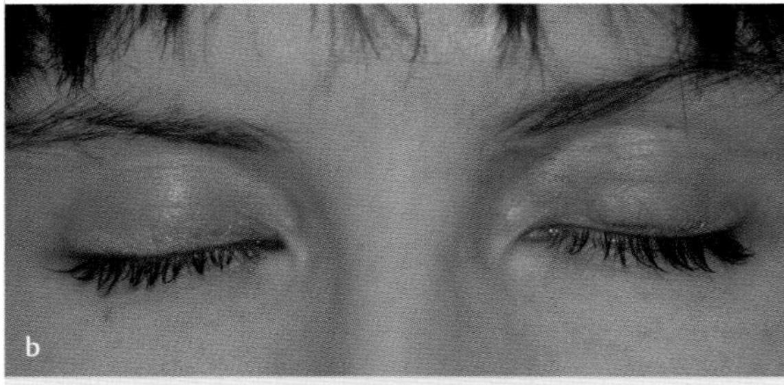

Fig. 24.9 The patient shown in ▶ Fig. 24.8, after placement of platinum chain along left upper eyelid. **(a)** Eyes open. **(b)** Eyes closed; lagophthalmos resolved.

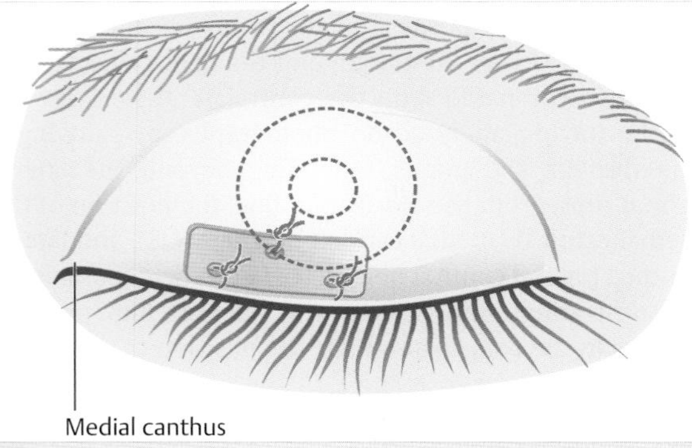

Fig. 24.10 Typical placement of weight over upper lid tarsus. (Adapted with permission from Gassner HG, Moe KS. Injury of the facial nerve. In: Eisele DW, Smith RV, eds. Complications in Head and Neck Surgery. 2nd ed. Philadelphia: Mosby; 2009:633–653.)

resection. This is suboptimal, because it does not allow precise measurement of the appropriate implant size. If the weight chosen is either too large or too small, the surgeon performing the revision is again unable to precisely measure the appropriate weight since an implant is already in place. Any high-risk patients (i.e., loss of corneal sensation, lack of Bell's phenomenon, diminished tear production) should have early surgical implantation to prevent complications.

Patient Information and Consent

Until recently, gold was the primary material used for upper lid implants. These are now being replaced by platinum implants (▶ Fig. 24.10 and ▶ Fig. 24.11). Platinum implants have an advantage over gold of being of a higher specific weight so that a smaller-volume implant can be

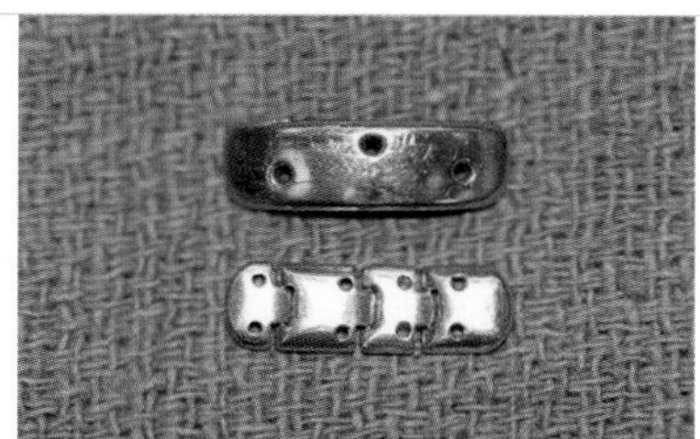

Fig. 24.11 Gold weight and platinum chain implants.

used with the same effect.[1] Berghaus et al developed a platinum chain implant that can flex and conform to the changing radius of the tarsus.[7] In a prospective study of more than 60 patients, those authors found a lower rate of complications with the platinum chain implant as compared with the fixed gold weight, and they noted excellent biocompatibility. An additional benefit of this may be a decrease in the incidence of postoperative astigmatism and improved cosmetic appearance (▶ Fig. 24.12).

Patients should be aware of the surgical risks, which include dissatisfaction with performance of the implant, extrusion, excessive lid ptosis, persistent lagophthalmos, unfavorable scarring, hematoma, and rarely infection or rejection. It is possible that the implant will need to be exchanged if the weight is not adequate. During any oculoplastic surgery there is risk of corneal abrasion or visual change.

Anesthesia and Positioning

Upper eyelid weight implantation is performed in the supine position, typically under local anesthesia with sedation.

Surgical Steps

In the preoperative setting, the patient is fitted for the appropriate weight. After cleansing the upper eyelid and eyebrow skin with an alcohol wipe, the weight is adhered to the upper eyelid with either tape or a topical adhesive. A set of nonimplantable measuring weights is used for this purpose. The weight is placed immediately superior to the upper eyelashes, centered at the point of maximal lagophthalmos (this is typically superior to the pupil or medial limbus; ▶ Fig. 24.10). It is important to place the weight as inferior as possible (without damaging the lashes) so that its mass is borne by the eyelid and not by resting on superior aspect of the globe. The authors typically begin with a 1.2 or 1.4 g weight. The patient then attempts eye closure and blinking, and should wear the weight for several minutes to determine comfort. Other weights are trialed based on this response. The weight is chosen that provides full, nearly natural lid closure with 1 mm or less of ptosis when in place. The patient must be comfortable with the weight in place.

With the patient supine on the operating table, the upper lid skin is examined and the dominant superior lid crease is marked. A small amount of local anesthetic containing epinephrine is injected subcutaneously. After the face is cleansed and draped, ophthalmic lubricant is placed on the cornea. An incision is made in the skin crease through the skin and orbicularis muscle. Dissection continues inferiorly in a preseptal plane onto the surface of the tarsus, until the follicles of the lashes are visible. The dissection should be approximately twice the width of the implant.

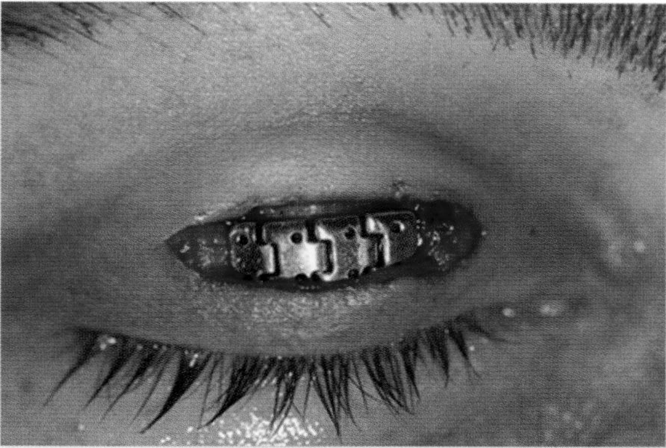

Fig. 24.12 Platinum chain smoothly contouring to the tarsus. Prelevator fat grafts were harvested and used to camouflage the medial and lateral borders of the chain.

The implant is then placed as inferior as possible on the surface of the tarsus, centered on the previously noted point of maximal lagophthalmos. The weight is then sutured to the tarsus at a minimum of four fixation points, using 7–0 resorbable or permanent monofilament suture on a spatulated ophthalmic needle. The suture is placed partial thickness in the tarsus, taking care not to penetrate the deep lamella of the lid. Less-experienced surgeons may want to place a lubricated corneal protector prior to this step to prevent corneal injury. After the sutures are placed, the upper lid is everted to confirm that the sutures do not contact the deep surface of the lid.

Platinum implants are denser than gold, and are thus smaller and less visible. Platinum chain implants have the additional advantage of being able to flex with the eyelid, which appears to decrease astigmatism and may have a lower incidence of extrusion. The weight should be placed as low on the tarsus as possible, centered at the point of maximum lagophthalmos.

If desired, 2-mm pieces of prelevator fat can be harvested from the upper lid deep to the septum. These can be placed on the lateral margins of the weight to soften the borders and help camouflage the weight. If it is noted preoperatively that there is excess upper lid skin that might interfere with function of the weight, the extra skin is excised at this point of the procedure as described in Upper Lid Blepharoplasty. The wound is then closed in two layers with resorbable 6–0 sutures through the orbicularis muscle, and interrupted 6–0 resorbable or permanent monofilament sutures through the skin.

Complications

The most common complication seen in patients referred after placement of an upper lid weight is positioning too high on the lid. As described previously, this prevents the full weight of the implant from being applied to the tarsus. Another error is attachment of the weight to the orbital septum. In the latter case, the weight is borne by the septum, which is attached to the orbital rim, rather than being transmitted to the levator aponeurosis through the tarsus. If the weight is placed too far medially or laterally, away from the point of maximal lagophthalmos, it will fail to close the lid fully. Improper weight selection may result in extrusion, lid ptosis, or persistent lagophthalmos. Weights may also migrate but this should be limited if placed directly on the tarsus deep to the orbicularis muscle, allowing it to be sealed in a circumferential muscular envelope.

Postoperative Care

Patients are asked to use at least twice daily ophthalmic ointment and frequent ophthalmic drops for at least 1 week. Patients may still need to continue using drops and ointment long-term to help with dry eyes. Sutures, if present, are removed at the postoperative visit 1 week later. Wearing dark glasses may ease the discomfort of bright light and offer protection from wind.

Outcomes

Patient outcomes are generally very good, with a significant improvement in quality of life when the weight is implanted appropriately. Patients should know that they may continue to be somewhat sensitive to wind and airborne particulate matter, and they should take appropriate precautions in those circumstances, which may be particularly problematic for some occupations.

Upper Lid Blepharoplasty

Patient Selection

Periocular facial nerve paralysis often accentuates preexisting upper eyelid skin laxity or redundancy for the reasons described previously. Since patients with paralytic lagophthalmos will have an upper eyelid weight placed through a blepharoplasty incision, performing a blepharoplasty simultaneously, when indicated, adds very little morbidity or recovery time. The preaponeurotic orbital fat can also be harvested and used to camouflage the borders of upper lid weight. Blepharoplasty of the nonparalyzed eyelid should also be considered in order to achieve symmetrical results. The patient should be evaluated for eyelid ptosis, which can be repaired at the same time as the blepharoplasty. Preoperative photographs should be taken to document dermatochalasis.

Indications

Upper eyelid blepharoplasty is indicated for patients with upper eyelid skin and or muscle laxity, which can cause functional visual impairment or aesthetic concerns. Many patients also have preaponeurotic fat herniation that requires contouring. Visual field testing with the eyelids untapped and taped should be performed to quantify the degree of visual field obstruction.

The decision to offer blepharoplasty should be the same as for the patient with aging face complaints; if the patient would be a candidate for the procedure had the facial paralysis not occurred, the same is true with facial paralysis. A critical caveat, however, is that care must be taken not to overexcise the lid skin on the paralyzed side, which could make the lagophthalmos and dry eye worse.

Patient Information and Consent

Patients should be informed of the risks of the procedure, which are listed in Complications. The most common complications include asymmetry, chemosis, and ecchymosis. Dry eye syndrome should be discussed, and preexisting symptoms of this type should be investigated.

Anesthesia and Positioning

In the preoperative area, incision markings are made with the patient sitting upright. The supratarsal crease is dotted with a marker instead of drawing a linear line to avoid excess markings. Generally, the supratarsal crease is 6 to 8 mm above the lash line in men and 8 to 10 mm in women. The medial incision border is at the level of the lacrimal punctum and laterally the incision remains within the orbital subunit. The lateral incision may be extended along a crow's foot rhytid in cases with lateral hooding. The amount of skin to be excised is determined by pinching the skin with forceps and the surgeon should see slight eversion of the lash line. In general at least 20 mm of skin should be preserved between the brow and the upper lid lash line. Markings should be made along the planned superior incision.

Upper eyelid blepharoplasty may be performed under local anesthesia, but procedure is preferably performed with the patient under conscious sedation. The patient lies in the supine position.

Surgical Steps

A small amount of local anesthetic (approximately 1 mL) with epinephrine is infiltrated into a subcutaneous plane and given about 10 minutes to take effect. An incision is made along the supratarsal crease through skin and orbicularis oculi muscle. The muscle is undermined in an inferior to superior direction with scissors and then the skin muscle flap is draped over the supratarsal crease. The amount of excess skin and muscle to be removed is again assessed to confirm that the amount of soft tissue removed will not be excessive. Fine-tipped monopolar cautery is used to trim the excess skin and orbicularis. Care should be taken not to injure the levator palpebrae and tarsus.

Next, the septum and preaponeurotic fat is contoured with the bipolar cautery as needed. Excess preaponeurotic orbital fat can be excised deep to the orbital septum if necessary, although the authors generally prefer to gently cauterize the septum to support the fat, rather than excising tissue. It is critical that meticulous hemostasis be performed to prevent postoperative hematoma. The orbicularis muscle is reapproximated with 6–0 absorbable suture making sure not to incorporate the orbital septum with the closure. The superficial skin is closed with a 6–0 resorbable or permanent monofilament suture in a subcuticular fashion. The most lateral aspects of the blepharoplasty incision are closed with simple interrupted sutures for additional support.

> Blepharoplasty is indicated in the patient who would benefit from the procedure for cosmetic or functional reasons on the innervated side. Aesthetic outcomes are best if the procedure is performed bilaterally. Skin excision should be conservative to avoid worsening lagophthalmos; the appropriate skin excision will lead to mild vertical rotation of the eyelashes without changing the position of the lid.

Complications

Postoperative complications include lid asymmetry, ecchymosis, hematoma, lid ptosis, lagophthalmos, dry eye, and chemosis. Corneal injuries may occur during the procedure or in the postoperative period from eye rubbing. Dissection deep to the orbital septum may injure the levator palpebrae if it is not correctly identified. Furthermore, incorporating the orbital septum in the closure may result in malposition of the supratarsal crease and possible lagophthalmos. Diplopia from extraocular muscle injury and direct injury to the globe is rare and should not occur with careful dissection. In the rare but devastating cases of retrobulbar hemorrhage, increased pressure in the orbital compartment may lead to vision loss if immediate surgical decompression by lateral canthotomy and cantholysis is not performed.[6]

Postoperative Care

Patients are asked to frequently apply ophthalmic drops and twice daily ophthalmic ointment for at least 1 week. Patients may continue to use drops and ointment to help with dry eyes. The patient should ice the operative site as tolerated for the first 48 hours and should avoid rubbing eyelid for 2 weeks. Sutures are removed at the postoperative visit 1 week later.

Outcomes

Generally, patients have excellent outcomes. As stated, although prospective studies of this technique have yet to be performed, the authors believe that conservative blepharoplasty, when indicated, can substantially improve upper lid weighting outcomes for patients with paralytic lagophthalmos. The performance of bilateral blepharoplasty will significantly improve the patient's appearance.

24.3.2 Correction of Lower Lid Malposition

Dysfunction of the lower eyelid may contribute substantially to the morbidity of facial paralysis. Unlike the upper lid, however, gravity exacerbates paralytic lower lid malposition. This contributes to exposure of the cornea and conjunctiva, and exacerbates evaporation of the tear layer.

As a result of excessive drying, there may be reflex hypersecretion of tears. This, along with failure of the lower lid to conduct tears to and through the lacrimal system, can lead to lateral dripping of tears that may prevent the patient going out in public or doing activities such as reading books. In a prospective evaluation of ophthalmologic complaints of patients with facial paralysis, epiphora was found to be the chief ophthalmologic complaint in 75% of patients with facial paralysis.[8]

> !
>
> Whereas upper lid loading is often considered, the patient's complaints with the dysfunction of the lower lid might be underestimated. In point of fact, this can be a major problem for the patients that should be addressed.

Thus, correction of lower lid malposition is frequently required for patients with facial paralysis. In facial paralysis, the atonic orbicularis muscle fails to raise and support the lower eyelid and maintain its resting position adjacent to the globe. Furthermore, it becomes part of the problem by adding weight to the lower eyelid and its support structures. Surgical correction seeks to reinforce the support structures of the lower eyelid so that they can both handle the soft tissue weight and maintain the eyelid in its normal position. Inferior lacrimal punctum repositioning against the lacrimal lake will also improve the passive flow of tears into the nose.

Lower lid laxity presents as a spectrum of lid malposition that may vary depending on the patient's age and underlying skin quality. The lateral canthal tendon is

Table 24.1 Ectropion Grading Scale

Grade	Description	Grade	Description
0	Normal eyelid appearance and function	L	Predominantly lateral
I	Normal eyelid appearance but minimally symptomatic; laxity present on examination	M	Predominantly medial
II	Scleral show without eversion of the eyelid	t	Previous tarsorrhaphy or blepharorrhaphy
III	Ectropion without eversion of the inferior lacrimal punctum		
IV	Advanced ectropion with eversion of the punctum from the lacrimal lake		
V	Ectropion with a complication (e.g., conjunctival metaplasia, retraction of the anterior lamella, or stenosis of the lacrimal system)		

Source: Reproduced from Moe KS, Kao C-H. Precaruncular medial canthopexy. Arch Facial Plast Surg 2005;7(4):244–250.

longer and weaker than the medial canthal tendon. As such, milder laxity presents as increased corneal exposure in the lateral lid, and spreads medially with more advanced pathology. In severe cases, the lateral and or medial lid actually falls away from the globe. When this occurs in the medial lid, the inferior lacrimal punctum falls away from the lacrimal lake, rendering the already passive drain system completely incompetent. The goal of surgical repositioning should therefore be to restore that lateral lid to its original or a somewhat more elevated position, so that it can guide tears inferomedially toward the inferior punctum. In addition, the procedure should restore the position of the medial lid so that the inferior punctum is rotated posteriorly to coapt with the lacrimal lake where it can syphon tears into the drainage system.

Patient Selection

The choice of the appropriate canthopexy procedure to treat the medial and lateral canthus is based on the correct diagnosis. The Ectropion Grading Scale (EGS) describes the degree and location of medial and lateral canthal pathology. The use of EGS aids in the selection of the proper technique for correction (▶ Table 24.1, ▶ Fig. 24.13 and ▶ Fig. 24.14).[8,9] A canthoplasty (lateral tarsal strip) may be performed when the horizontal length of the lid was excessive in the premorbid state, as judged by the contralateral lid tone. In the majority of cases when horizontal lid shortening is not necessary, lateral transorbital canthopexy (LTC) should be used.

For EGS LIII or higher, medial canthopexy is often required in addition to LTC. Restoration of medial canthal position must be performed in a manner that restores the appropriate three-dimensional position of the medial canthus, tightening medially, posteriorly, and superiorly. This cannot be achieved by tightening the anterior limb of the medial canthus; rather, the posterior limb (Horner muscle) must be tightened. This, like LTC, is performed

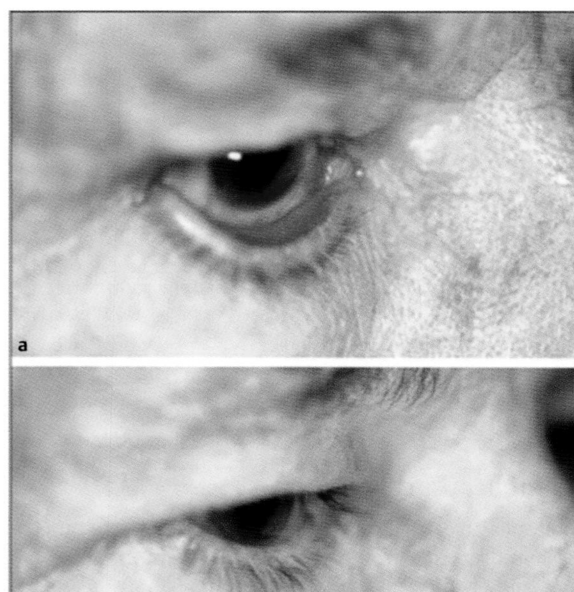

Fig. 24.13 Oblique views of paralytic ectropion in the right eye. **(a)** Preoperative appearance shows Ectropion Grading Scale grade LIV, MIV. Note that the lower eyelid has fallen away from the globe medially and laterally. **(b)** Appearance after lateral transorbital canthopexy and precaruncular medial canthopexy shows Ectropion Grading Scale grade LI, MI. Note the return of the medial canthus to the normal position against the lacrimal lake. (Reproduced from Moe KS, Kao C-H. Precaruncular medial canthopexy. Arch Facial Plast Surg 2005;7(4):244–250.)

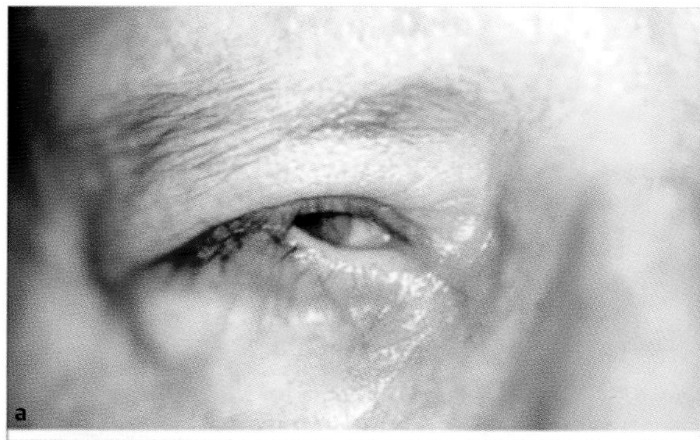
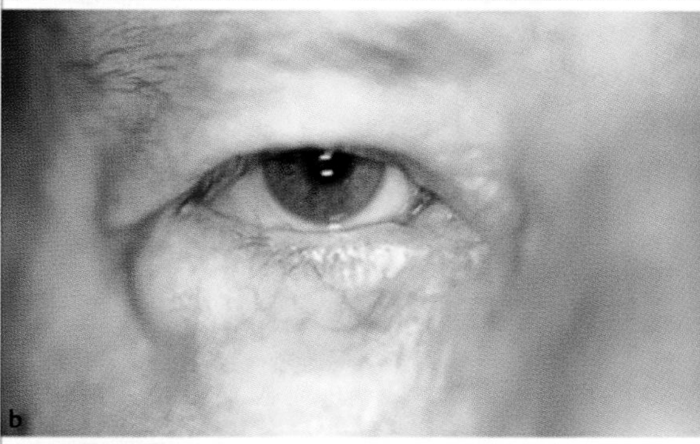
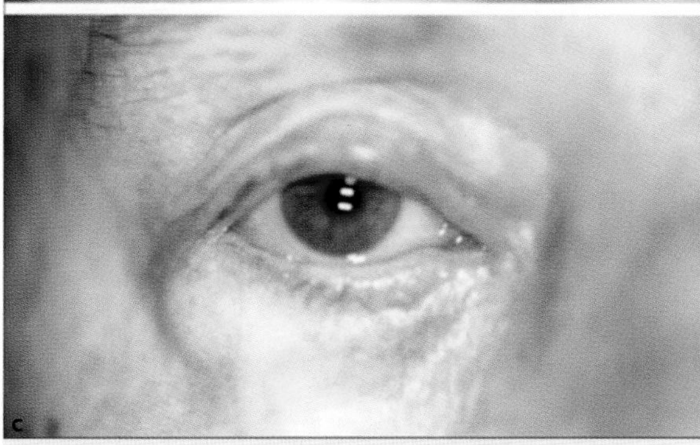

Fig. 24.14 Anterior views of ectropion in the right eye. **(a)** Preoperative appearance shows Ectropion Grading Scale grade Lt, MIV. Note the lateral tarsorrhaphy with blockage of the visual fields. Gold weight is present in the upper eyelid but is not visible. The medial canthus is displaced anteriorly, and the inferior lacrimal punctum does not contact the lacrimal lake. **(b)** Appearance after reversal of the lateral tarsorrhaphy, with lateral transorbital canthopexy to correct lateral laxity, shows Ectropion Grading Scale grade LI, MIII. Note the inferior displacement of the medial canthus that occurs after reversal of the tarsorrhaphy, resulting in excessive medial canthal height. **(c)** Appearance after precaruncular medial canthopexy, brow-lift, and upper blepharoplasty shows grade LI, MI. The medial canthal position and medial canthal height are now normal. Gold weight in the upper eyelid is now visible. (Reproduced from Moe KS, Kao C-H. Precaruncular medial canthopexy. Arch Facial Plast Surg 2005;7(4):244–250.)

from an approach deep to the canthus, leaving the canthal structures intact, and restoring their original position through a procedure termed precaruncular medial canthopexy (PMC).

Preoperative photographs should be examined closely to rule out other abnormalities of eyelid position. If a negative lower lid/maxilla vector is present, then patients may require a midface lift in addition to LTC of the lateral canthus.

Patient Information and Consent

Any oculoplastic procedure carries a small risk of corneal abrasion, or temporary or permanent visual loss. There is typically a mild amount of edema over the lateral orbital rim, most of which subsides over 1 week. At times there is a small amount of hooding of the upper lid skin over the incision, but this resolves as well.

Anesthesia and Positioning

These procedures can be performed under local anesthesia with sedation. However, as the procedures are performed deep to the canthus and may require drilling, the patient and surgeon may prefer the administration of general anesthesia. Patients lie supine throughout the procedures. If the procedures are to be performed under local or sedation, anesthetic drops are placed on the conjunctiva.

Surgical Steps

Medial Canthopexy

Lower lid paralysis with loss of active support from the orbicularis oculi muscle may lead to laxity of the medial canthal complex with anterior, inferior, and lateral displacement of the medial lower lid and canaliculus (▶ Fig. 24.13). Anatomic correction of the medial canthus can be difficult because of the presence of the lacrimal system and the proximity to the orbital contents. There are many techniques described to reposition the medial canthus including wedge excisions, medial tarsal strip tightening, and medial or lateral tarsorrhaphy. Some of these techniques can actually worsen the position of the medial canthus and pull the eyelid away from the globe or block vision (▶ Fig. 24.14). Most procedures increase horizontal or vertical eyelid tension but fail to address the anteroposterior vector. PMC is able to tighten the medial eyelid in all necessary three vectors (horizontal, vertical, and anterioposterior) and effectively reposition the inferior punctum without damaging the lacrimal system (▶ Fig. 24.15).[9]

First, a corneal shield is placed followed by injection of 1 to 2 mL local anesthetic with epinephrine in the region of the medial canthus medial to the caruncle. Superior and inferior lacrimal probes are inserted to protect the lacrimal system and fine scissors are used to make a precaruncular incision between the skin and caruncle

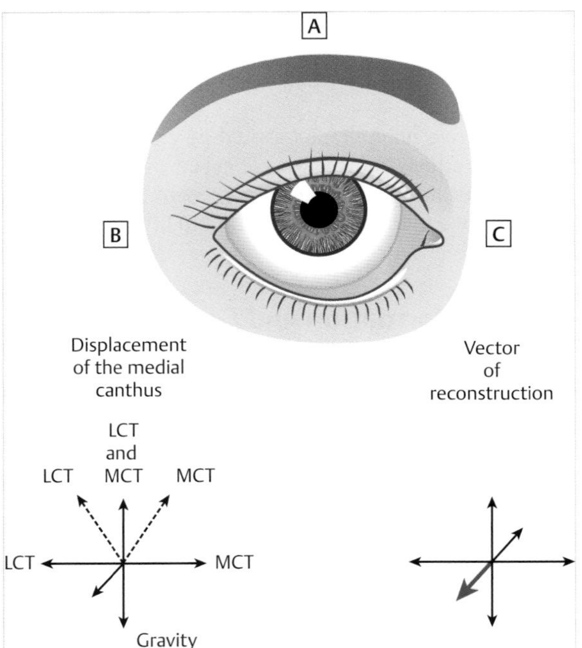

Fig. 24.15 The forces of displacement and reconstruction in medial ectropion. (A) Anterior, inferior, and lateral displacement of the medial canthus and the inferior canaliculus. (B) Eyelid support in medial ectropion. The thick solid arrow demonstrates the net force on the lower eyelid; the horizontal solid line, the support of the medial (MCT) and lateral (LCT) canthal tendons before repositioning; the dashed lines, how the forces of the MCT and LCT can be repositioned superiorly, horizontally, and posteriorly; and the vertical solid line, the condition after reconstruction when the net sum of the forces exerted by the repositioned canthus counteract the force exerted by gravity. (C) The red arrow demonstrates the direction of displacement before surgery, and the black arrow depicts the net counteracting force when the medial canthus has been properly repositioned in a posterior, superior, and lateral position. LCT, lateral canthal tendon; MCT, medial canthal tendon. (Adapted from Moe KS, Kao C-H. Precaruncular medial canthopexy. Arch Facial Plast Surg 2005;7(4):244–250.)

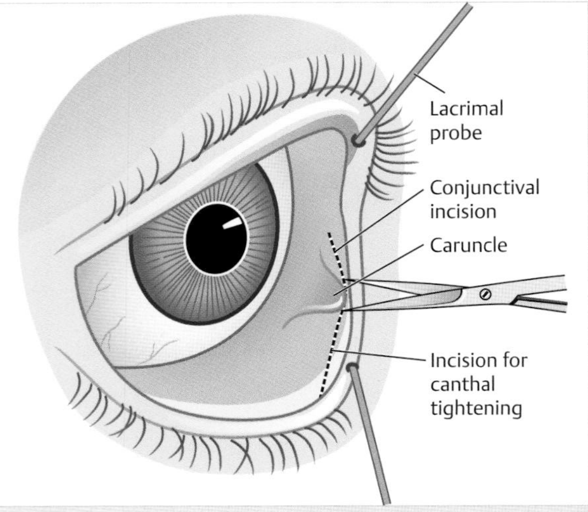

Fig. 24.16 Conjunctival incision for the precaruncular approach. Lacrimal probes are placed in the superior and inferior lacrimal puncta. The scissors demonstrate the initial conjunctival incision. The incision may be continued laterally for additional access to the orbital floor (*dark dashed line*) or anteriorly for full access to the medial canthal tendon and tarsal plate (*light dashed line*). (Adapted from Moe KS, Kao C-H. Precaruncular medial canthopexy. Arch Facial Plast Surg 2005;7(4):244–250.)

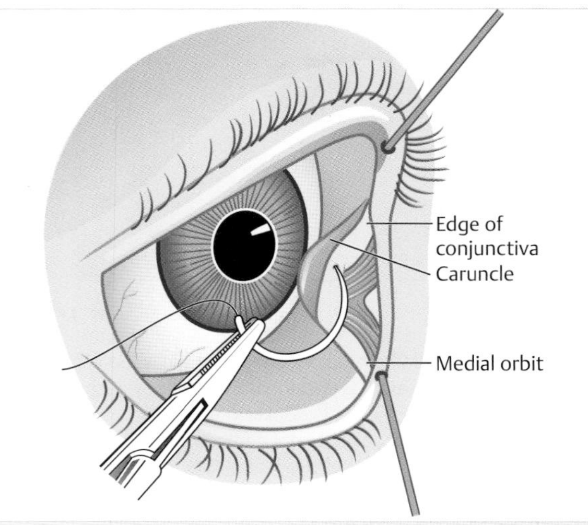

Fig. 24.17 Completed precaruncular approach to the medial orbit. The caruncle and adjacent conjunctiva are retracted laterally. A suture is placed along the posterosuperior lacrimal crest. (Adapted from Moe KS, Kao C-H. Precaruncular medial canthopexy. Arch Facial Plast Surg 2005;7(4):244–250.)

(▸ Fig. 24.16). To prevent damage to the lacrimal canals, monopolar cautery should be avoided in this area.

Dissection continues medially along the posterior limb of the medial canthal tendon (Horner muscle) to its attachment on the posterior lacrimal crest. A 5–0 permanent monofilament suture is then passed through the periosteum at the superior aspect of the posterior lacrimal crest, superior to the lacrimal sac. Previously the authors placed a resorbable screw in this area, but have since found fixation to the periosteum to be adequate (▸ Fig. 24.17 and ▸ Fig. 24.18). The lacrimal probes and corneal shield are then removed, and the other end of the suture is anchored deeply to the medial end of the tarsal plate as close to the eyelid margin as possible, immediately lateral to the lacrimal punctum (▸ Fig. 24.18). If the suture is placed too low, the punctum will remain everted, causing epiphora. Positioning of the suture as high as possible on the tarsus is essential.

If PMC is performed without LTC, the suture is then tied on itself, providing the appropriate tension to raise, medialize, and posteriorly tighten the medial canthus as

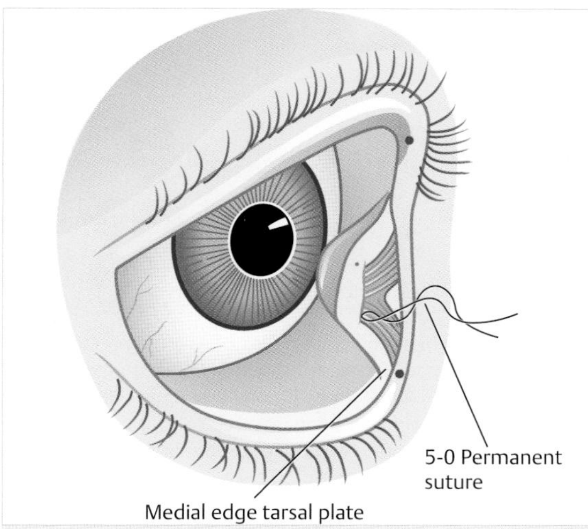

Fig. 24.18 A 5-0 permanent suture spans from the medial edge of the tarsal plate (immediately lateral to the lacrimal punctum) to the posterosuperior lacrimal crest. (Adapted from Moe KS, Kao C-H. Precaruncular medial canthopexy. Arch Facial Plast Surg 2005;7(4):244–250.)

desired. Slight overcorrection (1 mm) is desirable. The inferior punctum should be checked for proper inversion and elevation. The incision is closed using a 5–0 absorbable suture placed between the apex of the caruncle and the medial eyelid.[9]

If PMC and LTC are undertaken together, the sutures for the lateral and medial canthi are both placed before either canthus is tightened. Tension can then be placed on the sutures to determine how best to position the lid. When the appropriate amount of tension has been determined, the medial canthus sutures are fixated first, followed by the lateral canthal sutures. There is a tendency to begin by tightening the lateral sutures, but this may pull the entire lid laterally, exacerbating malposition of the inferior punctum. By repositioning the medial lid first, this problem is avoided.

Lateral Tarsal Strip

A 1 cm lateral canthotomy is made followed by cantholysis. The lid is positioned optimally and then a mark is made at the desired resection point. The superior eyelash margin is excised with scissors and then the skin of the anterior lid is dissected and removed. The posterior conjunctiva is de-epithelialized with the bipolar cautery. The canthal tendon is trimmed to the appropriate length. Q-tips are used to create a visible pocket along the lateral orbital wall, while preserving periosteum. Two 5–0 permanent monofilament sutures are placed to secure the lid to the lateral orbital wall. The superior and inferior grey lines are reapproximated with 5–0 polyglactin suture which is secured to the lateral orbital wall (lateral to the tarsal strip sutures). The skin incisions are closed with 6–0 permanent monofilament suture.

Transorbital Lateral Canthopexy

The authors prefer transorbital lateral canthopexy to wedge resections and the tarsal strip procedures, as the latter commonly result in asymmetry and an overriding appearance of the upper lid over the lower lid. Furthermore, it is more difficult to judge and create the appropriate lid tension when a portion of the lid is resected. Because LTC does not disrupt the lateral canthus or transect components of the lid, this judgment is simpler. With an EGS LIII or greater, PMC is typically indicated in addition to LTC.

Precise analysis and diagnosis is critical. The lid position should be staged with the Ectropion Grading Scale, as described. Care should be taken to treat the medial canthus when indicated; an attempt to correct the lid by a lateral procedure alone may pull the inferior canaliculus laterally, worsening the lid position and function. Grade IIIL or higher malposition should undergo precaruncular medial canthopexy (PMC) in addition to lateral transorbital canthopexy.

When performing PMC, it is important to place the fixation suture as high on the medial aspect of the tarsus as possible to ensure that the entire lid margin rotates up and against the lacrimal lake.

After local anesthetic with epinephrine is injected, a 1 cm incision is made lateral to the canthus over the lateral orbital rim. The orbital aspect of the orbicularis oculi muscle is transected, and the periosteum of the arcus marginalis is incised. The insertion of the lateral canthal tendon is identified and sharply elevated off of the orbital rim in one unit. Size 4–0 monofilament permanent sutures are placed through the medial aspect of the lateral canthal tendon at the canthal angle and through the lateral inferior tarsal plate. Two 1-mm holes are drilled through the orbital rim approximately 2 mm posterosuperior to Whitnall's tubercle in the region of the zygomaticofrontal suture so that the eyelid can be elevated (▶ Fig. 24.19). The sutures are placed through the holes and tightened until the desired eyelid position is achieved. The wound is then closed in layers.[1] If desired, previously performed tarsorrhaphies can be reversed using LTC if the patient has normal corneal sensation and Bell's response.

Complications

These procedures are quite safe. The most common complications of lower eyelid repositioning include temporary chemosis and failure to resuspend the canthal

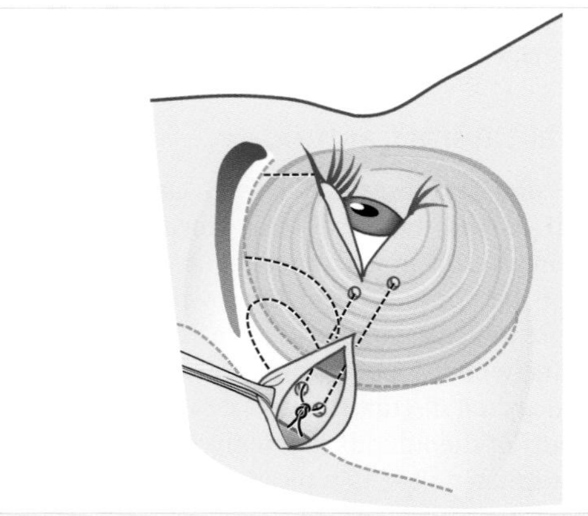

Fig. 24.19 Lateral transorbital canthopexy. (Adapted with permission from Gassner HG, Moe KS. Injury of the facial nerve. In: Eisele DW, Smith RV, eds. Complications in Head and Neck Surgery. 2nd ed. Philadelphia: Mosby; 2009:633–653.)

tendon appropriately. Corneal injuries may occur during the procedures or postoperatively from patients rubbing their eyes. Complications of lower eyelid repositioning include possible diplopia from extraocular muscle injury, or direct injury to the globe from traction or instrumentation. If a retrobulbar hemorrhage occurs, the increased in orbital pressure can lead to compartment syndrome and vision loss.[6]

Postoperative Care

The patient should place iced saline sponges on the operative site as tolerated for the first 48 hours and should avoid rubbing eyelid for 2 weeks. Ophthalmic drops and lubrication should be used as indicated. Patients are seen back in the clinic 1 week after surgery.

Outcomes

Most patients experience significant improvement in their symptoms and aesthetic appearance with lower eyelid repositioning (▶ Fig. 24.20; compare ▶ Fig. 24.1). Patients may complain of pruritus and erythema, and they will experience a degree of continued epiphora as long as the orbicularis oculi muscle is paralyzed. There is risk of malposition recurrence and need of revision. The risk of infection and scarring is rare.[9]

24.3.3 Midface Lift

Patient Selection

In the patient with significant paralytic ptosis of the midfacial soft tissue structures, more aggressive measures beyond canthal tendon resuspension are necessary. In these patients, active midface support is lost and a component of this support is transferred to the medial and lateral canthal tendons. Midface lifts can esthetically and functionally restore facial symmetry while adding support of the lower eyelid and improving nasal function.

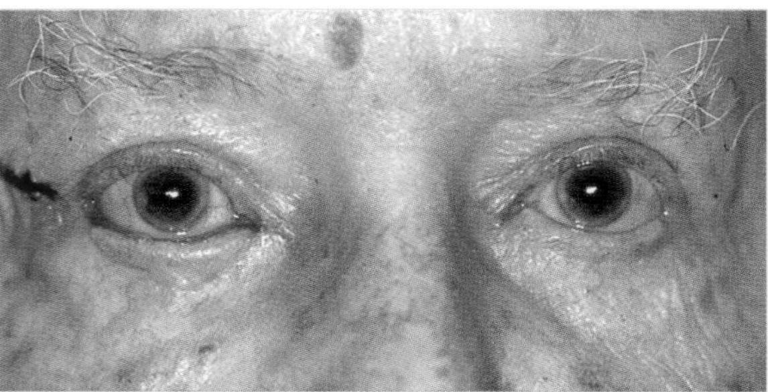

Fig. 24.20 The patient shown in ▶ Fig. 24.1, after lateral transorbital canthopexy, precaruncular medial canthopexy, upper lid weight, bilateral brow lift, bilateral upper blepharoplasty. Metaplasia of lower lid margin resolving. Note that the left brow has relaxed and descended to normal position after repositioning the paralyzed side.

!

In patients with facial palsy, dysfunction of the lower eyelid may not end at the inferior border of orbital rim and lower eyelid, but involve also the midface. Treatment of the midface might be necessary to receive optimal functional results for lower eyelid reanimation.

Patient Information and Consent

Patients should be aware of the goals of the surgery. The risks of the procedure are explained in Complications. Substantial elevation of the midface will support the lower eyelid. Due to intentional mild overcorrection, in the procedure may result in temporary asymmetry of the midface unless bilateral procedures are performed.

Anesthesia and Positioning

The midface lift is performed under general anesthesia, or local anesthetic with intravenous sedation, with the patient lying supine.

Surgical Steps

An incision is placed in the gingivobuccal sulcus, and subperiosteal dissection is used to elevate the soft tissues to the orbital rim and malar eminence. The infraorbital nerve is identified and preserved. An oblique incision is made a few centimeters behind the temporal hairline (as described for the endoscopic browlift). An avascular plane deep to the temporoparietal fascia and superficial to the superficial layer of the deep temporal fascia is developed. As the dissection proceeds anteriorly toward the course of the frontal branch of the facial nerve, the dissection transitions deep to the superficial layer of the temporal fat. This dissection proceeds over the zygomatic arch in a subperiosteal plane, and connects with the previous sublabial dissection. Two or three 3–0 polydioxanone sutures are placed in the inferior aspects of the dissected malar periosteum, pulled through the zygomatic tunnel into the temporal fossa, and fixed to the temporalis fascia. Alternatively, the Endotine (Coapt Systems, Inc.) can be used for elevation and fixation.

Another technique involves the use of a transconjunctival or subciliary incision with preorbital septal dissection that can be performed instead of the temporal incision. In these approaches, the dissection is connected with the previous sublabial dissection. Four 1-mm drill holes are burred along the rim making sure to protect the globe with a retractor. Three 3–0 permanent monofilament sutures suspend the midface periosteum, suborbicularis oculi fat, and orbicularis muscle to the burred holes. It may be difficult suspend the midface soft tissues to the superior orbital rim periosteum, especially if there is inadequate periosteal integrity, such as in irradiated orbits. It can also be difficult to find adequate orbital rim or floor periosteum to anchor to via a transconjunctival incision. Failure to permanently fixate the soft tissue may lead to further descent of the lower eyelid.

Finally a conservative excision of the skin at the lid–cheek junction is performed. The authors prefer to leave more skin and allow the bunching to improve with time rather than close the skin incision under any tension.

Postoperative Care

A significant component of the pathology underlying lower lid malposition is often descent of the midfacial soft tissue. Restoration of this will improve appearance and allow restoration of lid position by lateral transorbital canthopexy and precaruncular medial canthopexy. As for the other procedures described herein, bilateral surgery will have the optimal outcome.

A follow-up visit is made 1 week after surgery when sutures are removed. Patients are asked to not partake in strenuous activity that may lead to hematoma formation in the weeks after surgery.

Complications

Complications of midface lift procedures include failure to adequately resuspend the lid–cheek soft tissues. Most common symptoms include asymmetry, edema, and chemosis, which may last for several months. Injury to the facial nerve may occur, which would be symptomatic on the nonparalytic side. Patients may palpate the buried Endotines for months, which can also be a source of pruritus. Dissection through the temporal fat pad may lead to fat atrophy and temporal soft tissue wasting. Infections are rare but are a real possibility especially when an oral approach is also used. Patients need to be monitored for possible hematomas.

Outcomes

In general, midface lift outcomes are good. Patients need to be made aware that it may take several months for the edema to resolve. Asymmetry can be avoided by performing the procedure bilaterally.

24.4 Adjuvant Measures

24.4.1 Botulinum Toxin

Chemodenervation with botulinum toxin type A can be used to improve facial symmetry by treating the paralyzed side of the face; more details are given in Chapter 25. Patients have excellent improvement in their facial symmetry and quality of life with a single treatment, which lasts up to 6 months.[10] Botulinum toxin type A can also be used to improve synkinesis by treating nonparalyzed face. Treatment of synkinesis can be a challenging issue since it requires weakening the muscles in the paralyzed side, which may worsen symptoms of paralysis. It is important to not overtreat the synkinetic side. The recommended dose for Botox (onabotulinumtoxinA) is less than 8 international units (IU) into the paretic orbicularis oculi muscle, which is far less than what is injected in the nonparalyzed face to improve symmetry.[11] It is important to report the off-label use of botulinum toxin type A to patients. The conversion of Botox to Dysport (abobotulinumtoxinA) has been reported 3:1, but providers will need to determine the correct dosage at their own discretion.[12]

Generally, anesthesia is not necessary especially when using a small 30-gauge needle and tuberculin syringe. If patient is intolerant of pain, consider preinjecting with a local anesthetic, icing, or applying a topical anesthetic 30 minutes before treatment. Patients usually sit up right for the procedure. Typically, 10 to 20 IU botulinum toxin type A is injected into the frontalis, procerus, and corrugator muscles. Reconstitution of botulinum toxin type A with 5 mL 1% lidocaine can produce immediate paralysis of the injected musculature, which allows the provider to see the outcome. Patients are asked to not lie down for 4 hours following treatment to prevent transmission to unwanted areas such as the levator palpebrae muscle. Usually the results are observed 2 to 3 days after the injection.

Outcomes are generally excellent and patients will require repeated injections approximately every 3 months. Most common complications include bruising and mild edema, and rarely is lid ptosis or infection seen. It is best to wait 10 to 14 days prior to reinjecting areas that need more treatment.

24.4.2 Fillers and Fat

Patients whose facial nerve function is expected to return may undergo temporary procedure with hyaluronic acid (HA) fillers; see also Chapter 25. These fillers typically last between 9 to 15 months and are reversible with hyaluronidase. HA fillers have been used for upper lid loading to manage paralytic lagophthalmos.[13,14] Fillers may be considered in patients who are poor surgical candidates or would not tolerate placement of upper lid weight under local anesthetic. However, most patients do tolerate the gold standard upper lid weight implantations under local anesthesia. Filler injections in the upper lid may cause lid ptosis, irregularities, infection, erythema, edema, and rarely skin necrosis or blindness.

Autologous fat grafts and HA filler can be considered when lower lid support is necessary because of ectropion.[15,16] Most of these patients would benefit from a midface lift, which offers a more definitive outcome, but is associated with postoperative morbidity and long recovery times. Fat grafts and HA fillers can be considered for post-midface lift touch up work. HA fillers are temporary and reversible but autologous fat grafting may provide good long-term outcomes.

24.5 Key Points

- Unilateral facial palsy can be a bilateral problem for the eyes. Compensatory contralateral hypertonicity can affect the facial muscles of the contralateral eye.
- Unilateral facial paralysis patients should have the forehead addressed bilaterally so that symmetry can be obtained.
- The brow position should be examined when performing upper lid loading. Failure to address brow ptosis can lead to suboptimal function of the lid loading.
- Platinum implants have been shown to be superior to the commonly used gold weights. Platinum chain implants have the additional advantage of being able to flex with the eyelid.
- Blepharoplasty is indicated in patients who would benefit from the procedure on the innervated side, either for cosmetic of function concerns. Aesthetic outcomes are best if blepharoplasty is performed bilaterally. Skin excision should be conservative to avoid worsening lagophthalmos.
- Unlike the upper eyelid, which is commonly addressed with a loading weight, the dysfunction of the lower lid is many times underestimated. Lower eyelid dysfunction can be a major problem for the patients that should be addressed.
- The Ectropion Grading Scale (EGS) describes the degree and location of medial and lateral canthal pathology. Use of EGS aids in the selection of the proper technique for correction.
- A midface lift may optimize functional results of a lower lid surgery in facial palsy patients.

References

[1] Gassner HG, Moe KS. Injury of the facial nerve. In: Eisele DW, Smith RV, eds. Complications in Head and Neck Surgery. 2nd ed. Philadelphia: Mosby; 2009:633–653

[2] Pepper J-P, Kim JC, Massry GG. A surgical algorithm for lower eyelid resuspension in facial nerve paralysis. Oper Tech Otolaryngol 2012; 23: 248–252

[3] Bergeron CM, Moe KS. The evaluation and treatment of upper eyelid paralysis. Facial Plast Surg 2008; 24: 220–230

[4] Henstrom DK, Lindsay RW, Cheney ML, Hadlock TA. Surgical treatment of the periocular complex and improvement of quality of life in patients with facial paralysis. Arch Facial Plast Surg 2011; 13: 125–128

[5] Hartstein ME, Holds JB, Massry GG. Pearls and Pitfalls in Cosmetic Oculoplastic Surgery. New York: Springer; 2010

[6] Sykes JM, Kim J-E, Papel ID. Facelift complications. In: Capone RB, Sykes JM, eds. Complications in Facial Plastic Surgery Prevention and Management. New York: Thieme; 2012

[7] Berghaus A, Neumann K, Schrom T. The platinum chain: a new upper-lid implant for facial palsy. Arch Facial Plast Surg 2003; 5: 166–170

[8] Moe KS, Linder T. The lateral transorbital canthopexy for correction and prevention of ectropion: report of a procedure, grading system, and outcome study. Arch Facial Plast Surg 2000; 2: 9–15

[9] Moe KS, Kao C-H. Precaruncular medial canthopexy. Arch Facial Plast Surg 2005; 7: 244–250

[10] Salles AG, Toledo PN, Ferreira MC. Botulinum toxin injection in long-standing facial paralysis patients: improvement of facial symmetry observed up to 6 months. Aesthetic Plast Surg 2009; 33: 582–590

[11] Salles AG. Discussion: quantitative measurement of evolution of post-paretic ocular synkinesis treated with botulinum toxin type A. Plast Reconstr Surg 2013; 132: 1265–1267

[12] do Nascimento Remigio AF, Salles AG, de Faria JCM, Ferreira MC. Comparison of the efficacy of onabotulinumtoxinA and abobotulinumtoxinA at the 1: 3 conversion ratio for the treatment of asymmetry after long-term facial paralysis. Plast Reconstr Surg 2015; 135: 239–249

[13] Mancini R, Taban M, Lowinger A et al. Use of hyaluronic acid gel in the management of paralytic lagophthalmos: the hyaluronic acid gel "gold weight". Ophthal Plast Reconstr Surg 2009; 25: 23–26

[14] Martín-Oviedo C, García I, Lowy A, Scola E, Aristegui M, Scola B. Hyaluronic acid gel weight: a nonsurgical option for the management of paralytic lagophthalmos. Laryngoscope 2013; 123: E91–E96

[15] Caviggioli F, Klinger F, Villani F, Fossati C, Vinci V, Klinger M. Correction of cicatricial ectropion by autologous fat graft. Aesthetic Plast Surg 2008; 32: 555–557

[16] Fezza JP. Nonsurgical treatment of cicatricial ectropion with hyaluronic acid filler. Plast Reconstr Surg 2008; 121: 1009–1014

25 Adjuvant Treatment with Botulinum Toxin and Fillers

Claus Wittekindt

25.1 Introduction

Botulinum toxin (BTX) and injectable cosmetics have become very popular to treat lines on the face. The neurotoxin is preferred for active facial lines, and dermal fillers are used mainly to treat firmly established wrinkles (▶ Fig. 25.1). Cosmetic procedures with BTX account for approximately one-third of all cosmetic procedures, frequently in conjunction with dermal filler therapy. Despite excellent records on safety and efficacy in published studies, injectable agents do carry risks of severe complications. These procedures require in-depth knowledge of facial anatomy and injection techniques to ensure patient satisfaction. Hands-on-training is crucial in learning how to provide both treatments.

25.2 Botulinum Toxin

BTX inhibits presynaptic acetylcholine release from nerve terminals causing temporary paralysis of targeted skeletal muscles. In glandular tissue it inhibits cholinergic parasympathetic nerve function. It causes the fatal disease botulism, and a single gram of crystalline toxin might be able to kill more than one million people.[1] *Clostridium botulinum*, from which the toxin is derived, was first isolated at the end of the 19th century. The ability of its toxin to block neuromuscular transmission was discovered in 1949. Pioneering work was published from Scott who established the use of BTX for the treatment of strabismus over 25 years ago.[2] In 1989 BTX was approved for blepharospasm, hemifacial spasm, torticollis, and strabismus. In 2002 it was approved for cosmetic treatment of moderate-to-severe glabellar lines. Today use of BTX has become the number one cosmetic procedure and it is widely used for the treatment of rhytids of the glabella, forehead, and eyelids. For many indications related to facial palsy, BTX is not approved, i.e., for such indications it is applied as an off-label use.

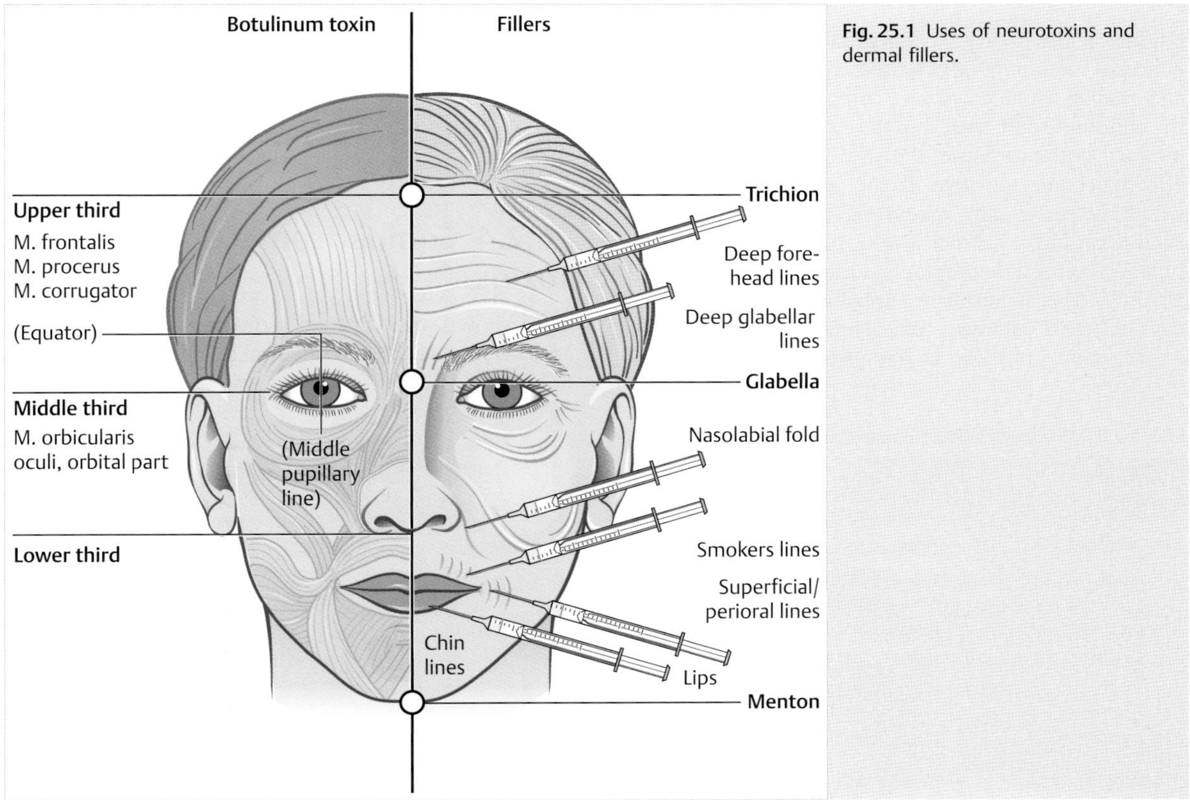

Fig. 25.1 Uses of neurotoxins and dermal fillers.

> **!**
>
> Use of botulinum toxin for patients with facial palsy is typically an off-label use. Informed consent from the patient is recommended. In the United States, treatment of synkinesis and hyperkinesis is frequently covered by most insurance carriers given submission of proper documentation.

25.2.1 Serotypes and Structure

Based on immunological properties, the neurotoxins of the bacterium *Clostridium botulinum* have been grouped into seven serotypes: types A, B, C1, D, E, F, and G. Human botulism is caused mainly by types A, B, E, and (rarely) F. Types C and D cause toxicity in animals only. The toxins are produced as protein complexes consisting of a core neurotoxin molecule with a molecular mass of 150 kilodaltons and associated proteins. The catalytic domain of the neurotoxin enters the neuronal cytosol after binding and translocation. The content of neurotoxin-associated proteins, originally produced by bacteria for protection of the neurotoxin, e.g., in the digestive tract, typically differs in respective BTX products.

25.2.2 Mechanism of Action and Recovery of Acetylcholine Release

Binding of the toxin to a cell-surface ganglioside on the neuronal membrane keeps the toxin around the neuron and enables endocytosis and compartmentalization into the endosome and, later, into the cytosol. The toxin finally interacts with proteins of the SNARE complex (soluble *N*-ethylmaleimide-sensitive factor attachment receptor), which normally aids exocytosis of neurotransmitters. Each toxin has a distinct SNARE protein substrate, with type A cleaving a membrane-associated protein known as SNAP-25. This mechanism explains why it takes 2 to 3 days before BTX shows a clinical effect, normally reaching its maximum after 7 to 14 days. Nerve terminals recover their normal function after reproduction of the SNAP-25 protein. In skeletal muscle, weakening will last 3 to 4 months. In contrast, the autonomic nerve system will recover after 6 months or even later.

> **!**
>
> Effects of botulinum toxin start after 3 days and activity usually persists in the face for 3 to 4 months before treatment has to be repeated.

25.2.3 Immunogenicity

Antibodies may be formed against the neurotoxin and other proteins added as components to the drug. Only the antibodies formed against the neurotoxin that inhibit its function leading to nonresponse are relevant. Botox (Allergan) has been studied for neutralizing antibodies in a pooled analysis: 2 of 718 patients who received 20 mouse units (MU) into the glabella developed antibodies but retained an objective clinical response to Botox. Notably, neutralizing antibody formation was not found to be associated with skin reactions upon injection.[3] Primary or secondary nonresponders resulting from the development of antibodies are only rarely seen when BTX is used in the face. The dosages used in the face are much lower than those used in other regions of the body. The risk of antibody development is dependent on the dosages used and on the frequency of the application of BTX. As a general rule, the patient should not receive the next BTX treatment before the disappearance of the effect of the last treatment. Therefore, facial injection intervals of less than 3 months should be avoided.

25.2.4 Comparison of Botulinum Toxins

Of all known seven distinct serotypes (A–G), only type A and B are available for medical use (▶ Table 25.1). All

Table 25.1 Overview of botulinum toxin preparations

Trade name	Manufacturer	Active component	Toxin type	Dose conversion in relation to Botox
Botox/Vistabel	Allergan	Onabotulinum toxin A	A	
Xeomin/Bocouture	Merz	Incobotulinum toxin A	A	1:1
Dysport/Azzalure	Ipsen	Abobotulinum toxin A	A	1:3–4
BTXA	Lanzhou Institute of Biological Products	Unknown	A	Unknown
Neuronox/Siax	Medy-Tox	Unknown	A	Unknown
Myobloc/Neurobloc	Solstice Neurosciences	Rimabotulinum toxin B	B	1:40–50

types are antigenically and serologically distinct, but structurally similar concerning the core neurotoxin molecule. Respective doses in mouse units are not interchangeable, and reported dose conversion ratios are controversial. For instance, in a 2013 study on the biological activity of four BTX preparations in mice, the dose conversion ratio between Botox and Dysport was reported to be considerably lower (1:2.6) in comparison with previous reports.[4] Local and systemic effects and safety margins of serotype A and B preparations have also been studied in mice, indicating a longer duration of muscle weakness and lower safety margins relating to a lethal dose in BTX type A.[5] Several blinded studies have compared the efficacy of BTX formulations in humans, with unequivocal results. For example onabotulinum and abobotulinum toxins have been studied in human mimic muscles, indicating a better and longer efficacy with 20 MU Botox (onabotulinum) in comparison with 50 MU Dysport (abobotulinum); apparently the conversion rate was rather low for Dysport.[6] To summarize, botulinum toxin preparations show comparable effects, duration of activity, and safety margins; however, because of the poor comparability between different commercial formulations, it is recommended to use the same manufacturer once an ideal dose is established.

The "unit" as a measure of BTX type A has been standardized by in vitro mouse assays. Specifically, 1 U BTX type A corresponds to the amount of toxin required to kill 50% of a group of female Swiss-Webster mice weighing 18 to 20 g (LD_{50}). This is the reason why the measurement unit, mouse units or units, was established. In its clinical application in humans, BTX type A has proven to be extremely safe. Extrapolating the data from mouse experimentation, it can be estimated that a adult male of 104 kg would sustain a lethal dose of BTX type A at amounts exceeding 3,500 U, a dose that far surpasses any dosing regimen used when treating mimic muscles.

!

Though several toxins are currently available on the market, each of these products is unique, with each having distinct biological characteristics, which can impact their efficacy. Practically this means that experience with a dosage with one preparation cannot be transferred directly to a preparation from another manufacturer.

25.3 Clinical Use

25.3.1 Aging Face

The clinical profile of BTX in cosmetic medicine has been studied intensively since the first report for the treatment of glabellar lines in 1990. With 20 U onabotulinum toxin, a response rate of approximately 80% can be estimated (▶ Fig. 25.2), and a median duration of efficacy of 90 to 120 days can be expected.[7] The safety of BTX has been reviewed in a meta-analysis including 1,678 subjects, and similar adverse events were observed in both placebo-treated and BTX-treated groups.[8] Eyelid ptosis (1.8%) and eyelid sensory disorders (2.5%) were the only adverse events that were significantly higher in the onabotulinum toxin groups. When treating glabellar lines, 20 to 40 U onabotulinum toxin resulted in a longer duration and lower relapse rate. In comparison to 10 U, using 30 or 40 U showed no statistical difference between the doses in women.[9] A comparable study with 20 U versus 40 to 80 U was undertaken in men.[10] Cumulative benefits upon regular treatment have been reported, with glabellar line severity not returning to baseline levels, and upon cessation of 20 months of treatment the patients retained improvements over baseline.[11] The approval of BTX formulations in facial lines varies based on the

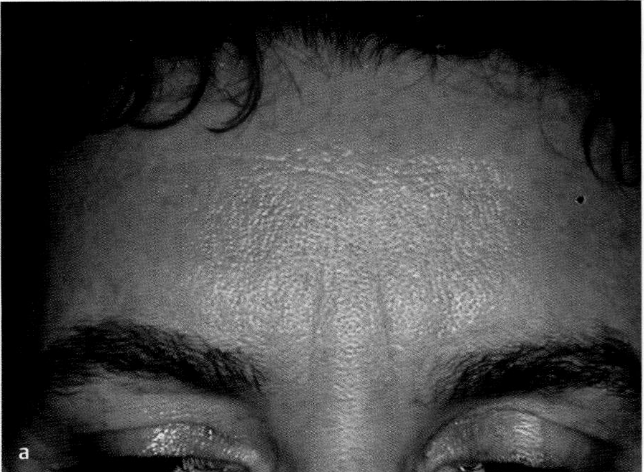

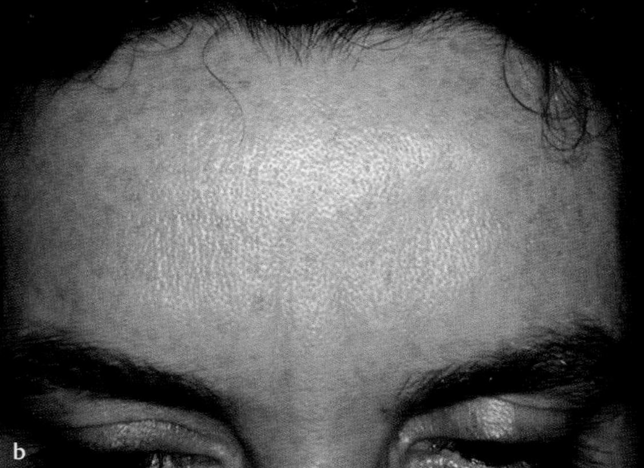

Fig. 25.2 Reduction of glabellar lines: **(a)** before, and **(b)** 4 weeks after injection of 20 U onabotulinumtoxin A into the glabellar region. Five sites have been injected: one into the procerus muscle at the midline and two injections laterally into each corrugator supercilii muscle on both sides.

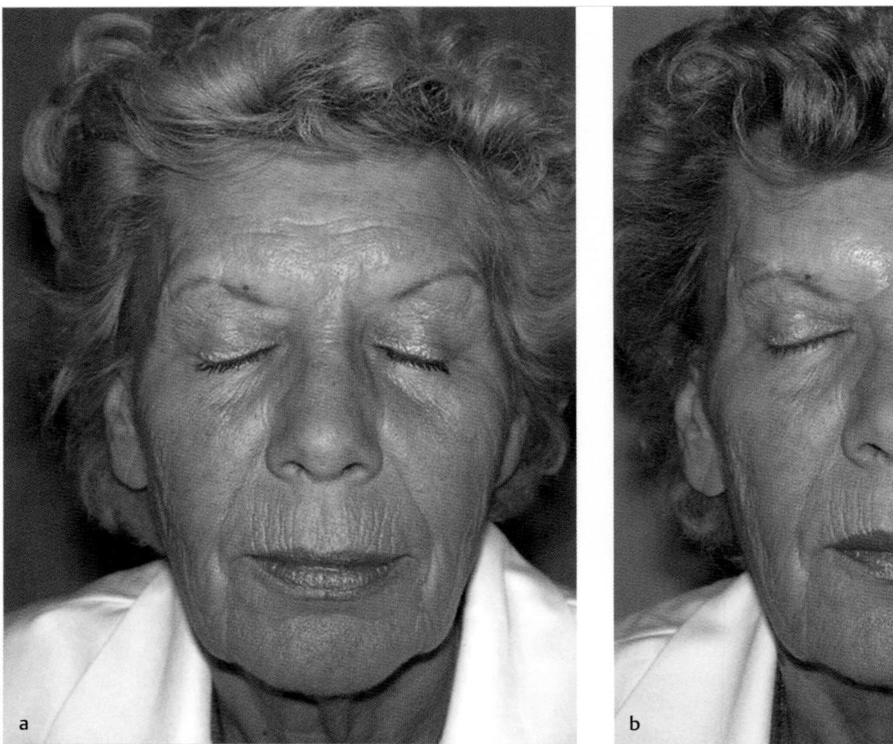

Fig. 25.3 A 62-year-old woman: **(a)** before, and **(b)** 3weeks after treatment with a total dose of 25 U onabotulinum toxin injected into five sites of the forehead region.

country, with the most widely approved indications being for glabella, frontal lines, and crow's feet in descending order.

The main goal in the management of the forehead is to attenuate wrinkles while maintaining patient facial animation. The lowest effective doses of BTX should therefore be used. Residual lines can be treated with soft tissue fillers; see Types of Fillers. Depending on the severity of rhytids, the forehead should be treated with doses of onabotulinum toxin ranging from 10 to 30 U in three to eight sites (▶ Fig. 25.3). Placement of the neurotoxin should be superior to the equator of the forehead in order to preserve an inferiorly based short segment of the frontalis muscle intact to ensure maintenance of brow position and frowning. Periorbital crow's feet are typically treated with a dose of 10 to 15 U onabotulinum at three to six sites for each side.

The middle one-third of the face is treated primarily with dermal fillers. BTX may be used with caution in the apex of the nasolabial folds in patients with excessive gingival show (gummy smile). The lower third of the face is treated mainly with injectable fillers. Possible targets of BTX are irregular contours of the chin, the depressor anguli oris muscles to improve the downturn of the oral commissure, and platysmal banding.[12]

!

Botulinum toxin is an established effective treatment for upper facial lines in cosmetic medicine.

- Beneficial effects will last 3 to 4 months.
- Safety has been established in many clinical trials.
- Dose-ranging studies have found 20 U BTX or equivalent to be recommended when treating glabellar lines.
- Units are not simply interchangeable among products from different manufacturers.

25.3.2 Facial Synkinesis

Facial synkinesis is abnormal involuntary movement of one set of facial muscles accompanying a voluntary movement of a different facial muscle. These unintended movements stem from misdirected reinnervation after facial nerve damage, and they affect daily activities such as smiling, chewing, and blinking. Individuals suffering from this condition can be affected aesthetically and might experience social isolation; see Chapter 3. The most common presentation of facial synkinesis is oculo-oral synkinesis (▶ Fig. 25.4). Other presentations of facial synkinesis include midfacial muscle contraction during

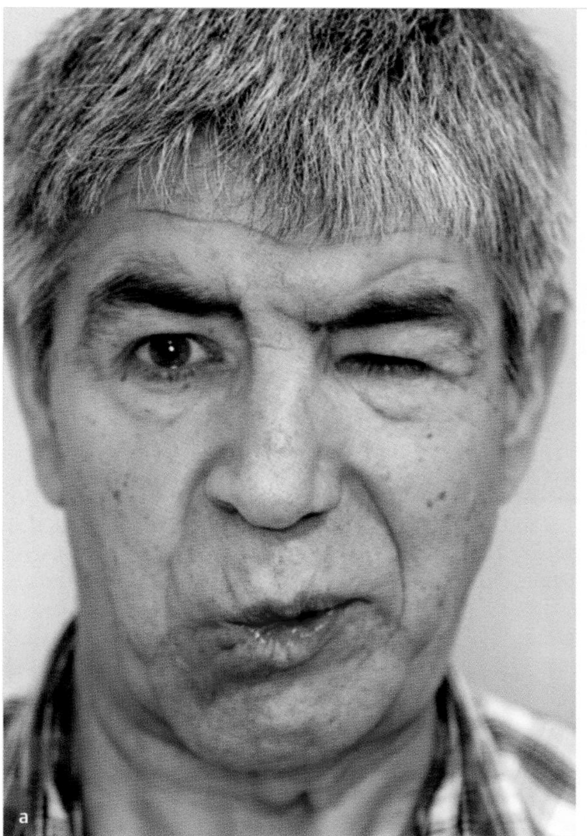

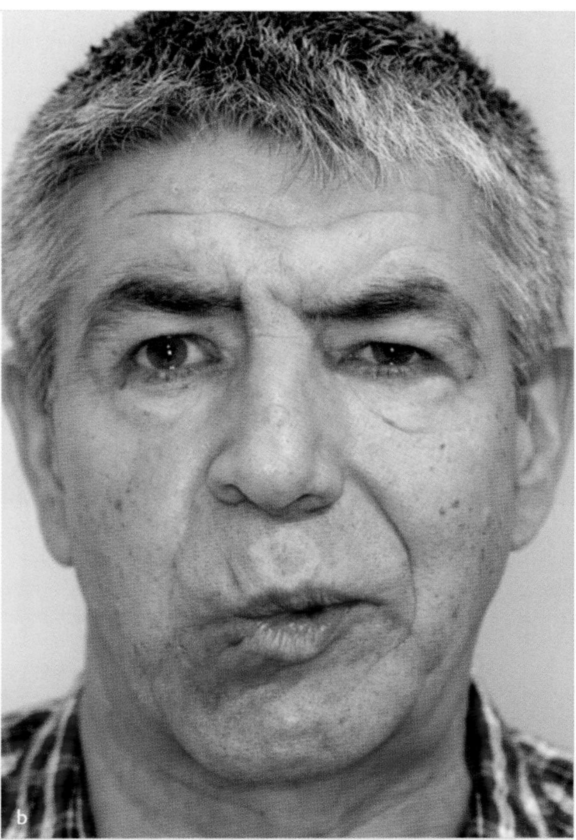

Fig. 25.4 (a) Patient with defective healing after resection of vestibular schwannoma, showing oro-ocular synkinesis. **(b)** Two weeks after injection of 15 U of incobotulinum toxin into the ocular sphincter, eye opening shows marked improvement.

voluntary closure of the eye, narrowing of the eye, lifting the brow, lifting the corner of the mouth, and platysma contraction.[13,14]

> **!**
>
> Treatment of facial synkinesis with botulinum toxin (BTX), especially of oculo-oral synkinesis, is well established and frequently used. For this type of synkinesis, BTX is injected into the affected orbicularis oculi muscle.

The most common therapeutic modality is infiltration of BTX (▶ Fig. 25.5); alternative treatments comprise mime therapy,[15] neuromuscular retraining,[16] biofeedback rehabilitation,[17] as described in Chapter 26, or surgery. The first reports of treatment for facial synkinesis with BTX were published in 1990.[18] Most of the reports show improvement of facial synkinesis within a few days after injection, remaining effective for 3 to 7 months. Complications are minor except for ptosis. It is worth noting that lower dosages, for instance 10 U onabotulinum toxin for the orbicularis oculi muscle, might be recommended when treating synkinesis instead of the 20 U usually required for blepharospasm.

Dose-related complications are generally mild and transient. Higher dosage offers no significant advantage over lower dosage in cosmetic improvements.[19] One placebo-controlled trial assessing the efficacy of BTX in 36 patients showed subjective and objective improvements, and lower doses were reported to be as effective as higher doses.[20] In conclusion, BTX is safe, easy to use, and effective in the management of facial synkinesis.

25.3.3 Hyperlacrimation

Aberrant regeneration of nerve fibers after facial nerve palsy may lead to increased lacrimation of the affected eye. Secretomotor fibers of the facial nerve reach the lacrimal gland through the greater superficial petrosal nerve. During recovery from facial nerve palsy, aberrant visceromotor fibers, originally innervating salivary glands, may regrow towards the lacrimal gland, causing hyperlacrimation whenever the patient salivates; this phenomenon is called crocodile tears. As the fibers to the lacrimal gland also use acetylcholine as a transmitter,

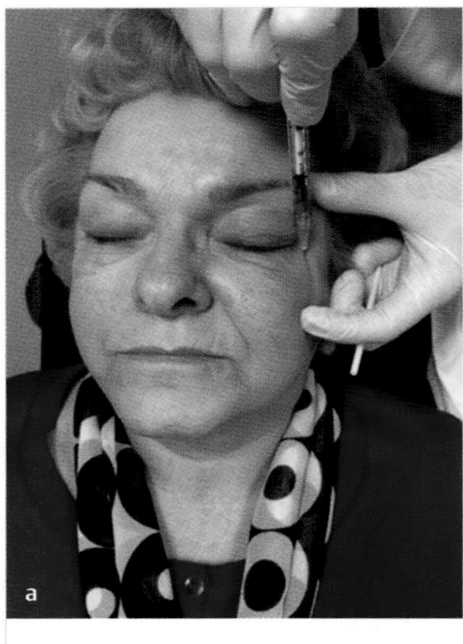

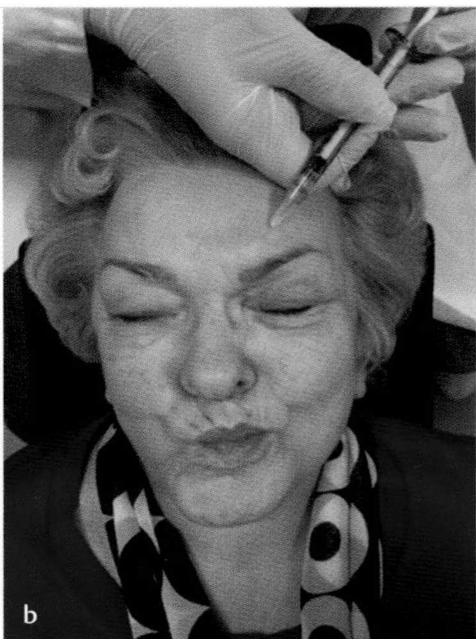

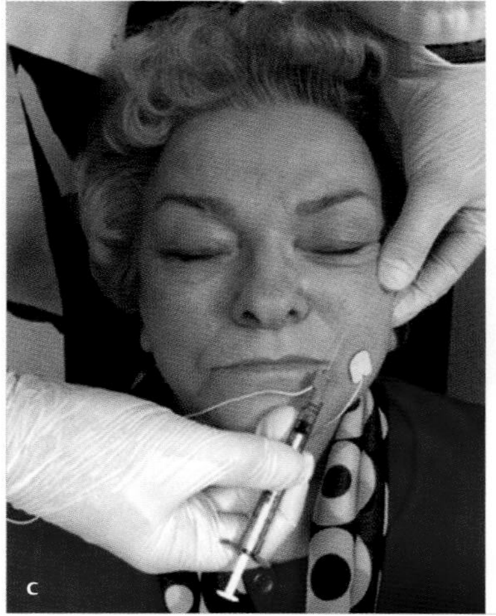

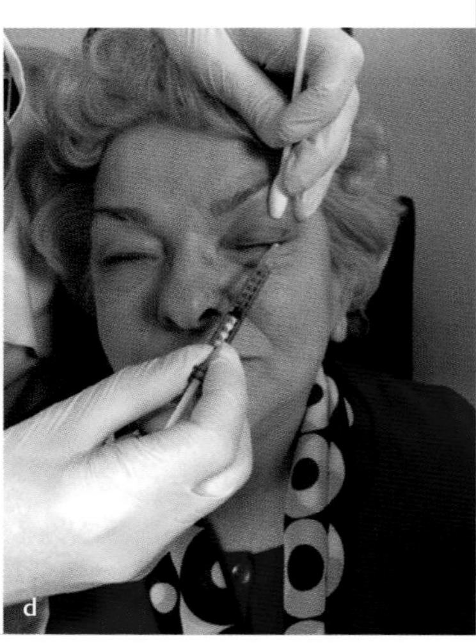

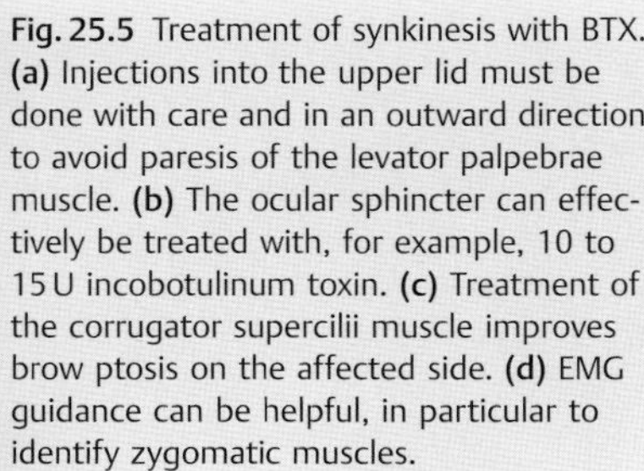

Fig. 25.5 Treatment of synkinesis with BTX. **(a)** Injections into the upper lid must be done with care and in an outward direction to avoid paresis of the levator palpebrae muscle. **(b)** The ocular sphincter can effectively be treated with, for example, 10 to 15 U incobotulinum toxin. **(c)** Treatment of the corrugator supercilii muscle improves brow ptosis on the affected side. **(d)** EMG guidance can be helpful, in particular to identify zygomatic muscles.

local injections of BTX into the gland may solve this symptom.[21] A dose of 2 to 5 U onabotulinum toxin injected directly into the lacrimal gland using topical anesthesia may lead to marked reduction of gustatory lacrimation. The effect lasts typically for 6 months. The risk of ptosis is high, and ultrasound guidance might prevent this side effect from occurring.

> **!**
>
> Injections of botulinum toxin in the lacrimal gland can treat crocodile tears effectively.

25.3.4 Gustatory Sweating (Frey's Syndrome)

Auriculotemporal syndrome, or gustatory sweating after traumatic lesions of the auriculotemporal nerve and aberrant regeneration of cholinergic fibers to sweat glands of the skin, is best known as a sequela after lateral parotidectomy. The syndrome was named after the Jewish physician Lucja Frey. She was murdered by the Nazis during the World War II, and would have been forgotten if not for the eponym Frey's syndrome.[22] The reported incidence of Frey's syndrome after parotidectomy varies considerably depending on the method of assessment. Gustatory sweating can be detected to a varying degree in almost 100% of cases, when evaluated by means of a postoperative iodine-starch test (Minor test). There have been no reports of a reliable surgical method for the prevention of Frey's syndrome after parotidectomy. Various forms of treatment, both medical and surgical, for Frey's syndrome, have been tried with varying degrees of success. Intracutaneous injection of BTX is a safe and effective treatment (▸ Fig. 25.6). Higher dosages (e.g., 5 U Botox instead of 2.5 U per cm^2) will lead to a longer-lasting effect, up to 18 months.[23] Relapse from gustatory sweating may be difficult to predict, and it may occur at different time points and in different areas. Reduced

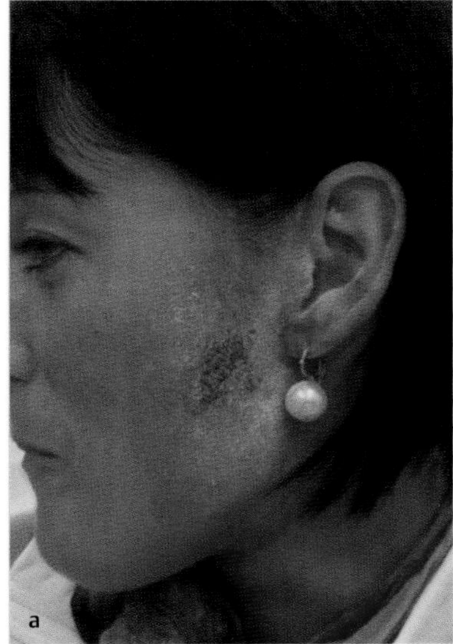

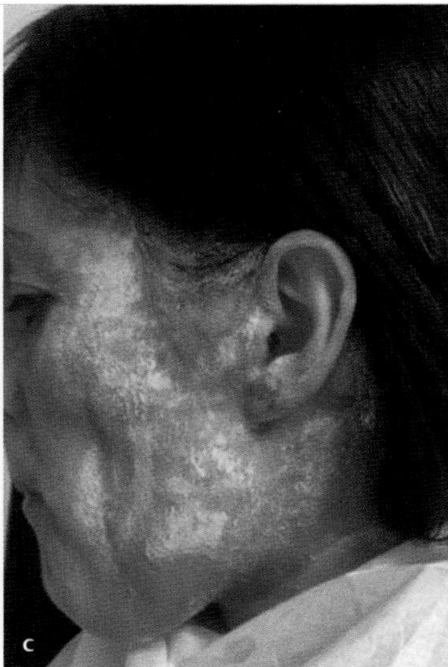

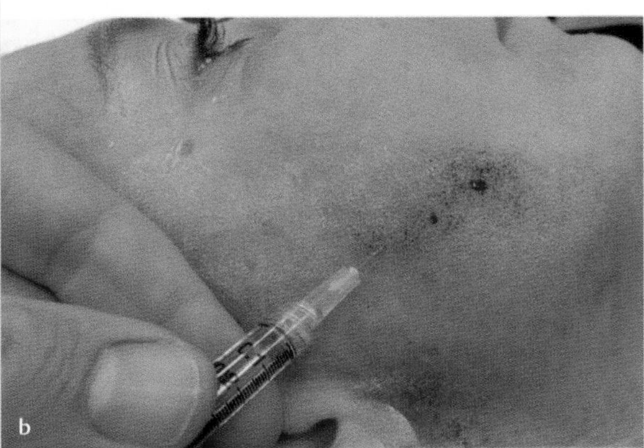

Fig. 25.6 (a) Frey's syndrome can be shown by using an iodine-starch test and simultaneous chewing. **(b)** BTX is injected into the subdermal plane, with 2 to 5 U at each injection point. Dissolving 100 U of Botox in 2 mL saline, for example, will cover approximately 1 cm^2 at each injection point. **(c)** Control after one week.

symptom scores, decreased area size, and increased duration of the effect have been reported after repeated injections of BTX.[24] Care has to be taken not to reach mimic muscles with the neurotoxin, e.g., by drawing lateral borders of zygomatic muscles and oral and ocular sphincters.

25.3.5 Facial Asymmetry

Paralysis of muscles on the affected side of the face results in loss of forehead lines and the nasolabial fold, lagophthalmos, brow droop, and drooping of the corner of the mouth. The application of BTX to the healthy side of the face in patients with long-standing facial paralysis has been used to improve facial symmetry at rest and during facial motion.[25] Patients not suitable for reanimation surgery are also candidates for BTX treatment, in order to improve facial symmetry (▶ Fig. 25.7). BTX might also be helpful in acute cases of facial paralysis.[26] The effect is more noticeable and the benefit is better in younger patients, and also in patients with partial recovery who are less likely to undergo facial reanimation surgery. BTX treatments have also been reported in patients with hypertrophic masseter muscle–induced facial asymmetry.[27] Rare indications include patients with congenital unilateral hypoplasia of the depressor anguli oris muscle or eyebrow asymmetry.

!

In patients with facial palsy, botulinum toxin treatment of the healthy side to weaken areas with strong creases during mimic muscle movement can enhance facial symmetry.

→•

- Electromyographic guidance can be helpful, particularly to identify zygomatic muscle belly.
- The tip of the needle should be directed away from the eye.
- Avoid overdosing with botulinum toxin in the upper eyelid and eyebrow to avoid brow droop, ptosis, or a diplopia.

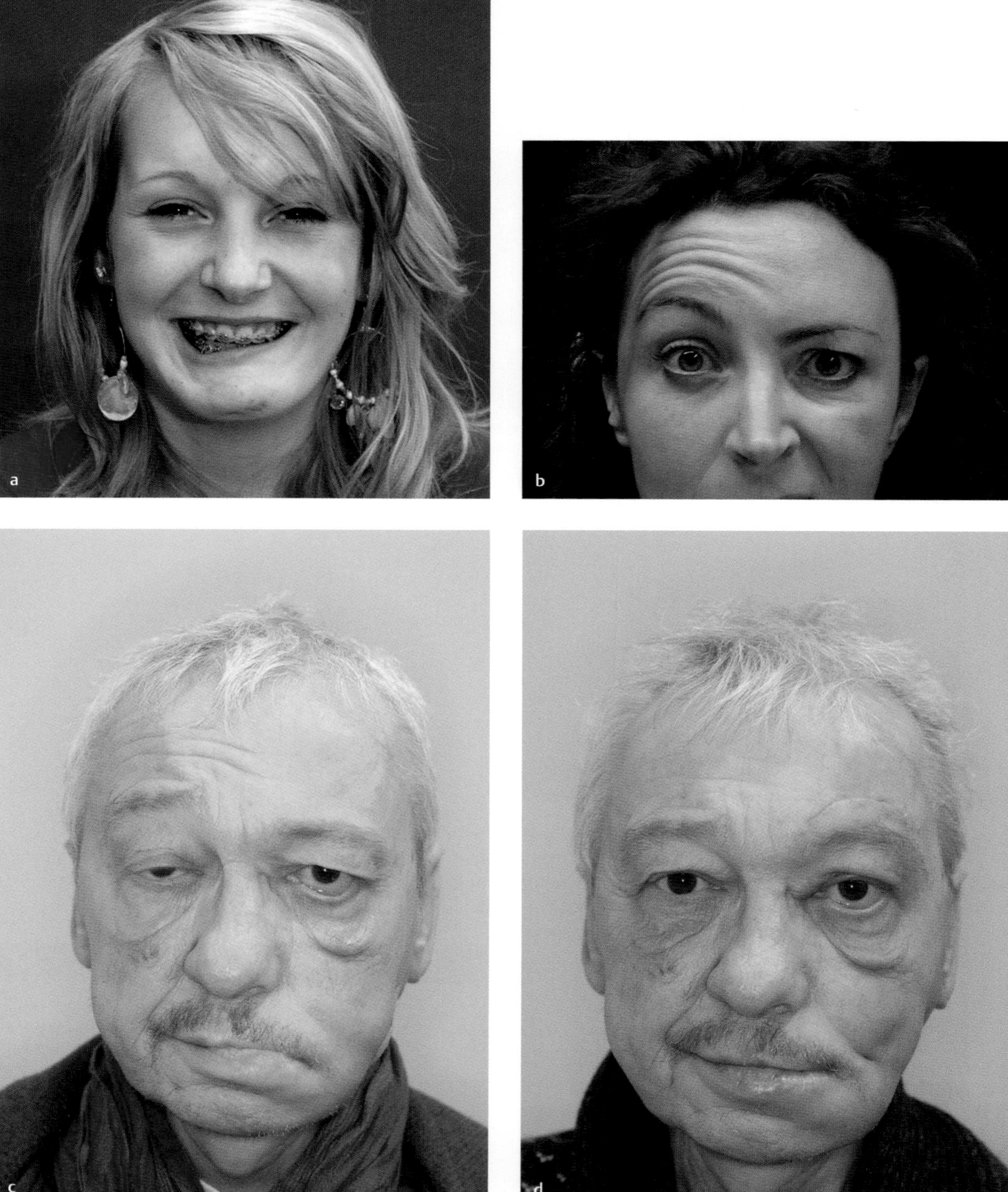

Fig. 25.7 Possible indications for BTX treatment. **(a)** Agenesis of the depressor anguli oris muscle. **(b)** Facial asymmetry during frowning. **(c,d)** BTX therapy of the unaffected side as an adjunct to surgery for definitive facial palsy.

Table 25.2 Examples of temporary and permanent facial fillers

Type of filler	Product	Peculiarities
Xenogenic	Bovine (Zyderm) or porcine collagen (Evolence)	Skin testing and overcorrection needed
	Avian hyaluronic acid (Hylaform)	Withdrawn from the US market
Allogenic	Human collagen (Cosmoderm, Cosmoplast)	Overcorrection needed
Bacterial	Hyaluronic acid from streptococci (Restylane, Juvederm, Belotero, etc.)	Gels and particulate gels are available; result lasts 6–12 months
Synthetic	Calcium hydroxylapatite (Radiesse)	Long-lasting effect; not suitable for use in lip enhancement
	Polyacrylamide (Aquamid)	Permanent filler with known disadvantages
	Polylkylimide (Bio-Alcamid, Perform)	Permanent filler with known disadvantages
Combined	Hyaluronic acid + dextranomeres (CRM DEX)	Available in Europe only
	Poly-L-lactic acid (Sculptra, New-fill)	Semipermanent filler; expensive
	Polymethylacrylate (Artecoll, Artefill)	Collagen included; semipermanent filler

25.4 Fillers

Clinical indications and the portfolio of facial fillers on the market have grown rapidly in recent years. Fillers may be used for all kinds of facial contouring, not only for treatment of nasolabial folds. The plethora of injectable fillers on the market makes it difficult to select appropriate products in practice. Facial fillers consist of various temporary to long-lasting substances. Each is designed with one or several specific purposes, such as wrinkle reduction or lip augmentation.

25.4.1 Types of Fillers

Soft tissue fillers can be described in different categories for classification. These include xenogenic (from a different species), allogenic (same species but antigenically distinct), bacterial, synthetic, or combinations of materials (▶ Table 25.2). Free fat grafting was described late in the 19th century, and in the late 1970s collagen was introduced for soft tissue augmentation. Since then numerous fillers have been developed for soft tissue augmentation. Many of the substances have limitations, such as a need for testing, a lack of durability, and inflammatory reactions, to name a few.

Collagens

The first dermal fillers were collagen products (Zyderm, Zyplast) from cattle. Before they were replaced by hyaluronic acid, collagen fillers were used intensively for treating facial wrinkles and folds. Overcorrection was required, and 3% of the population is allergic to bovine collagen, and hence skin testing was needed prior to injection. Bioengineered collagen derived from human tissue, with no need for skin testing, received approval in 2003 (Cosmoderm). However, a need for overcorrection, short (3–6 months) residence time in tissues, and side effects led to unpopularity.[28]

Hyaluronic Acid

Hyaluronic acid (HA) has become the gold standard for dermal enhancement in recent years. It is a natural biocompatible polysaccharide with high molecular weight that is ubiquitous in the extracellular matrix of all animal tissues. This led to the development of HA from avian and bacterial sources. Since natural HA undergoes quick degradation, dermal fillers are modified by cross-linking to form a water-insoluble hydrogel. As results normally last 6 to 12 months, it is preferable for use in patients who are a seeking longer-lasting result than is available with collagen. Differences in preparations include concentration, cross-linking, and galenics (cohesive gel or particles). Most products contain HA from biofermentation of *Streptococcus equus bacteria* and are available in volumes from 0.5 to 3.0 mL in syringes. Monophasic products are viscoelastic gels that do not contain particles (e. g., Juvederm). Gels containing particles (e.g., Restylane or Perlane) are biphasic. Larger particles or products with a higher concentration of cross-linked HA are generally injected deeper into the dermis for deep-fold correction and are reported to have higher residence times.[29]

Synthetic Materials

BioForm Medical first developed microspheres from calcium hydroxylapatite (Radiesse) as a bulking agent for urinary incontinence. Radiesse consists of long-lasting calcium hydroxylapatite microspheres suspended in water. The mechanism of action of Radiesse centers on the product being incorporated by the surrounding tissue and then being replaced by it collagenosis—it is broken down by hydrolytic enzymes into calcium and phosphate. It was approved in December 2006 for the correction of facial folds and facial lipoatrophy associated with HIV. It stimulates only a minor foreign body reaction, and granuloma formation or osteoneogenesis is unlikely.[30] Results last for up to 2 years. Use in lip augmentation is routinely discouraged because there have been reports of labial nodules resulting from the product clumping together.

Polyacrylamide is an injectable water-based gel (Aquamid) that has been recommended for skin sculpturing and facial atrophy. Reports have indicated that it is not effective for fine wrinkles, but should be injected into the deeper subcutaneous tissues.[31] While acrylamide itself is a neurotoxin, polyacrylamide is an inert polymer and nonbiodegradable. Since it is nondegradable, the augmentations are permanent. Hence, poorly administered treatment or complications are difficult to correct. Bacterial infections of the material have also been reported.

Polyalkylimide is a synthetic polymer used for deep dermal correction. The material is also used for contact lenses. The material is too large to become phagocytosed. Suspensions of the polymer are used to treat soft tissue defects, such as facial fat loss, acne, and scars, or to build up facial volume as needed in areas such as the cheeks, chin and lips. Numerous reports of adverse events have been reported since its invention, including infections and migration resulting in facial deformity.[32]

25.4.2 Complications

Obvious complications such as needle marks, pain, and swelling can be expected immediately after the injection. Asymmetry associated with overcorrection or undercorrection is expected within the first 2 weeks and may resolve without intervention. Should overcorrection from HA persist, successful treatment with hyaluronidase has been reported.[33] Specific to particulate HA is the Tyndall effect: a bluish discoloration that occurs when HA is placed too superficially. Hypersensitivity reactions are reported with bovine-derived fillers in up to 3% of patients. Infections are rare and might be associated with improper technique. Serious complications from nonpermanent injectable fillers have also been reported and include anaphylaxis, skin necrosis, and even blindness.[34] The idea of permanently correcting a defect in the face by injection is appealing. Bearing in mind that aging is a dynamic process and that complications of permanent fillers are generally more severe and more difficult to solve, the use of permanent fillers remains a subject of controversy.

25.4.3 Choosing the Right Filler

A wide variety of fillers is available on the market, and there is an endless flow of new products emerging. Understanding the biology of the components is crucial for treatment selection. HA fillers have become the gold standard in most countries. Less viscous products are preferred for superficial lines and fine wrinkles, such as in the lips and around the eyes. More-viscous HA products are chosen for deeper subcutaneous placement, e.g., correction of nasolabial folds and facial contouring. Calcium hydroxylapatite provides excellent structural support making it preferable for the correction of deep folds and nonsurgical nose shaping or cheek bone enhancement. Local restrictions and availability, injector experience, and the particular indication and location in the face where filling is required are only some of the more important factors to be considered for decision-making.

- A thorough understanding of filler products and the respective biology of ingredients is necessary.
- Permanent filler should be used with caution.
- Hyaluronic acid products have become the gold standard of fillers.
- Combination with chemodenervation (botulinum toxin) might prolong the effect of dermal fillers.
- Fillers might be of interest in patients with facial palsy and a structural defect on the affected side of the face.

25.4.4 Injection Technique

Local anesthesia may be provided alone or in combination with ice, topical numbing cream, or local anesthetic for regional nerve blocking. Choose the smallest needle that can deliver the filler. Injection techniques can be categorized into serial puncture, threading, fanning, and cross-hatching.[35] When the defect has been adequately augmented, the product is then firmly massaged into place.

- Serial puncture involves injecting small portions of the filler along the length of the defect.
- Threading involves tunneling the needle beneath the defect at the appropriate depth and injecting the product as the needle is withdrawn.
- Fanning means multiple threads are injected radially by changing direction without withdrawing the needle.
- Cross-hatching is a series of threads perpendicular to one another in a grid and is suitable for larger defects.

Upper Third

There might be supplementary lines remaining in the upper third of the face after treatment with BTX, and these need to be addressed. HA fillers might be used for enhancement of deep glabellar and forehead lines using

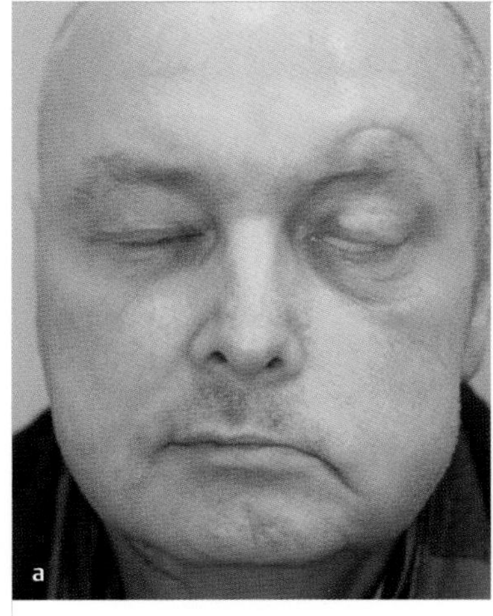

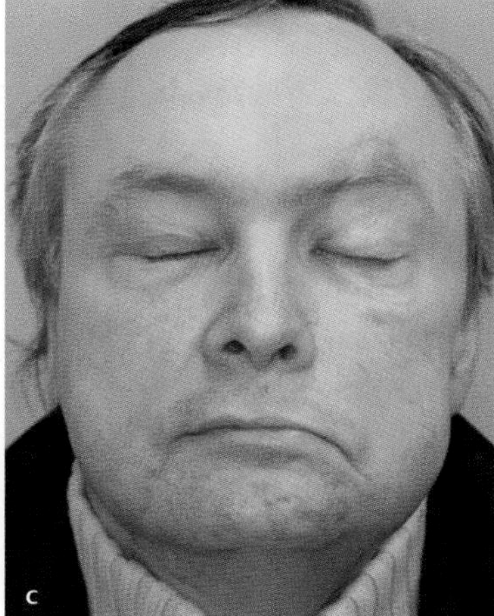

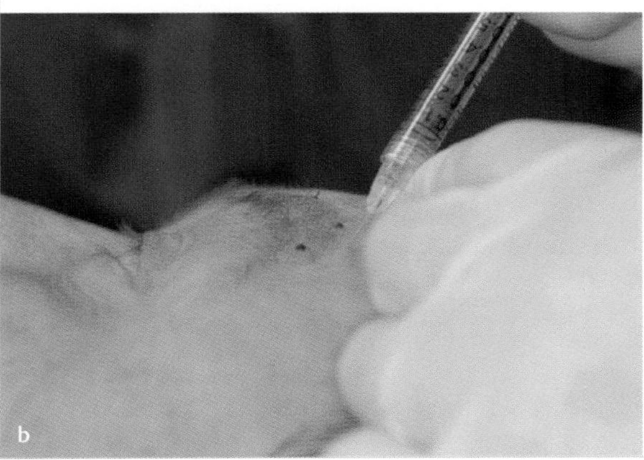

Fig. 25.8 (a) Skin defect above the left eyebrow after facial reanimation surgery, including browlift and lid loading. **(b)** Injection of HA using the serial puncture technique in the forehead. **(c)** Result after dermal filling on the left side in combination with BTX treatment of the contralateral side.

the threading technique; however, be aware that the glabellar region, in particular, carries a risk of skin necrosis regardless of the type of filler used. Crow's feet might be treated by combinations of BTX and fillers using the serial puncture technique or multiple linear threading technique. Pretreatment with BTX might increase the longevity of soft tissue fillers. Filler therapy is also suitable for use in defects resulting from surgery, if it is applied in combination with BTX (▸ Fig. 25.8).

The Middle and Lower Thirds

The middle third is primarily treated with fillers. The nasolabial folds are best treated with firm substances that provide structural support. The fanning technique or application via an intraoral approach might be used in this region. HA fillers are suitable for lip enhancement and perioral lines (▸ Fig. 25.9). BTX in low doses may complement volume augmentation. Irregular contours of the chin may also benefit from chemodenervation and fillers used in combination. Platysmal banding in the neck region can easily be addressed with BTX injections.

25.5 Key Points

- Botulinum toxin (BTX) (for dynamic wrinkles) and fillers (for subcutaneous volume loss) are powerful tools for selected patients in the management of the aging face or defects resulting from disorders of the facial nerve.
- Cosmetic improvements can be achieved with minimally invasive procedures using injections.
- Synergistic effects of BTX and filler treatments can be utilized.
- A thorough understanding of the respective product biology and experience of using it is critical to achieve a successful outcome.
- Scientific data are unambiguous for BTX and wrinkle improvement.
- Distinct medical indications exist, e.g., BTX for facial synkinesis and fillers for surgery defects.
- Complications can be severe and difficult to reverse, e.g., infection or skin necrosis after inadvertent intravascular injection.

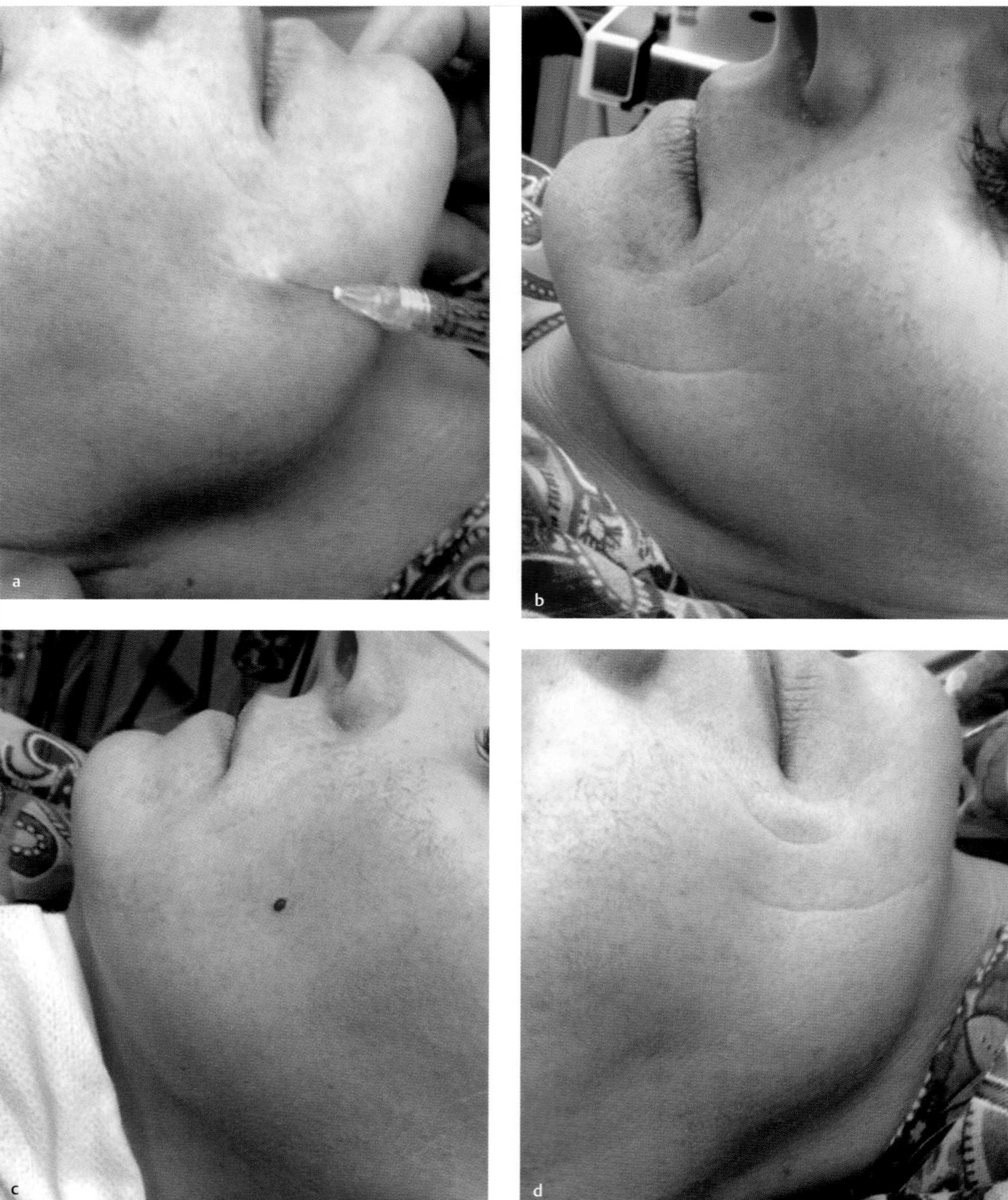

Fig. 25.9 (a,c) Augmentation of perioral lines with HA filler. The product is deposited as the needle is withdrawn from the tissue (threading method). **(b)** If the skin moves up and down with pressure, then the needle is in the dermis. If the needle can be visualized through the skin, it is too superficial. **(d)** The immediate result postprocedure.

References

[1] Arnon SS, Schechter R, Inglesby TV et al. Working Group on Civilian Biodefense. Botulinum toxin as a biological weapon: medical and public health management. JAMA 2001; 285: 1059–1070

[2] Scott AB. Botulinum toxin injection of eye muscles to correct strabismus. Trans Am Ophthalmol Soc 1981; 79: 734–770

[3] Naumann M, Carruthers A, Carruthers J et al. Meta-analysis of neutralizing antibody conversion with onabotulinumtoxinA (BOTOX®) across multiple indications. Mov Disord 2010; 25: 2211–2218

[4] Chung ME, Song DH, Park JH. Comparative study of biological activity of four botulinum toxin type A preparations in mice. Dermatol Surg 2013; 39: 155–164

[5] Aoki KR. Physiology and pharmacology of therapeutic botulinum neurotoxins. Curr Probl Dermatol 2002; 30: 107–116

[6] Lowe PL, Patnaik R, Lowe NJ. A comparison of two botulinum type a toxin preparations for the treatment of glabellar lines: double-blind, randomized, pilot study. Dermatol Surg 2005; 31: 1651–1654

[7] Carruthers A, Carruthers J. Botulinum toxin type A for the treatment of glabellar rhytides. Dermatol Clin 2004; 22: 137–144

[8] Brin MF, Boodhoo TI, Pogoda JM et al. Safety and tolerability of onabotulinumtoxinA in the treatment of facial lines: a meta-analysis of individual patient data from global clinical registration studies in 1678 participants. J Am Acad Dermatol 2009; 61: 961–70.e1, 11

[9] Carruthers A, Carruthers J, Said S. Dose-ranging study of botulinum toxin type A in the treatment of glabellar rhytids in females. Dermatol Surg 2005; 31: 414–422, discussion 422

[10] Carruthers A, Carruthers J. Prospective, double-blind, randomized, parallel-group, dose-ranging study of botulinum toxin type A in men with glabellar rhytids. Dermatol Surg 2005; 31: 1297–1303

[11] Dailey RA, Philip A, Tardie G. Long-term treatment of glabellar rhytides using onabotulinumtoxina. Dermatol Surg 2011; 37: 918–928

[12] Wise JB, Greco T. Injectable treatments for the aging face. Facial Plast Surg 2006; 22: 140–146

[13] Moran CJ, Neely JG. Patterns of facial nerve synkinesis. Laryngoscope 1996; 106: 1491–1496

[14] Beurskens CH, Oosterhof J, Nijhuis-van der Sanden MW. Frequency and location of synkineses in patients with peripheral facial nerve paresis. Otol Neurotol 2010; 31: 671–675

[15] Beurskens CH, Heymans PG. Mime therapy improves facial symmetry in people with long-term facial nerve paresis: a randomised controlled trial. Aust J Physiother 2006; 52: 177–183

[16] Brach JS, VanSwearingen JM, Lenert J, Johnson PC. Facial neuromuscular retraining for oral synkinesis. Plast Reconstr Surg 1997; 99: 1922–1931, discussion 1932–1933

[17] Nakamura K, Toda N, Sakamaki K, Kashima K, Takeda N. Biofeedback rehabilitation for prevention of synkinesis after facial palsy. Otolaryngol Head Neck Surg 2003; 128: 539–543

[18] Roggenkämper P, Laskawi R, Damenz W, Schröder M, Nüssgens Z. Botulinum toxin treatment of synkinesia following facial paralysis [in German] HNO 1990; 38: 295–297

[19] Armstrong MW, Mountain RE, Murray JA. Treatment of facial synkinesis and facial asymmetry with botulinum toxin type A following facial nerve palsy. Clin Otolaryngol Allied Sci 1996; 21: 15–20

[20] Borodic G, Bartley M, Slattery W et al. Botulinum toxin for aberrant facial nerve regeneration: double-blind, placebo-controlled trial using subjective endpoints. Plast Reconstr Surg 2005; 116: 36–43

[21] Keegan DJ, Geerling G, Lee JP, Blake G, Collin JR, Plant GT. Botulinum toxin treatment for hyperlacrimation secondary to aberrant regenerated seventh nerve palsy or salivary gland transplantation. Br J Ophthalmol 2002; 86: 43–46

[22] Moltrecht M, Michel O. The woman behind Frey's syndrome: the tragic life of Lucja Frey. Laryngoscope 2004; 114: 2205–2209

[23] Guntinas-Lichius O. Increased botulinum toxin type A dosage is more effective in patients with Frey's syndrome. Laryngoscope 2002; 112: 746–749

[24] de Bree R, Duyndam JE, Kuik DJ, Leemans CR. Repeated botulinum toxin type A injections to treat patients with Frey syndrome. Arch Otolaryngol Head Neck Surg 2009; 135: 287–290

[25] de Maio M, Bento RF. Botulinum toxin in facial palsy: an effective treatment for contralateral hyperkinesis. Plast Reconstr Surg 2007; 120: 917–927, discussion 928

[26] Kim J. Contralateral botulinum toxin injection to improve facial asymmetry after acute facial paralysis. Otol Neurotol 2013; 34: 319–324

[27] Park MY, Ahn KY, Jung DS. Botulinum toxin type A treatment for contouring of the lower face. Dermatol Surg 2003; 29: 477–483, discussion 483

[28] Alam M, Dover JS. Management of complications and sequelae with temporary injectable fillers. Plast Reconstr Surg 2007; 120 Suppl: 98S–105S

[29] Kablik J, Monheit GD, Yu L, Chang G, Gershkovich J. Comparative physical properties of hyaluronic acid dermal fillers. Dermatol Surg 2009; 35 Suppl 1: 302–312

[30] Sklar JA, White SM. Radiance FN: a new soft tissue filler. Dermatol Surg 2004; 30: 764–768, discussion 768

[31] Breiting V, Aasted A, Jørgensen A, Opitz P, Rosetzsky A. A study on patients treated with polyacrylamide hydrogel injection for facial corrections. Aesthetic Plast Surg 2004; 28: 45–53

[32] Karim RB, Hage JJ, van Rozelaar L, Lange CA, Raaijmakers J. Complications of polyalkylimide 4% injections (Bio-Alcamid): a report of 18 cases. J Plast Reconstr Aesthet Surg 2006; 59: 1409–1414

[33] Brody HJ. Use of hyaluronidase in the treatment of granulomatous hyaluronic acid reactions or unwanted hyaluronic acid misplacement. Dermatol Surg 2005; 31: 893–897

[34] Carle MV, Roe R, Novack R, Boyer DS. Cosmetic facial fillers and severe vision loss. JAMA Ophthalmol 2014; 132: 637–639

[35] Buck DW, II, Alam M, Kim JY. Injectable fillers for facial rejuvenation: a review. J Plast Reconstr Aesthet Surg 2009; 62: 11–18

26 Feedback Training and Other Training Programs

Wolfgang H. R. Miltner, Thomas Weiss, and Eva Maria Miltner

26.1 Introduction

This chapter provides a review of published articles on the rehabilitation of chronic peripheral facial palsy. The presentation is based on a literature search using Thomson Reuters' Web of Science (WOS) and the PubMed databases for the years 1950 to 2013. Included are only papers that have been published in peer-reviewed journals and realized the following additional features:

- Patients have been diagnosed prior to the start of the training program by neurological or otolaryngological experts as suffering from acute or chronic peripheral facial palsy.
- The acute condition had to have been present for at least 4 days, and patients were considered chronic if 3 months or greater had elapsed prior to initiating rehabilitation.
- Special emphasis was placed on randomized controlled trials (RCTs) that used random or quasirandom assignment of patients to the treatment program or a control procedure (waiting list, conventional treatment).
- The articles had to contain a comprehensive description of the treatment concept(s) applied.
- Studies were included only when the outcome measures applied were based on published procedures or presented in the publication in a comprehensive way.

It is estimated that about 12 to 40 individuals out of 100,000 people will experience Bell's palsy in industrialized countries each year.[1–4] Out of these subjects, about 70% will recover completely within the first 4 to 6 months of the disease. In about 25% of these subjects, Bell's palsy will become chronic.[5–7] Moreover, facial palsies of other etiologies, for instance, caused by trauma or a neoplasm, although rarer, are of interest as these etiologies are more likely to have permanent sequelae.

> **!**
>
> It is unknown what percentage of patients with acute or chronic facial palsy is referred for physiotherapy or any other training program.

Currently, there is no overview of how many subjects with chronic facial palsy receive professional rehabilitation treatment. Referral for rehabilitation, and its quality and duration, varies considerably between countries as a function of the education of referring professionals, the density of professional services available in urban and rural areas, and the coverage of rehabilitation services by health insurances.

> **!**
>
> There are no current standards for facial nerve rehabilitation concerning indication, type of training program, frequency, duration, and goals of therapy.

The literature search of WOS and PubMed indicates that research efforts on the effects and effectiveness of different methods of rehabilitation for chronic facial palsy are still rather small. Between 1958 and 2001 only three RCTs were published,[8] and since then not many additional studies have followed. A recent update of a Cochrane review[9] on physical therapy for idiopathic facial paralysis (Bell's palsy) found 65 potentially relevant articles indexed in the Cochrane Database of Systematic Reviews, the Cochrane Central Register of Controlled Trials of 2011, or other world databases (MEDLINE, EMBASE, etc). Twelve papers were identified, with a total of 872 subjects, that fulfilled the basic principles of RCT. Patients were analyzed as acute (i.e., treatment commencement either immediately after initial diagnosis of facial palsy or within a period of 3 weeks post initial diagnosis), postacute (i.e., treatment commencement > 3 weeks and up to 3 months post initial diagnosis), and chronic (i.e., treatment commencement > 3 months post initial diagnosis). Since then, three more studies have been published.[10–12]

> **!**
>
> There are a lack of controlled trials concerning the effectiveness of training programs for facial palsy.

Since the 1950s, publications on rehabilitation measures have covered:

- Electrical stimulation and physical therapy including mirror training.
- Mime therapy, proprioceptive neuromuscular facilitation, and/or neuromuscular reeducation.
- Electromyographical (EMG) biofeedback with or without a combination of the methods listed in the previous two points.

For the present review, first some of the studies that have investigated the efficacy of biofeedback, and trials that have tested electrical stimulation, physical therapy, and mirror training, will be presented. An overview of the most frequent therapy concept is given in ▸ Table 26.1.

Table 26.1 Overview of the most common training programs for patients with facial palsy

Type of therapy	Key characteristics
Neuromuscular biofeedback training	Mostly uses EMG surface-recording Visual and acoustic facial muscle feedback Individual selected muscles can be trained Can exercise specifically weak muscles, symmetry, hyperactivity, or synkinesis Needs EMG recorder, most used in outpatient setting; home devices are available but reliability has not been tested Effectiveness has been shown
Proprioceptive neuromuscular facilitation	Stimulates the development of complex patterns of coordinated muscular actions, the normalization of muscle tone, muscle stretching, and strengthening of muscle force Not many RCTs for facial palsy available
Mirror treatment	Another type of feedback training in front of a mirror Outpatient training necessary, but often used to continue at home Standardization of movement not as controllable as with EMG Effectiveness has been shown EMG feedback seems to be more effective
Mime therapy	Based on mime training for actors Stimulation of facial emotional expression and functional movements Focuses on symmetry of the face at rest and during movement Effectiveness has been shown
Home training	No standards defined Mostly facial movement exercises according to photographs, often in front of a mirror
Acupuncture	Popular for treatment of Bell's palsy in China Effectiveness has not been shown
Electrical stimulation	No standards defined Needs a special device for training in office or at home Effectiveness has not been shown

Abbreviations: EMG, electromyography; RCTs, randomized controlled trials.

> !
>
> The most frequent types of training, sometimes combined, are: physical therapy, mirror therapy, electrical stimulation, mime therapy, and electromyographic biofeedback therapy.

26.2 Neuromuscular Biofeedback Training

Neuromuscular biofeedback training represents a common approach in the rehabilitation of neuromuscular disorders, pain, and other disorders.[13–16] According to a consensus of three scientific and professional organizations concerned with biofeedback, biofeedback is defined as "a process that enables an individual to learn how to change physiological activity for the purposes of improving health and performance. Precise instruments measure physiological activity such as brainwaves, heart function, breathing, muscle activity, and skin temperature. These instruments rapidly and accurately "feed back" information to the user. The presentation of this information—often in conjunction with changes in thinking, emotions, and behavior—supports desired physiological changes. Over time, these changes can endure without continued use of an instrument."[17]

> !
>
> Biofeedback in facial palsy is the process that enables the patient to learn how to change physiological activity in the affected side of the face for the purposes of improving health and performance.

26.2.1 Technique

Neuromuscular biofeedback of facial palsy is based on EMG surface-recording techniques and the feedback of subject's muscle activity through visually or acoustically symbolized information. It is focused on the training of facial muscles that are paralyzed, or show weak activation, overactivation (hyperkinesis), or involuntary movements (synkinesis) in response to movements of other facial muscles on the palsy-affected part of a patient's face. For EMG recording, a variety of systems are available that represent standalone instruments or complex systems composed of electrophysiologic recorders (EMG signal amplifiers). These are interfaced to computers with software for data analysis/selection and the control of output devices such as video monitors for visual feedback or loudspeakers/headphones for acoustic feedback.[18]

> **!**
>
> Facial biofeedback training focuses on paralyzed, hyperkinetic, or synkinetic muscles.

Input to the biofeedback instruments is provided by at least two electrodes, i.e., an active electrode and a reference electrode. In contrast to needle electrodes that are able to record the activity of single muscle units, most applications of EMG biofeedback use surface electrodes with a variety of small diameters. This surface EMG signal is a quasirandom train of motor unit action potentials evoked by the contraction of striate muscles. Since facial muscles often are layered, the recorded train of muscle activity commonly does not represent the activity of a single striate muscle, but the summed activity of groups of layered muscles. Its frequency can range from a few hertz to over 2 kHz, and the amplitudes can vary from fractions of a microvolt to several hundred microvolts. As a result of the amplitude and frequency characteristics, detection of high-quality EMG signals requires conscientious application of noise-reduction and grounding practices.[19] In order to record the surface EMG signals, the surface electrodes are commonly fixed to the skin above the belly of a single muscle and referenced to an electrode at a muscularly inactive part of the subject's face against which the muscle activity of the active electrode is derived and amplified. In some conditions, several active electrodes above different muscles or groups of overlapping muscles are used that can be referenced to the same reference electrode. The latter is the case, for example, when synkinesis is treated or when complex patterns of facial expressions are being trained. A typical example of a biofeedback setup with an amplifier, electrode positions, feedback signals displayed on a screen, and the simultaneous mirror image of a subject on the feedback screen is presented in ▶ Fig. 26.1 and ▶ Fig. 26.2.

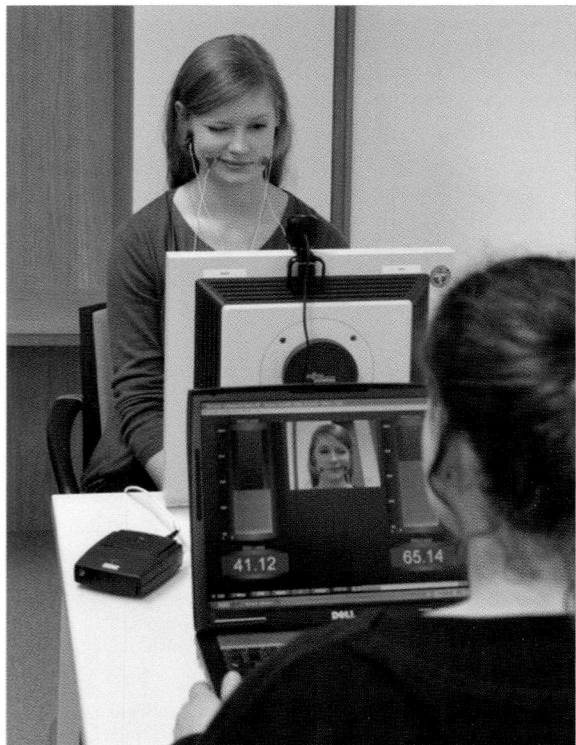

Fig. 26.1 A typical example of a biofeedback setup with amplifier, electrode positions, and feedback signals displayed on a screen.

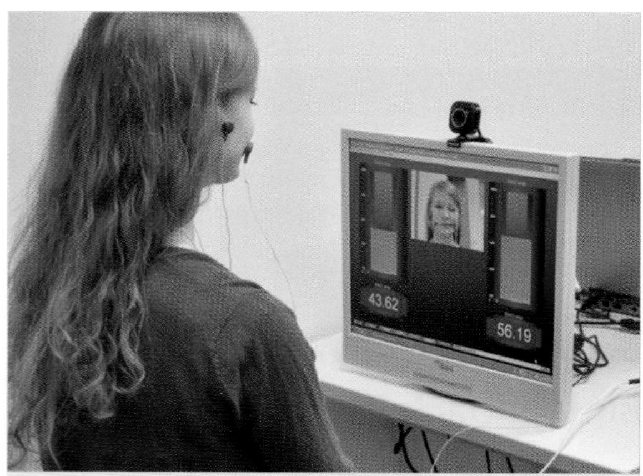

Fig. 26.2 A biofeedback setup showing a simultaneous mirror image of a subject on the feedback screen.

Although the course of EMG biofeedback training differs as a function of the patient's palsy condition, in most treatment conditions training of a single muscle, or group of overlapping muscles, follows some common patterns. In case of weak or absent muscle activation, subjects are encouraged to activate the target muscle lightly in a first step and keep the activation for several seconds, and then to deactivate the muscle again as much as possible. Care is taken that the threshold for feedback is kept low enough, so that even the weakest activation can be fed back to the patient. In standalone instruments, this feedback is mostly composed of a band of small LED lights. In computer-controlled systems, feedback can be composed of many different types of visualization; for example, increasing/decreasing hatch bars, circles, or rectangles. Some programs have elaborate visual reinforcement strategies such as use of waterfalls, opening or closing flowers, cars, or objects that move, walk etc. The increase/decrease of these feedback signals is a function of the recorded muscle activity, i.e., the more or less activity the muscle in question shows, the larger/smaller the feedback signal. When small activities of a target muscle can be reliably observed/recorded, training trials are commonly repeated until the patient has gained control of the requested level of activation/deactivation. Subsequently, the target intensity of activation/deactivation is increased and training with the new intensity is repeated until its control is mastered.

> !
>
> In feedback training of paralyzed or weak muscles, the activity of the muscle in exercise correlates to the strength of the feedback signal.

Treatment of overly activated muscles is aimed at reducing muscle activation. The number of repetitions of single training trials, the intensities, and duration of succeeding target activations/deactivations, as well as the frequency and duration of the total training session per day and muscle, have to be adopted to the diagnosis of the palsy and the patient's physical, motivational, and cognitive conditions.

> !
>
> In feedback training of overly activated muscles, the deactivation of the muscle during exercise is depicted as a reduction of the strength of the feedback signal.

In addition to the training of single target muscles, surface EMG feedback also provides options for the control of synkinesis or the balance between two or more muscles. In this case, patients are trained to activate one muscle unit while another target muscle is being deactivated, or to activate/deactivate a muscle while another target muscle is trained to keep its activity at a predefined level.

26.2.2 Efficacy

Few studies have presented data about the effectiveness of EMG biofeedback in patients with facial palsy(details of these studies are given in the following paragraphs). Almost all of these interventions were carried out as outpatient programs. With the exception of one study that employed RCT, all other studies identified with the literature search were retrospective and nonrandomized in nature, or did not include control procedures, or represented mainly a series of case studies with rather descriptive and anecdotal research quality. Since RCT studies are widely lacking for EMG biofeedback for facial rehabilitation, details will also be included of some of the non–RCT studies that at least used comprehensive methods of baseline and post-treatment assessments of facial muscular functioning and a comprehensible description of the intervention methods.

In a study by Hammerschlag and colleagues,[20] EMG biofeedback was used to evaluate the effects of biofeedback training in a group of 16 patients who underwent hypoglossal–facial nerve anastomosis with and without postoperative EMG rehabilitation. Treatment effects were reported only descriptively, based on the analysis of facial activities videotaped before surgery and after the application of an EMG biofeedback training that took part in a period between 5 and 42 months following the hypoglossal–facial nerve anastomosis. Facial movement capacities were assessed by four observers, who were unaware of the patients' rehabilitation therapy, using a precursor of the House–Brackmann facial nerve grading system.[21] EMG feedback training started as soon as quantifiable change of monitored EMG activity could be demonstrated in the reinnervated muscles. The training addressed the asynchronous muscle activities to achieve synchrony and symmetry of function and spontaneity of expression. Selective muscle contraction was trained with the zygomatic muscle to produce identical amplitudes and duration of muscle activities on both sides of the mouth, and assisted by volitional tongue motion to facilitate contractions of muscles reinnervated by the hypoglossal nerve. This was realized until the onset and termination of such contractions became synchronous with those occurring on the unaffected side (e.g., risorius muscle) while smiling. Also, inhibition of undesired activity on the reanimated side (gating of hypoglossal motor system outflow) was trained in separate training trials and reinforced throughout the sessions. Success was based on the patient's ability to progressively inhibit the EMG activity during increasingly more demanding tongue movements. The average course of training took 4 to 6 months with two half-hour training sessions per week. In order to maintain the muscular control, monthly EMG feedback reinforcement sessions were provided. The descriptive effects of this training indicated good clinical success of motor control with this approach of EMG feedback.

In a follow-up study of the same group[22] with 30 patients who had lost coordinated control of facial muscles after nerve anastomosis of the seventh and twelfth nerves, the same EMG feedback training procedures as used in the preceding study were successfully applied in order to reduce the high muscular tone and the mass contraction.

> !
>
> Biofeedback training can also be applied to patients with hypoglossal–facial nerve suture. In such cases the training must include training of the hypoglossal nerve.

Brach and coworkers[23] presented a special EMG biofeedback program that focused on the rehabilitation of synkinesis. Fourteen patients with chronic unilateral facial nerve paralysis received physical therapy for retraining of oral synkinesis between 5 and 336 months after paralysis onset (mean 78.3 months). Eight of the patients were affected on the right half of the face; the remaining patients were affected on the left side of the face. All 14 patients showed ocular to oral synkinesis and 13 patients had brow to oral synkinesis. Patients' facial impairment was rated as House–Brackmann grade IV. In five of these subjects, facial palsy was diagnosed as Bell's palsy, while in four patients the palsy was iatrogenic due to treatment of an acoustic neuroma or other tumor. In the remaining subjects, the origin of palsy was multifactorial. The intensity and pattern of synkinesis was assessed before and at several time points during the rehabilitation program by means of video analysis. Quantification of synkinesis of the mouth was based on the horizontal and vertical displacement of the right and left corner of the mouth and the horizontal displacement of the center of the upper lip (measured in millimeters) during a series of five voluntary maximal brow raises and eye closure movements and during a rest condition. Treatment consisted of EMG biofeedback of voluntary and unintended movement areas simultaneously with electrodes from one channel being placed over the frontalis muscle, and electrodes from the second channel placed over the oral muscles involved in the synkinesis (i.e., the zygomaticus, the depressors, or levator labii muscle groups). Patients were instructed to watch the visual display of facial muscle activity while trying to raise the eyebrows without moving the mouth. Additionally, they were asked to increase the activity of the frontalis muscle while keeping the activity from the oral musculature to a minimum in order to decrease the synkinesis. A similar technique was used to reduce oral synkinesis with eye closure; however, instead of visual feedback regarding the mouth movement, the patient was given auditory feedback concerning the activity of the oral muscles. The mean number of physical therapy sessions comprised 12.8 sessions offered within an average period of 6.7 months, with one weekly session for most patients and a monthly session for a small number of patients. Each treatment session took 45 to 60 minutes and consisted of a brief reassessment, training, and instruction in a home facial movement exercise program. In addition to the clinical training sessions, each patient was instructed to foster the desired facial movement patterns during home training. The home facial movement exercise program consisted of some combination of movement exercises, stretching for passive lengthening of facial muscles in contracture, exercises to increase the excursion of facial expression, and instruction in self-administered cross-friction massage. The exercise program usually consisted of 5 to 10 repetitions of 3 to 5 exercises to be done twice daily. Statistical analysis of movement parameters showed that 12 of 13 patients with brow to oral synkinesis and 12 of 14 patients with ocular to oral synkinesis showed a significant reduction of synkinesis. This effect was especially observed in patients with chronic synkinesis that had been present for more than 1 year. Although the mean reduction of synkinesis was between 30 and 65%, the EMG biofeedback treatment did not affect the House–Brackmann facial rating.

In a subsequent study by the same group,[24] 66 patients with moderate-to-severe synkinesis or mild-to-moderate synkinesis were treated. Patients with aberrant regeneration secondary to removal of acoustic neuroma or other tumors, trauma, Bell's palsy, or hemifacial spasm were enrolled in a similar facial neuromuscular reeducation training program as described for the previous study. For synkinesis assessment and grading, the Ross et al system of facial grading[25] of facial movements at rest and during voluntary movement was used before and after treatment. The training involved intermittent EMG biofeedback training supervised by a professional, and individualized home exercise programs of specific facial movements that addressed the patient's synkinesis and promoted the recovery of desired patterns of muscle activation for selected facial expressions and functions. Patients did not use the EMG biofeedback at home, but it was suggested that they use a mirror for feedback. Data analysis included multivariate analysis of variance with repeated measures to evaluate the changes in synkinesis and movement. Analysis revealed significant improvements of facial synkinesis and an increase of intended facial movement following treatment.

> **!**
>
> Most biofeedback training programs combine training with a therapist and home training programs.

Cronin et al[26] retrospectively investigated the effectiveness of an individualized neuromuscular facial retraining program with EMG biofeedback in 24 patients with mixed chronic facial paralysis due to Bell's palsy, trauma, nerve anastomosis, nerve infection (Guillain–Barré syndrome and Ramsey Hunt syndrome), or treatment of acoustic or facial nerve schwannoma. Twelve of these patients complained of synkinesis. The program included education of patients on the basics of facial anatomy and physiology and dual-channel EMG biofeedback treatment to compare and train the weak side of the face using the normal functioning side for comparison. In addition to EMG biofeedback, patients were instructed in eye care, vibration, massage, and functional isolated specific exercises to develop selective muscle control and decrease synkinesis. To decrease synkinesis, one EMG electrode was placed over the muscle to be contracted while a second electrode was placed over the synkinetic muscle of the same side of patient's face. Observing the graphs, the patient was asked to slowly contract and to hold the target muscle, while simultaneously relaxing the synkinetic muscle. Patients were treated on an outpatient basis 2 to 4 times per month. Facial reeducation was assisted by mirror training at home and some patients also received home EMG biofeedback units to deepen the feedback training on a daily basis. Treatment outcomes were assessed by tests of facial symmetry on EMG, percentages of facial function before and after intervention, changes in synkinesis, and measurements of other residual facial dysfunctions of dry eye, excessive tearing, drooling, lip droop on the affected side, and eye size asymmetry. After training all patients showed significant improvements in function, including an increase in facial symmetry and facial movements. Synkinesis was also reduced by at least two levels in patients who initially demonstrated synkinesis.

Following a retrospective control-group approach, Dalla Toffola and colleagues[27] investigated the effectiveness of physical therapy in comparison with EMG biofeedback methods in 28 and 37 patients, respectively, who had Bell's palsy. Assessment of facial functions was undertaken between 12 and 23 days after onset of the palsy and repeated every 2 weeks during the rehabilitation program, with the last assessment at 12 months postonset. Clinical assessment included evaluation of static and dynamic facial asymmetry, manual muscle strength of the frontalis, corrugator, orbicularis oculi, palpebral muscles, zygomaticus, canines, and orbicularis oris muscles, and of synkinesis within palpebral–zygomatic and orbicularis oculi–palpebral muscles. Additionally, tics and synkinesis during facial mimicry were examined. When present, synkinesis was defined as mild, moderate, or severe, and further facial motor dysfunctions were based on the House–Brackmann scale. Furthermore, EMG and electroneurographical (ENoG) evaluation was carried out between 3 and 4 weeks after paralysis onset in each patient, with clinical motor deficits with ENoG being assessed for the palpebral and orbicularis oculi muscles. Clinical treatment was offered during a subacute to chronic period after the onset of the palsy (minimum 1 month) after the first signs of motor recovery and included either physical therapy or EMG biofeedback. In the physical therapy, stretching of paretic muscles and transcutaneous electrical stimulation were performed to establish submaximal muscle contractions and supplemented with exercises to affect synkinesis. On average this treatment was offered for 24 sessions. Biofeedback therapy was applied for 17 sessions on average and aimed to teach control over the palpebral, zygomatic and risorius muscles, with threshold levels established on the basis of possible muscle activity. Acoustic stimuli were utilized as biofeedback. Inhibition of synkinetic movement was the primary goal, with biofeedback signals applied as soon as the patient showed synkinetic activity. Subsequently the patients were instructed in functional movements and pronunciation of words with continued care to avoid synkinesis. Treatment in both groups initially comprised three to five 1-hour sessions per week followed by one to two therapist-driven sessions per week, during which patients continued exercises autonomously at home. Comparison of muscle activities before and after the treatment indicated that EMG biofeedback treatment showed superior muscle recovery and minor reduction of synkinesis over physical therapy. After therapy, all patients showed clinical improvement, and neither treatment group had a patient receiving a House–Brackmann score greater than III. The biofeedback group had more patients with complete recovery or mild dysfunction than patients of the physical therapy group. Clinical evaluation of synkinesis indicated that synkinesis was always present in both groups of treatment but patients in the biofeedback group had fewer and less severe synkinesis following treatment than those in the physical therapy group.

In one of the few prospective RCTs, Ross and coworkers[28] investigated the efficacy of EMG biofeedback compared with that of mirror feedback in the treatment of chronic (18 months minimum) facial nerve paresis. Twenty-five patients were randomly assigned to an EMG biofeedback program with mirror feedback (11 patients) or to mirror feedback alone (13 patients). Seven patients served as controls without treatment. Treatment procedures included supervised mirror exercises of activation/deactivation of small graded isolated movements and controlling symmetrical muscle function and relaxation of muscles by a physical therapist, and an instructed and individualized home program aided by the use of a mirror for 30 to 60 minutes daily. Patients were requested to keep a diary about the exercises and observations of the daily home training. The training schedule consisted of two sessions per week for 2 weeks, one session per week for 6 weeks, and two sessions per month for 10 months, for total treatment duration of 1 year. The other treatment included the same procedure plus a single 0.5 hour of EMG biofeedback. Facial muscle activities were assessed at the beginning of training and at 6 and 12 months following treatment onset by quantification of facial movement with linear measures of surface anatomic landmarks, visual assessment of voluntary movement, and facial nerve response to maximal electrical stimulation. Statistically significant improvements were noted in both EMG biofeedback and mirror-feedback groups with respect to symmetry of voluntary movement and linear measurement of facial expression indicating positive effects of both treatment procedures. Effects of the biofeedback group trended toward stronger responses over those of the mirror-feedback group; however this difference did not reach significance.

!

In one of the few prospective randomized control trials [29] both electromyographic (EMG) biofeedback and mirror feedback improved synkinesis. There was a trend for a stronger effect of EMG biofeedback.

Nakamura and coworkers[29] presented one of the few RCTs on synkinesis. In this study, 27 patients with complete facial paralysis due to Bell's palsy (10) or herpes zoster oticus (17) were randomly assigned either to mirror treatment or to an untreated control group. Patients were instructed to avoid strong and random contractions of the facial muscles and to try to keep their eyes open symmetrically during three mouth movements (pursing one's lip, baring one's teeth, and puffing out one's cheeks) while watching their face in a mirror. Training was organized as home training for 30 minutes daily for a period of 10 months. The degree of synkinesis was evaluated while the patients performed several facial movements, by computing the percent asymmetry of the intrapalpebral width when performing the oral movements. One year after initial diagnosis, results showed a significantly smaller asymmetry in the width of eye opening, between both eyes, in the biofeedback treatment group compared with the control group.

Also this series of studies indicated positive outcomes of different physical therapy procedures that—in most cases—were composed of a few professionally supervised sessions that were extended by home training procedures.

26.3 Rehabilitation of Facial Paralysis following Different Treatment Concepts of Physical Therapy without Concurrent Biofeedback Methods

Physical therapy of facial paralysis *without biofeedback* includes a complex and rather mixed family of different treatment approaches, including thermal methods, electrotherapy/electrical stimulation, massage, acupuncture, facial exercises, and mirror training. All these methods have been often applied as combined professionally supervised outpatient interventions and have spanned different periods following the onset of facial paralysis. Furthermore, they have covered different periods of time, with different durations of single sessions, and different numbers of sessions and rhythms of sessions across time. Additionally, most of these interventions supplemented the physical treatments with home training programs, where patients were instructed to exercise selected and instructed facial movements in front of a mirror or without mirror assistance, or applied muscle stretching and other muscular measures. Since for this family of treatments, prospective RCTs have been conducted more often than for the biofeedback approach, the following review only includes studies on facial exercises and mirror training that applied prospective RCTs. For studies that did not follow such design, see other recent reviews.[9] Likewise, studies on thermal methods, electrotherapy/electrical stimulation, massage, and acupuncture are not presented, since critical reviews of these methods have indicated no clear positive results for facial paralysis (for extended reviews see the two systematic Cochrane reviews[9,30] that contain all studies that have claimed to follow RCT paradigms).

!

Studies on facial exercises and mirror training, thermal methods, electrotherapy/electrical stimulation, massage, and acupuncture without a feedback element lack proof of efficacy.

26.3.1 Proprioceptive Neuromuscular Facilitation

The efficacy of physiotherapy based on the Kabat concept was investigated by Barbara et al[31] in a prospective, randomized study with 20 consecutive patients who had postacute Bell's palsy that started 4 days before admission to therapy. In short, the Kabat concept, also called proprioceptive neuromuscular facilitation, is a complex method that aims to stimulate and assist the development of complex patterns of coordinated muscular actions, the normalization of muscle tone, and muscle stretching and strengthening.[32,33] The aim of muscle stretching is to increase the range of motion. Stretching of the muscle is induced by a shortening contraction of the opposing muscle. It is commonly applied in the treatment of peripheral nerve and spinal disorders and after trauma of the motor system. It was applied with one session per day for 6 days, and continued for 15 days. Effects of this treatment were compared with those on a waiting list for treatment who did not receive physical rehabilitation. Assessment of initial and post-treatment facial impairment was based on the House–Brackmann grading system applied at the beginning of intervention and again at days 4, 7, and 15 after onset of facial palsy. Additionally, the compound motor action potential was recorded with needle electrodes at the orbicularis oculi, frontal, and orbicularis oris muscles on the same days as the House–Brackmann grading. The intervention led to a change of the House–Brackmann grade from an initial IV to a II at the end of intervention. No change was obtained in the amount of the compound motor action potential.

26.3.2 Mime Therapy

Another concept for facial training is called mime therapy and this was examined in a series of three studies by Beurskens and Heymans.[34–36] Reports of other centers using this method are lacking. Mime therapy consists of a combination of training of facial emotional expression and functional movements. It focuses on the promotion of symmetry of the face at rest and during movement, and supports the patient to control synkinesis or mass movements of the paralyzed face. Treatment is offered 10 times with one session per week and each session lasting approximately 45 minutes. The therapy trains patients to align the two facial halves (to control and to reduce synkinesis) and to establish reintegrated emotional expressions. Training is organized as home training with daily exercises, assisted by a homework manual. The manual includes information concerning treatment and prognosis. The therapy includes automassage of the face and neck, breathing and relaxation exercises, and specific exercises for the face to coordinate both halves and to decrease synkinesis (for examples see ▶ Fig. 26.3); exercises in lip movement for eating, drinking, and rinsing of the mouth; letter and word pronunciation exercises; emotional expression exercises; and guidance in communication possibilities. Study one[34] represents a RCT including an outpatient mime group with 25 subjects suffering from chronic unilateral facial paralysis existing for a period of at least 9 months with a mean House–Brackmann score of grade IV. Effects of therapy were evaluated by changes observed in the stiffness of the face, lip mobility according to lip length and pout, and by the Facial Disability Index[37] whose effect was compared with that of a control group who were on a waiting list for treatment and did not receive treatment. Results showed that stiffness of the face, lip mobility in regard to lip length and pout indices, and the disability and participation level of the Facial Disability Index changed significantly in the mime group as compared with the group on the waiting list. Similar positive effects were obtained in a retrospective study on the effects of mime therapy that included 155 patients with subacute facial paresis (21% with Bell's palsy, 33% following surgical removal of an acoustic neuroma, 8% following herpes zoster, 15% after operative trauma, 6% with otitis media, 7% due to congenital facial nerve paresis, and the remaining 10% of unknown diagnoses). The retrospective evaluation indicated significantly improved facial symmetry at rest. Although the average severity of the asymmetry in all movements decreased, the severity of synkinesis increased for three out of eight movements. Substantially fewer patients reported disabilities in eating, drinking, and speaking; and quality of life improved significantly. The effects of the first study were replicated by the same group,[36] and thus this represents one of the few rehabilitation concepts for which direct replication is available.

> **!**
>
> The innovators of mime therapy have shown in a series of studies that the treatment improves symmetry at rest and during movements. It will be important for this work to be replicated in another center.

26.3.3 Mixed Home Training

Lindsay et al[38] tested quantitative improvements of facial function after facial rehabilitation in a large retrospective series of 160 consecutive subjects with facial paralysis. Facial rehabilitation included education, neuromuscular training, massage, meditation relaxation, and an individualized home program. After 2 months of home exercises, the participants were re-evaluated, and the home program was tailored as necessary. All participants were evaluated before the initiation of facial rehabilitation, and 160 participants were re-evaluated after receiving treatment with the Facial Grading Scale (FGS).[37] The FGS represents a quantitative instrument to evaluate facial function by scoring resting symmetry, active motion, and synkinesis. All participants underwent the initial evaluation at least 4 months after the onset of facial paralysis; for 49 participants, the evaluation took place more than 3 years after onset. Results of this retrospective analysis revealed statistically significant increases in FGS scores after treatment.

26.3.4 Neuromuscular Reeducation Versus Conventional Therapeutic Measures

A further RCT by Manikandan and coworkers[39] investigated the effects of a complex facial neuromuscular reeducation program in comparison with conventional therapeutic measures in the treatment of facial asymmetries in 59 patients with Bell's palsy. Patients were randomly assigned to one of these treatments. Unfortunately, the study did not provide information as to whether treatment started immediately, or shortly after, the onset of Bell's palsy or during the subacute or chronic state of the disorder. Electrical stimulation served as a control procedure, and the treatment tested was composed of gross facial expression training and massage. Electrical stimulation was provided in three sessions per day and included stimulation of the facial muscles and the facial nerve trunk and major divisions. Each muscle was stimulated 90 times in three sessions and 10 pulses were given to each facial nerve division and the main trunk. Intensity of the current was increased until minimal visible contraction of the muscle was observed. Electrical stimulation was given for 6 days a week for a period

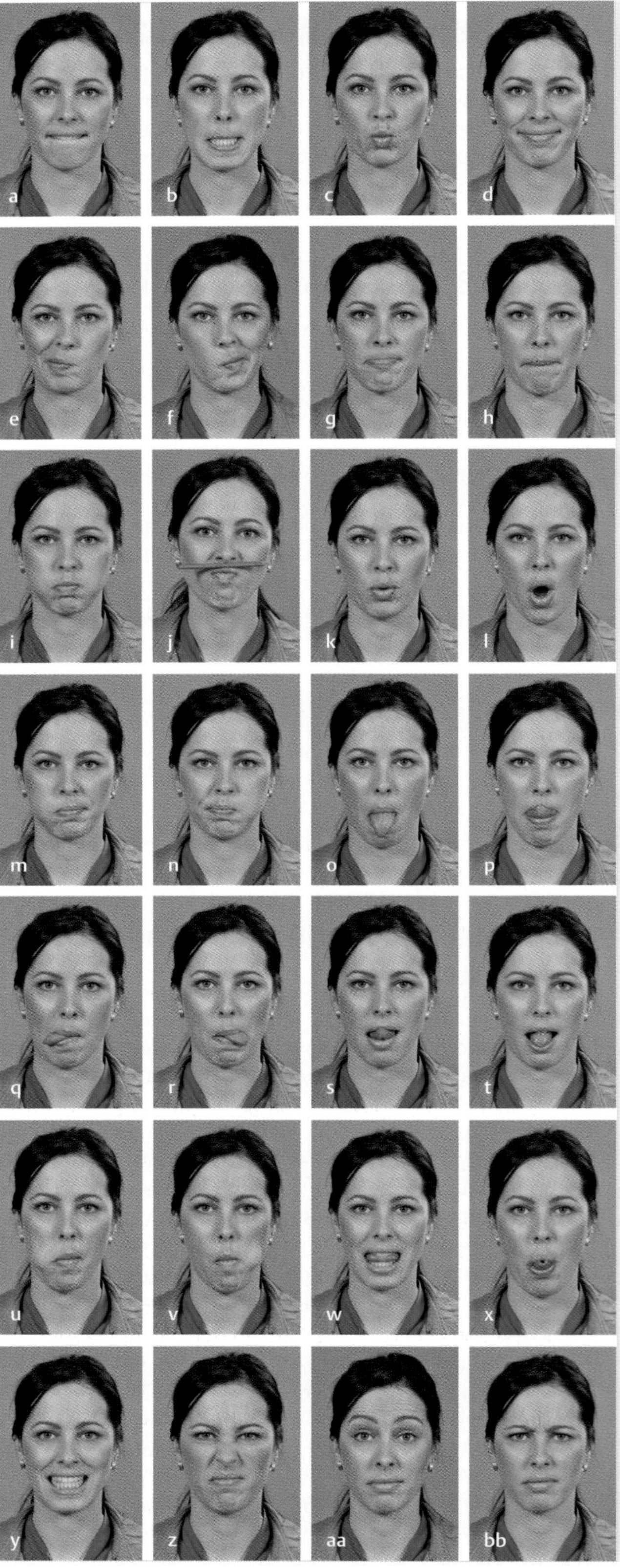

Fig. 26.3 Facial exercises to coordinate both halves of the face and to decrease synkinesis. **(a)** Bite lower lip. **(b)** Bite upper lip. **(c)** Purse lips. **(d)** Stretch lips. **(e)** Pull lips to the right. **(f)** Pull lips to the left. **(g)** Pull lower lip above upper lip. **(h)** Pull upper lip above lower lip. **(i)** Blow both cheeks. **(j)** Hold pencil. **(k)** Express small "O." **(l)** Express open "O." **(m)** Blow up right cheek. **(n)** Blow up left cheek. **(o)** Put out tongue. **(p)** Lift tongue toward tip of nose. **(q)** Move tongue into the right corner of mouth. **(r)** Move tongue into the left corner of mouth. **(s)** Touch upper lip with tongue. **(t)** Touch lower lip with tongue. **(u)** Press tongue to right cheek. **(v)** Press tongue to left cheek. **(w)** Put tip of tongue behind upper teeth. **(x)** Roll tongue. **(y)** Show teeth. **(z)** Turn up nose. **(aa)** Frown. **(bb)** Pucker.

of 2 weeks. The neuromuscular reeducation treatment consisted of facial expression exercises, which included eye closure, eyebrow raise, frowning, smiling, puckering and pouting, balloon blowing, chewing gum on the paralyzed side, and using a straw and pronouncing vowels to strengthen the cheek muscles. Each patient received a tailored program of these methods and was requested to do only 5 to 10 repetitions of facial exercises three times a day and to be careful that facial movements were performed symmetrically without allowing the voluntary movement of the uninvolved side to distort the movement. The effects of both interventions were assessed and evaluated using the FGS before and 3 months after treatment. Results revealed significant improvement of the FGS scores that assessed facial movements in both groups, with significantly better improvement in the neuromuscular program than in the control program. Other grading scores were not affected by either therapy.

26.4 General Status of Current Rehabilitation Outcome

Although facial paralysis has a dramatic effect on the patient's quality of life,[4,5,40] the literature search revealed only a small number of empirical studies that have evaluated the effects of current physiotherapeutic rehabilitation procedures. There are only 15 RCTs. The remaining literature consists of 80 case reports and a small number of case series and retrospective analysis of treatment between 1958 and 2013. Given the small level of scientific support, it is no wonder that, according to Husseman and Mehta,[8] a lot of patients are often recommended simply to await spontaneous recovery or are suggested to accept treatments whose clinical effect has never been tested by adequate scientific inquiry. Compared with other muscular disorders, such as motor disorders following stroke, aphasia, and other neurological traumata, real data are lacking. Nevertheless, to summarize the present evidence for facial palsy rehabilitation based on the papers reviewed here and on the earlier reviews mentioned previously, the situation does offer some hope. There exists a series of treatment methods that indicate a promising clinical outcome for many patients with a broad range of acute and chronic facial paralysis. Among these promising methods, surface EMG biofeedback, with and without additional mirror therapy, and facial exercises at home represent methods that have positively affected different aspects of facial paralysis and facial synkinesis and asymmetry. Similarly, mime therapy and facial exercises with and without mirror therapy are advisable concepts of rehabilitation.

> **!**
>
> Although it is difficult to compare the studies in this field, electromyographic biofeedback, with and without additional mirror therapy, and facial exercises at home represent the most effective methods to treat patients with facial palsy.

26.5 Methodological Problems

Of course, there are also many problems and open research questions that have to be solved in the future to further improve the provision of facial rehabilitation. This includes questions about the adequate assessment of motor function (grading) and of therapeutic progress and follow-up. Questions also remain about the intensity and duration of treatment. Also there are no data on the optimal relationship between supervised training and nonsupervised home training, and the amount, repetition rate, and duration of supervised and nonsupervised single muscle exercises. No research exists on the best structure of treatment components and the ideal sequence. Compared with other rehabilitation measures, is also seems that rehabilitation of facial paralysis has benefited from the use of new technologies to improve inpatient and, especially, home training; for example, by teletraining, computer-assisted training, or robotics. Finally, one must consider problems of study design and data analysis, and questions about manualization of treatment procedures[41,42] for proper administration and scientific replication.

26.5.1 Assessment of Motor Dysfunction

The House–Brackmann grading system[21] and the Facial Disability Index (FDI)[37] have dominated the assessment of motor dysfunction in many of the studies presented here, although both systems have almost never been used simultaneously. In addition, several further movement parameters such as vertical or horizontal displacement of the facial areas during dynamic movements or EMG measures of muscle functions have been used to quantify the amount of facial asymmetry or synkinesis. According to VanSwearingen,[43] the House–Brackmann grading system and the FDI account for about 72% of facial and social problems of patients with facial nerve disorders. While the House–Brackmann system assesses overall facial function and assigns a grade that reflects the overall severity of facial paralysis and secondary effects simultaneously, ENoG measures are regional and not able to assess the overall severity of muscular facial disorders. The psychometric properties of the House–Brackmann grading system have been evaluated as being sufficient in terms of its inter-rater reliability and its construct validity.[21] However, its disadvantage lays in the fact that it cannot differentiate finer pathological dysfunctions and fails to distinguish subtle differences in facial nerve recovery. On the other hand, psychometric properties of regional measures and ENoG measures have not been well assessed so far.

The FDI is a self-reported questionnaire for the assessment and quantification of the general disabilities of patients suffering from facial motor disorders.[37] It contains two subscales that determine the: (1) physical disability, and (2) the social consequences that are experienced due to the disorder. Its reliability and validity are considered to be good.[37] It is therefore difficult to decide which is the best measure to reflects the therapeutic effect of a treatment procedure. For the researcher, it might be less relevant whether a treatment procedure has gross effects, but more relevant whether it induces clinical change in principle. In contrast, the patient and the practitioner might put much more emphasis on the fact that a treatment affects functional change in the overall facial function and significantly affects the individual and social consequences and the response to the face by others.[4] Since the FDI supplements the gross grading of the House–Brackmann system, the application of both measures might represent an important advantage for the evaluation of the overall condition of a patient. Therefore, the application of both systems before and after rehabilitation treatment might provide valuable information about the effects of treatment.

!

When evaluating the effects of a training program, a standardized grading of the motor function and a standardized assessment of the facial nerve and specific quality of life should be performed. Although the House–Brackmann system is a global instrument with good inter-rater reliability, it is a gross measure and does not allow for measurement of fine changes in treatment outcomes.

26.5.2 Evaluation of Stability of Treatment Effects Beyond the Termination of Rehabilitation

Another critical aspect relates to the fact that no study mentioned in this chapter applied proper methods for the assessment of treatment effects beyond the termination of intervention. Some of the studies have used fixed follow-up measures, i.e., applied the assessment at the commencement of treatment or at the initial diagnosis of the facial disorder after a fixed period of time; for example, after 12 months succeeding the onset of the paralysis. Such a procedure carries many biases that might counteract a methodological sound empirical design. Using such a procedure might imply that treatment has happened at very different time periods in relation to the beginning and termination of the anamnestic and catamnestic time points. That a different period between initial diagnosis and the start of treatment will differentially affect a patient's motivation and compliance, and the reasoning of subjects about the disease and its potential treatability, was well documented in a series of studies.[44] There is clear evidence that long waiting periods until the start of treatment diminishes patients' motivation and compliance significantly. Additionally, variance between treatment termination and the time of catamnestic examination of patients affects additional biases and incalculable risk that the patient was provided with other additional treatments etc. None of the studies that used such a design reported that the subjects were carefully tracked during this waiting period with respect to additional treatments or additional complications in the course of recovery since initial diagnosis at the start of training or since treatment termination at the follow-up assessment. Thus, whether the treatment effects reported account for the treatment offered, or whether additional interventions and processes came into play, remains unresolved in these studies.

!

How long periods of waiting for the training affect the outcome is unknown. But it is clear that long waiting until the start of treatment diminishes patients' motivation and compliance significantly.

26.5.3 Sequencing of Treatment Components, Manualization

Many of the reviewed studies offered mixed treatment components that were partly provided in the practitioner or researcher's institution or at home. How these components were distributed between institutional or home training environments, and how frequently and intensively they were applied in what sequence, and how much time was spent for each component of treatment during each treatment session was not reported properly in any of the articles. This not only makes a proper application of the therapies for any practitioner rather difficult, but also prevents a direct replication of the studies. Replication is one of the most important prerequisites of methodological sound science and an indispensable condition for the progress of any interventional concept.[45–47]

Therefore, future studies should pay as much attention as possible to describing the treatment procedures as explicitly and exactly as possible in order to improve the proper and successful application of promising treatment procedures. Additionally, recent studies in psychotherapy have demonstrated that manual-based treatments with very close and detailed descriptions of the daily treatment procedures (called manualization of treatment procedures) are indispensably useful to improve and progress the outcome of interventions.[41,42,48]

26.5.4 Intensity of Daily Training and Total Duration of Training

A last point that was most astonishing to the authors as researchers who have spent years in the development and evaluation of motor rehabilitation programs for patients following stroke, and who have gained considerable practical and scientific experience with the administration and evaluation of constraint-induced movement therapy for these patients, is the fact that most treatments reviewed used rather short intervention periods (mostly maximal 30 to 60 minutes) per day and only a few sessions per week. Almost all articles of the review emphasized that facial paralysis represents a complicated neuromotor disorder where the treatment affords the systematic and intense exercising of new motor patterns. However, as our own motor development and almost all sports and the training of other complex movement patterns teaches us day by day, motor learning is one of the slowest types of learning that requires much more exercise, effort, attention, and persistence than the acquisition of any verbal or sensory information and competence.[49] One of the most important innovations of constraint-induced movement therapy[50–53] was the discovery that intensive motor training plays a key role for the immense clinical effects of this intervention.[51,54] Since the initial animal experiments on the recovery of motor suppression following somatosensory deafferentation in monkeys by means of "forced use,"[50,55] it has been repeatedly demonstrated that complex motor disorders, such as paretic arm or leg dysfunctions, can be overcome reliably only when the affected extremity is trained extensively and for several hours per day with a high degree of intensity, and that this training is offered for a minimum period of 2 to 3 weeks.[56] The most effective constraint-induced movement interventions have been demonstrated to be those that followed an intensive training regime with a daily training session of at least 3 to 6 hours.[56,57] According to this scientifically well-supported experience, it is suggested that most of the rehabilitation procedures for facial paralysis reviewed in this chapter would be significantly improved with better outcomes in a much shorter period following therapy onset, if treatment sessions were to be extended. Data suggest that taking therapy from 30 to 60 minutes daily to 3 to 4 hours per day of intensive exercise with only a few breaks would be more beneficial.

> **!**
>
> Most treatments reported in the literature use short intervention periods of 30 to 60 minutes per day and only a few sessions per week. Since facial paralysis represents a complicated neuromotor disorder, it can be hypothesized that longer training periods per day at least for a minimum period of 2 to 3 weeks would be much more effective, as has been shown for modern rehabilitation methods for stroke patients.

At the moment the authors' research group at the Facial Nerve Center of the Department of Otolaryngology at the University of Jena is testing such a concept in patients with chronic palsy. Patients participate in an inpatient program of massed facial practice that follows the principles of constraint-induced movement therapy. Training follows a manual that details the daily exercises and methods of assessment. Training is provided for a period of 2 weeks with daily-supervised facial motor training, as visually depicted in a treatment booklet by Hartwig,[58] by means of surface EMG biofeedback-assisted facial exercises. Supervised training occurs for 3 hours per day and focuses on facial asymmetries and synkineses. Additionally, patients participate in a nonsupervised training in the hospital ward for additional 2 hours per day. Here, patients are requested to repeat the facial movement exercises of the morning, assisted by mirror feedback and the training booklet of Hartwig,[58] and to record the type and duration of the muscle training with a diary. The study design corresponds to a prospective RCT with a wait for facial palsy patients of an average of 2 months prior to the start of treatment and a follow-up assessment after 6 and 12 months post-treatment. Assessment of motor functions includes quantification of facial impairments by means of the FGS. The FDI and other instruments have been additionally applied to examine the psychological consequences of the disorder, such as depression and anxiety, and the social consequences of the facial disorder. Furthermore, the quality/impairment of muscle activation is examined by ENoG and sonographical methods; see Chapter 4, Chapter 5, and Chapter 6. Facial asymmetry and synkinesis are additionally evaluated by a computer-based analysis of video recorded dynamical facial movements of 12 facial muscles. Data from the first 16 patients indicate[59] excellent recovery of facial motor functions and significant muscular plasticity of the most important target muscles for facial expressions. According to the preliminary pilot evaluation, this approach represents a new and promising extension of many of the reviewed rehabilitation concepts, and takes advantage of experiences gained with current research on the constraint-induced motor therapy concept.

26.6 Key Points

- Facial paralysis is a complex, psychologically, and socially highly disturbing neuromotor disorder of the face.
- The rehabilitation of this disease has long been widely neglected.
- However, several studies have demonstrated that the health care system possesses a series of methods that can make a positive impact on this impairment.
- Rehabilitation helps individuals to regain control of their facial muscles and emotional expressions in a way that social interaction with others becomes less stigmatizing, and patients can return to a normal, more satisfying life.

References

[1] Shaw M, Nazir F, Bone I. Bell's palsy: a study of the treatment advice given by Neurologists. J Neurol Neurosurg Psychiatry 2005; 76: 293–294

[2] Schiefer J. Bell's palsy. Akt Neurol 2013; 40: 37–48

[3] Morris AM, Deeks SL, Hill MD et al. Annualized incidence and spectrum of illness from an outbreak investigation of Bell's palsy. Neuroepidemiology 2002; 21: 255–261

[4] Dobel C, Miltner WHR, Witte OW, Volk GF, Guntinas-Lichius O. Emotional impact of facial palsy [in German] Laryngorhinootologie 2013; 92: 9–23

[5] Brach JS, VanSwearingen J, Delitto A, Johnson PC. Impairment and disability in patients with facial neuromuscular dysfunction. Otolaryngol Head Neck Surg 1997; 117: 315–321

[6] De Diego-Sastre JI, Prim-Espada MP, Fernández-García F. The epidemiology of Bell's palsy [in Spanish] Rev Neurol 2005; 41: 287–290

[7] Nunokawa Y, Shimada T. Prognosis of patients with peripheral facial palsy. J Phys Ther Sci 2011; 23: 49–52

[8] Husseman J, Mehta RP. Management of synkinesis. Facial Plast Surg 2008; 24: 242–249

[9] Teixeira LJ, Valbuza JS, Prado GF. Physical therapy for Bell's palsy (idiopathic facial paralysis). Cochrane Database Syst Rev 2011; 12: CD006283

[10] Azuma T, Nakamura K, Takahashi M et al. Mirror biofeedback rehabilitation after administration of single-dose botulinum toxin for treatment of facial synkinesis. Otolaryngol Head Neck Surg 2012; 146: 40–45

[11] Dalla Toffola E, Tinelli C, Lozza A et al. Choosing the best rehabilitation treatment for Bell's palsy. Eur J Phys Rehabil Med 2012; 48: 635–642

[12] Nicastri M, Mancini P, De Seta D et al. Efficacy of early physical therapy in severe Bell's palsy: a randomized controlled trial. Neurorehabil Neural Repair 2013; 27: 542–551

[13] Schwartz MS, Andrasik F, eds. Biofeedback: A Practitioner's Guide. London: Guilford Press; 2005

[14] Fischer JG, ed. Biofeedback: Studies in Clinical Efficacy. Soft cover reprint of the original 1st ed. 1987. Heidelberg: Springer; 2013

[15] Puckhaber HL. New Research on Biofeedback. Hauppauge, NY: Nova Science Publishers; 2006

[16] Rief W, Birbaumer N, eds. Biofeedback: Grundlagen, Indikationen, Kommunikation, praktisches Vorgehen in der Therapie. Stuttgart: Schattauer; 2006

[17] The Association for Applied Psychophsiology and Biofeedback, Inc. About Biofeedback. 2011. Available at: www.aapb.org/i4a/pages/index.cfm?pageid=3463. Accessed April 24, 2015

[18] The Association for Applied Psychophysiology and Biofeedback, Inc. 2011. Why you need to know how biofeedback devices work. Available at: www.aapb.org/i4a/pages/index.cfm?pageid=3292. Accessed April 24, 2015

[19] Fridlund AJ, Cacioppo JT. Guidelines for human electromyographic research. Psychophysiology 1986; 23: 567–589

[20] Hammerschlag PE, Brudny J, Cusumano R, Cohen NL. Hypoglossal-facial nerve anastomosis and electromyographic feedback rehabilitation. Laryngoscope 1987; 97: 705–709

[21] House JW, Brackmann DE. Facial nerve grading system. Otolaryngol Head Neck Surg 1985; 93: 146–147

[22] Brudny J, Hammerschlag PE, Cohen NL, Ransohoff J. Electromyographic rehabilitation of facial function and introduction of a facial paralysis grading scale for hypoglossal-facial nerve anastomosis. Laryngoscope 1988; 98: 405–410

[23] Brach JS, VanSwearingen JM, Lenert J, Johnson PC. Facial neuromuscular retraining for oral synkinesis. Plast Reconstr Surg 1997; 99: 1922–1931, discussion 1932–1933

[24] VanSwearingen JM, Brach JS. Changes in facial movement and synkinesis with facial neuromuscular reeducation. Plast Reconstr Surg 2003; 111: 2370–2375

[25] Ross BG, Fradet G, Nedzelski JM. Development of a sensitive clinical facial grading system. Otolaryngol Head Neck Surg 1996; 114: 380–386

[26] Cronin GW, Steenerson RL. The effectiveness of neuromuscular facial retraining combined with electromyography in facial paralysis rehabilitation. Otolaryngol Head Neck Surg 2003; 128: 534–538

[27] Dalla Toffola E, Bossi D, Buonocore M, Montomoli C, Petrucci L, Alfonsi E. Usefulness of BFB/EMG in facial palsy rehabilitation. Disabil Rehabil 2005; 27: 809–815

[28] Ross B, Nedzelski JM, McLean JA. Efficacy of feedback training in long-standing facial nerve paresis. Laryngoscope 1991; 101: 744–750

[29] Nakamura K, Toda N, Sakamaki K, Kashima K, Takeda N. Biofeedback rehabilitation for prevention of synkinesis after facial palsy. Otolaryngol Head Neck Surg 2003; 128: 539–543

[30] He L, Zhou MK, Zhou D et al. Acupuncture for Bell's palsy. Cochrane Database Syst Rev 2007; 4: CD002914

[31] Barbara M, Antonini G, Vestri A, Volpini L, Monini S. Role of Kabat physical rehabilitation in Bell's palsy: a randomized trial. Acta Otolaryngol 2010; 130: 167–172

[32] Sharma KN. Handbook of Proprioceptive Neuromuscular Facilitation: Basic Concepts and Techniques. Saarbrücken: LAP Lambert Academic Publishing; 2012

[33] Knott M, Voss DE. Proprioceptive Neuromuscular Facilitation: Patterns and Techniques. 2nd revised ed. Amsterdam: Bailliere Tindal; 1968

[34] Beurskens CHG, Heymans PG. Positive effects of mime therapy on sequelae of facial paralysis: stiffness, lip mobility, and social and physical aspects of facial disability. Otol Neurotol 2003; 24: 677–681

[35] Beurskens CHG, Heymans PG. Physiotherapy in patients with facial nerve paresis: description of outcomes. Am J Otolaryngol 2004; 25: 394–400

[36] Beurskens CHG, Heymans PG. Mime therapy improves facial symmetry in people with long-term facial nerve paresis: a randomised controlled trial. Aust J Physiother 2006; 52: 177–183

[37] VanSwearingen JM, Brach JS. The Facial Disability Index: reliability and validity of a disability assessment instrument for disorders of the facial neuromuscular system. Phys Ther 1996; 76: 1288–1298, discussion 1298–1300

[38] Lindsay RW, Robinson M, Hadlock TA. Comprehensive facial rehabilitation improves function in people with facial paralysis: a 5-year experience at the Massachusetts Eye and Ear Infirmary. Phys Ther 2010; 90: 391–397

[39] Manikandan N. Effect of facial neuromuscular re-education on facial symmetry in patients with Bell's palsy: a randomized controlled trial. Clin Rehabil 2007; 21: 338–343

[40] Bradbury ET, Simons W, Sanders R. Psychological and social factors in reconstructive surgery for hemi-facial palsy. J Plast Reconstr Aesthet Surg 2006; 59: 272–278

[41] Heimberg RG. Manual-based treatment: An essential ingredient of clinical practice in the 21st century. Clin Psychol Sci Pract 1998; 5: 387–390
[42] Wilson GT. Manual-based treatment and clinical practice. Clin Psychol Sci Pract 1998; 5: 363–375
[43] Vanswearingen J. Facial rehabilitation: a neuromuscular reeducation, patient-centered approach. Facial Plast Surg 2008; 24: 250–259
[44] Martin LR, Haskard-Zolnikrek KB, DiMatteo MR eds. Health Behavior Change and Treatment Adherence: Evidence-Based Guidelines for Improving Healthcare. Oxford: Oxford University Press; 2010
[45] Koole SL, Lakens D. Rewarding replications: a sure and simple way to improve psychological science. Perspect Psychol Sci 2012; 7: 608–614
[46] Pashler H, Harris CR. Is the replicability crisis overblown? Three arguments examined. Perspect Psychol Sci 2012; 7: 531–536
[47] Pashler H, Wagenmakers EJ. Editors' introduction to the special section on replicability in psychological science: a crisis of confidence? Perspect Psychol Sci 2012;7(6):528–530
[48] Marques C. Manual-based treatment and clinical practice. Clin Psychol Sci Pract 1998; 5: 400–402
[49] Weiss T, Miltner WHR. entralnervale Aktivierung und motorisches Lernen. In: Krug J, Minow HJ, eds. Messplatztraining. Sankt Augustin: Academia Verlag; 2004:47–57
[50] Taub E, Miller NE, Novack TA et al. Technique to improve chronic motor deficit after stroke. Arch Phys Med Rehabil 1993; 74: 347–354
[51] Taub E. Constraint-induced movement therapy and massed practice. Stroke 2000; 31: 986–988
[52] Miltner WHR, Bauder H, Sommer M, Dettmers C, Taub E. Effects of constraint-induced movement therapy on patients with chronic motor deficits after stroke: a replication. Stroke 1999; 30: 586–592
[53] Bauder H, Taub E, Miltner WHR. Behandlung motorischer Störungen nach Schlaganfall Göttingen: Hogrefe; 2001
[54] Wolf SL, Winstein CJ, Miller JP et al. Retention of upper limb function in stroke survivors who have received constraint-induced movement therapy: the EXCITE randomised trial. Lancet Neurol 2008; 7: 33–40
[55] Taub E, Harger M, Grier HC, Hodos W. Some anatomical observations following chronic dorsal rhizotomy in monkeys. Neuroscience 1980; 5: 389–401
[56] Taub E. The behavior-analytic origins of constraint-induced movement therapy: an example of behavioral neurorehabilitation. Behav Anal 2012; 35: 155–178
[57] Taub E, Uswatt G. Constraint-induced movement therapy: answers and questions after two decades of research. NeuroRehabilitation 2006; 21: 93–95
[58] Hartwig M. Fazialisprogramm: Gesicht-Mund-Zunge. Bad Honnef: Hippocampus Verlag; 2011
[59] Miltner WHR, Miltner EM, Volk GF, Guntinas-Lichius O. EMG biofeedback and massed practice in the rehabilitation of chronic facial paralyses. A prospective, randomised clinical trial. submitted

Part VII

Diseases Other Than Peripheral Facial Palsy

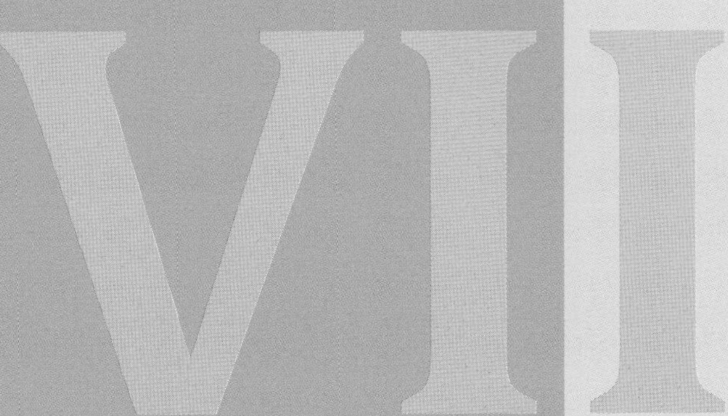

27 Central Facial Palsy

Carsten M. Klingner and Otto W. Witte

27.1 Introduction

The first and most important question that has to be answered when a patient complains about facial weakness is whether the lesion is of a peripheral or a central origin. This distinction is important because the course of treatment differs significantly between these causes. Specifically, if a central facial palsy is mistakenly identified as peripheral, the harm to the patient can be enormous because of a failure to request testing for potential life-threatening conditions (e.g., intermittent atrial fibrillation or endocarditis may be overlooked, which may lead to further and potentially deadly strokes). This chapter reviews the characteristics and causes of central facial palsies, as well as their treatment.

27.2 Definition

A central facial palsy is caused by an intracerebral, mostly contralateral, pathology that affects the facial upper motor neurons. The lesion can be spatially localized or can be diffuse in any region between the cerebral cortex and the synapses on the facial motor nucleus in the brainstem.

27.3 Epidemiology and Etiology

There are no data available about the epidemiology of central facial palsies. However, the most common etiology of a central facial palsy is stroke, which has an incidence of about 300 in 100,000 (Europe).[1] Stroke rates increase exponentially with age.[1] Approximately two-thirds of stroke patients have a facial palsy. Other etiologies such as neoplasia or cerebral inflammation are far less frequent causes of central facial palsy.

27.3.1 Causes of a Central Facial Palsy

Stroke

A stroke that involves the corticobulbar fibers is the most common cause of a central facial palsy. A localized lesion within the brainstem can cause symptoms of a central facial palsy if the lesion is proximal to the facial motor nucleus, or symptoms of a peripheral facial palsy if the lesion affects the facial motor nucleus (see ▶ Table 27.1 for brainstem syndromes of the pons with impaired facial function). Due to the general vascular supply territories a single localized lesion in the cortex is a rare event (▶ Fig. 27.1 and ▶ Fig. 27.2). However, it might be possible that a localized cortical ischemia is the first sign of an incomplete occlusion of a major cerebral artery or the result of a small vessel thrombosis. Therefore suspicion of a central origin of a facial palsy has to be handled like every other suspected stroke. The lesion can be caused by hemorrhage or ischemia and needs an emergency evaluation and diagnosis. This involves cardiac monitoring, intravenous access, and an emergency imaging of the brain. The most common effects of stroke are altered sensation (80%), difficulty of arm movement (70%), aphasia (33%), and visual problems.

> **!**
>
> Stroke that involves the corticobulbar fibers is the most common cause of a central facial palsy.

An ischemic stroke that causes an isolated central facial palsy is not an indication for administration of an intravenous recombinant tissue plasminogen activator. However, by using computed tomography (CT) angiography and CT perfusion, or magnetic resonance imaging (MRI) angiography, perfusion, and diffusion imaging, including measures of infarct core and penumbra, it is possible to judge the risk of an enlargement of the infarcted area.[2] These techniques provide additional information that may improve insights into diagnosis, mechanism, and severity of an ischemic stroke, and allow more informed clinical decision-making. In patients with a small infarct but an extended perfusion deficit because of an incomplete occlusion of a major cerebral artery, even a clinically isolated facial palsy may be considered for acute reperfusion therapy beyond the formal approval for intravenous fibrinolysis.

Table 27.1 Brainstem syndromes of the pons with impaired facial function

Syndrome	Ipsilateral symptoms	Contralateral symptoms
Foville's syndrome	Horizontal gaze palsy, facial palsy	Hemiparesis
Brissaud-Sicard syndrome	Hemifacial spasm	Hemiparesis
Gasperini syndrome	Palsy of the abducens nerve and facial nerve, impaired trigeminal function	Hemihypesthesia

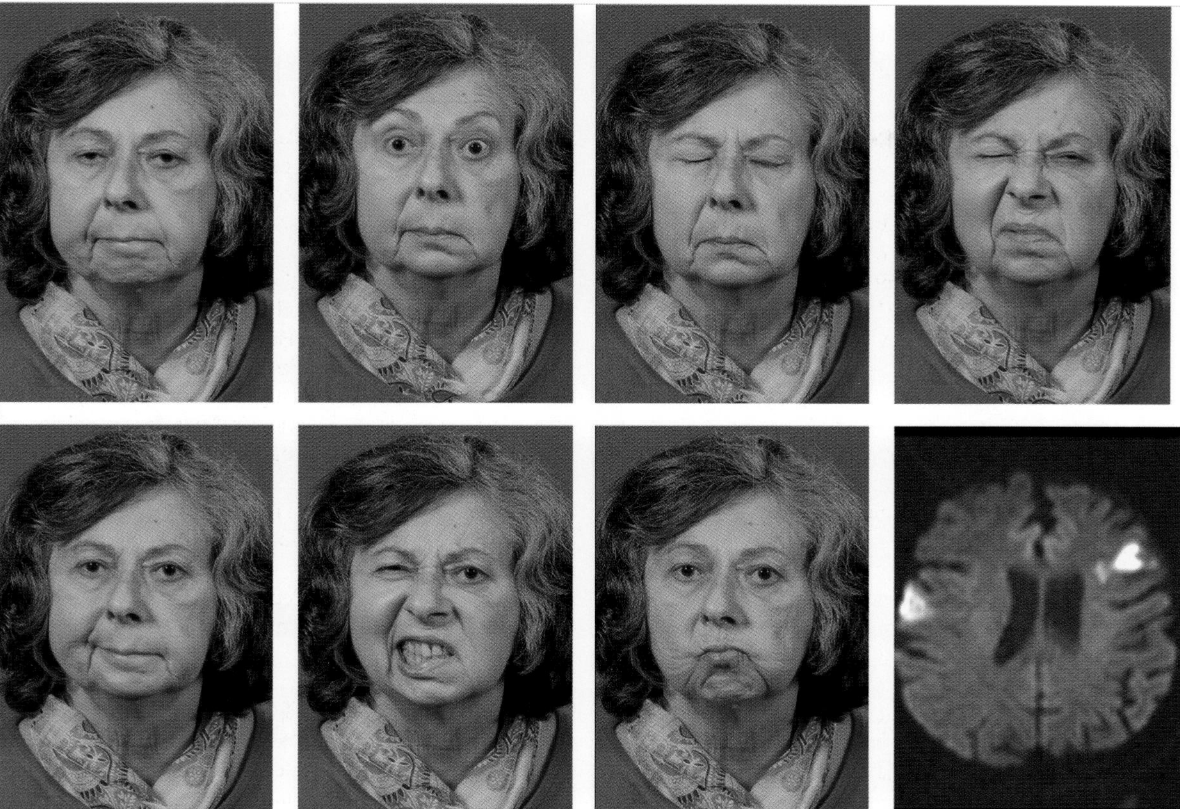

Fig. 27.1 Illustration of a left, central facial palsy, with the corresponding diffusion-weighted MRI. The 71-year-old woman presented to the emergency department with an acute facial weakness of the left face. She did not notice any symptoms until her skewed face was observed by her husband. The neurologic examination revealed a left-sided facial palsy, an ipsilateral hypesthesia of the left face, and an ipsilateral pronator drift. The additional left hemispheric frontal ischemia caused no symptoms noticeable in the neurologic examination.

A central facial palsy caused by a stroke should always be monitored in a stationary setting, which requires a specialized stroke unit.[3] The stroke unit is designed to care for patients with all types of stroke (ischemic, intracerebral hemorrhage, or subarachnoid hemorrhage), and those requiring specific interventions.

> **!**
>
> A central facial palsy caused by a stroke is best managed in a dedicated stroke unit.

Whatever the type of stroke, clarification of the etiology of the stroke is required for every patient. In patients in which ischemia has been verified as the cause of the symptoms, assessment for potential cardiac or vascular sources of the stroke is an important part of the urgent evaluation of the ischemic stroke, as it often has an impact on treatment decisions and is essential for reducing recurrent cerebrovascular events. In each patient, a cardiovascular history and examination, an electrocardiogram, and 24-hour telemetry monitoring should be performed to identify those with clinical evidence of heart disease. Patients with clinical evidence of heart disease or imaging that suggests a cardiac source of embolization should undergo a transthoracic echocardiogram and a transesophageal echocardiogram. Additionally, each patient should undergo ultrasonography of the intracranial and extracranial arteries that supply the brain (carotid, vertebral, posterior cerebral, anterior cerebral, middle cerebral, and basilar arteries). Ultrasonography can detect atherosclerotic carotid stenosis as well as less common etiologies, such as arterial dissection and vasculitis. However, magnetic resonance angiography has higher sensitivity and specificity than ultrasonography.[4] Patients with greater than 70% carotid stenosis on the side of the neurologic deficit benefit from a carotid endarterectomy, preferably within 2 weeks of the ischemic event, as it reduces the risk of future stroke.[5,6] Ischemic infarction is frequently accompanied by petechial hemorrhage without associated neurologic deterioration.

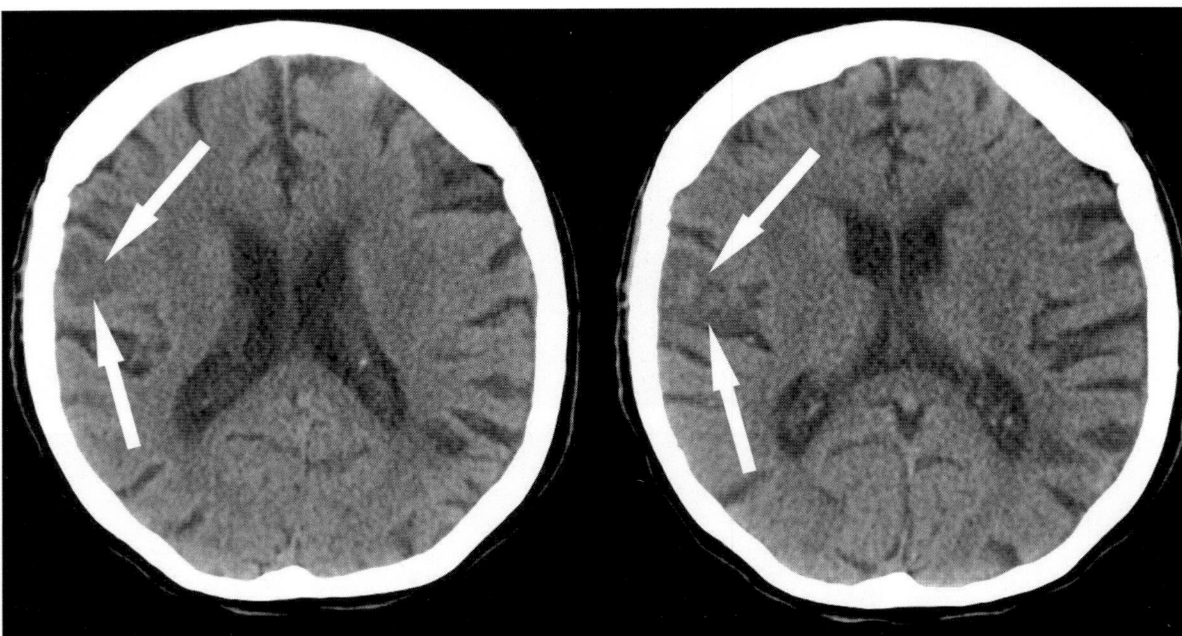

Fig. 27.2 CT of a left facial palsy due to a small cortical ischemia (*arrows*). A 77-year-old woman presented to the emergency department with an acute facial weakness of the left face. She noticed difficulties drinking (the drink had dribbled out of the left corner of her mouth). Her daughter had subsequently noticed her skewed face. The neurologic examination revealed an incomplete left-sided facial palsy without any other symptoms, particularly no hypesthesia and no ipsilateral pronator drift. The upper face was not completely spared, but it was involved to a lesser degree than the lower face. The corrugator and frontalis muscles were not involved.

For secondary prevention of future ischemic strokes, antiplatelet therapy with aspirin and a statin medication should be initiated within 24 hours of ischemic stroke in all patients who do not have contraindications, and should be continued long term. Although permissive hypertension is initially warranted, antihypertensive therapy should begin within 24 hours.

In patients with a verified intracerebral hemorrhage, care includes basic medical care, prevention of hematoma expansion, and treatment of potential secondary complications. Prevention of hematoma expansion is of outmost importance and requires a strict antihypertensive therapy protocol. Guidelines recommend a mean arterial pressure of lower than 130 mm Hg during the acute phase.[7] Procoagulant agents for hemostasis[8] and surgical evacuation[9] do not improve clinical outcomes in most cases. However, surgical intervention is necessary if an expanding hematoma causes a rapid rise in intracranial pressure, which may reduce cerebral perfusion pressure causing the development of a secondary injury.

Patients with a subarachnoid hemorrhage typically suffer from a thunderclap headache that develops over seconds. Most cases of subarachnoid hemorrhage are due to trauma, while most cases of spontaneous subarachnoid hemorrhage (without trauma) are due to the rupture of a cerebral aneurysm. Each patient with a suspected subarachnoid hemorrhage needs CT in the acute stage, while MRI is the more sensitive method after several days. If imaging is negative while a subarachnoid hemorrhage is suspected, a lumbar puncture should be performed (search for xanthochromia). In patients with a verified atraumatic subarachnoidal hemorrhage, its origin needs to be determined by angiography. The treatment involves general measures to stabilize the patient, prevention of vasospasm, and prevention of rebleeding. The therapeutic approach to prevent any rebleeding depends on the etiology of the subarachnoid hemorrhage. A cerebral aneurysm can be treated by clipping or coiling. The decision between clipping and coiling is made on the basis of the location of the aneurysm, its size, and the condition of the patient, and it is typically made by a multidisciplinary team.

Significant causes of morbidity and mortality following all kinds of stroke include venous thromboembolism, infection, and delirium. Patients suffering from impaired facial function often complain of difficulties in swallowing and speaking. Therefore, an evaluation for aspiration risk, including a swallowing assessment, should be performed, and nutritional, physical, and speech therapy should be initiated.

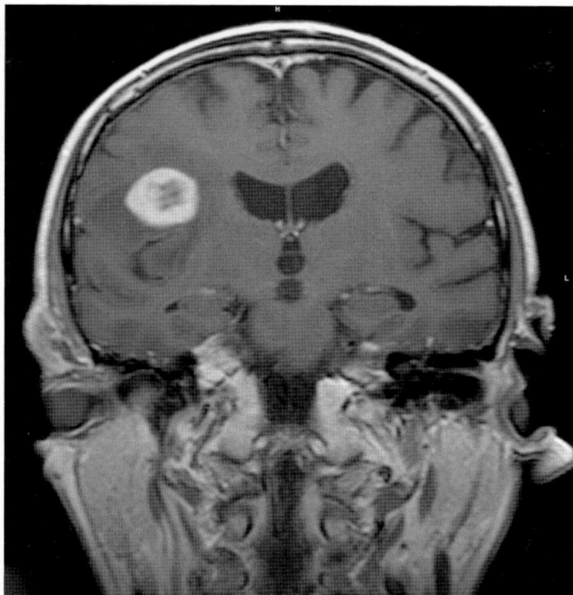

Fig. 27.3 Coronal contrast-enhanced T1-weighted MRI shows a solitary metastasis originating from prostate cancer. A 76-year-old man, with a history of nonmetastatic prostatic cancer, presented to the emergency department with a 2-week history of facial asymmetry. Two months previously, the patient had systemic restaging, which showed no evidence of metastatic cancer. The facial weakness of the left face was described as slightly progressive. The neurologic examination revealed a partly compensated left-sided facial palsy, an ipsilateral hypesthesia of the left face, and an ipsilateral pronator drift.

Neoplasia

Initial symptoms of brain tumors are typically headaches or other symptoms resulting from increased intracranial pressure, including seizures, focal deficits (related to particular brain regions), or affected cranial nerves. Focal deficits may be indicative of an isolated facial palsy if the tumor mainly affects the cortical representation of facial function (▶ Fig. 27.3). Patients commonly report a slow progression of symptoms; however, a sudden onset of symptoms may also occur as a result of tumor hemorrhage. In patients experiencing slow development of symptoms, the brain mechanisms for cortical reorganization and compensation often lead to a divergence between a strong resting facial asymmetry and a lighter facial weakness during voluntary movement. This pattern is difficult to distinguish from an old central lesion (e.g., a past ischemia) that has been incompletely compensated. However, this pattern is easily distinguishable from a lesion that occurs suddenly, where the facial weakness dominates the resting asymmetry during voluntary movement.

!

Suddenly occurring symptomatic tumor leads to impaired voluntary movements mainly, and decreased resting tone to a lesser extent.

Slow-growing tumor with symptoms developing slowly leads to decreased resting tone mainly, and impaired voluntary movements to a lesser extent.

⚠

Is there severe facial asymmetry but lighter facial weakness during voluntary movement? This can result from an old central lesion that has been incompletely compensated.

Brain tumors are rare compared with ischemic strokes; however, the onset of neurologic symptoms in a patient with a known tumor should prompt imaging of the neuroaxis to search for metastatic tumors. However, although MRI might be indicative of a brain tumor, the definitive diagnosis can only be confirmed by histological examination of tumor tissue samples obtained either by means of brain biopsy or by open surgery. There are various types of treatment available depending on the type of neoplasm and location (surgery, chemotherapy, radiotherapy).

Inflammation

Inflammatory diseases of the brain can be generalized, such as encephalitis/meningitis, or localized, such as inflammation of a specific part of the brain. The clinical hallmark of acute encephalitis is the triad of fever, headache, and altered mental status. Common neurologic features include: disorientation or depressed level of consciousness; disturbances of behavior, speech, or executive function; and diffuse or focal neurologic signs, such as cranial nerve dysfunction, hemiparesis, or seizures. More localized inflammatory diseases, such as multiple sclerosis, affect the white matter of the corticobulbar tract, including the brainstem. The inflammation causes damage to the myelin of the axons of neurons. Symptoms depend on the location of the inflammatory lesions and can present as facial palsy, but they are usually associated with other symptoms. Intracranial inflammation that leads to a facial palsy can affect all parts of the neuronal pathway between the cortex and the peripheral facial nerve. A relatively selective unilateral weakness of facial movements is more often caused by inflammation within the brainstem as opposed to inflammation of the cerebrum. The involvement of the facial motor nucleus in the brainstem, in particular, may result in a relatively selective unilateral weakness of facial movements. This phenomenon can present as a complete unilateral facial palsy, including the upper face, as well as an isolated weakness of eyelid closure due to the postsynaptic location of the lesion. Brainstem lesions that cause facial palsies often also affect the ipsilateral sixth cranial nerve due to the close spatial neighborhood of both nuclei.

Etiologies of acute cerebral inflammation are manifold and include infectious agents (bacterial, fungal, parasitic) as well as noninfectious etiologies (parainfectious, postinfectious, autoimmune, paraneoplastic). It is challenging for the clinician to make rapid diagnostic and therapeutic decisions when considering the specific symptoms of the patient.

MRI is the modality of choice for demonstrating the pathologic changes associated with structural inflammatory damage. However, imaging can remain normal in a subset of cases and changes can be extremely subtle, particularly at the early stage of the disease. Functional imaging (e.g., fluorodeoxyglucose positron emission tomography) can be helpful and might show hypermetabolism in the absence of structural MRI abnormalities in cases of generalized encephalitis.[10,11] However, in patients with an isolated abnormality of the brainstem, functional imaging is not helpful.

In addition to imaging, analysis of cerebrospinal fluid (CSF) is of utmost importance to reveal combinations of findings that suggest ongoing acute or chronic inflammation of the central nervous system (CNS). The white cell count, lactate concentration, and total protein levels are usually available very quickly even from nonspecialized laboratories, and a combination of these parameters often provides sufficient information for decision-making in emergency cases. Typical findings in the CSF are pleocytosis, oligoclonal bands, antineuronal antibodies, and intrathecal immunoglobulin synthesis (IgM, IgG).

!

The chameleon of neuroinflammation: a disseminated inflammation can mimic many neurological syndromes. Magnetic resonance imaging and analysis of cerebrospinal fluid are key to diagnosis.

27.3.2 Anatomy of the Central Facial Pathway

Patients with central facial nerve pathology can have loss of either volitional or emotional control. That is to say, the patient with certain central lesions cannot move their mouth muscles voluntarily; however, they are able to use those same facial muscles to produce a smile in response to a positive emotional event.[12–14] The concept of two motor systems, an emotional and a voluntary system, has been suggested as a possible mechanism of controlling these motor neurons.[15] Studies have shown that these different control systems do not use the same pathways to reach the mouth muscle lower motor neurons.[13] In the following section, the two pathways are described.

!

Two separate cortical motor systems, the voluntary facial movement system and the emotional facial movement system, control the facial muscles.

27.3.3 Voluntary Facial Movements

A voluntary facial motor command is generated by the interaction of at least five different brain areas: the primary motor cortex, the ventral lateral premotor cortex, the supplementary motor cortex, the rostral cingulate motor cortex, and the caudal cingulate motor cortex. The primary motor cortex is localized in the precentral gyrus and is the most crucial area involved in gross movements. Lesions that are localized in the facial representation of the precentral gyrus result in a paralysis of the contralateral face. The ventral lateral premotor cortex is localized immediately anterior to the facial representation of the primary motor cortex.[16] Lesions of the ventral lateral premotor cortex also result in paralysis of the contralateral face, but to a lesser extent than lesions in the primary motor cortex. The supplementary motor cortex is localized in the superior frontal lobule of the medial surface, caudal to the presupplementary motor area.[17] Lesions of the supplementary motor area do not cause paralysis, as this area is not crucial for the execution of simple motor tasks.[18] However, the supplementary motor area does appear to play an important role in the elaboration of voluntary movements involving a high degree of complexity.[19] Two further areas involved in facial expression reside in the cingulate cortex: the rostral cingulate motor cortex and the caudal cingulate motor cortex.[20] Studies in nonhuman primates have demonstrated that all these brain areas are tightly interconnected by corticocortical projections.[21] Studies using facial movement paradigms in humans have demonstrated enhanced metabolic activity in these cortical areas,[20] while studies of nonhuman primates have demonstrated enhanced neuronal activity determined by single-unit recording.[22] All of these brain areas have been found to project directly to the facial motor nucleus by the corticobulbar tract. The corticobulbar tract travels through the internal capsule and the upper midbrain to the lower brainstem where it synapses in the facial nerve nucleus (▸ Fig. 27.4).[23] There is some evidence from studies in nonhuman primates that each cortical motor facial area preferentially influences different sets of facial muscles.

27.3.4 Emotional Facial Movements

The cerebral generation of emotional facial movements is far more complex than that of voluntary movements. The brain areas responsible for voluntary facial movements are only one part in the generation of emotional facial movements. Crucial parts of the emotional facial control system reside in the extrapyramidal system.[24] Its pathways and pathophysiology are not well understood. It maintains wide interconnections by multisynaptic pathways with many parts of the brain. Additional brain regions that have been shown to be involved in the generation of emotional facial responses are the periaqueductal gray, the amygdale, and the striatum.[12–15] There is further evidence for a lateralized asymmetry of corticobulbar projections to the muscles of facial expression in the lower face,[25] favoring the left side. This asymmetry has been suggested because the right hemisphere has an advantage in processing emotional input and because emotions are expressed more intensely on the left side of the face.[26–28]

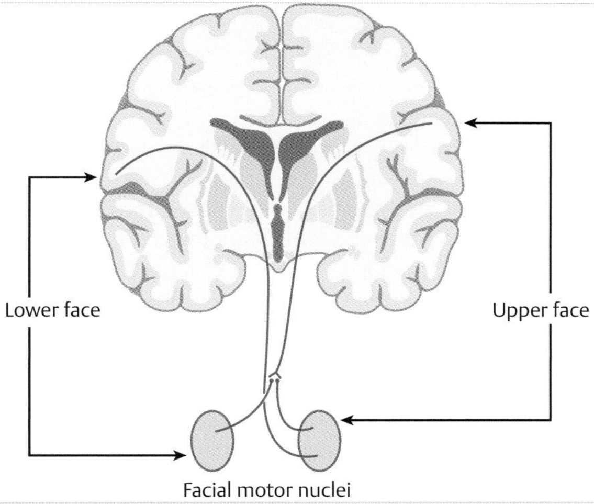

Fig. 27.4 Diagram of the corticobulbar pathway serving the facial motor nuclei in the brainstem. The lower face receives mainly contralateral projections, while the upper face receives bilateral polysynaptic projections.

27.3.5 The Facial Nucleus

The anatomy is described in detail in Chapter 1. Briefly, the facial nerve nucleus is located in the ventrolateral region of the caudal pons (▶ Fig. 27.5) and it is histologically composed of at least four distinct subnuclei: the lateral, the dorsal, the intermediate, and the medial subnuclei (▶ Fig. 27.5).[23,29] The facial nerve nucleus is musculotopically organized. It was long assumed that motor neurons in the upper half of the facial nucleus innervate the lower facial muscles (mainly muscles of the mouth), whereas neurons in the lower half of the facial nucleus supply the upper facial muscles (forehead).[30–33] However, studies in nonhuman primates have suggested that the musculotopic organization of the facial nucleus is arranged in longitudinal columns.[34–36] As a result of this organization it is possible that small lesions confined to various subsections of the facial nucleus cause deficits in isolated groups of facial muscles. The lateral and medial subnuclei receive direct, predominantly contralateral motor projections that are responsible for controlling lower facial muscles; hence the contralateral predominance. Studies in monkeys have also revealed a small number of descending corticofacial fibers from the ipsilateral motor cortex that innervate these subnuclei.[23]

The dorsal and intermediate subnuclei receive mostly bilateral, indirect (polysynaptic) projections through the pontine reticular formation and are responsible for

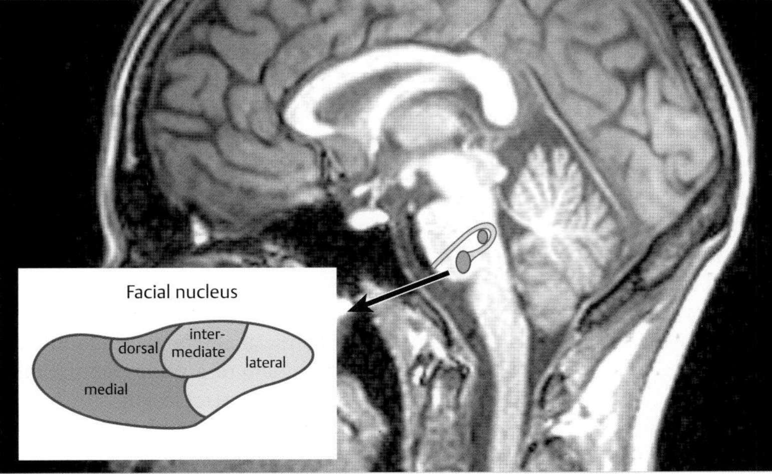

Fig. 27.5 Location of the facial nucleus within the pons (right). The inset shows a diagram of the subdivisions of the facial nucleus.

controlling upper facial muscles (forehead and orbicularis oculi).[37] In order to explain reports of central facial palsy caused by brainstem lesions caudal to the facial nucleus, it has been proposed that an aberrant pyramidal tract loops down into the ventral part of the upper medulla, crosses the midline, and ascends through the dorsolateral medullary region to the facial motor nucleus.[37–39]

27.4 Clinical Features

The most important difference between a peripheral and a central facial palsy is that the muscles of the forehead are less involved in the central facial palsy.[31,40] This difference is because the facial nucleus that innervates the muscles of the forehead receives bilateral upper motor neuron input (► Fig. 27.4). Also, the musculus orbicularis oculi receives mostly bilateral upper motor neuron input, but also some lower motor neuron input. Therefore, a central facial palsy can elicit a slight weakness of the musculus orbicularis oculi. However, patients with a central palsy are always able to close their eyes completely. Modest weakness of eyelid closure has been found to be associated with anterior cerebral artery stroke, in particular.[41] In contrast, the pattern of facial weakness caused by a peripheral facial palsy can vary widely, with a sparing or diminished involvement of the upper face. While a complete facial palsy suggests a peripheral cause, a palsy of the lower face makes distinguishing between a peripheral and central origin more difficult.

> !
>
> Eye closure is never completely lost in central facial palsy.

Although the complete clinical examination of facial function is described in Chapter 4, a few typical properties of facial functions that are helpful in differentiating between a central and peripheral palsy are described here.

Careful and thoughtful observation is the key to discerning subtle signs that help in the differentiation between a peripheral and central palsy. Asymmetry is the clue to unilateral weakness and is best perceived during conversation, when the patient is unaware of being observed. Note especially the blink, nasolabial folds, and corners of the mouth. Often a patient will present with a skewed face but will be able to perform facial movements that are equal on both sides. This pattern indicates a (mostly peripheral) facial palsy and a history of compensation. A skewed face accompanied by slight facial weakness (a dominant skewed face with slight facial weakness) can be an indication of a slowly evolving, and therefore partially compensated, central process.

The mimetic (involuntary) facial function should be examined indirectly during the interview (i.e., spontaneous laughter). Otherwise, this function can be tested directly. The examiner should not ask the patient to smile, as this usually elicits a voluntary response. In the authors' experience, the following questions are often successful "Do you yawn in your sleep?" or "Do you wake up or open your eyes first?" Weakness that is greater during an involuntary response than during a voluntary contraction ("Show me your teeth") indicates a deep-seated lesion that is often localized near the ventricles. In contrast, when the weakness is greater during a voluntary response than with an involuntary response, the lesion is localized cortically, in the gyrus praecentralis, or it affects the corticobulbar tract in the proximity of the cortex. In each case, it is important to note that a reliable divergence between voluntary and involuntary facial weakness is strong evidence for a central facial palsy.[12–14]

> →•
>
> Provoke spontaneous laughter to examine emotional facial nerve function.

As a result of the complex interconnection of various functions in the brain, facial palsy caused by a lesion of the upper facial motor neurons is, in most cases, associated with other neurologic symptoms. A detailed neurologic examination is therefore indispensable to enable differentiation between a peripheral and a central facial palsy.

Symptoms associated with facial palsy are largely dependent on the anatomical location of the pathology. Typical neurologic symptoms associated with a central facial palsy are summarized in ► Table 27.2. The most important symptom is weakness of the upper limb, ipsilateral to the facial palsy. This symptom is frequently associated because the cortical representations as well as the corticobulbar tract for both body regions are located next to each other. Moreover, the cortical representation of the lower face and the upper limb share the same vascular supply, mainly from the medial cerebral artery. A subtle weakness of the upper limb is often not reported by the patient but can be detected in a detailed neurologic examination.

Patients with mild central lesions may show normal strength in routine testing, but the neurologic deficit may be observed using ancillary maneuvers. The most important of these maneuvers is an examination for pronator drift (Barré's sign). The patient has to stretch out the upper extremities towards the front with palms up and their eyes closed, and hold this position for 20 seconds. The pronation of one hand (possibly with additional downward drift) is an indication of a subtle hemiparesis and therefore an indication of a central lesion.

In rare cases, a small and localized cortical or subcortical lesion may be represented as facial palsy, mainly of

Table 27.2 Symptoms that suggest a central facial palsy

Location	Clinical symptoms	Possible diagnosis
Cortex and internal capsule	Loss of voluntary movement with intact spontaneous expression, dysarthria, hemiparesis on side of the facial palsy	Lesion of motor cortex or internal capsule contralateral to the facial palsy. Most often ischemia caused by a problem of the middle cerebral artery
Opercular syndrome	Impaired voluntary facial, lingual and glossopharyngeal movements, preserved emotional movements. Dysarthria. Often involvement of the upper face (more pronounced than by motor cortex lesions)	Lesions of the opercular cortex surrounding the insula, caused by vascular, neoplastic, encephalitic or traumatic origin
Extrapyramidal	Impaired emotional movements, voluntary movements intact, hemifacial spasm, symptoms similar to Parkinson's disease	Lesion of various causes of the basal ganglia. Parkinson's disease
Midbrain	Impaired facial movements combined with ocular symptoms (strabismus, oculomotor paresis)	Vascular or neoplastic lesions
Pons	Impaired facial movements combined with loss of the abducens nerve function on the same side. Contralateral hemiparesis, ataxia, cerebellar signs	Vascular or neoplastic lesions
Pseudobulbar paralysis	Inability to control facial movements. Difficulty in chewing and swallowing. Uncontrolled emotional outbursts. Increased reflexes and spasticity in tongue and the bulbar region, slurred speech	Degeneration involving neurons of the bilateral corticobulbar pathways mostly caused by viral or toxic diseases

the lower portion of the face (with a slight impairment of eyelid closure, ▶ Fig. 27.1) without an accompanying neurologic deficit.

Whether a paresthesia of the face is a sign of a central or a peripheral lesion is a matter of debate. Some authors have reported this symptom to be an indication of a central lesion. However, in the authors' experience, a detailed interview and clinical examination of patients with a peripheral facial palsy often also reveals a paresthesia of the paralyzed face. It is assumed that the paresthesia of the paralyzed face is caused by a disturbed interaction between motor command and sensory feedback at the cortical level, and may represent the plasticity of the sensory–motor interaction.[42,43] The loss of brainstem reflexes indicates a central lesion in the brainstem. As part of the neurologic examination, the brainstem reflexes, as well as the function of all cranial nerves, should be investigated.

27.5 Diagnostic Work-Up

27.5.1 Medical Interview

Patients often visit the emergency department with the acute symptom of a skewed face. They report functional problems while eating or drinking and occasionally report dysarthria. Approximately half of these patients believe that they have suffered a stroke or fear an intracranial tumor. This initial account by the patient does not allow the physician to differentiate between a peripheral and central palsy. The interviewer must enquire about the specific typical anamnestic differences. The anamnestic characteristics of a central versus a peripheral palsy depend mainly on their cause. Therefore, the physician should have extensive knowledge of the anatomy, the differential diagnoses, and the typical clinical presentation of a wide variety of disorders.

Time Course

Patients with Bell's palsy, which is described in detail in Chapter 8, typically report that they notice their symptoms in the morning, when they look in a mirror, or they report that their symptoms have evolved slowly throughout the course of the day. A progression of symptoms over more than 2 days is rare, although a secondary progression of symptoms is sometimes reported. Other inflammation-associated causes for a peripheral facial palsy, such as neuroborreliosis, show a similar progression of facial weakness. This time course is rare for central facial palsies, but can occur as a result of similar causes, such as brainstem encephalitis or multiple sclerosis. Most central facial palsies occur suddenly because of an ischemic or hemorrhagic stroke. A gradual onset of symptoms (over a period of weeks) can be caused by both peripheral and central lesions, and thus has to be clarified with further diagnostic tests. In conclusion, a time course that is atypical of Bell's palsy indicates to the interviewer that further diagnostic tests are needed, particularly to exclude a central cause.

> !
>
> Most central facial palsies occur suddenly and do not show a progressive time course, as peripheral facial palsies often do.

Reported Symptoms

Any report of symptoms outside of the facial nerve function is highly suggestive of a central cause and, particularly, if the involved function is represented centrally near the facial function (e.g., a weakness of the ipsilateral hand that accompanies the facial weakness is almost conclusive for a central etiology). The involvement of other cranial nerves suggests damage to the brainstem or a more diffuse (mostly inflammatory) process in the CNS that affects the intracranial portion of the cranial nerves. The inability to close the eyelids is rarely reported by the patient, but it is nearly conclusive of a peripheral etiology. Further reported symptoms that suggest a peripheral etiology are a loss of the sense of taste on the ipsilateral side of the anterior two-thirds of the tongue, problems with lacrimation and salivation, or altered hearing. Symptoms such as ataxia or complaints of dizziness/vertigo are indicative of the involvement of the brainstem/cerebellum and must be investigated by further diagnostic tests.

> !
>
> Diagnosis of the location of the facial paralysis is aided by accompanying symptoms. A lesion of the pons is likely to involve cranial nerve VI. Problems in the internal auditory canal indicate a combination of cranial nerves VII and VIII. If the lesion is in the temporal bone, patients may have issues with taste, lacrimation, and salivation. Patients with Bell's palsy may also have numbness of the face (cranial nerve V), but symptoms involving the ipsilateral arm or other cranial nerves suggest a central etiology.

27.5.2 Imaging

Imaging is not routinely indicated for cases of peripheral facial palsy. MRI is considered to be the gold standard for assessment of the location of a central facial palsy; more details are given in Chapter 5. The MRI protocol should include diffusion-weighted imaging, gradient-recalled echo, fluid attenuated inversion recovery, magnetic resonance angiography, and perfusion-weighted imaging. In particular, MRI is preferable to CT for patients with an assumed brainstem lesion, as well patients with small lesions.[44,45] The brainstem should be measured by a separate sequence in thin layers. Also, in patients with brain tumors or metastases, contrast-enhanced MRI is the imaging modality of choice. CT is often utilized as the first-pass screening modality for cases of skull fracture and hemorrhage, and these are better diagnosed by CT than by MRI.

> !
>
> Magnetic resonance imaging with gadolinium is the gold standard for the localization of lesions responsible for a central facial palsy.

27.5.3 Electrophysiology

There are multiple electrophysiologic investigations that may be beneficial for the investigation of facial nerve function. The tests described in the following sections may be relevant for patients with a suspected central facial palsy.

Auditory Evoked Potentials

Auditory evoked potentials can be used to trace the signal generated by a sound through the ascending auditory pathway, including the brainstem. An auditory evoked potential is extracted from ongoing electrical activity in the brain via scalp electrodes. The resulting recording is a series of at least five waves. The first wave (I) is generated by cranial nerve VIII, the second wave (II) is generated by the cochlear nucleus, the third (III) by the superior olivary complex, the fourth (IV) by the lateral lemniscus, and the fifth (V) by the inferior colliculus. The auditory brainstem response is interpreted with respect to the wave amplitude, the latency, interpeak latency, and interaural latency. A brainstem lesion is characterized by a normal latency of waves I to III, while waves IV to V have an increased latency.[46]

> !
>
> Auditory evoked potentials are helpful in the detection of a brainstem lesion.

Somatosensory Evoked Potentials

Somatosensory evoked potentials can be used to trace the signal generated by a somatosensory stimulus through the ascending somatosensory pathway. The tibial nerve and the median nerve are most commonly electrically stimulated.[47] The response is then recorded from the cervical spine at the level of the fifth to the seventh cervical vertebrae (median nerve stimulation) or from the lumbar spine at the level of the first lumbar vertebrae (tibial nerve stimulation). In both stimulations (median and tibial nerve stimulation) the response is then recorded from the patient's scalp above the primary somatosensory cortex. It is also possible to record the somatosensory evoked potentials by stimulating the trigeminal nerve. However, because of frequent stimulus artifacts, trigeminal evoked potentials are often difficult to evaluate.[48]

The two most important aspects of the somatosensory evoked potentials are the amplitude and the latency of the recorded peaks. An increased latency or decreased amplitude is an indicator for a lesion of the sensory tract.[49] The assessment and comparison between the spinal and the cortical potentials also helps in the differentiation between a peripheral and a central lesion. Somatosensory evoked potentials are far more sensitive than the clinical examination for somatosensory deficits and can therefore reveal clinically silent lesions. In a patient with a suspected central origin of a relatively isolated facial palsy, pathologic findings will indicate a lesion within the brainstem.[50]

!

Somatosensory evoked potentials are helpful to differentiate between central and peripheral facial nerve lesions.

Motor Evoked Potentials

Motor evoked potentials are used to investigate the motor pathway from the primary motor cortex to the muscles. These potentials are evoked by a transcranial magnetic stimulation of the motor cortex and recorded from muscles of the lower face, and the upper and lower extremities. The orbicularis oculi muscle is not suitable for use, as the R1 component of the simultaneously evoked eye-blink reflex interferes with the cortical evoked potential because of a similar latency.

To differentiate between central and peripheral lesions, a second measurement is performed by stimulating at the level of the facial canal (face), the cervical spine (upper extremity), or the lumbar spine (lower extremity).[51]

The two most important aspects of the somatosensory evoked potentials are the amplitude and the latency of the recorded potentials. These parameters provide indicators of the functional integrity and excitability of the corticomotor pathway and make it possible to evaluate a related motor impairment. The assessment and comparison between potential due to cortical stimulation and that due to stimulation of the facial canal allows for differentiation between a peripheral and a central facial palsy.

Multiple studies have demonstrated that motor evoked potentials might predict motor recovery after stroke.[52–55] These motor evoked potentials allow one to determine whether the lesion that causes a facial palsy also affects the motor pathway to the upper or lower extremities. Normal motor evoked potentials exclude a major impairment of the corticospinal tract.

!

Motor evoked potentials are helpful to differentiate between central and peripheral facial nerve lesions.

27.5.4 Cerebrospinal Fluid Testing

An atypical peripheral facial palsy or meningeal signs require the analysis of CSF. Further indications are a suspected central facial palsy with a negative MRI, or signs of inflammation. Signs of inflammation might include unexplained increased inflammatory markers in the blood, fever, contrast-enhanced lesions on MRI, or the involvement of multiple cranial nerves. Altered mental status or the presence of immunosuppression should also draw attention to an infection in the CNS.

!

Atypical peripheral palsy? Signs of inflammation? In such cases analysis of cerebrospinal fluid is required.

The analysis of CSF is essential for establishing a diagnosis and tailoring therapy. The tests to be performed depend on the clinical symptoms, but they always include: a cell count; an analysis of the protein, glucose, and lactate levels; and in most cases a quantitative and qualitative analysis for different antibodies. Antibodies may be helpful in diagnosing autoimmune conditions, e.g., Devic's syndrome (autoimmune inflammation and demyelination of the optic nerve and the spinal cord), and anti-*N*-methyl-D-aspartate mediated encephalitis. A Gram stain should be performed in cases of suspected bacterial meningitis. If viral meningitis is suspected, viral polymerase chain reaction assessment for herpes simplex virus types 1 and 2 and varicella zoster should also be performed. In cases of a suspected malignancy, a histologic analysis (cytology) should be performed. Additionally, an extra CSF sample may be collected and stored in case further CSF tests are required later.

The CSF is considered to be normal if there are fewer than five white blood cells/μL, the CSF/serum glucose ratio is less than 0.5, the CSF protein level is less than 500 mg/L, and no organisms are seen in the Gram stain.[56] The most important parameter during the acute management of the patient is the number of white blood cells. An elevation of in the number of white blood cells to 10–100/μL is indicative of viral meningitis while greater than 1,000/μL white blood cells suggests bacterial meningitis. The finding of elevated numbers of red blood cells might be caused by iatrogenic contamination and highest numbers should be found in the first CSF tube. If the number of red blood cells continues to be elevated without reduction in consecutive tubes, xanthochromia is detected, and the patient is likely to have a subarachnoid hemorrhage that was not detected on CT.

27.6 Treatment

The most important therapy for patients with a central facial palsy is treatment of the cause of the lesion, which requires a precise diagnostic evaluation, as described previously. This therapy can be, for example, immunomodulatory therapy in autoimmune-mediated inflammatory lesions, elimination of the aneurysm that has led to the hemorrhage, or oral anticoagulation, which addresses the tendency for thrombosis due to atrial fibrillation.

The treatment of the symptoms of central facial weakness is similar to the treatment of a peripheral facial palsy. The focus of treatment is the physiotherapy of the diminished function. Patients with damage to the CNS and corresponding neurologic symptoms usually undergo neurologic rehabilitation in which the facial motor performance can be trained. Furthermore, physiotherapy approaches can also be attempted in specialized facilities; for example, sensory or electromyographical feedback or mirror training, as described in Chapter 28. Rehabilitation is usually effective in cases of central facial palsy.

27.7 Key Points

- Patients with a central facial palsy are nearly always able to close their eyes completely.
- A reliable divergence between symptoms of voluntary and involuntary facial weakness is strong evidence for central facial palsy.
- A central facial palsy is mostly associated with other neurologic symptoms.
- Suspicion of a central origin of a facial palsy should be handled as for a suspected stroke.

References

[1] Truelsen T, Piechowski-Jóźwiak B, Bonita R, Mathers C, Bogousslavsky J, Boysen G. Stroke incidence and prevalence in Europe: a review of available data. Eur J Neurol 2006; 13: 581–598

[2] Fisher M, Albers GW. Advanced imaging to extend the therapeutic time window of acute ischemic stroke. Ann Neurol 2013; 73: 4–9

[3] Jauch EC, Saver JL, Adams HP, Jr et al. American Heart Association Stroke Council. Council on Cardiovascular Nursing. Council on Peripheral Vascular Disease. Council on Clinical Cardiology. Guidelines for the early management of patients with acute ischemic stroke: a guideline for healthcare professionals from the American Heart Association/American Stroke Association. Stroke 2013; 44: 870–947

[4] Latchaw RE, Alberts MJ, Lev MH et al. American Heart Association Council on Cardiovascular Radiology and Intervention, Stroke Council, and the Interdisciplinary Council on Peripheral Vascular Disease. Recommendations for imaging of acute ischemic stroke: a scientific statement from the American Heart Association. Stroke 2009; 40: 3646–3678

[5] Randomised trial of endarterectomy for recently symptomatic carotid stenosis: final results of the MRC European Carotid Surgery Trial (ECST) Lancet 1998; 351: 1379–1387

[6] Rothwell PM, Eliasziw M, Gutnikov SA, Warlow CP, Barnett HJ Carotid Endarterectomy Trialists Collaboration. Endarterectomy for symptomatic carotid stenosis in relation to clinical subgroups and timing of surgery. Lancet 2004; 363: 915–924

[7] Morgenstern LB, Hemphill JC, III, Anderson C et al. American Heart Association Stroke Council and Council on Cardiovascular Nursing. Guidelines for the management of spontaneous intracerebral hemorrhage: a guideline for healthcare professionals from the American Heart Association/American Stroke Association. Stroke 2010; 41: 2108–2129

[8] Mayer SA, Brun NC, Begtrup K et al. FAST Trial Investigators. Efficacy and safety of recombinant activated factor VII for acute intracerebral hemorrhage. N Engl J Med 2008; 358: 2127–2137

[9] Mendelow AD, Gregson BA, Fernandes HM et al. STICH investigators. Early surgery versus initial conservative treatment in patients with spontaneous supratentorial intracerebral haematomas in the International Surgical Trial in Intracerebral Haemorrhage (STICH): a randomised trial. Lancet 2005; 365: 387–397

[10] Basu S, Alavi A. Role of FDG-PET in the clinical management of paraneoplastic neurological syndrome: detection of the underlying malignancy and the brain PET-MRI correlates. Mol Imaging Biol 2008; 10: 131–137

[11] Provenzale JM, Barboriak DP, Coleman RE. Limbic encephalitis: comparison of FDG PET and MR imaging findings. AJR Am J Roentgenol 1998; 170: 1659–1660

[12] Holstege G. Emotional innervation of facial musculature. Mov Disord 2002; 17 Suppl 2: S12–S16

[13] Hopf HC, Müller-Forell W, Hopf NJ. Localization of emotional and volitional facial paresis. Neurology 1992; 42: 1918–1923

[14] Trosch RM, Sze G, Brass LM, Waxman SG. Emotional facial paresis with striatocapsular infarction. J Neurol Sci 1990; 98: 195–201

[15] Holstege G. The emotional motor system. Eur J Morphol 1992; 30: 67–79

[16] Luppino G, Rizzolatti G. The organization of the frontal motor cortex. News Physiol Sci 2000; 15: 219–224

[17] Mitz AR, Wise SP. The somatotopic organization of the supplementary motor area: intracortical microstimulation mapping. J Neurosci 1987; 7: 1010–1021

[18] Laplane D, Talairach J, Meininger V, Bancaud J, Orgogozo JM. Clinical consequences of corticectomies involving the supplementary motor area in man. J Neurol Sci 1977; 34: 301–314

[19] Tanji J. New concepts of the supplementary motor area. Curr Opin Neurobiol 1996; 6: 782–787

[20] Picard N, Strick PL. Motor areas of the medial wall: a review of their location and functional activation. Cereb Cortex 1996; 6: 342–353

[21] Morecraft RJ, Cipolloni PB, Stilwell-Morecraft KS, Gedney MT, Pandya DN. Cytoarchitecture and cortical connections of the posterior cingulate and adjacent somatosensory fields in the rhesus monkey. J Comp Neurol 2004; 469: 37–69

[22] Rizzolatti G, Camarda R, Fogassi L, Gentilucci M, Luppino G, Matelli M. Functional organization of inferior area 6 in the macaque monkey. II. Area F5 and the control of distal movements. Exp Brain Res 1988; 71: 491–507

[23] Jenny AB, Saper CB. Organization of the facial nucleus and corticofacial projection in the monkey: a reconsideration of the upper motor neuron facial palsy. Neurology 1987; 37: 930–939

[24] Iwase M, Ouchi Y, Okada H et al. Neural substrates of human facial expression of pleasant emotion induced by comic films: a PET Study. Neuroimage 2002; 17: 758–768
[25] Triggs WJ, Ghacibeh G, Springer U, Bowers D. Lateralized asymmetry of facial motor evoked potentials. Neurology 2005; 65: 541–544
[26] Borod JC, Haywood CSE, Koff E. Neuropsychological aspects of facial asymmetry during emotional expression: a review of the normal adult literature. Neuropsychol Rev 1997; 7: 41–60
[27] Güntürkün O. The Venus of Milo and the dawn of facial asymmetry research. Brain Cogn 1991; 16: 147–150
[28] Sackeim HA, Gur RC, Saucy MC. Emotions are expressed more intensely on the left side of the face. Science 1978; 202: 434–436
[29] Kuypers HGJ. Corticobulbar connexions to the pons and lower brainstem in man: an anatomical study. Brain 1958; 81: 364–388
[30] Afifi AK, Bergman RA. Functional neuroanatomy: text and atlas. New York: McGraw-Hill; 1998
[31] Blumenfeld H. Neuroanatomy Through Clinical Cases. Sunderland, MA: Sinauer Associates; 2002
[32] Kingsley RE. Concise Text Of Neuroscience. Baltimore: Williams & Wilkins: 1996
[33] Wilson-Pauwels L, Akesson EJ, Stewart PA. Cranial Nerves: Anatomy and Clinical Comments. Toronto, Philadelphia: B. C. Decker; Saint Louis, MO: Mosby; 1988
[34] Satoda T, Takahashi O, Tashiro T, Matsushima R, Uemura-Sumi M, Mizuno N. Representation of the main branches of the facial nerve within the facial nucleus of the Japanese monkey (Macaca fuscata). Neurosci Lett 1987; 78: 283–287
[35] VanderWerf F, Aramideh M, Otto JA, Ongerboer de Visser BW. Retrograde tracing studies of subdivisions of the orbicularis oculi muscle in the rhesus monkey. Exp Brain Res 1998; 121: 433–441
[36] Welt C, Abbs JH. Musculotopic organization of the facial motor nucleus in Macaca fascicularis: a morphometric and retrograde tracing study with cholera toxin B-HRP. J Comp Neurol 1990; 291: 621–636
[37] Terao S, Miura N, Takeda A, Takahashi A, Mitsuma T, Sobue G. Course and distribution of facial corticobulbar tract fibres in the lower brain stem. J Neurol Neurosurg Psychiatry 2000; 69: 262–265
[38] Puvanendran K, Wong PK, Ransome GA. Syndrome of Dejerine's Fourth Reich. Acta Neurol Scand 1978; 57: 349–353
[39] Urban PP, Wicht S, Vucorevic G et al. The course of corticofacial projections in the human brainstem. Brain 2001; 124: 1866–1876
[40] Adams RD, Victor M, Ropper AH. Principles of Neurology. 6th ed. New York: McGraw-Hill; 1997
[41] Cattaneo L, Saccani E, De Giampaulis P, Crisi G, Pavesi G. Central facial palsy revisited: a clinical-radiological study. Ann Neurol 2010; 68: 404–408
[42] Klingner CM, Volk GF, Maertin A et al. Cortical reorganization in Bell's palsy. Restor Neurol Neurosci 2011; 29: 203–214
[43] Klingner CM, Witte OW, Günther A. Sensory syndromes. Front Neurol Neurosci 2012; 30: 4–8
[44] Schulte-Altedorneburg G, Brückmann H. [Imaging techniques in diagnosis of brainstem infarction] Nervenarzt 2006; 77: 731–743, quiz 744
[45] Majoie C. Magnetic resonance imaging of the brainstem and cranial nerves III-VII. Mov Disord 2002; 17 Suppl 2: S17–S19
[46] Sand T, Kvaløy MB, Wader T, Hovdal H. Evoked potential tests in clinical diagnosis. Tidsskr Nor Laegeforen 2013; 133: 960–965
[47] Allison T, McCarthy G, Wood CC, Jones SJ. Potentials evoked in human and monkey cerebral cortex by stimulation of the median nerve. A review of scalp and intracranial recordings. Brain 1991; 114: 2465–2503
[48] Valls-Solé J. Neurophysiological assessment of trigeminal nerve reflexes in disorders of central and peripheral nervous system. Clin Neurophysiol 2005; 116: 2255–2265
[49] Mauguière F, Desmedt JE, Courjon J. Astereognosis and dissociated loss of frontal or parietal components of somatosensory evoked potentials in hemispheric lesions. Detailed correlations with clinical signs and computerized tomographic scanning. Brain 1983; 106: 271–311
[50] Schimsheimer RJ, Ongerboer de Visser BW, Bour LJ, Kropveld D, Van Ammers VC. Digital nerve somatosensory evoked potentials and flexor carpi radialis H reflexes in cervical disc protrusion and involvement of the sixth or seventh cervical root: relations to clinical and myelographic findings. Electroencephalogr Clin Neurophysiol 1988; 70: 313–324
[51] Barker AT, Jalinous R, Freeston IL. Non-invasive magnetic stimulation of human motor cortex. Lancet 1985; 1: 1106–1107
[52] Catano A, Houa M, Caroyer JM, Ducarne H, Noël P. Magnetic transcranial stimulation in acute stroke: early excitation threshold and functional prognosis. Electroencephalogr Clin Neurophysiol 1996; 101: 233–239
[53] König IR, Ziegler A, Bluhmki E et al. Virtual International Stroke Trials Archive (VISTA) Investigators. Predicting long-term outcome after acute ischemic stroke: a simple index works in patients from controlled clinical trials. Stroke 2008; 39: 1821–1826
[54] Pennisi G, Rapisarda G, Bella R, Calabrese V, Maertens De Noordhout A, Delwaide PJ. Absence of response to early transcranial magnetic stimulation in ischemic stroke patients: prognostic value for hand motor recovery. Stroke 1999; 30: 2666–2670
[55] Timmerhuis TP, Hageman G, Oosterloo SJ, Rozeboom AR. The prognostic value of cortical magnetic stimulation in acute middle cerebral artery infarction compared to other parameters. Clin Neurol Neurosurg 1996; 98: 231–236
[56] Süssmuth SD, Brettschneider J, Spreer A et al. Current cerebrospinal fluid diagnostics for pathogen-related diseases [in German] Nervenarzt 2013; 84: 229–244

28 Facial Dystonia and Facial Spasms

Claus Wittekindt

28.1 Introduction

This chapter describes involuntary movements of the face, such as facial dystonias and hemifacial spasm (HFS). It is well known that the mimic muscles of the face share a predisposition for involuntary excessive movements, which many people experience at some point of their life. Diseases with involuntary facial movements belong to the hyperkinetic movement disorders. Hyperkinetic movement disorders include tics, twitches, cramps, dystonia, and spasms, among others. Recognition of involuntary movements is an important diagnostic skill. Tics are suppressible paroxysmal, stereotyped muscle contractions. Unlike tics, the majority of muscle twitches are isolated occurrences, entirely involuntary, and cannot be controlled or suppressed. Dystonia and cramps have unwanted, involuntary, excessive muscle contractions in common and may be manifestations of underlying disorders. Spasms can be the result of irritated nerves; the most common example is HFS secondary to compression at the root exit zone of the facial nerve. Treatment of diseases with involuntary facial muscle movements varies, depending on what is appropriate for the condition, and may consist of oral medications, injections of botulinum toxin, or even surgery.

28.2 Definition

Dystonia describes movement disorders that cause involuntary muscle contractions. These contractions cause slow repetitive movements or abnormal postures. Different forms of dystonia can be distinguished, affecting only one muscle, groups of muscles (focal dystonia), or muscles throughout the body (generalized dystonia). Segmental dystonias affect two adjoining parts of the body. Some forms of dystonia are genetic but the cause for the majority of cases remains unknown. Women are more prone to dystonia than men. It may be painful, particularly when the neck muscles are involved. Primary dystonia is a dystonia without any other symptoms and no structural abnormality in the central nervous system. Secondary dystonia refers to dystonia with an identified cause, usually involving brain damage.

> **!** Dystonias in the face typically start as a focal dystonia but can spread later to other parts of the body.

HFS is characterized by involuntary, unilateral, intermittent, irregular, tonic, or clonic contractions of mimic muscles. HFS is a peripherally induced movement disorder, most probably caused by vascular compression of the root exit zone of the facial nerve in the cerebellopontine angle. However, other etiologies of unilateral facial movements should always be considered. HFS can occur with trigeminal neuralgia, a condition termed tic convulsive. HFS more frequently affects women.

> **!** Hemifacial spasm is not a dystonia but a disease of the peripheral facial nerve!

28.3 Dystonia Classification

The term dystonia describes a disorder characterized by repetitive involuntary movements and abnormal posturing of the neck, trunk, face, and extremities. Most commonly the condition is confined to a specific body part. Some of the more common forms of dystonia in the head and neck are cervical dystonia (torticollis), blepharospasm, and Meige's syndrome. However, dystonia may affect any of the voluntary muscles of the body. Commonly, dystonia is initiated by voluntary motion (action dystonia) but may later become sustained. Classically, stress or fatigue worsen dystonia, while relaxation or sensory stimulation reduce it.

> **!** Dystonia is an idiopathic neurologic movement disorder, which is characterized by repetitive involuntary muscular contractions that can affect any muscle of the body.

Primary dystonia describes a case in which dystonia is the only neurologic disorder of a patient. It includes some genetic forms, e.g. idiopathic torsion dystonia, or Oppenheim's dystonia, which is an autosomal dominant condition of variable penetrance seen most commonly in juvenile patients of Ashkenazi Jewish descent. Secondary dystonia is most commonly caused by medications, brain lesions, or brainstem pathology. Most such dystonias are segmental in distribution. Dystonic storm is an acute, generalized dystonic contraction that may include vocal cords or laryngeal muscles, leading to potentially fatal respiratory obstruction. Potential complications include rhabdomyolysis and renal failure.

Symptoms can be caused by specific tasks (for instance, writer's cramp) or may result from taking drugs that interact with central dopaminergic neurons. One example is tardive dystonia, which resembles multiple movement disorders, namely after exposure to neuroleptics.

Table 28.1 Focal dystonias affecting the head and neck

Dystonia	Symptoms
Blepharospasm	Abnormal contraction of eyelids, increased blinking
Oromandibular dystonia	Dystonic contractions of muscle groups of the jaw, tongue, lips, or lower face Commonly affects women > 60 years old, frequently in combination with blepharospasm (Meige's syndrome)
Cervical dystonia	Painful contractions of the neck muscles May deviate head laterally (torticollis), anteriorly (anterocollis), or posteriorly (retrocollis)
Spasmodic dystonia	Dysfunctional contractions of the vocal cords

Dystonia can be classified in several ways. One way is by location: for some patients the whole body may be involved (generalized), while for others only certain parts of the body (focal dystonias) are affected. Some focal dystonias typically involve cranial muscles (▶ Table 28.1). Alternatively, dystonia can be classified by age of onset, with early childhood dystonias more commonly genetic in origin. Most facial dystonias have a late onset, typically after the age of 30 years. Dystonia can also be classified according to its underlying cause, i.e., primary dystonia in which the only symptom is dystonia. Movements can be painful, and concomitant neurologic features such as tremor are common. Although dystonia is a neurologic disease, cognitive abilities, memory, and communication skills are not usually affected.

Primary dystonia is thought to be a disorder of the basal ganglia since the symptoms resemble those of patients who have structural lesions in the same region (secondary dystonia). Dystonia results from abnormal functioning of the basal ganglia, a deep part of the brain that helps to control coordination of movement, including the speed and fluidity of movement, and prevents unwanted movements. Pathophysiologic deficits include reduced inhibition at many levels of the motor system. Traditionally, dystonia has been regarded as a hyperkinetic movement disorder originating from abnormal sensorimotor integration within the basal ganglia thalamocortical circuit. Lesions within this pathway, particularly in the putamen, may lead to dystonic movements. Other hallmarks of dystonia have been proposed. The cocontraction of agonist and antagonist muscles that occurs in dystonia has been described to derive from disturbed surrounding inhibition of competing motor programs during voluntary movements. Finally, reduced sensory plasticity within the brain may also contribute to the development of dystonia.[1]

28.4 Blepharospasm

Blepharospasm is the term used to describe abnormal contractions, involuntary blinking, or spasm of the eyelids and the ocular sphincters. It is a true focal dystonia and can be either primary or secondary in occurrence. Mild twitching of the eyelids is usually not described as blepharospasm, but is more often referred to as a tic, twitch, or flicker of the eyelid. Most cases of blepharospasm occur spontaneously with no apparent cause. People with blepharospasm have normal vision; however, in severe cases, the person is rendered legally blind, because the muscular spasms force the eyelids shut, sometimes for hours. Treatment includes paralyzing the eyelid muscles with injections of botulinum toxin. Surgery to remove parts of the ocular sphincter has also been employed.[2]

28.4.1 Epidemiology and Etiology

Men and women of any age can be affected by blepharospasm, but middle-aged and older women appear to be particularly susceptible. The mean age of onset of blepharospasm is the fifth decade of life. As with HFS, a female preponderance exists, with blepharospasm affecting women to men in a ratio of 1.8:1. The prevalence of blepharospasm in the general population has been estimated at approximately 5 in 100,000.[3] Blepharospasm is a focal dystonia arising from pathology of an unknown cause in the basal ganglia. Most likely there is loss of control in the central regulatory or inhibitory neurons of blink activity, and this results in overloaded circuit activity, rather than a single neuronal or synaptic defect. Heredity may play a role in the development of some cases of blepharospasm, while some patients have a history of dry eyes or light sensitivity. Some drugs are known to induce blepharospasm, such as those used in estrogen-replacement therapy, benzodiazepine abuse, or alcohol detoxification. A frequent cause of dystonia in patients with Parkinson's disease is a secondary dystonia arising from the effect of treating Parkinson's disease using levodopa.

28.4.2 Clinical Features

Symptoms of benign essential blepharospasm usually appear without warning in mid-to-late adulthood and gradually worsen during follow-up. The first symptoms may be an increased frequency of blinking and eye irritation that is aggravated by sunlight or trigeminal stimuli. Sleep or concentration can make symptoms disappear. Blepharospasm may begin in one eye, but eventually both eyes are always affected. As the disease progresses, the involuntary winking and squinting leads to increased difficulty in keeping the eyes open (▶ Fig. 28.1 and

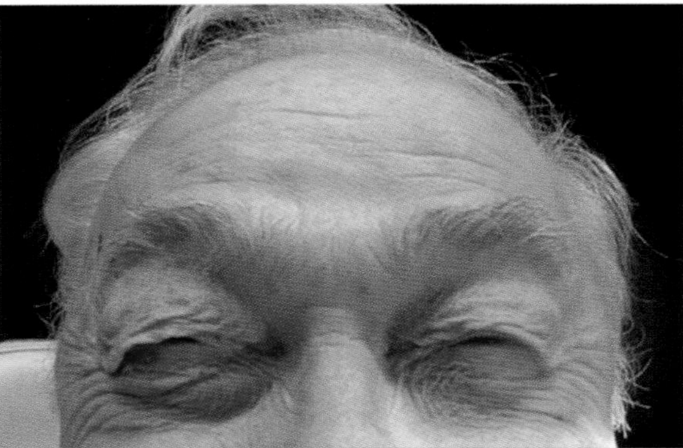

Fig. 28.1 Typical presentation of a patient with blepharospasm. The eyebrows are elevated because of apraxia of the lid opening.

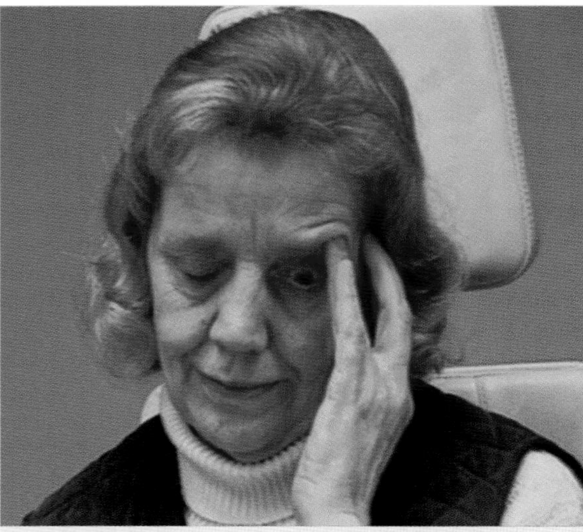

Fig. 28.2 A patient with blepharospasm. A finger is often used to assist eyelid opening.

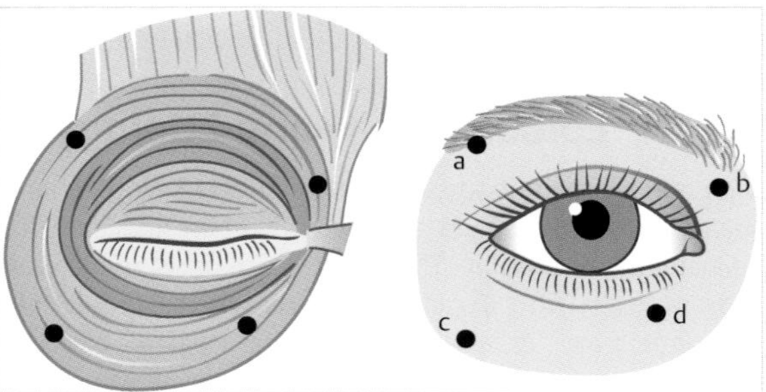

Fig. 28.3 Botulinum toxin injections for treatment of blepharospasm, step I. The orbital muscle (left side) is injected at points a, b, c, and d as shown in the diagram on the right side. (Adapted with permission from Albanese A, Bentivoglio AR, Colosimo C, Galardi G, Maderna L, Tonali P. Pretarsal injections of botulinum toxin improve blepharospasm in previously unresponsive patients. J Neurol Neurosurg Psychiatr 1996;60(6);693–694.)

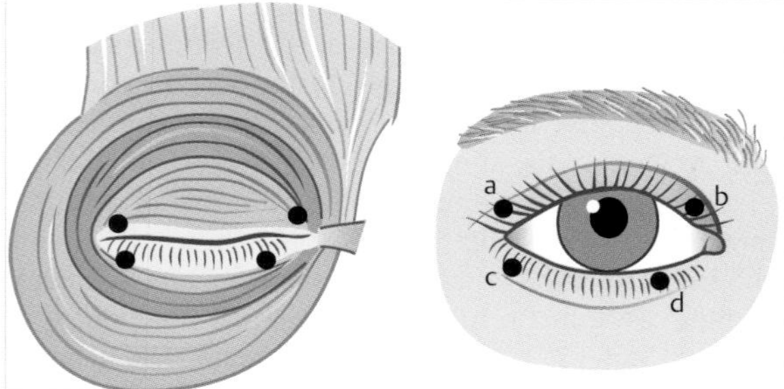

Fig. 28.4 Botulinum toxin injections for treatment of blepharospasm, step II. The preseptal muscle (left side) is injected at points a and b as shown in the diagram on the right side. Pretarsal injections can be advantageous, but need a lower dosage; these are injected at points c and d. This has to be decided individually. (Adapted with permission from Albanese A, Bentivoglio AR, Colosimo C, Galardi G, Maderna L, Tonali P. Pretarsal injections of botulinum toxin improve blepharospasm in previously unresponsive patients. J Neurol Neurosurg Psychiatr 1996;60(6);693–694.)

► Fig. 28.2). Excessive spasms of the ocular sphincter can lead to uncontrollable eyelid closure lasting minutes or even hours. In more than half of all patients with blepharospasm, the symptoms may spread beyond the eyes to affect other facial muscles or other areas of the body. Spasms affecting the tongue and jaw (oromandibular dystonia) in combination with blepharospasm is known as Meige's syndrome.

> **!**
>
> Although the clinical appearance is very specific, blepharospasm is often initially misdiagnosed, for instance as an allergic reaction or dry eye syndrome.

28.4.3 Diagnostic Work-Up

Blepharospasm is a clinical diagnosis. No imaging study is necessary and no laboratory studies are required.

28.4.4 Treatment

There is no cure for the primary blepharospasm. The mainstay of treatment is injections of botulinum toxin (► Fig. 28.3 and ► Fig. 28.4). Other drug therapy (for instance anticholinergic drugs, neuroleptic drugs, benzodiazepines) for blepharospasm has proved generally unpredictable, being helpful in only 15% of cases and usually of short-term benefit only. Botulinum toxin injections are generally administered every 3 months, with variations based on patient response, and they usually give immediate relief of symptoms; more details on botulinum toxin are given in Chapter 25. The necessary dose for effective symptom reduction tends to increase after many years of use and is higher than for treatment of synkinesis. The most common side effects are ptosis, lagophthalmos, and dry eye.[4]

- Use an injection dose of 20 units or less of Botox equivalent for each eye when starting treatment; the differences between the different botulinum toxin formulations are explained in Chapter 25.
- Start with 1 unit of Botox equivalent in preseptal muscles to avoid ptosis.
- The direction of the needle tip should always be in opposite direction from the globe.

The surgical removal of muscles (protractor myectomy) is also a possible treatment option.[2] This surgery has improved symptoms in about 50% of patients. Reasons to consider myectomy are apraxia of the eyelid opening, blepharospasm-associated deformities, or because the patient refuses injections with botulinum toxin. Benefits of alternative treatments (e.g., biofeedback, acupuncture) have not been proven.

28.4.5 Outcome and Prognosis

Botulinum toxin treatment is a safe and effective way of controlling blepharospasm. In a retrospective review of patients' long-term preferences, 72.1% of patients were still being treated with botulinum toxin after a follow-up time of more than 10 years.

28.5 Other Dystonias Affecting the Face

Cranial dystonia is a relatively broad description for dystonias affecting any part of the head. Involuntary spasms might involve the eyelid, facial, mandibular, oral, lingual, and laryngeal muscles. Synonymous terms for this entity include Meige's syndrome, Breughel's syndrome, idiopathic orofacial dystonia, blepharospasm–oromandibular dystonia, and cranial–cervical dystonia.

28.5.1 Meige's Syndrome

Blepharospasm associated with dystonic movements of other muscle groups in the face, neck, or limbs is known as Meige's syndrome. Involvement of lower cranial muscles is seen in a large number of such patients and is also referred to as oromandibular dystonia. Abnormal movements include retraction and forced opening of the mouth, tensing of the platysma, jaw clenching, pursing and tightening of the lips, flaring of the nostrils, dystonia of the tongue, and contractions of the soft palate and floor of the mouth (► Fig. 28.5). Eating, swallowing and speech may become impaired. Forced jaw closure may damage the lips and tongue. Teeth may become damaged and temporomandibular joint pain may occur, along with recurrent jaw dislocation. Other muscle groups that may also be affected by dystonic movements include muscles of the larynx, leading to spasmodic dysphonia. In general, the outcome has been poor after treatment with botulinum toxin to the muscles of the oral cavity and pharynx, and severe side effects (impact on swallowing) can result. Some reports on Meige's syndrome have shown that treatment with internal pallidum deep brain stimulation and unilateral pallidotomy has a favorable outcome.[5,6]

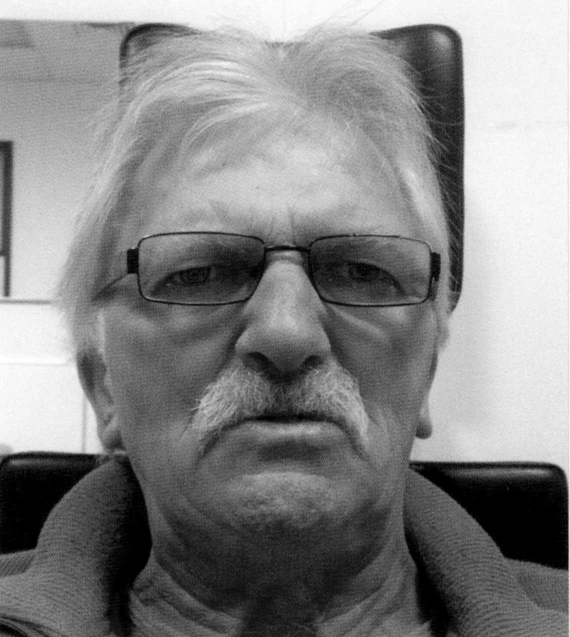

Fig. 28.5 In Meige's syndrome, blepharospasm is associated with dystonic movements of lower cranial muscles (tongue and platysma).

28.5.2 Oromandibular Dystonia

The term oromandibular dystonia is used to describe a focal dystonia that affects the mimic muscles, and the jaw and/or tongue causing difficulties in mouth opening or closing, affecting speech and chewing (► Fig. 28.6). Oromandibular dystonia might be associated with dystonia of neck muscles. The combination of the two is sometimes called cranial–cervical dystonia. In some patients, activities such as speaking and chewing can reduce the symptoms. A common aspect of oromandibular dystonia is difficulty in swallowing. Drug-induced dystonia frequently affects facial muscles. Cases of inherited cranial–cervical dystonia have been reported in the literature.

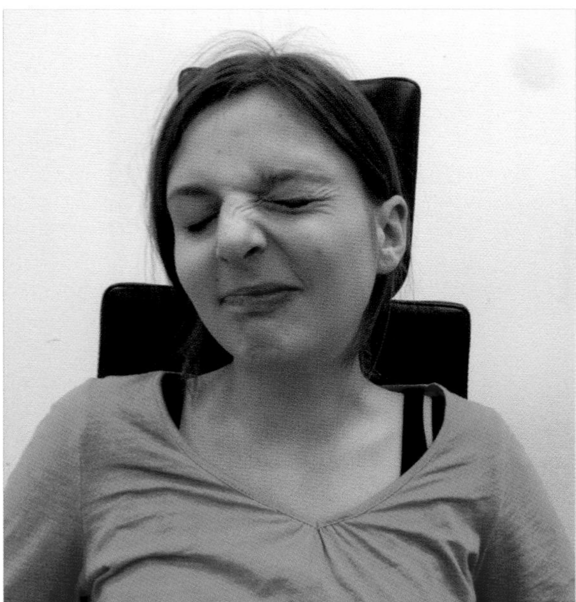

Fig. 28.6 Spasm of jaw closing, the left face, and lingual muscles in oromandibular dystonia.

Treatment is highly individualized, and about one-third of patients will respond to oral medications to some degree. Botulinum toxin has been applied and is most effective in jaw-closure dystonia, while treatment of the jaw-opening muscles is more challenging. Side effects are common when lingual dystonia is treated with botulinum toxin.[7]

28.6 Hemifacial Spasm

HFS is a disease characterized by irregular, involuntary contractions of mimic muscles on one side of the face, or rarely on both sides of the face.[8] Two main clinical scenarios have been described: typical and atypical forms. In the typical form, convulsion or twitching usually starts in the lower eyelid and continues to the ocular sphincter. Later, the oral sphincter and lip elevators are affected. The reverse of this progression is observed in atypical forms. Medication, surgery, and botulinum toxin injections are treatment options to stop the spasms and relieve discomfort.

28.6.1 Epidemiology and Etiology

The annual incidence of HFS has been estimated at somewhat below 1 in 100,000 people. The disease occurs in both men and women; however, middle-aged or elderly women are typically more often affected. The prevalence for women has been estimated at 14.5 in 100,000, and 7.4 in 100,000 for men.[9] The prevalence of HFS increases with age, reaching 40 per 100,000 for those aged 70 years and older.[10] An Asian over-representation among patients with HFS has been reported.[11]

The etiology of HFS and the location of the abnormality was the subject of debate for over a century. Although it now most frequently attributed to a vascular loop compression at the exit zone of the facial nerve, there are many other etiologies of unilateral facial movements that should be considered. The attention of the reader will be drawn to a marked heterogeneity of unilateral facial spasms, mimickers of HFS, and atypical presentations of nonvascular cases. The root exit zone of the facial nerve is where axonal isolation by glial cells ends and peripheral axonal myelination starts, and this is why it is felt to be most vulnerable to compression. Promising results have been reported since the 1970s when Janetta et al reported 47 patients who underwent facial nerve decompression surgery in the cerebellopontine angle. They reported nerve–vessel conflicts at the root exit zone of the facial nerve in all cases and underlined the theory that vascular compression is the primary cause of HFS.[12]

> **!**
>
> Hemifacial spasm is most likely caused by vascular compression at the root exit zone of the facial nerve; however, other etiologies should also be considered.

In a report on 215 patients referred for evaluation of HFS, 62% were classified as idiopathic HFS (presumably caused by vascular compression) and 2% had hereditary HFS. Secondary causes were found in 19%, including patients with Bell's palsy, facial nerve injury, demyelination, and brain vascular insults. There were an additional 18% of patients with HFS mimickers classified as psychogenic, tics, dystonia, myoclonus, and hemimasticatory spasm.[13] Ephaptic (nonsynaptic) transmission of electrical activity crossing from one neuron to another that is central to the site of vascular compression of the facial nerve, is another theory to explain HFS.[14] Abnormal activity of axons secondary to compression damage, and increased excitability of the nucleus of the facial nerve due to defective feedback from facial nerve damage have also been mentioned.

Magnetic resonance tomographic angiography imaging has been performed before microsurgery, revealing the anterior inferior cerebellar artery (AICA) to be the most common vessel compressed in HFS. Failure to identify neurovascular contact has been noted in cases with compression by veins or small arteries, thickened arachnoid tissue, or distal compression. It should be mentioned that neurovascular contact has also been observed in 15% of asymptomatic nerves.[15] In a further study using three-dimensional magnetic resonance imaging (MRI) in 25 patients with HFS, AICA was again identified as the most common vessel causing HFS. The posterior inferior cerebellar artery, vertebral artery, internal auditory artery, and veins at the root exit zone of the facial nerve have also been found to cause vascular contacts. In general, compression of the facial nerve by a blood vessel cross-compressing the facial nerve near the entry of the nerve into the brainstem is accepted to be the major cause of HFS.[16]

Families with hereditary HFS have been reported in the literature, suggesting an underlying genetic predisposition.[17] The inheritance pattern seems to be autosomal dominant with a low penetrance; these patients seem to be identified at a younger age of onset. No clinical differences have been seen in familial cases compared with sporadic cases, including response to surgery; this suggests that inherited cases and sporadic cases show a similar type of vascular compression.[18]

28.6.2 Clinical Features

Involuntary movement of mimic muscles is the only symptom of HFS. Spasms normally occur spontaneously but may be exacerbated by voluntary facial movement, stress, or anxiety. Nonmotor functions, such as lacrimation and salivation, are not usually affected. HFS typically occurs on one side of the face only, which differentiates this movement disorder from blepharospasm, which is typically a bilateral disorder.[13] In 1905, Babinski described paradoxical synkinesis in HFS, and this is known as "the other Babinski sign" (► Fig. 28.7). When the ocular sphincter contracts, the ipsilateral frontalis muscle contracts at the same time, resulting in an eyebrow lift during eye closure.[19]

The "other Babinski sign" is present in hemifacial spasm but not in blepharospasm, making it helpful in the differential diagnosis.[20]

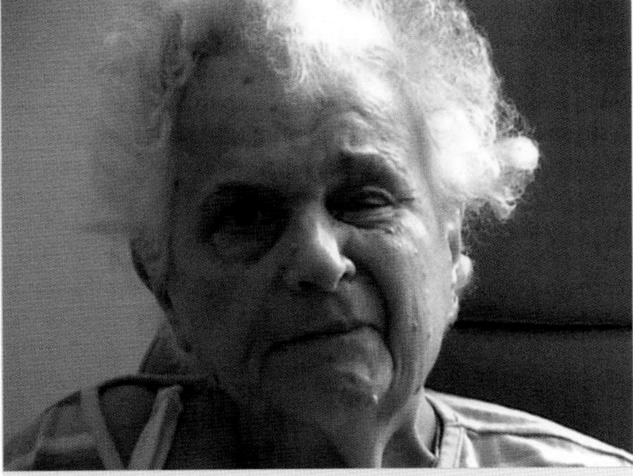

Fig. 28.7 Left hemifacial spasm. The eyebrow is raised during eye closure, known as "the other Babinski sign."

HFS tends to affect the left side of the face slightly more often than the right side. The first symptom is usually intermittent twitching of the lower eyelid that later leads to involuntary eye closure. Unlike tics, the majority of muscle twitches are isolated occurrences, not repeated actions. Muscle twitches are also known as myoclonic jerks. They are entirely involuntary and cannot be controlled or suppressed. This intermittent twitching of the eyelid later spreads to the muscles of the lower face, resulting in forced pulling of the corner of the mouth laterally. Spasms may also start in the lower part of the face, and move upwards (atypical form). Spasms can occur at a rate of 5 to 20 contractions per second and may also become continuous and affect all of the muscles on one side of the face. Twitching may increase under stress, and can even be present during sleep. Although benign and painless, twitching frequently leads to social embarrassment, with a remarkable impact on the patient's perception and satisfaction with various aspects of their life.[21]

!

Involuntary spasmodic movement of mimic muscles on one side of the face is the only symptom of hemifacial spasm. Women account for two-thirds of cases.

Concurrent trigeminal nerve dysfunction results in the syndrome called "painful tic convulsive." It has been estimated that 0.2 to 11% of patients with trigeminal neuralgia have associated HFS. Coexistence with blepharospasm has also been reported.[22] In a 2011 study of 95 patients, hand tremor accompanied HFS in 40% of cases,[23] in another study 15 to 65% of patients complained of symptoms of depression.[24] The spasms affect vision in about 60% of patients and interfere with work in about one-third of the patients. Finally, stapedius muscle contraction may be responsible for tinnitus in the ear. Although HFS is well known by neurologists and otorhinolaryngologists, a delay in diagnosis is frequent and may take several years. The mean lag time between onset and diagnosis was found to be 5.4 years in a Canadian study.[25] Onset is generally between in the fourth or fifth decades of life; however, about 7% of cases present before the age of 30.[26] Onset during infancy is extremely rare and may indicate an underlying brain tumor.

28.6.3 Diagnostic Work-Up

Diagnosing a case of HFS starts with a complete history and detailed neurologic examination, including electromyography (EMG); further details of EMG are given in Chapter 6. Early cases of HFS may be difficult to distinguish from tics, facial myokymia, or myoclonus (► Table 28.2). Needle EMG has a characteristic footprint and typically shows irregular, brief, high-frequency bursts

Table 28.2 Differential diagnosis of hemifacial spasm

Symptoms of hemifacial spasm	Comment
Oromandibular dystonia	Affects the lower facial musculature, jaw, pharynx, and tongue In conjunction with blepharospasm, the diagnosis is called Meige's syndrome Jaw opening, jaw closing, and jaw deviating dystonia are rare
Tics	Brief, repetitive, coordinated movements of grouped facial and neck muscles They may occur in encephalopathy Drugs may produce tics (anticonvulsants, caffeine, methylphenidate, antiparkinsonian agents)
Myoclonic movements	Symptomatic myoclonic movements may arise from brain lesions Movements tend to be more generalized; imaging may retrieve an underlying cause Typically respond to anticonvulsants
Hemimasticatory spasm	A segmental myoclonus with unilateral contractions of mastication muscles (usually the masseter)[27]
Facial chorea	Occurs in the context of a systemic movement disorder (e.g., Huntington's disease)
Facial myokymia	Appears as vermicular twitching under the skin. Electromyogram reveals bursts of motor unit potentials interrupted by periods of silence of up to a few seconds Consider a brainstem process
Craniofacial tremor	May occur in association with essential tremor, electrolyte dysfunction, Parkinson disease or thyroid dysfunction

(150–400 Hz) of motor unit potentials, which correlate with clinically observed facial movements, making neurophysiologic testing invaluable in cases where diagnosis is difficult.

> !
>
> High-frequency burst patterns on needle electromyography is nearly pathognomonic for hemifacial spasm.

MRI should be performed in every case, particularly if an underlying compressive lesion is suspected; for further details see Chapter 5. 3-Tesla MRI has been reported to be superior concerning anatomic conspicuity, delineation of cranial nerves, and assessment of small vessels.[28] Three-dimensional high-resolution MRI has been reported to offer a high predictive value in detecting offending vessels before surgery.[29] Cerebral angiography offers little additional diagnostic value in HFS. In the majority of cases, imaging of the brain is unable to reveal any specific cause of nerve irritation. A small vessel (usually an artery, but occasionally a vein) may be detected compressing the root exit zone of the facial nerve at the brainstem. However, this vessel may be too small to be demonstrated by means of cross-sectional imaging. Furthermore, it is often difficult to directly correlate vessels with the facial nerve.

28.6.4 Treatment

Decompression surgery and botulinum toxin injections are the current main treatments in HFS; further details on the application of botulinum toxin are given in Chapter 25. Mild cases of HFS may be managed with sedation or carbamazepine for noncompressive lesions. Carbamazepine, benzodiazepines, and baclofen may also be used in patients who refuse botulinum toxin injections or in those with secondary therapy failure to botulinum toxin.

> !
>
> In most patients with hemifacial spasm, the treatment of choice is injection of botulinum toxin. Decompression surgery is an alternative for definitive treatment.

Drugs

Carbamazepine, benzodiazepines, anticholinergics, or baclofen have been used, but all can cause sedation. The efficacy of oral medications is often transient and clinical trials have included only small numbers of patients. Gabapentin has been studied in HFS, and resulted in a significant reduction of facial spasms.[30]

Botulinum Toxin

Numerous open-label and some double-blind placebo-controlled studies have shown excellent symptom improvements after botulinum toxin injections.[31] The toxin solution is injected into the subdermal plane overlying the mimic muscles; details are given in Chapter 25. Despite variations in injection techniques, dilution volume of the toxin, or application of EMG guidance, favorable results can be expected in 75 to 100% of patients.[4] The mean duration of action is 3 to 6 months. Adverse effects include ptosis, dry eyes, eyelid and facial weakness, and diplopia. Side effects all are transient; serious systemic effects are not expected. Repeated injections are generally well tolerated, and benefit is maintained over the years of therapy. Immunoresistance due to antibody formation is rare in HFS since low doses of botulinum toxin are used.

Surgery

Favorable results have been reported after microvascular decompression surgery. Success rates of more than 90% have been reported in some series. However, recurrence rates of up to 20% also have also been reported in the literature.[32] After the invention of botulinum toxin treatment, which is safe, patients will often elect not to have surgery. Complications of surgery include cerebral infarction, hemorrhage, and temporary or persistent facial nerve weakness or hearing loss, with up to 25% of the patients experiencing hearing loss in some reports.[33] In a review of the experience of a single institution who carried out more than 4,400 operations, facial weakness, cerebellar injury (0.68%), hearing loss (1.44%), and cerebrospinal fluid leakage (1.95%) were the most frequently reported complications.[34] Patients with typical onset of symptoms show better results than those with atypical onset, and complications are more frequent in patients who undergo reoperation. Extracranial operations, including sectioning of peripheral nerve branches, removal of facial muscles, and injections of alcohol or phenol to injure the facial nerve, have been used with poor rates of success and they should no longer be performed.

28.6.5 Outcome and Prognosis

HFS is a progressive, but nonfatal, illness. The prognosis depends on the treatment and the respective response. Favorable outcome has been reported after treatment with botulinum toxin as well as after microvascular decompression surgery.

28.7 Key Points

- Blepharospasm is the most frequent feature of cranial dystonia.
- The cause of most forms of dystonia forms idiopathic.
- Hemifacial spasm (HFS) is characterized by involuntary movements of mimic muscles due to compression of the facial nerve at its exit from the brainstem.
- HFS and dystonia affecting the face may result in severe disability.
- Although HFS and blepharospasm are distinct in their pathophysiology, botulinum toxin is an effective first-line treatment for both disorders.

References

[1] Quartarone A, Hallett M. Emerging concepts in the physiological basis of dystonia. Mov Disord 2013; 28: 958–967

[2] Pariseau B, Worley MW, Anderson RL. Myectomy for blepharospasm 2013. Curr Opin Ophthalmol 2013; 24: 488–493

[3] Defazio G, Livrea P. Epidemiology of primary blepharospasm. Mov Disord 2002; 17: 7–12

[4] Ababneh OH, Cetinkaya A, Kulwin DR. Long-term efficacy and safety of botulinum toxin a injections to treat blepharospasm and hemifacial spasm. Clin Exper Ophthalmol 2013

[5] Reese R, Gruber D, Schoenecker T et al. Long-term clinical outcome in meige syndrome treated with internal pallidum deep brain stimulation. Mov Disord 2011; 26: 691–698

[6] Valálik I, Jobbágy A, Bognár L, Csókay A. Effectiveness of unilateral pallidotomy for meige syndrome confirmed by motion analysis. Stereotact Funct Neurosurg 2011; 89: 157–161

[7] Esper CD, Freeman A, Factor SA. Lingual protrusion dystonia: frequency, etiology and botulinum toxin therapy. Parkinsonism Relat Disord 2010; 16: 438–441

[8] Wang A, Jankovic J. Hemifacial spasm: clinical findings and treatment. Muscle Nerve 1998; 21: 1740–1747

[9] Kemp LW, Reich SG. Hemifacial Spasm. Curr Treat Options Neurol 2004; 6: 175–179

[10] Auger RG, Whisnant JP. Hemifacial spasm in Rochester and Olmsted County, Minnesota, 1960 to 1984. Arch Neurol 1990; 47: 1233–1234

[11] Wu Y, Davidson AL, Pan T, Jankovic J. Asian over-representation among patients with hemifacial spasm compared to patients with cranial-cervical dystonia. J Neurol Sci 2010; 298: 61–63

[12] Jannetta PJ, Abbasy M, Maroon JC, Ramos FM, Albin MS. Etiology and definitive microsurgical treatment of hemifacial spasm. Operative techniques and results in 47 patients. J Neurosurg 1977; 47: 321–328

[13] Yaltho TC, Jankovic J. The many faces of hemifacial spasm: differential diagnosis of unilateral facial spasms. Mov Disord 2011; 26: 1582–1592

[14] Gardner WJ. Concerning the mechanism of trigeminal neuralgia and hemifacial spasm. J Neurosurg 1962; 19: 947–958

[15] Fukuda H, Ishikawa M, Okumura R. Demonstration of neurovascular compression in trigeminal neuralgia and hemifacial spasm with magnetic resonance imaging: comparison with surgical findings in 60 consecutive cases. Surg Neurol 2003; 59: 93–99, discussion 99–100

[16] Rahman EA, Trobe JD, Gebarski SS. Hemifacial spasm caused by vertebral artery dolichoectasia. Am J Ophthalmol 2002; 133: 854–856

[17] Micheli F, Scorticati MC, Gatto E, Cersosimo G, Adi J. Familial hemifacial spasm. Mov Disord 1994; 9: 330–332

[18] Miwa H, Mizuno Y, Kondo T. Familial hemifacial spasm: report of cases and review of literature. J Neurol Sci 2002; 193: 97–102

[19] Devoize JL. "The other" Babinski's sign: paradoxical raising of the eyebrow in hemifacial spasm. J Neurol Neurosurg Psychiatry 2001; 70: 516

[20] Pawlowski M, Gess B, Evers S. The Babinski-2 sign in hemifacial spasm. Mov Disord 2013; 28: 1298–1300

[21] Setthawatcharawanich S, Sathirapanya P, Limapichat K, Phabphal K. Factors associated with quality of life in hemifacial spasm and blepharospasm during long-term treatment with botulinum toxin. Qual Life Res 2011; 20: 1519–1523

[22] Tan EK, Chan LL, Koh KK. Coexistent blepharospasm and hemifacial spasm: overlapping pathophysiologic mechanism? J Neurol Neurosurg Psychiatry 2004; 75: 494–496

[23] Rudzińska M, Wójcik M, Hartel M, Szczudlik A. Tremor in hemifacial spasm patients. J Neural Transm 2011; 118: 241–247

[24] Tan EK, Lum SY, Fook-Chong S, Chan LL, Gabriel C, Lim L. Behind the facial twitch: depressive symptoms in hemifacial spasm. Parkinsonism Relat Disord 2005; 11: 241–245

[25] Jog M, Chouinard S, Hobson D et al. Causes for treatment delays in dystonia and hemifacial spasm: a Canadian survey. Can J Neurol Sci 2011; 38: 704–711

[26] Tan EK, Chan LL. Young onset hemifacial spasm. Acta Neurol Scand 2006; 114: 59–62

[27] Cruccu G, Inghilleri M, Berardelli A et al. Pathophysiology of hemimasticatory spasm. J Neurol Neurosurg Psychiatry 1994; 57: 43–50

[28] Garcia M, Naraghi R, Zumbrunn T, Rösch J, Hastreiter P, Dörfler A. High-resolution 3D-constructive interference in steady-state MR imaging and 3D time-of-flight MR angiography in neurovascular compression: a comparison between 3 T and 1.5 T. AJNR Am J Neuroradiol 2012; 33: 1251–1256

[29] El Refaee E, Langner S, Baldauf J, Matthes M, Kirsch M, Schroeder HW. Value of 3-dimensional high-resolution magnetic resonance imaging in detecting the offending vessel in hemifacial spasm: comparison with intraoperative high definition endoscopic visualization. Neurosurgery 2013; 73: 58–67, discussion 67

[30] Daniele O, Caravaglios G, Marchini C, Mucchiut L, Capus P, Natalè E. Gabapentin in the treatment of hemifacial spasm. Acta Neurol Scand 2001;104(2):110–112

[31] Jost WH, Kohl A. Botulinum toxin: evidence-based medicine criteria in blepharospasm and hemifacial spasm. J Neurol 2001; 248 Suppl 1: 21–24

[32] Payner TD, Tew JM, Jr. Recurrence of hemifacial spasm after microvascular decompression. Neurosurgery 1996; 38: 686–690, discussion 690–691

[33] Sindou M, Fobé JL, Ciriano D, Fischer C. Hearing prognosis and intraoperative guidance of brainstem auditory evoked potential in microvascular decompression. Laryngoscope 1992; 102: 678–682

[34] McLaughlin MR, Jannetta PJ, Clyde BL, Subach BR, Comey CH, Resnick DK. Microvascular decompression of cranial nerves: lessons learned after 4400 operations. J Neurosurg 1999; 90: 1–8

Part VIII

Miscellaneous

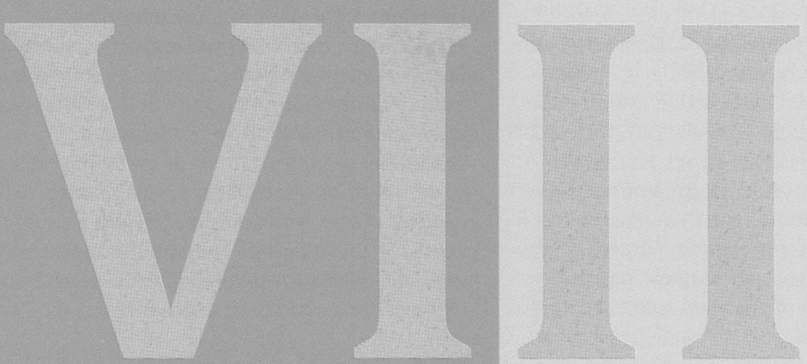

29 Medicolegal Aspects of Iatrogenic Facial Nerve Palsy

Eric L. Slattery and Jack M. Kartush

29.1 Introduction

Iatrogenic facial nerve injury is of the highest concern to surgeons operating near the facial nerve, including the specialties of otolaryngology, facial plastics, general surgery, and oral surgery. Surgery near the facial nerve can be a challenging task due to its tortuous course—from brainstem to facial musculature—and the delicacy of its surrounding anatomic structures. Consequently, the devastating complication of facial nerve injury can occur even in the most capable of hands. Injury may lead to a range of sequelae—from transient mild paresis to severe long-term impairment of both cosmesis and function. Severe injury will not uncommonly lead to claims of malpractice. This chapter will review both prevention and management of iatrogenic facial nerve injury.

29.2 Epidemiology of Iatrogenic Facial Nerve Injury

Facial nerve injury occurs in a wide variety of procedures. Recently a large-volume facial nerve center reported on 102 patients with iatrogenic injury seen over a 10-year period, originating from oral and maxillofacial surgery (40%), head and neck surgery (25%), otologic surgery (17%), cosmetic procedures (11%), and other procedures (7%).[1] Fifty percent of these patients presented over 3 months after the initial surgery with 36% of referrals being self generated.

29.2.1 Oral Surgery

Within oral surgery, temporomandibular joint (TMJ) procedures have the highest litigated occurrence with facial nerve injury. Reasons for surgery of the TMJ include overdevelopment and underdevelopment of the mandible, condylar growth problems, mandibular arthritis/ankylosis, and tumors of this region.[2] However, permanent facial nerve injury has decreased over time from 25 to 1.7% through evolved surgical technique.[3] Weinberg and Kryshtalskyj reported use of the preauricular approach to the TMJ demonstrating a 10.8% dysfunction rate in either the temporal or the zygomatic branches of the facial nerve.[4] All but one patient in their series had return of facial nerve function by 14 weeks postoperatively. One study of 32 patients reported that the frequency of facial nerve weakness (none with permanent paralysis) was related to degree of pathology and surgical procedure.[5] Patients with total ankylosis of the joint and those who underwent gap arthroplasty had the highest rates of temporary weakness of the nerve.[5] Facial nerve paralysis has been described after distraction osteogenesis of TMJ ankylosis.[6] Notably, often the surgical technique used for accessing the TMJ relies on avoidance rather than identification of the facial nerve.[2,7] Using avoidance rather than identification is suggested to lead to potentially higher injury rates in revision cases, as the anatomy is altered.[1]

!

Temporomandibular joint procedures have the highest litigated occurrence of facial nerve injury. It is not clear if the risk of facial nerve injury during these procedures can be mitigated with nerve identification versus avoidance.

29.2.2 Head and Neck Surgery

Injury to the facial nerve, including distal branches, is not uncommon following head and neck procedures. High rates usually surround oncologic procedures. Facial nerve injury with salivary gland surgery is a well-known complication; for more details see Chapter 19. Injury rates of the facial nerve differ based on the reasons for the procedure, ranging from potentially an expected outcome in some cases involving malignancy, to seldom in cases with benign pathology. Long-term rates of facial nerve injury from parotidectomy range from 0 to 19%.[8–12] Risk factors known for postoperative facial nerve injury include lesion size,[13] malignant tumors,[8] type of surgery,[11,14] inflamed tissue,[8,13] age,[15,16] extent of facial nerve dissection,[12] and length of procedure.[16] Stretching of the nerve, which occurs more frequently with deep lobe tumors and in total parotidectomy, has also been associated with increased injury rates.[13] Temporary paresis of segmental facial nerve branches is not uncommon based on the routine need to stretch tissue adjacent to the nerve during dissection of the gland and the pathology.

The ramus mandibularis branch is most commonly damaged during surgery of the submandibular gland. Permanent nerve injury occurs in 0 to 8% of cases following excision of the submandibular gland.[17]

Facial nerve injury can occur following neck dissection for removal of metastatic lymph nodes. Often distal branches of the nerve are injured. The rate of temporary paresis of the marginal mandibular nerve measured as lower lip weakness following neck dissection for head and neck cancer has been estimated at 14%, 2 weeks after surgery.[18] The same study noted higher rates when level I was dissected in the neck and permanent injury based on continued weakness at 1 year occurring in 7% of patients. A similar study examined smile asymmetry following neck dissection and found a weakness noted by the surgeon in 18% of patients 6 months after surgery.[19] Interestingly, 41% of these same patients described their smiling as changed at the same time point, suggesting that subtle nerve damage is underestimated by a clinician's physical examination. In cases of head and neck melanoma, low rates of facial nerve dysfunction postoperatively have been described following sentinel lymph node biopsy, although the rates are higher when nodes are mapped into the parotid gland (10% transient weakness).[20,21] Similarly, excision of cutaneous malignancies can lead to injury of the facial nerve as well. Often parotidectomy is performed for aggressive cases of cutaneous malignancies, with neurotrophic spread into the facial nerve not uncommon.[22,23]

29.2.3 Otologic Surgery

The course of the facial nerve within the temporal bone makes injury possible even during routine otologic surgery. Green et al[24] reviewed 22 cases of facial nerve damage from various otologic procedures: mastoidectomy (57%), exostosis removal (14%), tympanoplasty without mastoidectomy (14%), stapedectomy (5%), and cochlear implant (5%).

In contrast to other surgical procedures, when iatrogenic injury occurs in otologic surgery, there is a higher incidence of severe nerve injury versus neuropraxic or partial injuries. This is likely to represent the fact that injury here is typically due to direct trauma (often a high-speed drill) versus a stretch injury (e.g., parotid and thyroid surgery). Furthermore, the fallopian canal exacerbates the effect of edema, resulting in ischemic neuropathy.

The distal part of the tympanic portion of the facial nerve is the area most often damaged (55%).[24] Injury in revision cases (4–10%) is known to occur at higher rates than injury in primary cases (0.6–3.7%).[25] Injury rates increase when normal anatomy is altered by disease such as cholesteatoma or granulation tissue.[24,26] Of special note is otologic surgery for congenital abnormalities. Higher rates of anomalous location of the facial nerve occur in cases with congenital stapes fixation.[27] In cases of congenital aural atresia, the risk of injury to the nerve is markedly increased due to the aberrant lateral and anterior course that commonly occurs distal to the second genu.[28–30]

> !
>
> During ear surgery there is a higher incidence of severe nerve injury versus neuropraxic or partial injuries. Congenital malformations and revision surgery pose increased risks.

29.2.4 Neurotologic Surgery

Significant rates of facial nerve injury have long been associated with resection of skull base lesions such as cerebellopontine angle tumors. However, the application of binocular microscopy, various temporal bone approaches, and the use of intraoperative neurophysiologic monitoring, as described in Chapter 15, have dramatically improved facial preservation rates over the last few decades. Subspecialization with additional fellowship training beyond residency for both otologists and neurosurgeons has also undoubtedly contributed to better outcomes.

House and Leutje reported a 13.5% complete paralysis rate in their first 500 cases.[31] Pooled data from earlier studies suggest only a 53% normal or near normal facial nerve function after resection of tumors 2 cm or larger, demonstrating the effect of tumor size on prognosis.[32] Use of intraoperative electromyographic (EMG) facial nerve monitoring has been shown to increase preservation of facial nerve function and is now widely accepted and employed in resecting tumors of the cerebellopontine angle.[33–37] Furthermore, Kartush and others have demonstrated that staging very large tumors (two-stage surgery or surgery followed by stereotactic radiation) can significantly improve facial nerve outcomes with excellent facial function (House–Brackmann [HB] score I or II) reported as high as 78 to 82% of cases.[32,38,39]

> !
>
> Nerve monitoring and staging of large tumors has had a significant impact on improving long-term facial nerve function.

29.2.5 Plastic Surgery

Permanent injury to the facial nerve in cosmetic procedures occurs infrequently. Damage occurs in 0.53 to 2.6% of rhytidectomy cases.[40,41] Both the temporal and the marginal mandibular branches are at risk with rhytidectomy, with specific techniques injuring one branch or the other at higher rates. It has been estimated that greater than 85% of facial weakness is temporary and returns within months of the procedure.[42] The temporal branch is also at risk during forehead and browlift procedures, but permanent injury is thought to occur at very low rates (< 1%).[43]

> !
>
> The temporal and marginal mandibular branches are at greatest risk during rhytidectomy. The vast majority of these injuries is temporary.

29.3 Malpractice Claims, Litigation, and Facial Nerve Injury

It is estimated that most surgeons will face at least one lawsuit over their career.[44] Typically, malpractice is a claim of either negligence or improper consent.[45] Claims of negligence require four conditions to exist[46]:

- A duty was owed by a physician.
- The physician by acting outside standard of care breached this duty.
- The patient suffered a compensable loss.
- The injury resulted from the breach in duty.

Judgments focus on identifying the specific standards of care relative to the case at hand and whether these standards were breached. Standard of care is typically defined for the jury as the care that would have been provided by a similarly trained practitioner under similar circumstances. Until very recently, written standards of care or guidelines for clinical practice have rarely been available. Consequently, determining the standards of care in a particular case has relied on expert witness testimony, which often draws from personal experience, examination of literature, and professional guidelines. It should be noted that negligence differs from incompetence. Incompetence refers to the inability to perform necessary duties due to mental impairment, drug or alcohol use, or technical/knowledge deficit.[47] Competent individuals can be negligent. Consent is considered informed when alternative therapeutic approaches and likely risks are given to patients. The definition of informed consent varies from country to country or even from state to state in the United States.[45] Analysis of medicolegal action is complicated by most cases (approximately 85%) not reaching trial due to allegations being dismissed or settlements out of court.[48] Such cases not reaching trial are unfortunately difficult to access for study.

Res ipsa loquitur is a Latin expression meaning “the thing speaks for itself.” It is a phrase sometimes used during malpractice litigation by plaintiff's counsel to imply that an act or outcome is so obviously a breach of the standard of care that no further evidence is required. This strategy has sometimes been used in the past for iatrogenic facial nerve injury but experts for both plaintiff and defendant typically agree that even the most experienced and well-trained surgeon can inadvertently injure the nerve. Therefore, the mere fact of facial nerve injury does not itself impute malpractice.

Consequently, litigation focuses on whether the standard of care was breached by either incompetence or negligence not only during surgery but before and after an injury was identified: i.e., proper informed consent and proper management once an injury occurred. As noted previously, negligence indicates that the surgeon did have appropriate training but failed to follow standards that would have minimized or obviated the injury. Much of the time and expense related to malpractice litigation arises from trying to convince judge or jury on what particular standard was breached despite the absence of documented standards in clinical practice and surgical technique. As every physician knows: (1) expert recommendations often vary, and (2) each clinical circumstance may have unique or extenuating circumstances that might invalidate general recommendations being applied to the specific case.

> **!**
>
> Most frequently, litigation focuses on whether the standard of care was breached, or if there was a failure to obtain informed consent.

Because of these complicating factors, national medical organizations have been reluctant to publish clinical practice guidelines. Furthermore, another concern has been that such guidelines could be used unfairly against physicians during litigation. Nonetheless, in recent years with a new emphasis on patient safety, quality assurance, and reducing medical errors, there is an evolving belief that the benefits accrued from nationally accepted guidelines outweigh the potential disadvantages.

A notable example of the potential benefits of nationally recommended guidelines has been the “Standards for Basic Anesthesia Monitoring” first ratified by the American Society of Anesthesiology in 1984.[49] There was initial reluctance for having any society-recommended guidelines and, in particular, there was specific concern about declaring intraoperative oxygenation monitoring (pulse oximetry) as being mandatory. Just as with facial nerve monitoring, many anesthesia practitioners did not feel that this technology should be considered mandatory. Over the years, however, these guidelines have proved beneficial to both patients and anesthesia providers. Thirty years since those standards were accepted and published, there now appears to be a clear consensus by anesthesia providers that pulse oximetry should be used during every case.

Of interest, the American Academy of Otolaryngology–Head and Neck Surgery has begun publishing a series of clinical guidelines, which include how to manage ear wax—but no guidelines on when facial monitoring should be used nor what is the proper method to use it. It is hoped that this omission will eventually be corrected, but until then both the indications and the proper method of monitoring will remain debatable.

Facial nerve injury is distressing to patients and is a dreaded complication by physicians. Facial paralysis can have significant effects on eye protection, oral competence, and speech, and can result in social stigmatization of the patient. For these reasons, although the complication of facial nerve injury is often discussed preoperatively, medicolegal action may still be pursued. Claims for injury of the facial nerve make up a majority of all cases involving the cranial nerves, including the optic nerve, which ranked second.[50]

Lydiatt in 2003 examined all US civil cases between 1985 and 2000 that went to trial for facial nerve injury.[51] Fifty-three cases were identified involving otologic procedures (25%), cosmetic (23%), benign neoplasms of the parotid (17%), malignant neoplasms of the parotid (2%), non-neoplastic disease of the parotid or other head and neck benign pathology (28%), and TMJ procedures (6%). In 36 cases, the specialty of the defendant was known, with otolaryngologists comprising over 40%, plastic surgeons about 30%, and the rest divided among general practice, dermatology, neurosurgery, general surgery, and oral surgery. Allegations included failure to diagnose in 19%, lack of informed consent in 30%, and surgical misadventure in 89%. Verdict outcomes were broken down by specialty. In otology ($n = 13$) the verdict favored the plaintiff in 38% of cases, settlement in 23% of cases, and concluded for the defendant in 38% of cases. In the cosmetic group ($n = 12$), suits concluded for the plaintiff in 33% of cases, resulted in settlement in 25% of cases, and concluded for the defendant in 42% of cases. In the benign neoplasms of the parotid group ($n = 9$) 56% of cases concluded for the plaintiff, 11% settled, and 33% concluded for the defendant. In non-neoplastic disease and other benign pathology of the head and neck ($n = 15$) 33% of cases concluded for the plaintiff, 33% of cases were settled, and 33% of cases concluded for the defendant. Finally the defendant won in all three TMJ cases and the one malignant parotid case. The average amount paid for plaintiff awards was US $567,994, and the average settlement award was US $337,313. Notably, five of the six awards greater than US $1,000,000 were from the East Coast region of the United States.

Hong et al examined medical malpractice within salivary gland surgery in the United States between 1987 and 2011.[52] Twenty-six cases that went to trial or had formal settlements were examined, and 10 of the 26 cases involved the facial nerve. The parotid gland was involved in 62% of the total number of cases, and the submandibular and sublingual glands were involved in 38% of cases. All cases surrounding facial nerve injury came from the parotid surgery group: 6 of the 10 cases involving the facial nerve alleged improper surgical performance, 4 cases alleged error in diagnosis, and 4 cases involved consent problems.

Medicolegal aspects of facial nerve injury in relation to otologic surgery have been reviewed by several authors. Ruhl et al examined suits in the United States involving otologic procedures between 1983 and 2012.[53] Fifty-eight cases were identified with 14 cases involving facial nerve injury without hearing loss, and an additional five cases noted facial nerve injury with hearing loss. Blake et al also examined suits in the United States specific to otologic and neurotologic procedures between 1988 and 2011, and identified 47 cases.[54] Facial nerve injury existed in 27.7% of claims. Of the seven acoustic neuroma cases identified, reasons for claims included facial nerve injury in only one case. Similar trends have been noted in the United Kingdom. In one study, 137 cases of negligence claims from 1995 to 2002 were identified.[55] Similar to the United States studies, facial nerve injury was a main contributing factor to pursuing medicolegal action. The low incidence of malpractice claims for facial nerve injury following acoustic tumor resection is almost certainly due to the emphasis that both surgeon and patient place preoperatively on discussing this not uncommon complication.

Regardless of the type of surgery, inadequate informed consent is often cited in claims. The proportion of cases that claim lack of consent is surprising as facial nerve injury is a well-known complication of many of these procedures. Lydiatt noted that 30% of patients whose case went to trial for facial nerve injury claimed they were not properly informed.[51] It seems likely that discussions of this complication, as distressing as it is, had taken place in many of these cases. A major contributing factor for feeling uninformed includes poor patient retention of information following discussions with patients.[56] Strategies such as documentation, providing patients with written explanation of risks, and listing specific complications on the consent the day of surgery may aid in ensuring consent is informed.

A qualified expert witness is routinely needed to support a claim of negligence.[45] Lydiatt noted that in cases of facial nerve injury in which the specialty of expert witnesses is known, the expert witnesses of the defense and plaintiff were of the same specialty in 14 of 15 cases, with slightly higher than 50% being otolaryngologists, and plastic surgeons making up 25 to 30%.[51] A recent study compared plaintiff and defendant expert witness qualifications.[57] Plaintiff expert witnesses had significantly less experience than defendant expert witnesses (31.8 versus 35.4 years) and had lower scholarly impact measured by h-index (6.3 versus 10). A higher proportion of defendant expert witnesses were in academia (49.3% versus 31.7%).

!

The risk of a malpractice claim following iatrogenic facial nerve injury can be mitigated by:

- Preoperative discussion of facial nerve risks.
- Documentation of that discussion.
- Proper, timely handling of the postoperative complications.

29.4 Avoiding Error in Surgery near the Facial Nerve

Primum non nocere is a frequently used Latin aphorism meaning "first, do no harm." However, despite its popularity as a maxim in medical ethics, to truly *never* do harm would require one to never treat a patient. Although the medicolegal environment places emphasis on negligence as the reason for untoward outcomes, in reality there are many other reasons for error.[58] Like sports, surgery is not infrequently performed at the limits of human abilities. But in sports, star athletes earning millions of dollars a year are honored if they fail "only" 70% of the time, e.g., a top baseball player's batting average of .300. Clearly, a professional ball player's failure to "get on base" every time at bat does not bespeak incompetence or negligence—but is instead due to the *complexity of the task*. The same is typically true for the practice of surgery. Nonetheless, proper training and an understanding of the common causes of error can reduce the incidence of iatrogenic injury.

Surgery is an inherently difficult task, with even the most skilled and accomplished surgeons causing inadvertent injury to the facial nerve. Factors that contribute to error include time constraints, system and resource problems, technique, inexperience, and fatigue or other altered states.[59,60] It has been suggested that lower surgical volume, especially for high-complexity operations, and inexperience leads to increased error.[61,62] However, one report demonstrated that 84% of surgical errors occurred during routine operations and 73% of errors were made by experienced surgeons operating within the area of their expertise.[63]

"Slip" and "mistake" are two words for errors that are commonly used interchangeably. However, cognitive psychologists and systems analysts separate the words into two distinct types of error.[60] In brief, a *slip* is the correct plan that was not executed correctly. A *mistake* is the wrong plan—therefore the execution of that plan may or may not have even been relevant to the outcome. Of importance, certain mistakes will increase the chance of slips. Understanding the distinction between slips and mistakes is critical, not only for post hoc analysis of iatrogenic errors, but also for optimizing strategies to avoid similar errors in the future. An otologic example may be illustrative.

At the Michigan Ear Institute, fellows are taught fundamental temporal bone drilling rules:

1. Understand the likely direction that a slipped drill will take in order to predict and prevent harm.
2. "Leave natural protection" (e.g., bone) on delicate structures in order to reduce the chance of harm when a slips does eventually occur.
3. If natural protection must be removed from delicate structures, remove it as late in the dissection as possible.

In downhill snow skiing, catching the edge of a ski on a ridge of snow may lead to momentary loss of control—and the faster the skier is travelling, the greater the potential for harm from even a brief slip. Similarly, even the most skilled surgeon may have a surgical drill tip inadvertently skip out of control—and with common drill speeds of 80,000 rpm, injury to facial nerve, brain, or inner ear can occur in a fraction of a second.

When drilling the horizontal semicircular canal during a right labyrinthectomy or a translabyrinthine approach to the internal auditory canal, many surgeons first widen their surgical field by opening the facial recess and removing the incus. However, the standard clockwise-rotating burr will have a natural tendency to skip anteriorly (in a right ear) toward the genu of the facial nerve. Consequently, if the surgeon has removed the natural anatomic protection of the facial nerve, a skipped drill will have a higher likelihood of injuring the nerve.

If the enlightened surgeon is aware that this slip may occur despite their best intentions, then altering the surgical plan (e.g., *not* opening the facial recess and *not* removing the incus until after the labyrinthectomy) may mean that even if the drill slips, the facial nerve will not be injured because it was not surgically exposed earlier in the procedure. Thus, an optimized plan may not prevent slips—but it may prevent some slips from causing harm.

Unlike other practices of medicine, surgical error can take the form of manual or judgmental error. Publications such as that by Regenbogen[63] will note that the vast majority involves manual error to some degree—but, as detailed previously, a careful analysis is required to weigh the role of optimized planning and its effect on execution.

Many errors in medicine result from errors in attention. Unrecognized changes, fatigue, and disruption of automatic behavior are pertinent to errors of attention.[59] Employing standardized protocols and checklists can decrease the incidence of mistakes.[59,64]

Clearly, developing a mastery of anatomy and technique will reduce the chance of nerve injury—but such mastery is dependent upon the individual's skills, their training, and their diligence in temporal bone laboratory dissection. Visualization of the fallopian canal and/or its key adjacent landmarks is typically advised, especially in revision cases in which purposefully avoiding the nerve may lead to problems due to altered anatomy.[1] Injections of local anesthesia should be done carefully, because inadvertent applications adjacent to a dehiscent nerve can result in a temporary conduction block that will render intraoperative monitoring useless during the procedure. In otologic surgery, injection should not be performed inferior or medial to the mastoid tip. Local anesthetic in the middle ear can likewise cause a palsy, often entering the middle ear through a tympanic membrane perforation and then contacting the nerve through common dehiscences of the fallopian canal. As detailed in Chapter 15, placement of gelfoam to cover a perforation prior to injecting local anesthetic into the ear canal anticipates and prevents this complication. Incisions should be placed to avoid the nerve and its branches. Maintaining hemostasis during the procedure allows for better visualization of the operative field. If the nerve is exposed, minimizing traction and suction of the nerve is important. As previously noted, in otologic surgery, attention to burr rotation, direction, and orientation of drill handling will decrease injury to structures.[59] Drill bit control can be maximized by changing the orientation of the drill, using a drill bit sized optimally to the anatomic location, switching to a diamond burr, and maximizing exposure. Certain errors in otologic surgery may be difficult to justify, such as failing to find the nerve in an area of normal anatomy, and inexperience at finding key landmarks in the temporal bone.[55] Each surgeon must take an honest assessment of their skills and training when scheduling cases—as well as completing cases; on occasion, an inexperienced surgeon encountering marked anomalies or severe pathology may benefit both themselves and their patient by "backing out" of a procedure and referring the patient to someone with greater experience.

29.4.1 Intraoperative Monitoring

Intraoperative monitoring is discussed in detail in Chapter 15. One specific adjunct in facial nerve surgery worth detailing is use of intraoperative neurophysiologic monitoring (IOM) (▶ Fig. 29.1). Intraoperative monitoring has been recognized as standard during many neurotologic procedures since the 1991 National Institutes of Health consensus conference statement described the value of monitoring during acoustic tumor resection.[37] Monitoring aids in early identification of the nerve, detects nerve injury during dissection, and allows for assessment of nerve function when dissection has been completed.[65]

In contrast, routine facial nerve monitoring outside of neurotologic procedures of the cerebellopontine angle remains controversial. While nearly all surgeons agree there may be times that IOM is of value during tympanomastoid surgery (re: pathology, anomalies), some claim hesitance to use monitoring for every case. Extremely large prospective trials would be needed to show significant benefit of IOM in routine otologic cases given the low rates of injury in other types of surgery, and thus it is unlikely that they will ever be performed. Nonetheless, monitoring is being used with ever-increasing frequency in routine otologic procedures and there is an increasing body of literature that is advising that monitoring be routinely used during every middle ear and mastoid operation.[66–68] Wilson, Lin, and Lalwani found that monitoring was not only of clinical value for routine otologic surgery but was also cost-effective.[68]

In a recent survey by Kartush, nearly 90% of 230 North American otologists in the American Neurotology Society reported routine use of facial nerve monitoring during mastoid surgery.[69,70]

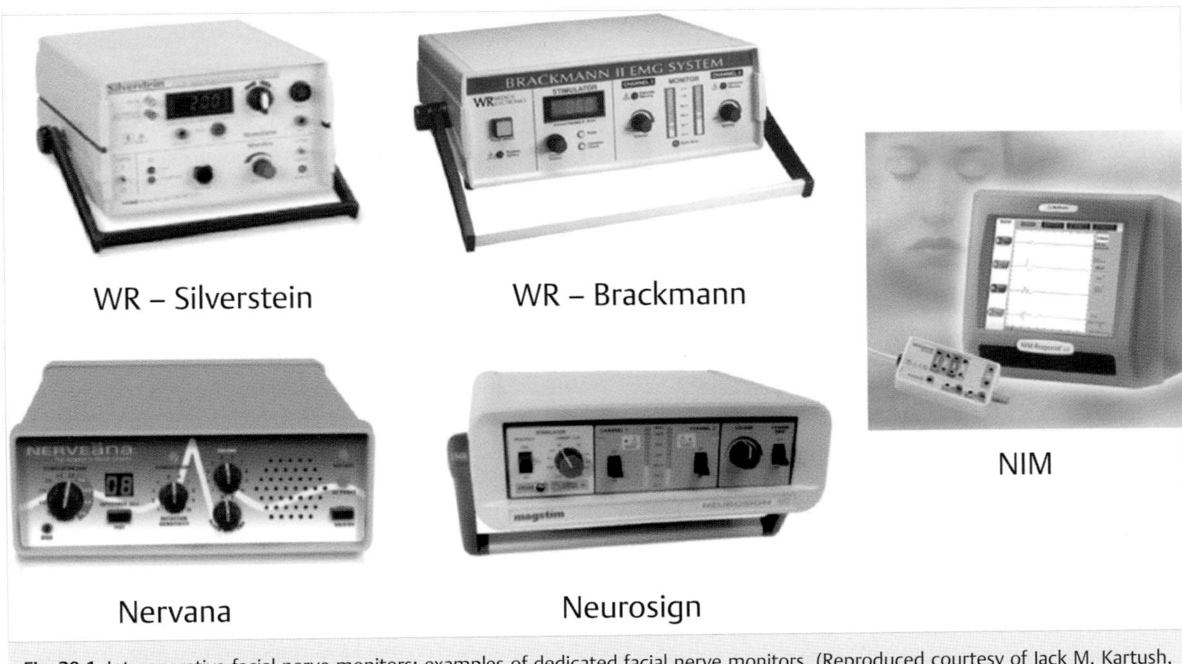

Fig. 29.1 Intraoperative facial nerve monitors: examples of dedicated facial nerve monitors. (Reproduced courtesy of Jack M. Kartush, MD.)

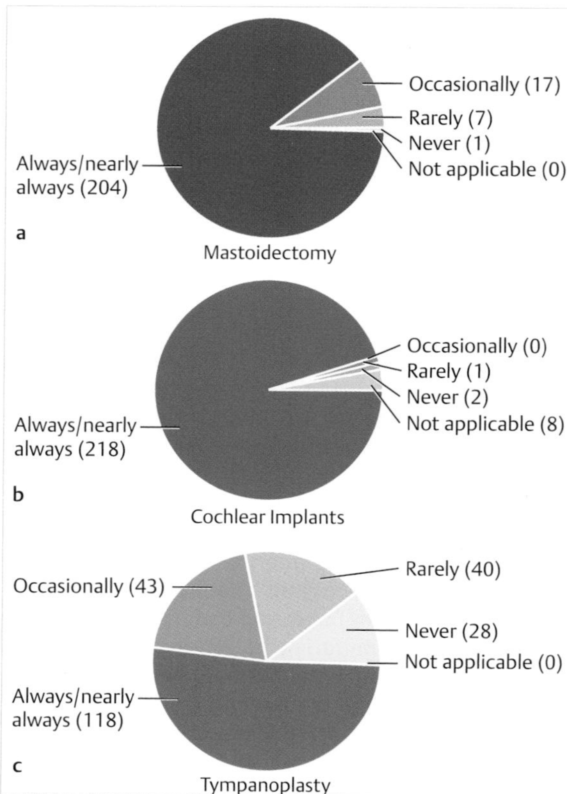

Fig. 29.2 Survey results of 230 otologic surgeons reporting on use of intraoperative monitoring during routine middle ear and mastoid surgery. Do you use intraoperative facial nerve monitoring for: **(a)** Mastoidectomy, **(b)** cochlear implantation, **(c)** tympanoplasty? (Reproduced courtesy of Jack M. Kartush, MD.)

Furthermore, 95% used monitoring during cochlear implant surgery. In contrast, monitoring was used in only 50% of tympanoplasties (▶ Fig. 29.2). Despite increasing use of monitoring, Kartush emphasized three caveats:

- Monitoring is not a substitute for knowledge of anatomy or surgical skills.
- Poor monitoring is worse than no monitoring.
- Monitors fail less frequently than do "monitorists."

Surgeons typically state that routine use of monitoring during all tympanomastoid cases assures that they and their operative team remain facile with monitoring—and that in the infrequent cases of an anomaly or greater pathology than expected, the monitor becomes of markedly greater value. Of interest, some surgeons use monitoring selectively only in what they perceive are high-risk cases—but injuries occur with a surprising frequency even in perceived low-risk procedures such as canaloplasty for exostoses.[24]

The role of routine intraoperative monitoring in parotid surgery to decrease postoperative facial nerve weakness has also been debated, even though decades ago McCabe proclaimed that stimulating the facial nerve electrically was in fact a sine qua non of parotidectomy.[71] At the time, McCabe referred to facial nerve stimulation with visual observation of the muscle contractions. Today, that method may still be used by some although, increasingly, facial nerve monitors are used to more accurately record and document small responses that may not be visible to the eye. Terrell et al reported a statistically significant difference in early facial weakness in monitored (33%) versus unmonitored (57%) patients[16]; however other reports suggest its usage does not decrease facial nerve injury.[71–73] Similarly no consensus on benefit of intraoperative facial nerve monitoring exists with otologic surgery.[66] Studies suggest that monitoring provides earlier identification of the nerve, and identification of fallopian canal dehiscences that occur with greater frequency in diseased ears.[66,74,75] As noted previously, intraoperative facial nerve monitoring has been shown to have higher quality-adjusted life years compared with unmonitored cases, suggesting higher cost-effectiveness of using monitoring.[68]

A study reported 10 cases of suits involving the salivary glands between 1987 and 2011; none cited lack of use of facial nerve monitoring as grounds for the suit.[52] Another report cites an otologic case with alleged improper performance solely due to lack of facial nerve monitoring, wherein the jury concluded that facial nerve monitoring was not standard of care.[53] Despite this, physicians often indicate that monitoring could have helped in cases that did result in injury, and describe using it in previous cases to help reduce injury. While defining a "standard of care" is difficult, clearly in the United States intraoperative monitoring is being used with increasing frequency during tympanomastoid and parotid surgery. In fact, litigation of iatrogenic nerve injury now often claims not a "failure to have monitored" but a "failure to have monitored *correctly.*"

This leads to a discussion of how surgeons are trained in monitoring. While some types of monitoring are quite complex and require technical assistance (e.g., spinal cord monitoring using somatosensory and motor evoked potentials), facial nerve monitoring is a relatively simple, single modality procedure that can be surgeon-directed. This nonetheless requires that the surgeon receive proper training in both the technical and the interpretive components of monitoring. Unfortunately, most academic residency teaching programs and private hospitals do not yet have in place a core curriculum and set of standards that should be met. Often, junior residents receive brief, spur of the moment instruction by senior residents whose knowledge base may also be questionable. Alternatively, some hospitals employ or contract neuromonitoring technologists. While this may transfer the burden of performing and understanding the EMG needle placement and monitoring device setup, a surgeon untrained in monitoring will have difficulty in correctly interpreting the EMG responses and knowing how to troubleshoot false-negative and false-positive errors.

As detailed in Chapter 15, poor monitoring is worse than no monitoring. It is analogous to a soldier using a broken minesweeper. In such circumstances, the device may not only be ineffective but lead the user into a false sense of security.[76,77] Key points in proper usage include[70,76]:

- Avoidance of long-lasting muscle relaxants.
- Judicial use of local anesthetic.
- Careful placement of electrodes.
- Impedance check of electrodes.
- Performance of tap test to ensure recording circuit continuity.
- Verification of stimulus current flow after incision.
- Early stimulation of the facial nerve to obtain a baseline response.
- Stimulation as needed during the procedure and prior to closing.

Video examples of the nerve monitoring protocol steps (▶ Video 15.1 to ▶ Video 15.15) are available at the Thieme MediaCenter.

According to the senior author's (JMK) experience, a common monitoring error is that some surgeons simply place the EMG electrodes and listen for possible spontaneous EMG responses caused by trauma. They assume that electrical silence during the operation means no trauma. Not only is this assumption false but failure to use electric stimulation during the procedure results in two problems. First, only by performing electrical stimulation during the procedure can the integrity of the nerve and monitoring system be verified by: (1) confirming current flow by stimulating any available soft tissue, and (2) stimulating near the nerve with sufficient current to achieve a baseline response. Second, while being alerted to trauma by a sudden burst of EMG activity is of value, optimized nerve monitoring has its greatest value in *preventing* or minimizing trauma by allowing early nerve identification especially in cases where disease, tumor, or scar may obfuscate standard anatomic landmarks. Kartush Stimulating Instruments (KSIs) are a unique variant of monopolar stimulators that allow *simultaneous* stimulation during surgical dissection (▶ Fig. 29.3; Neurosign Magstim). KSIs encourage frequent electrical stimulation by obviating the need to have the surgeon's work flow disrupted by repeatedly exchanging their conventional surgical instrument for a dedicated stimulator probe.

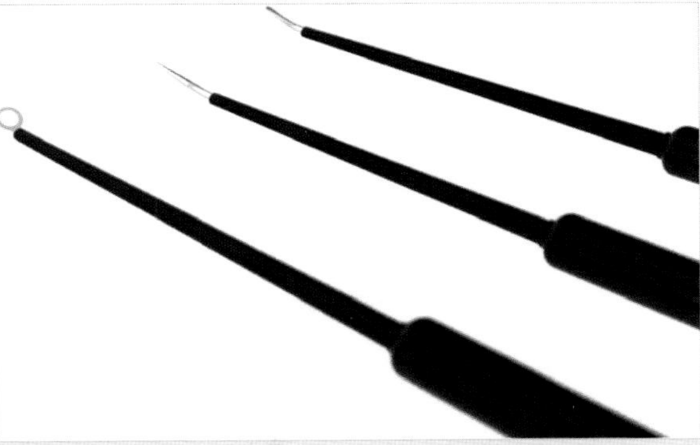

Fig. 29.3 Stimulating instruments. Kartush Stimulating Instruments (KSIs) are a variant of monopolar stimulators that allow simultaneous stimulation during surgical dissection (Neurosign Magstim, Carmarthenshire, UK). (Reproduced courtesy of Jack M. Kartush, MD.)

29.5 Management of Facial Nerve Injury

Management of Facial Nerve Injury is described in more detail in Chapter 20. When a postoperative facial palsy has been detected, the surgeon must consider a number of important factors:

- Should surgical re-exploration be considered and, if so, when and by whom?
- What is the likely site and severity of nerve injury?
- If surgical re-exploration is deferred, what tests and treatments should be considered, e.g., steroids, computed tomography scan, electrical testing, eye care (lubrication, taping, early gold weight eyelid implant)?

29.5.1 Initial Assessment

Assessing patients as soon as is feasible after surgery is important to determine if a facial palsy was immediate or delayed in onset. Delayed palsies have a higher likelihood of recovering and therefore may lead the surgeon toward observation rather than immediate re-exploration. However, the surgeon should not be misled by an inaccurate initial assessment, e.g., when the patient is still drowsy from anesthesia or relying on unreliable second-hand assessments by other healthcare personnel who are not adept at assessing facial weakness. Children typically have excellent facial tone that may be misinterpreted as representing only a partial weakness when in fact the nerve may be completely transected.

Of particular note is that even experienced examiners can be fooled into believing a complete paralysis is a partial paresis if the only movement observed is slow closure of the upper eyelid. However, eyelid closure occurs not only from active contracture of the orbicularis oculi muscle (innervated by the facial nerve), but also due to relaxation of the levator muscle (innervated by the oculomotor nerve). If this underlying neurophysiology is not understood, a surgeon can be misled into underestimating the severity of nerve injury. Thus, if the only facial movement visible is slow closure of the eyelid, it is important for the surgeon to carefully assess if there is active orbicularis oculi contraction rather than only passive relaxation of the levator muscle.

> **!**
>
> Slow closure of the eye after surgery does not rule out a complete facial palsy. This can be the result of a relaxation of the levator muscle masking a complete facial palsy.

A complete and immediate postoperative facial paralysis is always a matter of serious concern. If it persists for more than a few hours, then the temporary effect of local anesthetic on the nerve can be excluded and a more severe injury becomes likely. Iatrogenic facial nerve injuries should be managed promptly but with careful consideration of the pros and cons of possible surgical re-exploration (▶ Fig. 29.4 and ▶ Fig. 29.5). Whereas decades ago some claimed that "the sun should never set on an iatrogenic facial nerve injury," current consensus favors evaluating each instance separately.

29.5.2 Surgical Exploration and Repair

At times litigation focuses on failure to re-operate immediately. However, in addition to taking time to carefully assess the individual case, some studies have in fact claimed a benefit to delaying nerve repair. Under experimental conditions, neural transection initiates a cascade of metabolic changes that take 21 days before the regenerating nerve cells are best suited to crossing an anastomosis.[71] While from a practical perspective, an unequivocally transected nerve is typically repaired as soon as the injury is confirmed, the aforementioned metabolic changes are sometimes cited as justification not to rush into surgical repair.

Barrs has shown in an animal study that grafting the facial nerve can have successful results from 0 to 90 days post-transection.[78] There did not appear to be improved regeneration when repaired at 21 days, as the prior study speculated. Therefore, there appears to be no neurophysiologic imperative to operate on the same day or at day 21. Instead, the timing of possible

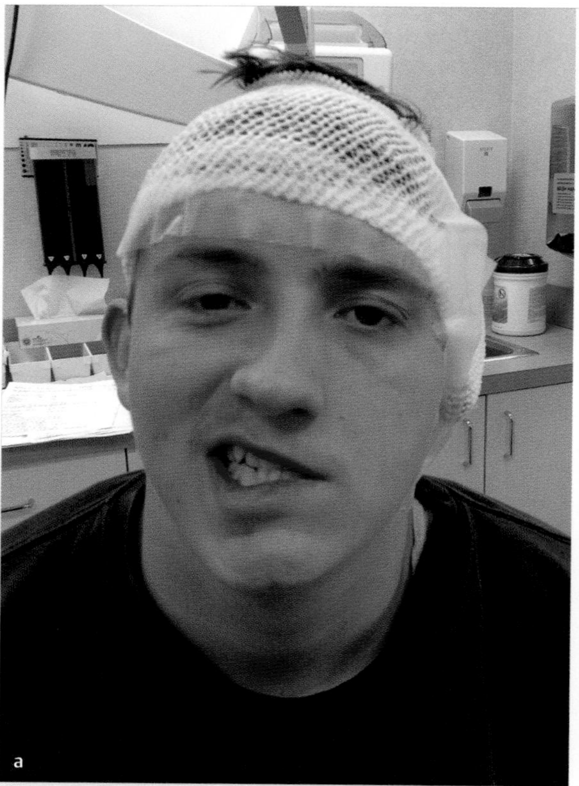

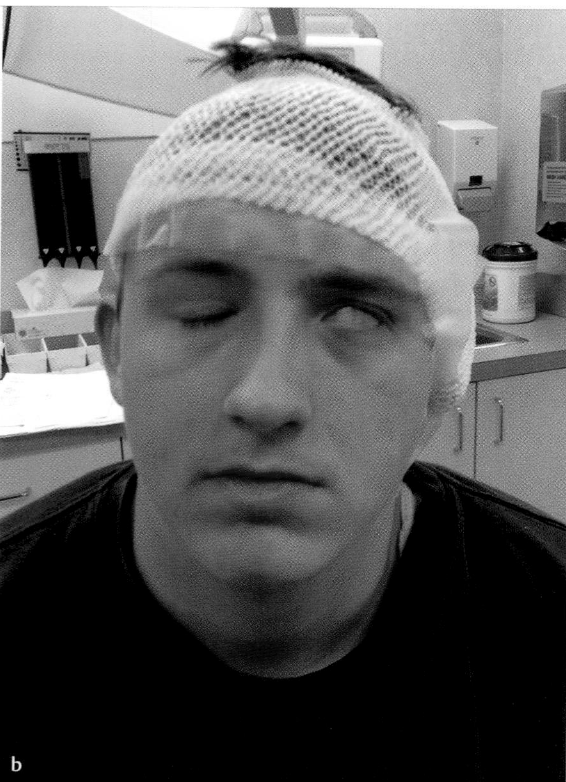

Fig. 29.4 Iatrogenic left facial nerve injury. A patient referred following mastoidectomy for cholesteatoma. **(a)** The patient was noted to have complete facial paralysis after surgery. **(b)** Bell's phenomenon with attempted eye closure. (Reproduced courtesy of Eric Sargent, MD.)

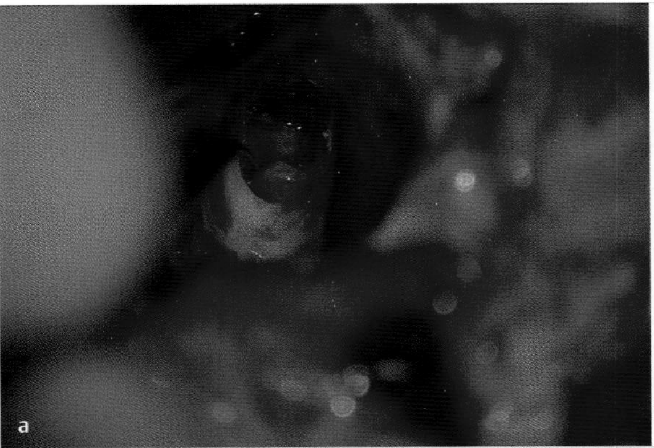

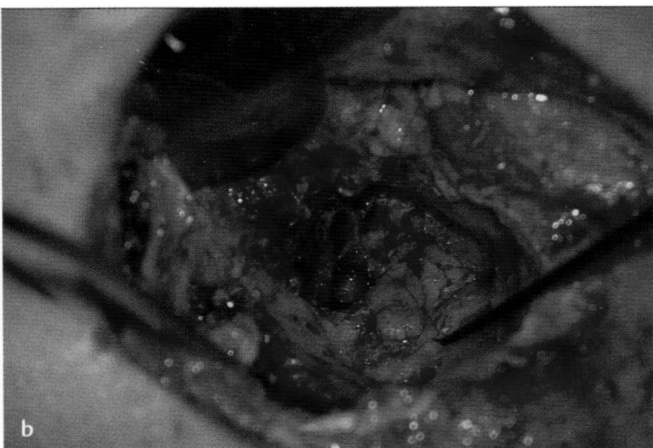

Fig. 29.5 Transected facial nerve. Intraoperative photograph of the patient shown in ▶ Fig. 29.4. **(a)** The nerve was transected at the second genu (instrument points to transected nerve). **(b)** Great auricular nerve graft was anastomosed for repair. An eyelid gold weight was also placed at the time of surgery. (Reproduced courtesy of Eric Sargent, MD.)

surgical re-exploration for repair should be based on other parameters including:

- Likely site of injury.
- Experience of the surgeon in facial nerve repair.
- Likelihood of neuropraxic versus axonotmetic/neurotmetic injury.
- Possibility of ischemic entrapment within the fallopian canal.
- Effects that waiting would have on granulation/scar tissue and distal nerve excitability.
- Risks incurred in surgical re-exploration.

In some circumstances, it is difficult to know if a postoperative facial palsy represents a mild neuropraxic injury that may recover spontaneously versus a more severe injury—i.e., during acoustic or parotid tumor resection, a nerve that has been stretched and is no longer responding to electric stimulation. If the nerve is known to be in anatomic continuity, observation rather than sectioning and grafting the nerve *may* be the best option. Conversely, facial palsy post parotid surgery might similarly represent a recoverable stretch injury—but if the nerve has in fact been unknowingly transected, delaying reoperation will make finding the nerve endings difficult, because of scar formation as well as the fact that following 2 to 3 days of Wallerian degeneration, the nerve monitor will no longer be of value to electrically identify the transected distal nerve.

If an injury is noted in the operating room, assessment of the severity of injury is critical. An accurate assessment may require expanding the surgical exposure of the nerve around the site of injury and precisely stimulating the nerve both proximal and distal to the injury.

In otologic surgery, injury to the nerve involves the main trunk. If contusion or partial transection of less than one-third of the diameter of the nerve is thought to have occurred, then decompression of the nerve 5 to 10 mm of both sides is often recommended.[79] It should be noted that the primary surgeon frequently underestimates the amount of facial nerve injury.[24] If injury is more extensive including total transection, neurorrhaphy or grafting is usually needed. Intraoperative monitoring certainly cannot prevent all facial nerve injuries, but if injury occurs monitoring may not only alert the surgeon to what might otherwise be an unrecognized injury, it can be used to map both the location and the severity of disruption by stimulating proximal and distal to the site of injury. Relatively high levels of current that are suitable for mapping would be too high to allow for precise conductivity assessments over a short nerve segment. Precision of electric stimulation can be enhanced by using low (suprathreshold) levels of stimulation with a monopolar stimulator—or switching to a bipolar stimulator.

If an unanticipated facial palsy is noted in the recovery room, one must consider at least three factors:

- Completeness of palsy.
- Onset of palsy.
- The experience and assessment of the primary surgeon.

Often the use of local anesthetic can cause a temporary palsy. Observation for several hours to see if the function returns is warranted. If no recovery occurs after several hours, consider consultation with an otologic subspecialist if the operating surgeon is not experienced in facial nerve repair. For injuries during parotidectomy, the surgeon performing the re-exploration should also have the capability and training to follow the proximal nerve into the mastoid. If facial nerve function is present but weak, observation with medical treatment aimed at decreasing swelling may be an option. Steroids and possibly antiviral therapy may be useful to decrease inflammation.[80] If complete paralysis continues after several hours, re-exploration should be considered especially in cases where:

- The nerve was not specifically identified.
- Monitoring was not used.
- Monitoring was used but a preclosure electrically evoked response was not obtained.
- The surgeon is not confident of the nerve's integrity.

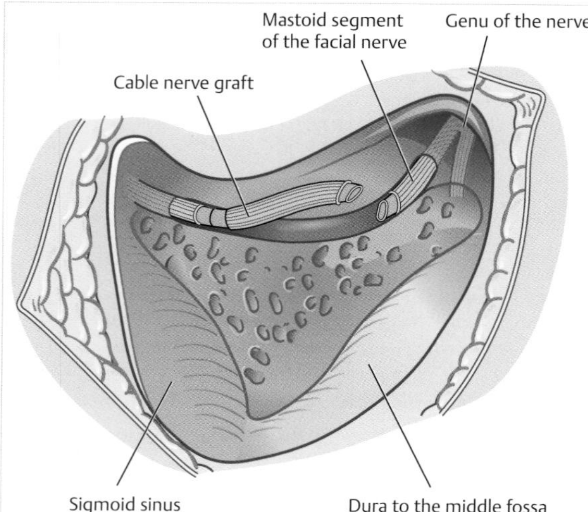

Fig. 29.6 Cable nerve graft. Illustration of nerve grafting for transected facial nerve in mastoid. Epineurium is trimmed to reduce ingrowth of scar into anastamosis. (Reproduced with permission from Kartush JM. Facial nerve surgery: an overview. In Jackler RK, Brackmann DE, eds. Textbook of Neurotology. 1st ed. St Louis: Mosby; 1994:1257–1269.)

As noted above, iatrogenic facial palsy should be handled promptly but a decision to re-explore surgically should not be made hastily. *If* the nerve ends can be found, waiting to perform neural repair up to 1 month after transection may have little effect on long-term outcome. Transected facial nerves promptly reanastomosed by experienced hands will typically obtain a HB grade III recovery (▶ Fig. 29.6). Before undergoing immediate same-day exploration and potential repair of an injury, the surgeon should take into account their expertise in facial nerve repair as well as their emotional state and level of fatigue. However, if immediate re-exploration is not elected, the surgeon must be cognizant that the nerve distal to injury will remain electrically stimulatable for only 2 to 3 days post injury. Therefore, with injury following parotidectomy, exploration after this time makes identification of distal ends more difficult and may require retrograde dissection. After 12 to 18 months, degeneration of the targeted facial muscles often occurs, making primary repair after this time of little value.

Additional testing may provide useful information following iatrogenic facial nerve palsy. If injury occurred in otologic surgery, a computed tomography scan shows the facial nerve with high precision in the osseous fallopian canal of the temporal bone and may be a useful adjunct in gauging potential violation of the nerve in this region. It may also detect concomitant injury to the semicircular canals and tegmen. When the severity of nerve injury is in doubt and surgical re-exploration is being deferred, intraoperative electrical testing can be extremely valuable in assessing the site and severity of injury; for futher details see Chapter 6, Chapter 9, and Chapter 15.

When a surgeon is faced with an iatrogenic facial nerve injury, it is understandable that they focus on whether or not to re-explore the surgical site—however they should remember the importance of eye care in order to avoid long-term corneal damage. In young patients with good skin tone, lubricant eye drops will typically suffice but for elderly patients in whom a lengthy recovery is expected, consideration of an early gold weight eyelid implant can provide superior corneal protection; see Chapter 24.[81] Unlike tarsorrhaphy, which can obscure peripheral vision, the eyelid implant is effective, well tolerated, and easily explanted with minimal, if any, residual scarring.

29.6 Key Points

- Iatrogenic facial nerve injury is a devastating complication for both the patient and the surgeon.
- Due to the high dissatisfaction of patients following facial nerve injury, medicolegal action will often ensue.
- Physicians should explain and document risks of injury to the facial nerve prior to procedures being performed to ensure informed consent.
- Proper training, attention to detail, and routine identification of the facial nerve and/or its adjacent landmarks help to minimize damage.
- Nerve monitoring can be a useful adjunct when the surgeon is properly trained in both the technical and the interpretive components of monitoring.
- When injury does occur, prompt and proper management of both the nerve and the care of the paralyzed eyelid are essential to optimizing outcomes.

References

[1] Hohman MH, Bhama PK, Hadlock TA. Epidemiology of iatrogenic facial nerve injury: A decade of experience. Laryngoscope 2014; 124: 260–265

[2] Candirli C, Celik S. Efficacy of deep subfascial approach to the temporomandibular joint. J Craniofac Surg 2012; 23: e126–e129

[3] Hall MB, Brown RW, Lebowitz MS. Facial nerve injury during surgery of the temporomandibular joint: a comparison of two dissection techniques. J Oral Maxillofac Surg 1985; 43: 20–23

[4] Weinberg S, Kryshtalskyj B. Facial nerve function following temporomandibular joint surgery using the preauricular approach. J Oral Maxillofac Surg 1992; 50: 1048–1051

[5] do Egito Vasconcelos BC, Bessa-Nogueira RV, da Silva LC. Prospective study of facial nerve function after surgical procedures for the treatment of temporomandibular pathology. J Oral Maxillofac Surg 2007; 65: 972–978

[6] Lypka MA, Urata MM, Yen S, Yamashita DD. Facial nerve paralysis: a complication of distraction osteogenesis of the mandibular ramus in the treatment of temporomandibular joint ankylosis. J Craniofac Surg 2007; 18: 844–848

[7] Politi M, Toro C, Cian R, Costa F, Robiony M. The deep subfascial approach to the temporomandibular joint. J Oral Maxillofac Surg 2004; 62: 1097–1102

[8] Bron LP, O'Brien CJ. Facial nerve function after parotidectomy. Arch Otolaryngol Head Neck Surg 1997; 123: 1091–1096

[9] Laccourreye H, Laccourreye O, Cauchois R, Jouffre V, Ménard M, Brasnu D. Total conservative parotidectomy for primary benign pleomorphic adenoma of the parotid gland: a 25-year experience with 229 patients. Laryngoscope 1994; 104: 1487–1494

[10] Ward CM. Injury of the facial nerve during surgery of the parotid gland. Br J Surg 1975; 62: 401–403

[11] Patey DH, Moffat W. A clinical and experimental study of functional paralysis of the facial nerve following conservative parotidectomy. Br J Surg 1961; 48: 435–440

[12] Gaillard C, Périé S, Susini B, St Guily JL. Facial nerve dysfunction after parotidectomy: the role of local factors. Laryngoscope 2005; 115: 287–291

[13] Dulguerov P, Marchal F, Lehmann W. Postparotidectomy facial nerve paralysis: possible etiologic factors and results with routine facial nerve monitoring. Laryngoscope 1999; 109: 754–762

[14] Mehle ME, Kraus DH, Wood BG et al. Facial nerve morbidity following parotid surgery for benign disease: the Cleveland Clinic Foundation experience. Laryngoscope 1993; 103: 386–388

[15] Mra Z, Komisar A, Blaugrund SM. Functional facial nerve weakness after surgery for benign parotid tumors: a multivariate statistical analysis. Head Neck 1993; 15: 147–152

[16] Terrell JE, Kileny PR, Yian C et al. Clinical outcome of continuous facial nerve monitoring during primary parotidectomy. Arch Otolaryngol Head Neck Surg 1997; 123: 1081–1087

[17] Springborg LK, Møller MN. Submandibular gland excision: long-term clinical outcome in 139 patients operated in a single institution. Eur Arch Otorhinolaryngol 2013; 270: 1441–1446

[18] Møller MN, Sørensen CH. Risk of marginal mandibular nerve injury in neck dissection. Eur Arch Otorhinolaryngol 2012; 269: 601–605

[19] Batstone MD, Scott B, Lowe D, Rogers SN. Marginal mandibular nerve injury during neck dissection and its impact on patient perception of appearance. Head Neck 2009; 31: 673–678

[20] Picon AI, Coit DG, Shaha AR et al. Sentinel lymph node biopsy for cutaneous head and neck melanoma: mapping the parotid gland. Ann Surg Oncol 2006 [Epub ahead of print]

[21] Chao C, Wong SL, Edwards MJ et al. Sunbelt Melanoma Trial Group. Sentinel lymph node biopsy for head and neck melanomas. Ann Surg Oncol 2003; 10: 21–26

[22] Lai SY, Weinstein GS, Chalian AA, Rosenthal DI, Weber RS. Parotidectomy in the treatment of aggressive cutaneous malignancies. Arch Otolaryngol Head Neck Surg 2002; 128: 521–526

[23] Schroeder WA, Jr, Stahr WD. Malignant neoplastic disease of the parotid lymph nodes. Laryngoscope 1998; 108: 1514–1519

[24] Green JD, Jr, Shelton C, Brackmann DE. Iatrogenic facial nerve injury during otologic surgery. Laryngoscope 1994; 104: 922–926

[25] Wiet RJ. Iatrogenic facial paralysis. Otolaryngol Clin North Am 1982; 15: 773–780

[26] Selesnick SH, Lynn-Macrae AG. The incidence of facial nerve dehiscence at surgery for cholesteatoma. Otol Neurotol 2001; 22: 129–132

[27] Carlson ML, Van Abel KM, Pelosi S et al. Outcomes comparing primary pediatric stapedectomy for congenital stapes footplate fixation and juvenile otosclerosis. Otol Neurotol 2013; 34: 816–820

[28] Jahrsdoerfer RA, Lambert PR. Facial nerve injury in congenital aural atresia surgery. Am J Otol 1998; 19: 283–287

[29] Dedhia K, Yellon RF, Branstetter BF, Egloff AM. Anatomic variants on computed tomography in congenital aural atresia. Otolaryngol Head Neck Surg 2012; 147: 323–328

[30] Bauer GP, Wiet RJ, Zappia JJ. Congenital aural atresia. Laryngoscope 1994; 104: 1219–1224

[31] Friedman RA, House JW. Acoutic Tumors. San Diego, CA: Singular Publishing Group; 1997

[32] Porter RG, LaRouere MJ, Kartush JM, Bojrab DI, Pieper DR. Improved facial nerve outcomes using an evolving treatment method for large acoustic neuromas. Otol Neurotol 2013; 34: 304–310

[33] Leonetti JP, Brackmann DE, Prass RL. Improved preservation of facial nerve function in the infratemporal approach to the skull base. Otolaryngol Head Neck Surg 1989; 101: 74–78

[34] Niparko JK, Kileny PR, Kemink JL, Lee HM, Graham MD. Neurophysiologic intraoperative monitoring: II. Facial nerve function. Am J Otol 1989; 10: 55–61

[35] Kartush JM, Lundy LB. Facial nerve outcome in acoustic neuroma surgery. Otolaryngol Clin North Am 1992; 25: 623–647

[36] Kartush JM. Electroneurography and intraoperative facial monitoring in contemporary neurotology. Otolaryngol Head Neck Surg 1989; 101: 496–503

[37] The Consensus Development Panel. National Institutes of Health Consensus Development Conference Statement on Acoustic Neuroma, December 11–13, 1991. Arch Neurol 1994; 51: 201–207

[38] Raslan AM, Liu JK, McMenomey SO, Delashaw JB, Jr. Staged resection of large vestibular schwannomas. J Neurosurg 2012; 116: 1126–1133

[39] Patni AH, Kartush JM. Staged resection of large acoustic neuromas. Otolaryngol Head Neck Surg 2005; 132: 11–19

[40] Baker DC, Conley J. Avoiding facial nerve injuries in rhytidectomy. Anatomical variations and pitfalls. Plast Reconstr Surg 1979; 64: 781–795

[41] Rees TD, Aston SJ. Complications of rhytidectomy. Clin Plast Surg 1978; 5: 109–119

[42] Kamer FM. One hundred consecutive deep plane face-lifts. Arch Otolaryngol Head Neck Surg 1996; 122: 17–22

[43] Javidnia H, Sykes J. Endoscopic brow lifts: have they replaced coronal lifts? Facial Plast Surg Clin North Am 2013; 21: 191–199

[44] Jena AB, Seabury S, Lakdawalla D, Chandra A. Malpractice risk according to physician specialty. N Engl J Med 2011; 365: 629–636

[45] Nepps ME. The basics of medical malpractice: a primer on navigating the system. Chest 2008; 134: 1051–1055

[46] Orosco RK, Talamini J, Chang DC, Talamini MA. Surgical malpractice in the United States, 1990–2006. J Am Coll Surg 2012; 215: 480–488

[47] American Medical Association. Code of Medical Ethics. Chicago, IL: American Medical Association 2014

[48] Jena AB, Chandra A, Lakdawalla D, Seabury S. Outcomes of medical malpractice litigation against US physicians. Arch Intern Med 2012; 172: 892–894

[49] American Society of Anesthesiologists. Standards for basic anesthetic monitoring. 2011. Available at: http://asahq.org. Accessed April 28, 2015

[50] Svider PF, Sunaryo PL, Keeley BR, Kovalerchik O, Mauro AC, Eloy JA. Characterizing liability for cranial nerve injuries: a detailed analysis of 209 malpractice trials. Laryngoscope 2013; 123: 1156–1162

[51] Lydiatt DD. Medical malpractice and facial nerve paralysis. Arch Otolaryngol Head Neck Surg 2003; 129: 50–53

[52] Hong SS, Yheulon CG, Sniezek JC. Salivary gland surgery and medical malpractice. Otolaryngol Head Neck Surg 2013; 148: 589–594

[53] Ruhl DS, Hong SS, Littlefield PD. Lessons learned in otologic surgery: 30 years of malpractice cases in the United States. Otol Neurotol 2013; 34: 1173–1179

[54] Blake DM, Svider PF, Carniol ET, Mauro AC, Eloy JA, Jyung RW. Malpractice in otology. Otolaryngol Head Neck Surg 2013; 149: 554–561

[55] Mathew R, Asimacopoulos E, Valentine P. Toward safer practice in otology: a report on 15 years of clinical negligence claims. Laryngoscope 2011; 121: 2214–2219

[56] Hutson MM, Blaha JD. Patients' recall of preoperative instruction for informed consent for an operation. J Bone Joint Surg Am 1991; 73: 160–162

[57] Eloy JA, Svider PF, Patel D, Setzen M, Baredes S. Comparison of plaintiff and defendant expert witness qualification in malpractice litigation in otolaryngology. Otolaryngol Head Neck Surg 2013; 148: 764–769

[58] Leape LL. Error in medicine. JAMA 1994; 272: 1851–1857

[59] Kartush JM. Errors in otology. Ear Nose Throat J 1996; 75: 710–712, 714

[60] Hamill N, Kartush JM. Errors in facial nerve surgery. Proceedings of the VIIIth International Symposium on the Facial Nerve, Matsuyama, Ehime, Japan, April 13–18, 1997; Matsuyama, Japan. The Hague, The Netherlands: Kugler Publications; 1998

[61] Luft HS, Bunker JP, Enthoven AC. Should operations be regionalized? The empirical relation between surgical volume and mortality. N Engl J Med 1979; 301: 1364–1369
[62] Birkmeyer JD, Siewers AE, Finlayson EV et al. Hospital volume and surgical mortality in the United States. N Engl J Med 2002; 346: 1128–1137
[63] Regenbogen SE, Greenberg CC, Studdert DM, Lipsitz SR, Zinner MJ, Gawande AA. Patterns of technical error among surgical malpractice claims: an analysis of strategies to prevent injury to surgical patients. Ann Surg 2007; 246: 705–711
[64] Arriaga AF, Bader AM, Wong JM et al. Simulation-based trial of surgical-crisis checklists. N Engl J Med 2013; 368: 246–253
[65] Hong RS, Kartush JM. Acoustic neuroma neurophysiologic correlates: facial and recurrent laryngeal nerves before, during, and after surgery. Otolaryngol Clin North Am 2012; 45: 291–306, vii–viii
[66] Heman-Ackah SE, Gupta S, Lalwani AK. Is facial nerve integrity monitoring of value in chronic ear surgery? Laryngoscope 2013; 123: 2–3
[67] Noss RS, Lalwani AK, Yingling CD. Facial nerve monitoring in middle ear and mastoid surgery. Laryngoscope 2001; 111: 831–836
[68] Wilson L, Lin E, Lalwani A. Cost-effectiveness of intraoperative facial nerve monitoring in middle ear or mastoid surgery. Laryngoscope 2003; 113: 1736–1745
[69] Bronstein D. Otologists report greater widespread use of intra-operative facial nerve monitoring. ENT Today. May 1, 2014. Available at: http://www.enttoday.org/article/otologists-report-greater-widespread-use-of-intra-operative-facial-nerve-monitoring/. Accessed April 28, 2015
[70] Kartush JM. Video Webinar: New practice guidelines in facial nerve monitoring. ASNM, June 2014. Available at: www.asnm.org/event/id/440608/Webinar- New-Practice-Guidelines-in-Facial-Nerve-Monitoring.htm. Accessed April 28, 2015
[71] McCabe BF. Injuries to the facial nerve. Laryngoscope 1972; 82: 1891–1896
[72] Grosheva M, Klussmann JP, Grimminger C et al. Electromyographic facial nerve monitoring during parotidectomy for benign lesions does not improve the outcome of postoperative facial nerve function: a prospective two-center trial. Laryngoscope 2009; 119: 2299–2305
[73] Meier JD, Wenig BL, Manders EC, Nenonene EK. Continuous intraoperative facial nerve monitoring in predicting postoperative injury during parotidectomy. Laryngoscope 2006; 116: 1569–1572
[74] Pensak ML, Willging JP, Keith RW. Intraoperative facial nerve monitoring in chronic ear surgery: a resident training experience. Am J Otol 1994; 15: 108–110
[75] Choung YH, Park K, Cho MJ, Choung PH, Shin YR, Kahng H. Systematic facial nerve monitoring in middle ear and mastoid surgeries: "surgical dehiscence" and "electrical dehiscence". Otolaryngol Head Neck Surg 2006; 135: 872–876
[76] Kircher ML, Kartush JM. Pitfalls in intraoperative nerve monitoring during vestibular schwannoma surgery. Neurosurg Focus 2012; 33: E5
[77] J. K. Lee A. Intraoperative monitoring. In: Babu S, ed. Practical Neurotology for the Otolaryngologist: Plural Publishing, Inc. 2012:165–191
[78] Barrs DM. Facial nerve trauma: optimal timing for repair. Laryngoscope 1991; 101: 835–848
[79] Weber PC. Iatrogenic complications from chronic ear surgery. Otolaryngol Clin North Am 2005; 38: 711–722
[80] Hadlock T. Facial paralysis: research and future directions. Facial Plast Surg 2008; 24: 260–267
[81] Kartush JM, Linstrom CJ, McCann PM, Graham MD. Early gold weight eyelid implantation for facial paralysis. Otolaryngol Head Neck Surg 1990; 103: 1016–1023

Index

Note: Page numbers set **bold** or *italic* indicate headings or figures, respectively.

N

O

P

Q

R

S

T

U

V

W

Y

Z